COMLEX* Level 1
Qbook

KAPLAN MEDICAL

Content Editor

James J. Cox, Jr., D.O.
Former Assistant Professor, Nova Southeastern University
Department of OPP
Former Instructor, Department of Family Medicine
Family Medicine Clinic
Osteopathic Medicine Clinic
College of Osteopathic Medicine

TEST-TAKING AND STRATEGIES GUIDE

Author

Steven R. Daugherty, Ph.D.
Director of Education and Testing
Kaplan Medical
Rush Medical College
Chicago, IL

Contributor

Judy A. Schwenker, M.S.
Director of Study Skills
Kaplan Medical

COMLEX LEVEL 1 QBOOK

Editors

Michael S. Manley, M.D.
Department of Neurosciences
University of California, San Diego
Director, Medical Curriculum
Kaplan Medical

Leslie D. Manley, Ph.D.
Department of Neurosciences and Pharmacology
University of California, San Diego
Director, Medical Curriculum
Kaplan Medical

Contributing Editor

Mary Ruebush, Ph.D.
Adjunct Professor of Microbiology
Montana State University
Bozeman, MT

OMM Questions

Author

Robert G. Savarese, D.O.
Resident Physician
Kessler Institute for Rehabilitation, NJ

Director of Medical Curriculum

Mark Tyler-Lloyd, M.D.

Associate Director of Medical Curriculum

Rita Gidwaney, M.D.

Production Manager

Michael Wolff

Medical Illustrators

Rich LaRocco
Christine Schaar

Cover Design

Ann Shin

Cover Art

Christine Schaar
Rich LaRocco

Contents

Biochemistry

Microbiology/Immunology

Pathology and Pathophysiology

Pharmacology

Behavioral Science and Biostatistics

OMM

Preface

This Qbook includes a Test-Taking and Strategy Guide followed by 950 COMLEX-USA Level 1–style questions divided into test blocks of 50 questions each. All questions represent only the current COMLEX Level 1 formats. Each test is followed by comprehensive explanations of both the correct answer choices, as well as all the wrong answer choices (distractors). By reviewing why each distractor is incorrect, you learn more than just the answer to that one question; you learn the information needed to answer multiple similar questions on the same topic. You'll also appreciate how the exam is constructed, and you'll begin to feel a greater sense of control over the exam. The key to exam day success is controlling the exam and not letting it control you!

First

Begin by reading the Test-Taking and Strategy Guide on pages 3–47. Use the strategies and approaches outlined as you work through the tests in this Qbook. Also reread the final sections of this guide (pages 33–47) as your exam approaches. This section gives you great advice on what to do during the weeks leading up to the exam, as well as on test day itself.

After Completing Subject Area Review

We recommend that you wait until you complete your review of a subject area before taking an exam. There are two exams each in Anatomy, Behavioral Science, Biochemistry, Microbiology/Immunology, Pharmacology, Physiology, and Osteopathic Manipulative Medicine. Because of the increasingly clinical nature of the exam, we have included five tests covering Pathology and Pathophysiology. Take each exam in the allotted one-hour time frame, and **do not** look at the answers until you've completed a test.

After Completing the Questions in This Book

If you have completed all of the practice questions and reviewed all of the explanations in this book and would like extra questions for review, consider adding one or both of our online Qbanks for an additional fee. The COMLEX Qbank offers 1,000 COMLEX-style questions (including OMM) in a database customizable by organ system or discipline or both. IV Qbank has 1,200 questions organized by chief complaint and focuses on the integration of basic-science concepts around a common disease entity. Both include our detailed feedback analysis and explanations. COMLEX and IV Qbank accounts can be opened at kaplanmedical.com.

Finally, we want to hear what you think about this Qbook. Please share your feedback by E-mailing us at **medfeedback@kaplan.com**.

Good luck on your COMLEX Level 1 exam!

Kaplan Medical

Test-Taking and Study Strategies Guide

Introduction

Preparing for and doing well on the COMLEX-USA Level 1 is an essential requirement on the road to becoming a practicing osteopathic physician. This guide is intended to help you with that process. The suggestions offered here come from two sources: *1*) the faculty of Kaplan Medical, who have experience helping students pass the COMLEX; and *2*) hundreds of other students who are eager to let you know what worked and what did not work for them as they prepared for the Level 1 exam.

This guide does not contain tricks or gimmicks. More than 30 years of experience helping students prepare for tests tells us that there is no magic way to help you achieve your best performance. Rather, we offer here some practical suggestions to help you make the most of your preparation time and to avoid common pitfalls on the exam itself. Preparing for and taking multiple-choice tests are skills in their own right. These skills have little to do with the day-to-day practice of medicine but are necessary hurdles that you must surmount to advance in your medical career.

Of course, how you prepare for and handle your exam are up to you. You may have your own methods of study or a way of taking the exam with which you are more comfortable. This guide is not intended as a rigid prescription to which everyone must adhere, but it does summarize the key study and test strategies that have helped thousands of students achieve their maximum scores. As you read this guide, think about the way that you study and the way that you take exams. Consider your options and make the choices that work best for you.

Take heart; there have been many ahead of you. The COMLEX Level 1 is not insurmountable. It only requires some knowledge of techniques, a little planning, a dash of impertinence, and above all, patience. By sharing the accumulated knowledge of the many students who have gone before you, we hope to prepare you to do your very best and to achieve a score that matches your goals.

I hope you find this book useful.

Steven R. Daugherty, Ph.D.
Director, Education and Testing
Kaplan Medical
e-mail: steve.daugherty@kaplan.com

The COMLEX-USA Level 1

THE PURPOSE OF THE EXAM

COMLEX-USA Levels 1, 2, 2-PE, and 3 are the only comprehensive licensing examinations used to certify candidates to practice osteopathic medicine in all states of the U.S. This exam is dedicated to and is specifically written for osteopathically trained medical students. The exam sequence is designed to allow candidates to demonstrate how well they understand and apply the concepts that are integral to the basic and clinical sciences. All osteopathic physicians must pass all levels of the COMLEX before they can practice osteopathic medicine. Level 1 tests their mastery of the basic science components of the medical sciences curriculum and their understanding of the scientific principles underlying quality medical care.

To reach this point, the students must have already demonstrated competence within the osteopathic curriculum or they would not be undertaking this exam. They have successfully taken standardized examinations for most of their academic life. They took them to get into medical school, and they marked their progress throughout medical school. Not to minimize this task, but this examination is just another step in a long series.

However, one must keep in mind that the COMLEX is different from and, in many ways, broader and more difficult than any exam ever taken in medical school. As such, it requires more preparation than most medical school exams.

Each question on the exam has been carefully written, screened, selected, and pre-tested before it is included for scoring in the examination. Out of all the questions submitted for inclusion on the exam, only a small fraction actually make it into the final test. The people who construct this exam know what they are doing. They are specialists and have attended to all the details.

Students must think about items on the exam not as questions to be answered but as problems to be solved. Good COMLEX questions test the student's capacity to think about important medical knowledge and apply it in specific presented situations. The COMLEX has evolved beyond an exam that tests recall of facts into one that assesses students' ability to use that knowledge in clinical situations. A good knowledge base is essential but is not sufficient. Students must know how to *use* the information they know.

As one takes the COMLEX, he or she will find question after question where there is uncertainty of the answer. Unlike most exams where, if one has prepared sufficiently, one has a fairly good idea what each question is about, most students report that on the COMLEX there is material that they are either unfamiliar with or never really fully understood. If one has this feeling, it should not cause worry. Even the brightest, best-prepared students report this experience. Everyone else is feeling the same way. The exam *feels* difficult because it is supposed to *be* difficult. The student's task is to get as many questions correct as possible within the allocated time limit.

One can do well on this exam, but doing one's best requires both forethought and preparation. This preparation must be on several levels. First, one must be familiar with the types of questions one will face, as well as the overall structure of the exam itself. Second, study time must be organized as efficiently as possible to get the most out of it. Third, the student must know how to use the content being tested, not just recognize it, and be able to apply it in hypothetical situations. Fourth, one must prepare physically and mentally for the task at hand. In short, one must know the exam, master the material tested, and be prepared to handle oneself during this often stressful time.

LEVEL 1 FORMAT AND CONTENT

In **May** of **2006**, the COMLEX-USA Level 1 ceased to be a 2-day, 16-hour, 750-question exam. Rather, **400** questions are administered as a 1-day, 8-hour, computer-based exam.

Note

The two optional 10-minute breaks deplete the total time allotted for taking the test.

COMLEX-USA Level 1 at a Glance

Examination length: One day; 8 hours

Question type and number: 400 multiple-choice questions

Allocated break times: Two optional 10-minute breaks (after first two sections of morning and afternoon sessions) and a lunch break

Tip: It is best to download and practice the computer software interface. A tutorial of the computer-based testing examination is available at http://www.nbome.org/CBT/cbe_intro.htm.

Exam Content/Blueprint

The content is structured into two distinct categories, Dimension I (subjects) and Dimension II (application). Table 1-1 shows the eight categories of Dimension I.

Table 1-1. COMLEX Level 1 Content Coverage (Dimension I Categories)*

Category of Study	Topics that May Be Included
Asymptomatic/General Symptoms	Abdominal/pelvic pain, AIDS, alcoholism, anemia, anesthesia, back pain, bacteriuria, cancer, chest pain, chronic pain syndrome, contraception, diabetes, ear pain, ECG abnormalities, electrolyte abnormalities, exercise/sports workup, extremity pain, eye pain, face pain, genetic screening, genital pain, head pain, heart sound abnormalities, hepatitis, HIV, hyperlipidemia, hypertension, hyperuricemia, immunologic disorders, osteoporosis, physical examination, scoliosis, somatic dysfunction
Symptoms and Disorders of Digestion and Metabolism	Absence seizures, alcohol abuse, appetite disturbances, brain concussion, coma, constipation, controlled substance abuse, delirium, diarrhea, dysphagia/feeding problems/odynophagia, encopresis, gallbladder dysfunction, nausea, nonprescription drug abuse, petit mal seizures, syncope, tobacco abuse, vomiting, weight gain/obesity, weight loss
Symptoms and Disorders of Sensory Alterations	Adjustment disorders, anxiety, behavioral disturbances, bereavement, confusion/disorientation, daytime sleepiness, dementia, depression, dizziness, eating disorders, fatigue, hearing disorders, insomnia, learning difficulties, libido decrease, marital discord, mental retardation, olfactory disorders, paralysis, paresthesia, seizures, sleep terrors, sleep/wake cycle disturbances, speech disorders, suicidal ideation, tactile disorders, taste disorders, tics, tremors, vertigo, visual disorders, weakness
Symptoms and Disorders of Motor Alterations	Fasciculations, fractures, gait disturbances/falls, muscle spasms, muscular atrophy, short stature, somatic dysfunction, spinal deformities, sprains/strains
Symptoms and Disorders Related to Human Sexuality and Urination	Anuria, delayed puberty, dyspareunia, dysuria, enuresis, impotence, incontinence, infertility, menopausal symptoms, menstrual disorders, oliguria, polyuria, precocious puberty, priapism, pyuria
Symptoms and Disorders of Respiration and Circulation	Airway obstruction, apnea, breathing rate/rhythm abnormalities, cough, cranial hemorrhage, dyspnea, hemarthrosis, hematemesis, hematochezia/melena, hematuria, hemoptysis, nasal bleeding, systemic or undefined bleeding, vaginal bleeding (abnormal)
Symptoms and Disorders of Thermoregulation	Fever, hypothermia
Symptoms and Disorders of Tissues and Trauma	*Masses/swelling:* abdominal, axillary, breast, chest/lung, child abuse, crash injury, edema, extremity, head/face, knee, neck, pelvic, rectal, scrotal/testicular *Discharge:* anal, ear, eye, nasal, neck, nipple, penile, skin, umbilical, urethral, vaginal *Skin/nail/hair/teeth disorders:* alopecia, baldness, blanching, burns, cyanosis, hirsutism, jaundice, lesions, nail disorders, pruritus, rash, vitiligo *Other:* domestic abuse, elder abuse, lacerations, lymphadenopathy, motor vehicle accidents, multiple traumas, rape, shock, wounds
Symptoms and Disorders of Human Development	Bleeding in pregnancy, labor and delivery process, lactation, neonatal complications, normal obstetrics, postpartum infections, pregnancy complications

Based on NBOME Level 1 Examination Guidelines and Sample Exam Booklet

Within these subject areas, five content areas are assessed:

Content Area (Dimension II)	Percentage of Questions
Scientific Understanding of Disease Mechanisms	75 to 85%
History and Physical Exam	5 to 12%
Management	3 to 7%
Diagnostic Technology	1 to 5%
Health Promotion/Disease Prevention	1 to 5%

The actual percentages listed in the table above will vary depending upon the particular exam, but these ranges should give you a sense of what is emphasized. Note that by far the largest section of the exam is scientific understanding of disease mechanisms. The Level 1 exam is a basic science exam. The test writers want to be sure you understand core medical concepts before proceeding to more complex clinical experiences.

Question format

Most of the questions will appear as one-best-answer, multiple choice questions, and a small number will be the matching type questions (see COMLEX Level 1 Question Types, in this chapter). You will also see a series of one-best-answer questions that reference a single question stem or clinical vignette.

Score reporting

The numerical score report will be translated into both two-digit and three-digit versions. You will also still receive a pass/fail designation and a graphical performance profile.

The COMLEX-USA measures performance with an accuracy of plus or minus 10 points. Your score (excluding the performance profile) will be sent to you.

Remember that each question counts the same, whatever the subject. An Anatomy question counts just as much as a Pathology question. You are not required to pass each discipline separately but to answer enough questions correctly to attain an overall passing score. Past experience has shown that you can do very poorly in one subject and still pass the exam. However, doing poorly in osteopathic medicine alone or any other two subjects combined makes passing very unlikely. And, of course, if your goal is to go beyond simply passing; you will need to do well in all of the subject areas.

Keep in mind that the COMLEX is a criterion-referenced test. This means that you are scored relative to a preset standard, not "on a curve" relative to other examinees. The COMLEX determines a minimal competency level, and everyone who achieves that level or above passes. Unlike medical school exams, you are not competing against each other on the COMLEX; you are competing against the test. This means that preparing with other students is likely to be your best method of study.

Note

The minimum three-digit passing score is 400. (The two-digit score, converted from the three-digit score, is 75.) Percentile rank will no longer be reported.

Along with your overall score, you will also receive a performance profile. This is an assessment tool to review your strong and weak areas. It will give you an indication of how you performed in each of the areas. A shortened example of what a score report might look like is shown in Table 1-2.

Table 1-2. Sample of Graphical Performance Profile

	Low Performance	Borderline Performance	High Performance
Physician Skills			
Health Promotion/ Disease Prevention			X
History and Physical			XXXXXXXXXXXXX
Diagnostic Technologies			X
Management			XXXXXXX
Scientific Understanding of Mechanisms			XXX
Topic Categories			
Osteopathic Principles and Practice			XXXXXXXXX
General Osteopathic Medicine			XX

Marks on the graph that tend toward the right indicate better performance. Marks on the graph that tend toward the left indicate performance that needs improvement. Notice that the score reported for subject is not given as a number but rather as a series of "X"s. These "X"s are confidence intervals intended to give you a general sense of how well you did in each area without attaching a specific number to the result. This is for two reasons. First, the people who prepare and score the COMLEX do not want students, schools, and residency directors to become too focused on specific numbers as indicators of performance. By not giving specific numbers, the Board hopes to reduce the general level of competitiveness in medicine. Second, the COMLEX is being honest in admitting that student scores can vary from one test taking to the next and that an exact score could be higher or lower on any given day. Thus, subsection scores are given as a range specifying a confidence interval. You can use these ranges to get a general idea of areas of strength and weakness, but they are not really useful for comparing with your friends and classmates.

Score Reporting for the COMLEX-USA Level 1

Scoring results will be given in the following forms:

- three-digit score
- two-digit score
- pass/fail designation
- graphical performance profile

Receiving results:

- After results are normalized, you should receive your results approximately 4 weeks after test is taken.

Note

It is strongly recommended that you take the tutorial computer simulation of the COMLEX available at www.nbome.org/CBT/cbe_intro.htm. Familiarity with the software interface is less anxiety-provoking.

Note

Remember, the examinee can only review and change answers within a section (50-question block).

Note

The time taken within the two optional breaks allowed after the morning and afternoon sessions will be deducted from your overall allotted time to complete the examination. You do not have to take the full 10 minutes of each break if you'd like to return to the examination.

About Computer-Based Testing

You will need to know how to click a mouse to select answers and to use other simple features. Only minimal computer knowledge is necessary for taking this examination, and how little or much you know about computers will not affect your exam performance.

However, this examination will *not* be computer adaptive in terms of difficulty level progression. In other words, the next question that the computer chooses will not be determined by how well you answered the previous question.

Interface functions

On the computer screen, an Exhibit button displays for the test-taker some graphic materials referring to specific questions. Also, a Lab values button providing normal adult laboratory values will be available on your screen throughout the examination.

The exam also features a "review page." This page is presented only for each block, and the examinee can review his or her answers and have the opportunity to change them with this feature.

Exam format

New types of questions involving multimedia will slowly be introduced into the COMLEX. Candidates will be notified in advance when such changes occur. Please be sure, also, to check for any updates on the NBOME website.

Breaks

Time allocated toward breaks on the COMLEX is divided into **two 10-minute optional** breaks and **one** optional lunch break. (The lunch break is 40 minutes and does not count against total exam time.) The first two breaks after each session (one in the morning and the other in the afternoon) deplete the time you have in completing the test.

You may begin your lunch break as soon as you finish the morning session. The time you take here is not deducted from the overall exam time. After the lunch break, the afternoon session of the examination will **automatically start**. This second session will start **exactly 280 minutes** after the commencement of the COMLEX, when the candidates view their first question in the morning session.

Fees and Scheduling

Unfortunately, the cost of administering a computer-based exam is higher; thus, the fee to take the examination has risen. Levels 1 and 2 will cost $465 each, and Level 3 will be $615.

However, the upside to having the COMLEX computerized is that it will be administered throughout the year, at least once a month, at more than 300 locations throughout the country.

Registration and scheduling information can also be found on the NBOME's website.

OSTEOPATHIC CONTENT

One of the most common questions from students is, "How many osteopathic questions are there on the Level 1 exam?" The best answer is that *all* of the questions are osteopathic questions. Osteopathic content is not only tested in separate questions but is included as a part of every question where the inclusion makes sense. (Students have reported that it is approximately 20 to 30% of exam questions.) This is accomplished in two ways:

1. *Osteopathic information included in a clinical case.* For example, if you are presented with the case of a woman suffering from an anxiety disorder, the physical finding of muscle tension will be included to facilitate the diagnosis.

2. *Osteopathic interventions included as answer choices.* For example, a woman is presented complaining of neck pain and students are asked what to do next. Direct action OMT will be presented as one of a number of options, which may also include administering NSAIDs or oral steroids.

Important: Just because an osteopathic intervention is included as an option, it does not necessarily mean it is the correct answer. The exam does not "favor" osteopathic interventions, but wants you to see them as an available choice alongside other medical interventions. Osteopathic information included may be essential or irrelevant to answering any given question. Your task is to read the question and assess the relevance of what is presented before selecting your answer.

Important: Not all of the questions on the exam will count. The examiners want to see how these questions perform, e.g., how many people get them correct and which of the distractors are selected. When you answer these questions (and you won't know which ones they are), you are helping the COMLEX examiners calculate question difficulty for future tests.

In addition, other questions may be eliminated from the scored pool after the exam results are reviewed. Questions that may be eliminated include those with more than one possible answer, those deemed ambiguous, or those that were more difficult than anticipated. The good news, then, is that not all of the questions on the exam count. The bad news is that you do not know which ones they are. Your best approach: Answer all questions as if they do count. But remember, if you find yourself unable to answer some questions, don't panic; they may not even count!

Additional information about the COMLEX, including any last-minute changes, can be found on the Internet at: http://www.NBOME.org, http://www.AACOM.org, and www.kapmedical.com.

COMLEX LEVEL 1 QUESTION TYPES

This study guide contains examples of each of the types of questions discussed below. As you practice and review these questions, pay attention to the way the questions are constructed, as well as to the content tested.

Single-Best-Answer Questions

Most of the questions presented on the Level 1 exam are of the single-best-answer type. This means that your job is to select from the given set of options the one answer that is clearly better than all of the others. Most commonly, questions will offer five answer options (A through E), although on recent exams an increasing number of options are presented.

The most important thing to remember is that these questions require you to select not only a good answer, but the *best* answer from the choices given. One answer is always considered clearly better than the others. Therefore, it is critical that you read through all of the options before making your choice. Remember, you don't get any points for selecting the second-best answer. If an answer choice seems partially correct, then it is entirely wrong. You are looking for the *one* best answer.

Be aware that the COMLEX has moved away from questions that require simple basic science recall, such as:

> Which of the following areas of the heart is supplied by the right coronary artery?

and toward questions that require an application of knowledge, such as:

> A 77-year-old woman is admitted with angina pectoris. An angiogram is performed and reveals a 90% blockage of the right coronary artery. Blood supply is most likely to be diminished to which of the following areas?

You'll notice the same objective lies within both questions. The first question is a direct request for a fact. The second question, the kind that is now more common, asks for the same fact in the context of a clinical presentation.

Question Subtypes

There are a number of different subtypes of single-best-answer questions. Most students find it useful to classify these subtypes with reference to the following criteria:

1. Positively worded questions ("most likely")
2. Negatively worded questions ("least likely")
3. Clinical case questions (long clinical cases)
4. Long matching questions
5. Two-step (double-jump) questions
6. Bait-and-switch questions
7. Conjunction questions
8. True/False (fast-recall) questions
9. Visual questions
10. Primacy and recency effects

There are overlaps among these types of questions, but this list provides a good framework for talking about issues you need to keep in mind. Note that clinical case questions may be of either the single-best-answer or the double-jump type.

Increasing numbers of Level 1 questions are designed to be clinically relevant and may be posed in the form of mini-case presentations, but don't be fooled. Although couched in clinical language and settings, the questions on Level 1 are intended to test your basic science knowledge. Students tell us that the most important cognitive step for doing well on these questions is to be able to uncover the core basic science issue being tested. Remember that, for the most part, the faculty writing questions for the Level 1 exam are Ph.D.s, not physicians, and the questions will reflect this bias.

Positively worded questions—the most common type of question

Positively worded questions ask you to select the answer that is "most likely" to be true. These are by far the most common type of questions on recent exams. Note that all of the options given may be *somewhat* likely. Your job is to select the one that is *most* likely. An example of this type of question follows:

> An 85-year-old man has had urinary frequency, difficulty initiating stream, and dysuria for the last two months. A rectal exam reveals an enlarged prostate. Prostate-specific antigen (PSA) is not elevated. Which part of the prostate is most likely affected in this patient's condition?
>
> (A) Peripheral zone
> (B) Prostatic capsule
> (C) Prostatic urethra
> (D) Posterior lobe of the prostate
> (E) Transitional/central zone
>
> Answer: A

Negatively worded questions—not on the exam

Negatively worded questions, those that ask for the option that is "least likely," are no longer used on the Level 1 exam. If you see this type of question in review books, you'll know either that the book has not been recently updated or that the author is not familiar with the current COMLEX question types. We recommend that you not waste your time mastering the techniques for handling negatively worded questions.

Clinical case questions—basic science in clinical clothing

Clinical case questions are distinguished by a fairly lengthy presentation of a patient's history, physical exam findings, and maybe even lab results. Your task is to read through this voluminous information and arrive at the best answer to the question being asked.

The most important part of the clinical case question is the last sentence. This is the sentence that actually poses the question. Until this point, you cannot be sure exactly what you will be asked. Many students are tempted to simply skip to this last line, and then skim the case looking for necessary information to formulate an answer. Generally, this is not the best strategy.

Clinical case questions are often constructed by first writing a classic case, and then including one or two extra details. These details, by themselves, may suggest one or the other of the given answer options. To answer these questions correctly, you must read the *whole* case and treat all the information given as a whole. The total gestalt of the case is what is crucial, not any one individual fact.

Question writers know that because of the length of the questions, candidates do not want to read the whole question if they can help it. They know that some test takers are scanning for that *one* critical piece of information. Because of this, single pieces of information may lead the examinee away from the right answer to one of the incorrect distractors. Avoid this trap. You need to focus on the meaning of the case as a whole, not merely a single piece of it.

When reading through the case, choose what is important. Paraphrase the question and note key factors and symptoms as they are presented. This will help you to remember them when formulating your answer. Then select the answer that best matches not just some but all of the facts presented. An example of this clinical case type of question follows:

> A 24-year-old female presents with a fever and myalgia. She experienced brief, self-limited diarrhea 24 hours after attending a barbecue two weeks earlier. She remained asymptomatic until the day prior to presentation when she developed a fever of 39.4°C (103°F), conjunctivitis, and severe muscle pain. On physical examination she appears acutely ill and has a fever of 39.4°C. There is a diffuse maculopapular rash and generalized muscular tenderness. Several hemorrhages are noted beneath the fingernails. Admission hemogram reveals a white blood cell count of 15,000 with 25% eosinophils. The infectious form of the most likely causative agent is a(n)
>
> (A) cyst
> (B) cysticerci
> (C) encysted larvae
> (D) ovum
> (E) rhabditiform larvae

Answer: C

Long matching questions—multiple-response options

Long matching questions are essentially basic, single best answer questions with a twist. Rather than being presented with a question followed by a set of options, the student is first presented with a list of options, followed by one or more questions that are answered by selecting from those options. As many as 9 options (A through I) may be presented.

(A) *Blastomyces dermatidis*

(B) *Chlamydia trachomatis*

(C) *Coccidioides immitis*

(D) Coxsackie A virus

(E) *Haemophilus ducreyi*

(F) *Haemophilus influenzae*

(G) *Histoplasma capsulatum*

(H) Influenza B virus

(I) *Neisseria gonorrhoeae*

A pair of brothers (35 and 38 years old) present with fairly dramatic pneumonias. On lung exam, rales are easily heard. Chest x-rays of both men reveal bilateral and diffuse infiltrates. The brothers spent a day together two weeks ago hiking in a mountainous area of Virginia where they entered a dusty cave. What is the most likely causative agent?

Answer: G

Some test-takers find that questions with numerous options produce anxiety. This need not be the case. In fact, many examinees feel that questions with many options are easier and actually take less time to do.

The real danger with long matching questions is that students will waste too much time reading back and forth through the list of options. *The correct method of approaching these questions is to think of an answer, look for that answer, and then pick it.* If none of the options looks appealing, then take a guess and move to the next question. Repeatedly reading over the options is not an effective strategy. This is the same strategy we recommend for all questions, but it is most critical when there are a large number of options.

One more thing: If several questions are asked using the same option set, it is important to remember that the same option *may* be used once, more than once, or not at all. If you think "D" is the answer to two questions in the same long matching set, then pick it each time.

Two-step (double-jump) questions

Two-step (also called double-jump) questions require several cognitive choices to arrive at a correct answer. Consider this two-step question where a correct answer requires you to formulate a proper diagnosis and then select the most appropriate pharmacologic treatment. Note that you get no credit for the intermediate step of diagnosis. The correct answer is found only by reasoning all the way through to the treatment.

A bright, energetic, overweight, 46-year-old man loves to talk and to give his opinion on the world around him. He is always quick with a joke and seems to love a good laugh. Yet whenever he has to talk in front of more than three or four people, he reports sweating, heart palpitations, and trembling hands. "My mind just goes blank," he says, "and I feel that I'm going to say something so stupid that I would rather die." The most appropriate treatment for this man would be

(A) alprazolam

(B) atenolol

(C) clonadine

(D) diazepam

(E) phenelzine

Answer: B

In this next question, you must reason with additional characteristics of the organism in mind by first correctly identifying what the organism is, based on the laboratory data. Again, you get no credit for identifying the correct organism but only for "two-stepping" to the additional characteristic.

A 71-year-old male was admitted from his extended care facility because of recent aggravation of an exfoliative skin condition that has plagued him for several years. He had been receiving a variety of antibiotic regimens, including many topical preparations over the last year or two. He now has a temperature of 38.9°C (102°F). The skin of upper chest, extremities, and neck shows erythema with diffuse epidermal peeling and many pustular lesions. Cultures obtained from these lesions were reported back from the laboratory as yielding a Gram-positive organism that is highly salt (NaCl) tolerant. This organism is also most likely

(A) bacitracin sensitive

(B) bile soluble

(C) coagulase positive

(D) optochin sensitive

(E) novobiacin sensitive

Answer: C

Note that you need to make *two correct decisions* to arrive at the correct answer; hence the name "two-step." The goal is to guide you away from simple memorization in your learning. Instead, the exam wants you to be able to use the information you have memorized to reason through to a correct answer.

The correct process for answering these questions is not "read, answer," but "read, think, answer." These two-step (and even three-step) questions are becoming more common on the Level 1 exam.

Bait-and-switch questions—misdirected attention

Sometimes what you first think the question is about is not what the question is really asking. Did you ever begin reading a question thinking that the core focus is Physiology and discover at the end of the question that the real issue is Pharmacology? Ever read a clinical case collecting evidence for a diagnosis and find that at the end of the question they give you the diagnosis, but want to know something about treatment options? If you have had these experiences, then you have run into the so-called bait-and-switch questions.

Bait-and-switch questions begin by presenting material that may lead you to think about content in one direction but then shift you to another line of thought at the end; a sort of mental sleight of hand. *The key question is always given in the last line of the stem.* Everything else before this is simply a setup. You cannot tell for certain what information is useful and what information is unnecessary until you get to the end of the stem and encounter the actual question.

Because of this, some students make a habit of reading the last line of the question stem, then scanning the rest of the presented information to look for pertinent material. This strategy may sometimes work, but it has pitfalls. If you have the discipline to read the question line and then return to read the rest of the stem in detail, this is not a bad strategy for this type of question. However, experience suggests that this is not the best strategy for most students.

There are two difficulties with reading the last line of the stem first:

1.   You do not know that you are faced with a bait-and-switch question until you read through the whole question first. In other words, you often can't tell that this strategy will work until you have already read the question. Sometimes reading the last line first helps, and sometimes it doesn't. You can't tell whether it will or will not help until you have read the entire question.

2.   Many people do not have the discipline to read the last line and then return to read through the rest of the question stem. Once they read the question line, many students move directly to the options without adequately evaluating the information presented in the question stem. Alternatively, students scan the question stem looking for one single piece of information to help them answer the question. *Looking for only one key fact often means you will miss some key detail and will therefore end up with a wrong answer.*

Given this, our best advice is to read the last line of the question first *only if* you then read through the rest of the question. Read the last line *before* reading the rest of the question, not *in place of* reading the rest of the question. Reading the last line first to avoid reading the entire question is a low-yield strategy and results in an increased error rate.

A generally healthy 65-year-old male was in a car accident and broke several ribs on his left side. His medical record shows a history of mild diabetes and treatment in the past year for gonorrhea. Approximately 12 days after the car accident, the patient developed a painful, well-circumscribed vesicular rash over his left rib cage. The rash persisted for several weeks. The rash is due to

(A) primary infection with herpes B virus

(B) primary infection with herpes simplex virus type 1

(C) primary infection with herpes simplex virus type 2

(D) reactivation of latent Epstein-Barr virus

(E) reactivation of latent varicella-zoster virus

Answer: E

A 59-year-old male with a history of hypertension and cigarette smoking survived a myocardial infarction two years ago. He has been reluctant to follow the diet prescribed by his physician, but as part of his recovery program, he has taken up running. Following an early morning run, he consumes a breakfast consisting of cereal, eggs and bacon, sausage, pancakes with maple syrup, doughnuts, and coffee with cream and sugar. Which of the following proteins will most likely be activated in his liver after breakfast?

(A) Glycogen phosphorylase

(B) PEP carboxykinase

(C) Hydroxymethylglutaryl-CoA reductase

(D) Glycogen synthase

(E) Carnitine acyltransferase

Answer: D

Conjunction questions—two questions in one

In the same manner as two-step questions, conjunction questions require two correct choices to arrive at the best answer. Options are presented as sets of terms or facts linked by a conjunction (usually the word "and"). The best answer is the one in which *both* parts of the option are correct.

By using this type of question, the examiners are able to move beyond asking for a single piece of information to asking instead which two pieces satisfy the question criterion. Most commonly, students are asked to detect two overlapping disease states or to determine which are the two best interventions to be done next.

A 66-year-old man is brought to his physician's office by his wife, who expresses concern that "something is just not right." During neurologic examination, both recent and long-term memory appear unimpaired. However, the patient seems to have difficulty concentrating. He asks repeatedly where he is and what he is doing there. He has difficulty with simple arithmetic and in writing simple sentences. He has no difficulty outlining or reproducing presented figures, but on a discrimination task, he confuses his right and left hands. This patient is most likely suffering from lesions affecting the

(A) dominant parietal and frontal lobes

(B) dominant parietal and dominant temporal lobes

(C) dominant temporal and frontal lobes

(D) non-dominant parietal and dominant temporal lobes

(E) non-dominant parietal and non-dominant temporal lobes

Answer: A

The best method for handling a conjunction question is to treat it as two separate questions. Answer the question twice, once for each part of the response option. Cognitively, it is difficult to hold the two parts of the option in mind at the same time. By splitting the task into two simpler choices, you are less likely to become confused or make mental mistakes. For example, in the latter question above, first notice that some of the symptoms are suggestive of a frontal lobe lesion; then, as a second step, focus on those symptoms that suggest a dominant parietal lobe dysfunction.

True/False questions—probing for basic recall of facts

True/False questions ask you to read a set of options and select the one that is most likely to be a true statement of fact. These questions, commonly found in older review books and on many medical school exams, are not on the COMLEX. They are useful for testing recall of basic facts but are less helpful in testing your capacity for reasoning and applying learned knowledge.

The basic form of the question is: "Which of the following is true?" You must select the statement that is likely to be the correct answer in most situations. Special care must be taken if the question describes a specific situation. In this case, you must select the option that is most likely true, not in general, but in the *specific situation presented*.

For true/false questions you must pay careful attention to the exact wording of the options. Faculty usually construct true/false questions by writing out a series of true statements and then changing a word or two to make all but one of the statements false. Here, unlike other COMLEX questions, your attention should be directed to the options (which is one reason why these questions are so rarely used).

It deserves emphasizing again: True/False questions are not on the COMLEX Level 1. Review books that feature a large number of these questions are probably outdated and should be treated accordingly.

The mechanism of action of heparin includes

(A) binding to antithrombin III and inducing a conformational change in it to potentiate its action

(B) binding to heparin and the complex activating antithrombin III

(C) enhancing the activity of antithrombin III with coagulation factors by acting as a template

(D) inhibition of regeneration of vitamin K quinone

(E) the formation of IgG antibodies, leading to thrombocytopenia

Answer: A

Two different manufacturers prepare ibuprofen 200-mg tablets. The two batches of tablets are said to be bioequivalent if

(A) they have the same shape and color

(B) the area under the curve is the same after a single dose

(C) the relative bioavailability = 1

(D) they have the same volume of distribution

(E) they have the same t1/2 and volume of distribution

Answer: B

Visual questions—know them when you see them

In the past year, COMLEX Level 1 has featured the increasing use of visual materials such as pictures, histology slides, EKGs, x-rays, skin lesions, fetal monitor strips, and MRI and CT scan results. Many students are uneasy about these types of questions but need not be. The images presented for the Level 1 exam will be of fairly common phenomena, things you have probably seen before.

Your first task when faced with a visual question is to stay calm. Deal with these questions just as you would any other question. When you come to a visual question, look at the presented image, but also *read any accompanying text*. Students tell us that a substantial portion of the visual questions can be answered from hints included in the text.

To prepare for visual questions, review images and then tell yourself what you are looking at. Many students study incorrectly by starting with a concept and then looking at the matching image. The exam always requires you to select the concept that matches the image, not to find the image that matches the concept. The key here is to know what you are looking at when it is presented.

Primacy and recency effects—getting the right cognitive set

Information that appears early in a question stem and information that appears at the end of the question stem exert a strong influence on the examinee. Early and late information form your cognitive set, which makes finding the correct answer either easier or harder. Information at the start of the question stem has a primacy effect, which controls your thinking by determining what you start thinking about. Information at the end of the question stem has a recency effect, which controls your thinking by providing the jumping-off point to select the correct answer.

If the key information for the question appears in the primacy or recency spots, you will be led to the correct answer. The difficulty comes when the key information lies somewhere in between. Primacy and recency information can blind you to other essential content. Examinees sometimes fixate on early or late information and in so doing miss other important information given in the question stem.

For example, if a question begins by describing a patient as having a generalized anxiety disorder, all of the information that follows will tend to be seen in that context, even though the anxiety disorder diagnosis may not be directly pertinent to the correct answer for the question.

Primacy or recency effects seem most pronounced when the beginning or ending information in a question stem is something with which you are unfamiliar. We all have a special tendency to fixate on unknown content.

If you suspect that primacy or recency information is distorting your reading of a given question, try changing the order in which you read the question. Skip the initial content, read the rest of the question first, and see if this changes your perspective. Simply, if reading the question forward seems confusing, try reading it backward. Remember, no one single piece of information is the key; you must deal with each question as a whole. Avoid fixating on one word or concept you do not know, and focus on the parts of the question you do know.

UNDERSTANDING DISTRACTORS

To deal most effectively with exam questions you need to have some understanding of how the questions are constructed. Getting a question correct means selecting the best answer. Incorrect options are called distractors. Their purpose is to distract; that is, to get you to pick them rather than the best answer. Each distractor will be selected by some examinees, or it would not be included as an option. Every option fools somebody. Your job is to not be misled.

In general, distractors will seem plausible and few will stand out as obviously incorrect. Distractors may be partially right answers but not the *best* answer. Common misconceptions, incomplete knowledge, and faulty reasoning will cause you to select a distractor.

The COMLEX examiners tell its question writers that their distractors must follow these six rules:

1. They must be *homogeneous*. For example, they will be all laboratory tests or all therapies, not a mix of the two.

2. They must be *incorrect or definitely inferior to the correct answer*. There will be enough of a difference between the right answer and the distractors to allow a distinction. For example, if estimating the percentage of a population with a disease, the options will differ by more than 5%.

3. They must *not contain any hints to the right answer*. Distractors are meant to induce you to make an incorrect choice, not give you clues to the correct one.

4. They must *seem plausible and attractive to the uninformed*. If you are not sufficiently familiar with a topic, you may well find that all of the options look good.

5. They must be *similar to the correct answer in construction and length*. Trying to "psych out" the question by looking for flaws in its construction is not a useful strategy.

6. They must use osteopathic distractors whenever possible. Because it is an osteopathic exam, you might be tempted to choose them; however, they may not always be the correct answer.

Questions that do not adhere to these rules are not used on the exam. All options are meant to distract you, but often one of the distractors will seem better than the others, the so-called preferred distractor. This is the wrong answer that is chosen most often. Preferred distractors are why you can often get yourself down to two choices: the correct answer versus the preferred distractor.

Selecting the correct answer is not a matter of splitting hairs. The correct answer will be clearly correct. If you think two answers are so close that you cannot reasonably choose between them, then the odds are that neither one is correct; you need to look carefully at a different option.

"Test-wise" strategies do not usually help with this exam. Test questions that are not carefully reviewed often contain subtle flaws that help the examinee discover the correct answer. While previous board exams may have contained items with these flaws, the current exam does not. The COMLEX has put great effort into eliminating these cues from the exam.

Many students have learned these test-wise strategies and used them effectively on their medical school exams, but these strategies will *not* help you on the COMLEX. Worse, focusing on these test-wise strategies actually hurts you because it distracts you from doing the mental work you need to do to recall the proper content and think through the question.

This means that you should break yourself of the habit of looking for:

1. *Grammatical cues*, where one or more of the distractors do not follow grammatically from the stem. For example, a stem ends in "an" and only some options begin with a vowel.

2. *Logical cues*, where a subset of options is logically exhaustive, indicating that the answer is one of the subset. For example, including the three options: greater than, same as, and less than in a five-option question. You will also not find logically exhaustive options when one of the options is nonsensical.

3. *Absolute terms*: Terms such as "always," "never," and "rarely," which wise test-takers avoid, will not be used in this exam.

4. *Long correct answers*: Options will be the same in construction and level of detail. Efforts are made to ensure that the correct answer is not longer, more specific, or more complex than the other options.

5. *Word repeats*, where the same word or phrase is included in both the stem and the correct answer.

6. *Word association links*, where the correct answer can be arrived at by simple word association without a deeper understanding of the topic. For example, Vietnam veteran and post-traumatic stress can be associated. However, in a diagnostic stem about a Vietnam veteran, the correct answer may well be some other condition.

7. *Convergence strategy*, where the correct answer includes most of the elements in common with the other options. For example, consider the following question:

Remember

No buzz words or trade drug names are used on the exam.

The 16th president of the United States was:

(A) Julius Lincoln
(B) Abraham Smith
(C) Abraham Lincoln
(D) Vladimir Lenin
(E) Andrew Jackson

By the convergence strategy, the correct answer is "C" (two Lincolns and two Abrahams).

8. *Negative phrasing terms*, such as "except," "least of all," "contraindicated," and "not likely," which wise test takers avoid, will not be used on the exam.

Remember, the COMLEX examiners spend a great deal of time and effort in constructing this exam. The COMLEX will not feature the types of flaws mentioned above. If you're thinking of using these strategies, don't. Tricks don't work on the COMLEX. They distract you from the high-power cognitive strategies that are much more likely to lead to a correct answer.

Study Techniques

MAKING CHOICES IS THE KEY TO SUCCESSFUL EXAM PREPARATION

Effective preparation for the COMLEX Level 1 is about making choices. At each stage of the preparation process you need to choose the strategies that will most likely lead you to success and stick with them.

Your first choice is to decide what your goal is. Are you simply trying to pass the exam? Is your goal to beat the mean? Or are you trying to attain one of the top scores in the country? Decide at the outset what is important to you and keep that goal constantly in mind. You have to decide on your personal definition of success.

After you are clear about what you are trying to achieve, it's time to plan how you will reach your goal. Everyone has a different way of studying. Some people prefer a quiet room and total focus on the work at hand; others can study with noise and confusion around them. However, there are some well-recognized ways to study any material effectively that will enable you to learn and retain the most information in the shortest time. The best way to retain information is to be *active* in your own learning process.

Active use of material that you learn increases retention and facilitates recall. Repetition makes memories. Each instance of recall produces a new memory trace, linking it to another moment of life and increasing the chance for recall in the future. Memory is dynamic. Recall actually changes neuronal structures. To be truly useful, a piece of information needs to be triangulated, connected to a number of other concepts, or better yet, experiences. Meaning, not mere information, is your goal.

Remember

Active use of the material is the key to successful studying.

Rereading textbooks from cover to cover and underlining—yet again, in a different color— every line on every page is *not* an efficient way to learn. You need to focus on the material most likely to be on the examination. Studying that material through active application is the best way to enhance your understanding and retention of the information.

The following study techniques will help you develop better ways to prepare for the exam—but remember, learning for retention and use requires active involvement.

CHOOSING WHAT TO STUDY (AND WHAT TO IGNORE)

How can you possibly know what is likely to be on your examination? There are a number of approaches.

1. First, talk to your medical school faculty. Often, they have seen past exams or have reviewed an item analysis and can tell you the topics most likely to appear on the examination. They should be able to direct you to what is essential knowledge in their field and what is less important.

2. Take advantage of the National Board of Osteopathic Medical Examiners' web site: www.NBOME.org and download the Level 1 Examination Guidelines and Sample Exam. Contained in the back of this sample exam will be Dimension I, which is a group of suggested Board topics. Although this isn't a comprehensive list, it has proven in the past to be a good starting point for structuring one's studying. These general topics should then be broken down in a differential diagnosis, comparing and contrasting all like diseases that would frequently be seen in a primary care setting. Dimension II indicates the basic parameters of knowledge that the student should know about each of the disease topics listed in Dimension I.

3. Talk to students and colleagues who took the examination in past years. Do they remember some topics being particularly "hard hit"? An example is molecular biology on recent examinations. Was there a "flavor" to the exam? For example, did there seem to be a lot of Pathology? Students who took the exam in the past cannot tell you what will be on the exam that you will take, but they can direct you to the high-yield content areas that you must make sure to master.

   - However, be cautious. Candidates typically overestimate how much of their weakest area was on the exam. They are most likely to recall tested content that they got wrong.

   - Also, beware of the trap of "studying for last year's exam"; exam content differs from year to year. This year's exams will be different from last year's, and within any given year, your exam will be different from that of others.

4. Take advantage of the resources offered by Kaplan Medical. Kaplan Medical is able to provide a wide range of diagnostic exams, review materials, practice questions, and courses to aid in your exam preparation. These resources are available at your local Kaplan Center, over the Internet at the Kaplan web site, and in live lecture courses offered across the United States. The Kaplan staff will be happy to help you find the information you need and the preparation resources that are right for you. You can also call us toll-free at (800) 533-8850.

5. Certain topics are standard. Others appear as trends. In general, topics begin to appear on the exam two to three years after they reach prominence in the scientific/lay community. Any interesting medical topic that appeared in the literature at least two years ago is a candidate for inclusion on the exam.

DECIDING HOW TO STUDY

Mastering the material you must learn for this exam is a three-stage process. These stages parallel the functional organization of memory.

1. You must learn *basic terms and definitions*. This provides the core vocabulary to understand the content being tested. This stage is a matter of simple recognition and memorization. Terms and definitions are learned by the use of *associational memory*. This is the level where mnemonics can be useful.

2. You must learn *central concepts* for each of the eleven subject areas. This stage is a matter of being able to explain the meaning of concepts, how they are used, and how they connect with other concepts. Understanding the cross-linkages within subjects and across subjects will serve you well over the course of the exam. Your basic mental task here is that of *reconstructive memory*, learning to recall concepts in terms of how things fit together. At this stage, the practice of recalling one concept facilitates the recall of other related ideas. Patterns begin to emerge. This is the level at which diagrams, tables, and pictures can be most helpful.

Remember

You do not have to study everything.

Remember

You must be able to recognize concepts, understand their importance, and apply them in presented situations.

3. You must be able to *apply the concepts* in presented clinical settings and to recognize what concepts are most important in mini-case presentations. This is the hardest stage of preparation, and the one that most students neglect. Remember that the exam will test not only whether you understand general concepts but also how well you can make use of them in specific situations. Achieving your best possible score depends on knowing not only what concepts mean but also how they are applied in a given medical situation. The task at this level is that of *reasoning*, understanding the implications of presented information, and being able to choose the appropriate action from the available options. At this level, study/discussion groups and doing practice questions can be most helpful.

Your method of study and your study schedule should be arranged to allow you to master each of these stages in turn.

Having the time to master the necessary material at all three of these levels requires some forethought and planning. The Kaplan Individual Diagnostic Profile and Exam can help you pinpoint your strong and weak areas and guide you in formulating a study plan.

As you make your decisions about how you will study, the following suggestions may be helpful:

1. *Be organized.* Set up an organized study schedule and adhere to it. The biggest danger when preparing for the exam is spending too much time on one area or ignoring one subject altogether. Decide how much time you will study each day and put your time in as if it were a paid job. Schedule regular breaks and keep them. Stick to your schedule. Plan your work and work the plan.

2. *Determine your weak areas* by taking pretests or a diagnostic exam, or by using information from your courses. Begin your study plan with your weak areas and plan to cover those at least twice before the exam.

   It is easy to discover your weak areas. In addition to the results of your diagnostic exam, watch your own reaction to each subject. The subject or subject areas you like the least are probably the ones in which you are the weakest. Do not completely neglect your strong areas, but allocate less time to them. This can be difficult. Research suggests that, left on their own, most students study what they know best and give less time to subjects that make them uncomfortable. This is basic reward and punishment—spending time on what makes us feel good and avoiding what makes us feel bad. *Doing well on the exam means reversing this process. Spend the most time on the subjects that make you the most uncomfortable.*

3. *Emphasize integration* by reviewing subjects together and/or by organ system. This will greatly aid your preparation for COMLEX, which emphasizes the integration of basic sciences. This type of review is best conducted in a group with other people. Other people may look at the same material differently than you do and may help you expand your perspective and understanding.

   Review materials in related clusters. For example, take the anemias and review how each one might present, the basic epidemiology, what lab tests would differentiate them, their underlying mechanisms, and the initial therapies for each. This strategy allows you to "preview" questions and anticipate both the correct answer and the most likely distractors.

4. *Keep your sessions short:* no more than an hour to an hour and a half before you take at least a 15-minute break. Your concentration declines significantly after an hour or so. Sitting longer will provide only minimal extra return. In addition, the break time allows the short-term memory to be consolidated into long-term memory, which, of course, is the goal. The key is not how long you spend studying, but how efficiently you study, getting the most out of your time.

Remember

You do not have to pass all of the subsections of the exam, but you do not want to be weak overall or very weak in two or three areas.

Remember

Do not entirely neglect your strong areas, but pay less attention to them when studying, leaving them later for review.

Remember

Your efficiency at the learning process decreases rapidly as the amount of study time increases.

5. *Do not reread textbooks such as Harrison's or Robbin's from cover to cover.* Use review books that consolidate the information for you.

6. *Study from our lecture notes. Limit the number of outside sources* from which you study. Trying to master several sources is confusing and time-consuming. If you have several books, use one as your primary study material and the others as backup to clarify points as needed. Especially as your exam gets closer, resist the temptation to buy each new review book you see your friends using. Too many study sources creates overload, and overload stifles comprehension.

Highly Effective Study Methods

Each person has her or his own preferred way of studying. You must decide what will work best for you. High-yield study methods all have one feature in common: *The more active you are with the material, the more content you will ultimately retain.* Remember, your goal in studying is not just to put in the most time, but also to be efficient, *to get the most out of your time.* Many of the best students use the following techniques:

1. One of the best study techniques is to *pose questions* to yourself as you review material. Perhaps you'll want to jot the questions down on index cards to share with others in your study group and to practice later. By asking yourself questions you are framing the material, challenging yourself to focus on key areas, and, in the long run, developing many of the questions you will see on the examination. Your goal is not to learn knowledge for general use but to be able to answer multiple-choice exam questions. Your study strategy should reflect this.

   The ultimate goal here is to move you from thinking like a student answering questions to thinking like a physician who is writing questions. By this process, you "get into" the heads of the question writers; you begin to understand what makes a good question and the basic science issues likely to be at the core of presented questions.

2. *Use graphs and charts* to enhance your comprehension of the material. A picture is worth a thousand words. Many common graphs and charts appear repeatedly on the exam. Practice reading graphs, charts, and tables because this is important for the COMLEX. Try abstracting the salient facts quickly from a graph or chart. This may be expedited by using a plain sheet of paper to cover unneeded information, lines, etc., and to focus your attention on selected information.

   Drawing the graph yourself seems to help you remember it more than just looking at it numerous times. Drawing the graph from memory will give you the confidence that you truly know it. The more active you are with the material, the more likely you are to both remember it and understand important nuances.

3. *Practice paraphrasing* material to highlight important information. Paraphrasing means processing the material you have read, telling yourself what is important and unimportant as you read through it, and summarizing the key content *in your own words.* Pretend that you are the teacher who is in charge of presenting the content. What would you choose to emphasize? What would you leave out if you were short on time? How would you explain the concept to someone new to the field? Remember, if you can say it *in your own words*, then you really know it. Second, the art of paraphrasing will allow you to answer questions with extensive information in the stem, such as case histories, much more efficiently. Many students say the most difficult part of the COMLEX is getting through the large volume of reading required for each question. When you are paraphrasing, you do not treat every piece of information with the same emphasis but decide what is important and what is not. Developing this skill will also be helpful as you progress through your medical career.

4. *Creating summary notes* is a good way to foster this paraphrasing process. Summary notes are your personal representation of key points organized in a way that makes sense to *you*. Summary notes should run parallel to your primary study material and should serve to annotate, illustrate, and amplify the key points of that material. The physical action of simply writing the notes tends to reinforce learning and aid long-term retention. Once completed, summary notes provide a ready guide for those times when you review the material again.

5. *Study with friends or colleagues in groups of four or five.* The best groups comprise people with a range of expertise. Try to form a group where each person's weakness is complemented by the strength of someone else in the group.

    The goal of these study groups is not to show your colleagues how much you know; rather, it's to find the holes in your knowledge while you still have time to correct those gaps. Don't be afraid to tackle the tough topics. With the aid of your study group, things will make sense much sooner than they will on your own. Challenge each other. Pose hypothetical situations and seek agreement as to the best answers.

6. *Plan your study time for a distributed practice review.* For the most efficient studying, avoid cramming and plan to re-review key material on a regular basis. Repeated exposure to material over time leads to more thorough retention than one massive concentrated exposure.

    As you re-review, remember that active learning is best. This means you should avoid simply reading the same page of notes over and over. Instead, use key words as mental triggers and tell yourself as much as you can about the issue you are studying. For example, don't simple reread the Krebs cycle. Rather, tell yourself about it as if you were explaining it to someone else, and then check yourself against your notes.

    Repeated review sessions are also the time to begin to make links among different sections of your material. What does your understanding of the physiology of the cardiovascular system tell you about common pathology or pharmacologic intervention? The threads of common diseases weave through each of the basic science subjects; tie them together and provide a framework that aids in retention.

7. *Doing practice questions* is essential in your preparation for taking a multiple-choice exam. Your goal here is to test yourself, but also to learn good question-answering habits. As you answer questions, examine whether you got them right, but more important, look at why you got the question right or wrong. Did you not know the content? That's your cue that more study is needed. Did you misread the question? Then evaluate how you misread it and learn how the question-writer wants you to read it.

Remember

If you can teach someone a topic, then you surely know it well enough for the exam.

Common problems on multiple-choice exams include:

Problem Type	Source of Errors
Format problems	Particular question subtypes
Anxiety problems	Questions that contain numbers or that are done early in the review session
Fatigue problems	Questions done late in the review session
Reading errors	More common in long questions
Directionality errors	Questions that ask prediction of consequences
Group delineation errors	Questions that present material in a unique context

When you do your practice questions, do them under a time limit similar to the actual exam. In general, your rule should be one minute per question. This is roughly the amount of time (66 seconds) you will have during the actual exam. Get used to the time constraint—it is one of the unchangeable realities of the COMLEX.

To diagnose mistakes you might be making in answering questions, try this:

1. First, do a set of 50 questions with the time limit of one minute per question. Use a clock to be sure that you stay within the time limit.

2. Next, before scoring the question set, go through the 50 questions again with no time constraint. Take as much time as you want to reflect on and think through each question.

3. Now, score yourself on both passes, timed and untimed. Your score on the untimed set is likely to be noticeably higher.

4. Finally, review the questions, paying close attention to the ones you got wrong under time pressure but which you got right when you had more time.

If you answered the questions correctly when you had more time, your problem is not a lack of knowledge but rather something you are doing when you first read and process the question. Look for patterns. What types of questions did you commonly miss? What mistakes did you make consistently? Consider what you can do to correct these bad habits.

When answering practice questions, avoid these common mistakes:

- *Do not just answer questions without preparatory studying.* Review the material first until you feel you know it, then use the questions to test yourself. Learning the answers to hundreds of questions that you may not see on the exam will not help you prepare. If you study by answering questions before you are ready, you will erode your self-confidence and fail to develop key linkages within the material.

- *Do not get into the habit of lingering over a question or thinking about it for an extended period of time.* You do not have this luxury on the real exam. Remember that you have just over one minute per question. You should spend about 75% of that time reading and analyzing the question stem, and the other 25% selecting an answer. Be honest when you do not know an answer; move on, and look it up when you are finished.

- So-called "retired questions" from the COMLEX and many published questions in review books are not representative of questions featured on the current COMLEX Level 1. They are a reasonable way to review content, but often do not reflect the length or form of the questions on the current exam. Kaplan practice exams are your best sample of true COMLEX-type questions.

- *Do not answer questions individually.* Do them in clusters under time pressure, with five to ten as a minimum. This will get you used to moving from question to question. Do not look up the answer after each question. Instead, check yourself after you have done the full set of questions.

When you start working on questions, *do not panic if you don't get the correct answers.* Learn from your mistakes. Questions are a part of the study process; they help you see what else you need to learn. You will get better at answering the questions as your studying continues.

Try this question-mastering exercise:

1. Cover the options to the question and read the question stem. Pause at each period and paraphrase what you have read.

2. When you finish reading the question, cover it and reveal the options. Select from the options without looking back at the question stem.

Remember

Passive learning will not increase your retention of information; you must work with the material.

With practice, you will get faster, and this strategy will become a habit. This strategy forces you to get the information out of the question as you read it and does not allow you to waste time by going back and rereading. Remember, you have time to read each question only once. Learn to use that time as efficiently as possible.

Tackling the Exam

3

THE WEEK BEFORE THE EXAM

During the last few days before the exam you should be tapering off your studying and getting into mental and physical shape.

This is not the time for cramming in new material, but time to organize and integrate what you already know. Work on making what you know more accessible.

1. Review key words, phrases, and concepts. Look over your summary notes one more time. This is the time to drill yourself on essential information. *The key is to practice recall*, not simply read over the material again. What you need to know is probably already in your head. Your task now is to train yourself to access it when you need it. Answering practice questions is a good way to reinforce your recall skills—but remember, practice questions are often harder than the questions on the real exam. Do not panic if you do not get them right. Use them to clarify your understanding of key details.

2. Have an honest conversation with yourself and decide what you will not know. No one can know everything that is asked on this exam. Be honest with yourself about what you do and do not know. Knowing that you do not know something gives you more of a sense of control on the exam and makes you less likely to panic when you encounter the material and/or waste time on questions you are not likely to get correct. When you come to a question that you know you do not know, simply mark your favorite letter and move on!

3. Get yourself onto the right time schedule. Wake up every day at the same time you will need to wake up on the day of the exam. This will get your circadian rhythm coordinated with the exam schedule. Do not nap between 8:00 AM and 5:00 PM. Otherwise, you will accustom your body to shutting down during critical exam hours. If you get up at the right time each day, you will also find it easier to fall asleep at night. By getting into the proper sleep–wake cycle, you will find it easier to get to sleep the night of the exam as well.

4. You should be getting a sufficient amount of sleep. For most people that means at least six to seven hours a night. Sleep is an essential time for your brain to consolidate what you have learned. You need sleep; it makes you a more efficient learner when you are awake.

5. Take some time each day to relax. Have a good meal. Take a walk in the fresh air. Find time for exercise. The change of pace will refresh you, and the physical activity will help you relax and sleep at night.

6. Consider the impact of your personal relationships. Family responsibilities and obligations can be very distracting. The week before the exam you should avoid family confrontations and any stressful relationships. Your focus should be on the exam and nothing else. The other parts of your life can wait.

Remember

Use the time before the exam for review, not for trying to learn new material.

Remember

No one gives you extra credit for suffering, so why do it?

Remember

- Use the time before the exam for review, not for trying to learn new material.

- Avoid "buzz words" as a means to recall material.

- Concentrate on common medical conditions. (When you hear hoof beats, think of horses, not zebras.)

THE DAY BEFORE THE EXAM

1. Take the day off from all studying. This is your day to relax and gather your strength before the main event. Get out of bed at the same time you will have to get up the next day, and then treat this day as a vacation day to reward yourself for all your hard work. If you must study, limit yourself to reviewing your own notes and flashcards.

2. Have some fun. Go for a walk. Listen to your favorite music. Go see a good comedy or an action movie that will allow cathartic release. Go shopping. Spend time with a significant other. Do whatever you like. You have worked hard and deserve it.

3. Make sure that you have checked out the basics for the exam.

   - Do you have alternative transportation if, for example, your car does not start?

   - Do you trust your alarm clock to wake you up in time? If not, make arrangements with friends as a backup. You want to be sure to wake up rested, refreshed, and on time.

   - Lay out what you'll need for your exam before you go to sleep. This includes your photo identification and pencils, as well as any personal items, such as eyeglasses. While you're at it, don't forget to pack a lunch!

4. Call your friends and classmates and make plans to celebrate after the exam is over. You'll need to blow off some steam anyhow, and talking with colleagues will remind you that you are not in this by yourself.

5. Be sure to do some physical activity. Just taking a walk for an hour will help you relax.

6. Get a good night's sleep. To help you sleep, consider a hot bath or warm milk. Avoid taking sleeping medication, as it may leave you groggy in the morning.

THE DAY OF THE EXAM

Remember

Choose to spend your time where it will do you the most good.

This is not the most important day of your career, but just another hurdle on your way to becoming a licensed osteopathic physician. Keep it in perspective. Treat the exam like what it is, a routine mechanical exercise. You are not a doctor for this day, but an assembly-line worker. Rather than making cars or toasters, you are answering questions. Deal with each question as you come to it, make your choice, and then move on.

No matter how well prepared you are for the COMLEX Level 1 exam, you will get many questions wrong. This is not an exam where you should expect to know every answer. Remember, 70% correct puts you well over the mean! Knowing this, your test-taking strategy should be somewhat different than it may be when you take other exams.

Doing well on this exam means spending your time on those questions you are most likely to get correct and not wasting time on questions you are likely to get wrong. Two minutes spent on a question that you get wrong is two minutes wasted. Approach every question assuming that you will be able to answer it correctly. If you discover that you cannot arrive at a clear answer, admit it, make a choice, and move on to the next question. The core idea is a simple one: You know you will get some questions wrong. Therefore, choose which ones they will be and spend your time on those questions for which your probability of a correct answer is higher.

TEST-TAKING TIPS

Try to arrive at the testing center 30 minutes early so you are not rushed and you have time to get organized. Remember that you have a total of eight hours each day to complete 400 questions in two booklets. You will have one hour for lunch after the first booklet is completed. You may be required to sign out when leaving the testing room.

But don't try to do an entire booklet without several breaks. Most people need a mental break of a minute or more every hour. A mental break means to look up from your test, put your pencil down, close your eyes, and just breathe for a minute. This minute off will return you to the exam refreshed and better able to concentrate for the next hour.

Some students have their own personal strategies for dealing with multiple-choice exams. If you have a method that you are comfortable with, stick to it. However, many people find the following recommendations helpful. Our experience shows that your best strategy is to follow this advice:

- *Scan the booklet*, making sure that all the pages are there and that there are approximately 200 questions. Take the time to identify where the single-item questions, case-scenario-set questions, and matching-set questions are located.

- *Start with the beginning* of the question booklet and work your way to the back of it. This means start with the first question and do each question, in order, until you come to the last question. The idea here is to get into a rhythm that will carry you through the exam. This rhythm will help create what one psychologist calls a "flow" experience. The flow experience is a state of optimal concentration and maximal performance.

- *Do not skip any questions*. Deal with each question as you come to it. If you don't know it when you come to it, you are not likely to know it later. Skipping around wastes time and can end up confusing you about where you are in the exam and how much time you have left. Answer each question as best you can and move on to the next one.

- *Deal with each question and then be done with it.* Our best advice is to read the question, decide on your answer, and then mark your answer on the answer sheet. Marking your answers in the test booklet first and then transcribing them as a block on the answer sheet takes more time and puts you at greater risk of filling in your answer to the wrong question. If you complete the answer sheet as you do each question, you are less likely to have this problem.

- *Be very cautious about changing answers*. In general, your odds of changing a correct answer to a wrong one are so much higher than the reverse that it is simply not worth the risk. If you change an answer, you are most likely making it wrong! Your first impulse is usually the correct one—stay with it unless some clear insight occurs to you. If you are not very sure, leave your first answer.

  If you finish a question booklet with time left over, go back and check only those answers that you have previously marked. Checking almost always leads to changing and tends to reduce your score. If you have a spare moment, make sure that you have entered an answer for every question in the block—and then relax. Sit, take a break, and mentally prepare yourself for the next booklet of questions. Focus on the questions to come, not the ones that are past.

- *Segment your time* so that you know how much you have left and so that you do not find yourself rushed at the end. You have just over one minute per question (66 seconds). Some questions will take more time, and some less. Work on your pacing from the beginning of the question block. Check your watch every 30 questions to make sure you are on the correct pace to finish. If you pace yourself throughout the booklet, you should not be squeezed for time at the end.

- *Do not spend a lot of time on individual questions.* Research has shown that students spend the most time on questions that they get wrong. If you find yourself spending a lot of time on a question, this is your indication that you do not know the answer. How will you know if you are spending too long on any one question? If you find yourself thinking, "Maybe I'm taking too long on this question," you are. As soon as you think this, stop, mark your best guess, and move on to the next question.

- *During your lunch break, try to relax and not think back over the exam.* (It's hard, but try!) The desire to recall questions is strong but not helpful. Those questions are in the past. Focus on relaxing and making the most of your break. Remember, you will always tend to recall those questions you got wrong. Thinking back over these questions will just convince you that you do not know anything. This puts you in a bad frame of mind and leads to negative thoughts that only make the remainder of the exam more difficult. Be glad one set of questions is behind you. Forget about them and think about something more pleasant.

- *The night between the first and second days of the exam, plan to spend no more than two hours reviewing.* Experience shows that the questions you are most likely to remember are the ones you got wrong; look these topics up within the span of your review. Resist the desire to look up every single question you can remember, and focus your review only on any minor weaknesses you may have on the major topics. Students have consistently reported that many of the topics already seen will be repeated multiple times throughout the exam.

- *Forget the first day.* Have a good meal. Relax. Get a good night's sleep and get up and do it all over again the next day.

A PROVEN ROUTINE FOR HANDLING EACH QUESTION

Increasingly, the exam is not just about regurgitating facts but about applying those facts in a clinical context. To handle these types of questions your response pattern must not simply be "read, answer," but "read, think, answer." You must train yourself to take this crucial moment of thought on each question. Give yourself time to reflect and call to mind the key facts that will help you answer the question. Many questions require you to make multiple determinations to arrive at a correct answer. You must take a reflective moment on each question to allow yourself the time for this cognitive processing. Read the question, call to mind what you know, and select an answer. Approach each question with the assumption that you know the answer, and then muster your knowledge to attack it.

The mental task of selecting an answer on a multiple-choice exam is different from the task you face when you make decisions in clinical medicine. In the day-to-day practice of medicine, when selecting a laboratory test, arriving at a diagnosis, or finding the best treatment option, you want to carefully consider all of the options and be sure about your choice. A patient's health, and perhaps life, is in your hands. Before making a choice, most people report that they want to feel as close to 100% certainty as they can. On the COMLEX, you do not have the time to wait for this level of certainty. You must train yourself to make your choice within the allotted time. This often means choosing an answer even when you are not completely sure. If you wait for that absolute feeling of inner certainty, you will take too long. Don't wait until you are sure. Make your choice as soon as you have identified a clear best guess. Then move on to the next question. Remember, there is always another question coming.

Remember

Effective time management during the exam is key to getting your best score.

Remember

Don't stall. Keep moving through the exam.

The Kaplan Method: Three Tries for an Answer

You have three chances to get each question right. If you cannot get a clear answer using these three attempts, you do not know the answer. In this case, mark your favorite letter and move on to the next question. The key to this strategy is that you always know what you are going to do next. This helps you feel in control and reduces anxiety.

Step 1: read the question

This may seem trivial, but studies have shown that most students look at the answers first. Questions cause anxiety and answers provide the solution, so many people go right for the solution. However, you cannot pick the correct answer until you know what you are being asked.

Superior students generally spend about 45 seconds reading the question and about 15 to 20 seconds choosing from the given options. Poorer students tend to reverse this time allocation, spending less time on the question and more on the options. Time reading the question is time well spent. More time on the question means more time spent thinking.

- Read the question and pick out and underline key words. Key words are diagnostic information, abnormal values, indications of gender or race, and any qualifying terms.
- Read carefully enough that you have to read the question only once. Going back over the question takes time. Read for comprehension the first time.

Paraphrasing is the key to effective reading. Superior test-takers continuously summarize the key information briefly while reading the question. This allows you to look at the options with a sharp focus on the key elements, and it lessens the need to go back and reread the question while examining the choices. Look at the following question to see how this is done.

Remember

Keep moving forward through the exam. There is always another question coming.

> A 75-year-old smoker and alcohol abuser is hospitalized for evaluation of a squamous cell carcinoma of the larynx. On his second hospital day, he complains of sweating, tremors, and vague gastrointestinal distress. On physical examination he is anxious, with a temperature of 101°F, heart rate of 104, BP of 150/100, and respiratory rate of 22 breaths per minute. Later that day, he has three generalized tonic-clonic seizures. Which of the following is the most likely cause of his seizures?
>
> (A) Alcohol withdrawal
> (B) Brain metastasis
> (C) Febrile seizure
> (D) Hypocalcemia
> (E) Subdural hematoma
>
> Answer: A

The mental paraphrasing for this question might be as follows:

An old man with laryngeal cancer who smokes and drinks too much has sweats, tremor, anxiety, and some GI problems—he has three seizures a few days after admission. What's causing the seizures?

Paraphrasing is the mental equivalent of underlining. It helps you select what's important and keep those key facts in mind while you are evaluating possible answers. Like most test-taking skills, it also takes practice. If you practice paraphrasing material when you study, you will find that you have developed the basics to answer questions. Paraphrase each time you work with questions to gain skill and confidence.

Remember

You can't give a correct answer to a question you haven't read.

Step 2: the prediction pass

After reading the question, stop. Before looking at the options, try to come up with an answer. We call this "the prediction pass" because you are trying to think like the question writer and predict the correct answer. By the COMLEX's own rules, questions are written so that any expert in the field can come up with the correct answer without having any options present.

With the correct answer in mind, you are less likely to be led astray by distractors. Remember, they are supposed to distract you and convince you to pick the wrong answer. If you see the answer you thought of, scan the other answers to be sure that your choice is the best. Then pick it and move on to the next question.

Step 3: the selection pass

After reading the question, look through all of the answer choices, in order (A, B, C, D, E, etc.). If you see a correct answer, pick it. This is "the selection pass." If the answer seems obvious and direct, good. Don't fool yourself into thinking the question must be tricky or more difficult.

Most answers will be clearly correct. If you find yourself making up a long story about why one option is better than another, stop yourself. You are probably wrong. The correct answer should be clearly correct. If two answers seem to be almost the same, then neither one is correct. Once you have identified what looks like the best answer, choose it and move on to the next question.

Step 4: the final pass

If you've read all the options and are still not sure of the answer, you have one final try: the "final pass". At this stage, rather than trying for a correct answer, you are eliminating those you know to be incorrect. Using this strategy, you can usually eliminate all but two of the options.

- When you have narrowed your choices down to only two options, you have arrived at the most crucial moment of the exam. The correct action at this point is to pick one of the two answers and move on to the next question. If you are really unsure of the correct answer, which one you pick does not matter. With two options to choose from you have a 50% chance of getting the question correct rather than the 20% chance you started with.

- Make a choice. Many people waste time at this point by not choosing. Some people, when they have eliminated all but two answers, go back and reread the question in hopes of finding some information that will help them choose between the two options. Interviewing students and observing their thought processes during the exam suggests that this is the wrong strategy. When students reread a question at this point, they tend to add to it or pick out single features that help them feel better about choosing one of the answers. *However, it does not help them pick the right answer.* By adding assumptions to the question students may feel more confident, but they are really mentally rewriting the question to be one that they feel more comfortable answering. The answer they pick is then the right answer to the question that they envision, but (perhaps) not for the actual question presented.

If you've made these three passes—prediction pass, selection pass, and the final pass—and you are still not sure of the answer, your best option is to guess. At this point, mark any letter and move on to the next question. *Marking no answer counts the same as a wrong answer.*

Remember, the key to doing well on this exam is to train yourself to make choices. If you do not know an answer, admit it, make your best guess, and move on to the next question.

- Don't be afraid to use common sense, but watch out for "myths." Myths are options that most people might think are true, but are not. You are supposed to know the truth, not the myth.

Remember

When you have the question down to two choices, pick one and move on. Lingering over the question tends to result in making the wrong choice.

Remember

You are not expected to know all the answers. A passing score consists of getting 55 to 65% of the questions correct.

- Questions with a large number of options should be handled the same way as all single-best–type questions. The only difference is that you do not get a Final Pass because it would eat up too much time. That means these questions usually take less time to handle if done correctly.

AFTER THE EXAM

Take the day off and have some fun. You deserve it. Forget about the exam and pay attention to the rest of your life, which you have likely put on hold while preparing for the exam. You will have plenty of time to think about the exam again when your scores come in. For now, however, take a holiday and treat yourself kindly.

Physical and Mental Preparation

4

Taking the COMLEX is a big event. Like an athlete preparing for a big race, you want to approach it fully prepared, both physically and mentally. The following information consists of test-taking training tips to help you prepare for your test-taking marathon.

PHYSICAL PREPARATION

All-day examinations are physically stressful. What can you do to help decrease this stress?

Get in training. At least one month before the exam, begin the plan described below.

1. *Get enough rest.* Although you may be tempted to study late into the night and right up to the moment before the examination, this strategy can backfire and hurt you. The brain needs rest. By shutting off factual input, you foster the assimilation of information into long-term memory and allow time for making connections that help the integration, retention, and recall of information. In the week before the exam, you should be getting at least 6.5 hours of sleep a night.

2. *Eat right.* While preparing for the exam, have good solid meals. Protein, carbohydrates, and some fats are all important. However, do not overeat or eat very late because this will impair your sleep. Breakfast on the big day should be no more than cereal with fruit, a bagel, toast, or other complex carbohydrate source. Avoid heavy breakfasts to avoid the subsequent "crash" that many people experience at a crucial time in the first or second question block. Likewise, keep sugar or simple carbohydrate equivalents, such as candy, to a minimum at this time. Hard candy, not chocolate, can be useful as a pick-me-up during the examination. If you normally drink coffee in the morning, drink coffee the morning of the exam. You don't want to trigger a caffeine withdrawal headache. Eat light lunches, salads, simple sandwiches, and nonalcoholic drinks to avoid after-lunch sleepiness.

    *   Some students report that taking a vitamin B complex, especially B_6, can help with stress reduction.

    *   Schedule and eat meals as a part of your study time. These meals serve as breaks that give you a chance to recharge and be more efficient in your studies.

3. *Get some exercise.* The exam requires you to be in good physical condition because you will be sitting for long periods of time and want to avoid muscle fatigue that results in neck, back, or leg aches. As part of your preparation, start an exercise program and stick with it, no matter how difficult. Your regimen should include stretching and aerobic exercise, such as brisk walking or bike riding. The night before the exam, exercise, but on a more moderate scale. Besides the physical benefit, exercise can also help decrease your anxiety.

MENTAL/EMOTIONAL PREPARATION

People differ tremendously in their reactions to test situations. Some appear to sail through, confident and calm, whereas others experience mental and physiologic symptoms of test anxiety, such as insomnia, nausea, muscle twitching, or increasing inability to concentrate. If you have serious concerns about test anxiety, don't wait until the day before the exam to seek help. There are safe and mild antianxiety medications that may help, but you need to have them prescribed early so the dosage and effects will be predictable. There are also therapists who can teach you self-hypnosis techniques, but these require practice, so again, don't wait. Deal with the problem so anxiety doesn't increase as exam day approaches and your options for dealing with it decrease to zero. This is a situational problem, and effective treatment is available.

Here are some suggestions for dealing with test anxiety and some exercises that may help you to cope.

1. *Avoid negative thoughts and feelings.* Negative self-talk, such as, "There is no way I can pass this exam" can be distracting and produce more anxiety about the test. Focusing on avoiding failure is a recipe for failure. Focus instead on achieving success.

2. *Make anxiety your friend.* A degree of anxiety on the day of the examination is not only natural but also beneficial. How often have you heard of people responding well beyond their daily abilities when pushed to the limits psychologically? There is no need for you to test your limits, but expect to be a little tense and anticipatory on exam day. Incapacitating anxiety will destroy your ability to pass. We have heard many individuals say, "I knew everything, I even taught my peers, but I didn't pass. I don't understand it." Anxiety may do this to you!

3. *Seek help if necessary.* If you find that your studying is being overwhelmed by your anxiety, the most useful action may be to seek counseling. Talking to someone about your anxiety is not a waste of time if your study time is unproductive due to that anxiousness. Get help to be more productive.

4. *Be aware of obsessive thoughts.* If you find yourself focusing on your inability to answer questions, the volume of material, or doubts about your ability to pass the exam, try giving yourself something else to think about. Keeping your mind focused on a small task at hand, such as the information you are currently studying, will help you avoid letting obsessive thoughts distract you.

5. *Make a study schedule.* Buy a calendar and write out which subjects you will study on each day and a time frame for each. Leave room for breaks and "free time." This helps you gain control over your life and your studying. Following a schedule gives you structure, which makes you more efficient and reduces stress.

6. *Improve your attention control.* Awareness is like a searchlight. Whatever you direct your attention to is pretty clear, but other things and events tend to fade into the periphery. Try focusing separately on sights, sounds, the feelings in your hands and feet, etc. Your awareness can shift very quickly from one focus to another; however, you can be fully aware only of whatever is in your realm of focus at that moment. Use this fact to redirect your wandering thoughts and feelings by focusing your attention. In time this will allow you to quickly de-emphasize extraneous thoughts by redirecting them to simple bodily functions. Keep in mind how attention works:

    - You can attend to only one thing at a time.
    - Attention is voluntary and immediate; focus on *now*. The future has no role to play.
    - You can monitor your own attention.
    - Attention can be redirected.
    - Focusing on other things that are more relevant can redirect irrelevant attention.
    - You cannot pay attention continuously to one thing without breaks.

7. *Use visualization.* Spend a few moments thinking back to a crisis situation that you handled beautifully. Perhaps it was a medical emergency or a family quarrel where you intervened and helped resolve the issue. It can be any type of crisis in which you took charge successfully. Recall how strong and in-control you felt, how effectively you handled a bad scene, and even what the setting was like. Reflect on the event to recall it in as much detail as you can. Each day while you are studying, spend five to ten minutes revisiting this past event until you are able to bring it to mind with great clarity and detail. Now, when you feel anxiety welling up, take a mental time-out and revisit this scene. When you do, all the emotions of that day will also return and replace that anxiety.

8. *Use an affirmation card.* Take 30 minutes or so to write a series of statements on an index card. The statements should describe what you believe are your greatest personal strengths, character traits, and talents. You might state that you are a deeply empathetic person or that you are very good at solving problems. It doesn't matter what you write down, as long as you believe each statement is true and that you are proud of that skill, personality aspect, or talent. Once you have created the card, keep it with you as you study and practice with test questions. When anxious feelings begin to intrude, take out the card and read through it slowly, realizing the truth of what you have written. With practice, this process will help you focus and lessen negative thoughts.

9. *Take a mental time-out.* If anxious or angry thoughts interfere while you are practicing questions, try this exercise. Close your eyes, take some slow, deep breaths, and flex. Then relax, first the muscles in your neck, then in your shoulders, then in your lower limbs. Use a 1-2-3 count for each inhaled and exhaled breath to keep your breathing deep and even. The whole process will take only a few minutes and will help you reduce the physical symptoms of anxiety, allowing you to return to the test with a calm, focused state of mind.

10. *Learn and practice deep-breathing techniques.* It can be difficult to focus your attention when you are anxious; however, deep breathing can help. With enough practice during stressful events, this technique will become second nature during the exam.

11. *Use time-outs during the exam.* If necessary, to break the anxiety loop during the exam, back away from the mouse and keyboard and take a few deep breaths. Thirty seconds of rest will seem like 30 minutes in the middle of the exam. Try timing yourself and see how long it feels. By taking very little time away, you get a lot of mental rest. When the exam becomes too much, the best strategy is not to push yourself to concentrate harder, but to back off and rest for a few moments. You will find that when you return to the exam, your anxiety will be reduced and the questions will make more sense.

Summary Pointers

5

The COMLEX is a long, two-day exam. These two days can seem endless and exhausting. You need to have a clear goal in mind and a clear plan for reaching that goal. You need to be in good mental and physical shape for the exam.

REMEMBER

1. Not every question counts (although you won't know which ones do and which ones don't.)

2. You need to, be prepared in all of the eleven core subjects: Anatomy, Behavioral Science, Biochemistry, Genetics, Microbiology, Immunology, Molecular Biology, Pathology, Pharmacology, Physiology, and Osteopathic Manipulative Medicine. A question in one subject counts just as much as one in another.

3. Become familiar with the basic single-best-answer question subtypes: positively worded, long matching, two-step, bait-and-switch, true/false, clinical case, and conjunction questions.

4. You must be able to answer questions regarding material presented either as basic knowledge or as applied to clinical tasks. Increasingly, for this exam, application of knowledge is the key.

5. Spend some time becoming familiar with what is likely to be tested, but be careful of the mistake of "studying for last year's exam."

6. Be organized and plan your study time. Kaplan has a variety of resources, ranging from home-study materials to live lecture review courses that you may find useful in this regard. Make a study plan and stick to it.

7. Seriously consider forming a study group and helping each other review information. Presenting to each other is one of the best ways to learn to use the material you have studied.

8. Practice questions only after mastering the underlying material. Always do questions in clusters and within a time limit.

9. Taper off your preparation before the exam to give yourself a chance to rest up mentally and physically.

10. During the exam, read each question and answer it in order. Never change an answer. Segment your time to be sure you are not rushed at the end of the exam.

11. Do not linger over questions you do not know. Make what seems the likely choice, move on, and use the time to answer questions you do know.

12. You have three chances to get every question right: prediction, selection, and final passes. If you can't get a good answer after these three tries, guess and move on.

13. Consider using any of the time-tested behavioral strategies, especially taking a time-out for coping with anxiety and distracting negative thoughts during the exam.

14. Take care of yourself. Suffering doesn't help anyone.

Remember

Make a plan and stay with it.

Remember

Doing well on this exam is the result of knowledge plus correct test strategy.

Know your material and how to handle the test. The most successful students have a mastery of both.

THE COMLEX LEVEL 1: DOs AND DON'Ts

DOs

DO remember that the content of COMLEX will be similar to previous exams, as will the amount of time per question (just over one minute).

DO be organized. Set up an organized study schedule and adhere to it. Plan your work and work the plan.

DO be sure to make up questions while you study (use index cards) and form a study group to review important content.

DO use graphs and charts in texts to speed up your comprehension of the material. A picture is worth a thousand words, and the exam will test you using similar images.

DO practice questions under a time limit similar to the actual exam. In general, your rule should be one minute per question.

DO understand that there is material on the exam that you either will be unfamiliar with or never really fully understood. Don't panic! Guess and move on.

DO know that you are not required to pass each subsection (Physiology, Biochemistry, etc.) of the exam separately, but to answer enough questions correctly to attain an overall passing score.

DO understand that you will need to get between 55 and 65% of the questions to receive a passing score.

DO realize that you'll probably see more pictures than in past exams. They are only intended to test you on core basic science content.

DO know that not all of the questions on the exam will count. Forty to 50 questions on the exam are included so they can be pre-tested and evaluated for use in later exams. In addition, as many as 20 to 25 other questions may be eliminated from the scoring pool after the exam results are reviewed.

DO make sure your selected answer on each question matches *all* the information presented in that question. All answers are somewhat likely; you want to pick the one *most* likely.

DO be prepared for two-step questions, where you will need to make two correct decisions to arrive at the correct answer (e.g., come up with a diagnosis, then decide what the treatment should be).

DO remember that when you have the question down to two choices, you need to pick one and move on. Lingering over the question tends to result in making the wrong choice.

DON'Ts

DON'T just practice questions without preparatory studying. Review material first until you feel you know it, and then use questions to test yourself.

DON'T do practice questions individually. Do them in clusters with five to ten as a minimum to get yourself used to moving from question to question. Also, don't look up answers after each question; look up answers after each cluster.

DON'T get into the habit of lingering over a question or thinking about it for an extended period of time. You do not have this luxury on the exam itself.

DON'T just memorize material! Learn and understand how to apply the content in presented scenarios. Very little of the exam will test rote memory for basic facts, and that's not enough to pass.

DON'T reread your textbooks from cover to cover. You need to focus on the material most likely to be on the examination. Talk to others who have taken the exam to see how they prepared, and talk to faculty.

DON'T be afraid to face your weak or least-liked areas. Take pretests and/or diagnostic exams to help you identify your strengths and weaknesses. Begin your study plan with your weak areas, and plan to cover those at least twice before the exam. Do not entirely neglect your strong areas, but leave them to a time closer to the examination.

DON'T expect traditional exam "tricks," shortcuts, or buzzwords to point you to the correct answer. The COMLEX has put great effort into eliminating these cues from the exam.

DON'T get caught by distractors. They may be partially right answers, but not the best answers. Common misconceptions, incomplete knowledge, and faulty reasoning will cause you to select a distractor.

DON'T substitute reading the last line of the question for reading the whole question. This can cause you to miss important information or point you to distractors intended to confuse the issue.

DON'T skip any questions. If you don't know it when you come to it, you are not likely to know it later. Deal with each question as you come to it, answer it as best you can, and move on to the next question.

DON'T change an answer. Your odds of changing a correct answer to a wrong one are so much higher than the reverse that it is simply not worth the risk.

A FINAL COMMENT

This exam is not a test of your intelligence or even of how good a doctor you will be. This is a test of your capacity to identify and apply core principles within the constraints of the multiple-choice format. Planning, preparation, practice, perseverance, and patience will lead you to your best score.

Good luck, and remember, we're here to help.

Qbook–Practice Tests

Anatomy (Gross Anatomy, Neuroanatomy, Embryology, and Histology)

1. A 75-year-old man with a 40-pack-year history of smoking and hypercholesterolemia is diagnosed with severe atherosclerosis. Physical examination reveals chronic tissue changes at T1-T8 bilaterally. Atherosclerotic occlusion of which of the following arteries would result in insufficient perfusion of the urinary bladder?

   (A) External iliac

   (B) Inferior epigastric

   (C) Internal iliac

   (D) Internal pudendal

   (E) Lateral sacral

2. A 36-year-old woman is hospitalized for treatment of a stomach ulcer that has been getting progressively worse over several months. Structural examination was significant for a chronic, left-sided somatic dysfunction at T5-T9. Radiographic studies reveal the site of involvement to be along the greater curvature, approximately 4 cm away from the pyloric sphincter. That night, the ulcer perforates, and there is considerable intra-abdominal bleeding. Surgery reveals that the ulcer has eroded through the stomach wall and has damaged the artery supplying the involved region of the stomach. Which artery was likely involved?

   (A) Left gastric

   (B) Left gastroepiploic

   (C) Right gastric

   (D) Right gastroepiploic

   (E) Short gastric

3. A woman who recently gave birth has elevated prolactin levels. The gland responsible for secretion of this hormone is derived from which of the following structures?

   (A) Cerebral vesicle

   (B) Infundibulum

   (C) Neurohypophysis

   (D) Proctodeum

   (E) Rathke's pouch

4. A structural examination reveals chronic somatic dysfunction at T1-T4 in a 72-year-old patient with left ventricular hypertrophy. Which of the following structures constitutes part of the ventricles of the heart?

   (A) Auricle

   (B) Crista terminalis

   (C) Fossa ovalis

   (D) Sinus venarum

   (E) Trabeculae carneae

5. A 49-year-old Vietnamese man is diagnosed with tuberculosis. On physical examination, large flocculent masses are noted over the lateral lumbar back, and a similar mass is located in the ipsilateral groin. Physical examination also reveals increased tenderness just medial to the upsilateral ASIS upon palpation. This pattern of involvement strongly suggests an abscess tracking along which of the following muscles?

   (A) Adductor longus

   (B) Gluteus maximus

   (C) Gluteus minimus

   (D) Piriformis

   (E) Psoas major

6. When viewing an MRI, the nucleus that lies immediately medial (and deep) to the uncus is the

   (A) amygdala

   (B) caudate nucleus

   (C) claustrum

   (D) hippocampus

   (E) putamen

7. A 2-year-old boy is brought to the pediatrician by his mother because he has had several episodes of rectal bleeding. Evaluation with a technetium-99m perfusion scan reveals a 3-cm ileal outpouching located 60 cm from the ileocecal valve. This structure most likely contains which of the following types of ectopic tissue?

   (A) Duodenal

   (B) Esophageal

   (C) Gastric

   (D) Hepatic

   (E) Jejunal

8. A 34-year-old man is examined in the prison infirmary after sustaining a superficial stab wound to the superolateral aspect of the thoracic wall at the level of the third rib. There is little bleeding and no difficulty breathing; however, the medial border of the scapula on the injured side pulls away from the body wall when the arm is raised. In addition, the arm cannot be abducted above the horizontal. Spencer techniques have failed to show improvement in the shoulder's somatic dysfunction. Which of the following muscles is paralyzed?

   (A) Levator scapulae

   (B) Pectoralis minor

   (C) Rhomboid major

   (D) Serratus anterior

   (E) Supraspinatus

9. A histologist is examining cells arrested at various stages of oogenesis. He discovers a follicle within the stroma of the ovary that has developed an antrum. This follicle would be classified as

   (A) Graafian

   (B) primary

   (C) primordial

   (D) secondary

   (E) tertiary

10. A 54-year-old man has cirrhosis, with obstruction of the portal circulation within the liver. There is chronic somatic dysfunction at T5-T9 on the right side. Portal blood could still be conveyed to the caval system via which of the following?

    (A) Azygos and hemiazygos veins

    (B) Gonadal veins

    (C) Internal iliac veins

    (D) Splenic vein

    (E) Vesical venous plexus

11. A 47-year-old man presents to his neurologist with an unsteady, broad-based gait and slow, slurred speech. Neurologic examination reveals dysdiadochokinesia, intention tremor, hypotonia, and nystagmus. The patient's lesion is in a brain structure that derives from which of the following embryonic structures?

    (A) Diencephalon

    (B) Mesencephalon

    (C) Metencephalon

    (D) Myelencephalon

    (E) Telencephalon

12. A 47-year-old woman with a history of rheumatic fever is examined by her physician. Physical examination is significant for a low-pitched, rumbling, diastolic murmur preceded by an opening snap. Structural examination reveals that T1-T4 have chronic tissue changes in the left paraspinal musculature. The affected valve can be best evaluated by auscultation at which of the following locations?

    (A) Left second intercostal space

    (B) Left fifth intercostal space

    (C) Left lower sternal body border

    (D) Right second intercostal space

    (E) Right fifth intercostal space

13. Examination of a patient's eye reveals a malformation of the ciliary body. This malformation is due to abnormal development of the

    (A) axons of retinal ganglion cells

    (B) choroid fissure of the optic stalk

    (C) mesoderm surrounding the optic cup

    (D) mesoderm surrounding the optic stalk

    (E) neuroectoderm of the optic cup

14. A neuroscientist decides to perform a study that requires him to increase the concentration of norepinephrine in the cortex of an animal subject. He does this by electrically stimulating a nucleus in the brain. Which of the following nuclei is the most important source of noradrenergic innervation to the cerebral cortex?

    (A) Basal nucleus of Meynert

    (B) Caudate nucleus

    (C) Locus coeruleus

    (D) Raphe nucleus

    (E) Substantia nigra

15. A surgeon tells a medical student to tap the side of the face of a patient who just had thyroid surgery. The surgeon is most worried about damage to which of the following vessels?

    (A) Common carotid artery

    (B) External carotid artery

    (C) Facial vein

    (D) Internal jugular vein

    (E) Superior and inferior thyroid arteries

16. A 45-year-old man comes into the emergency department with abdominal pain that has progressively worsened since the previous night. He also notes nausea and vomiting, but is afebrile. Upper gastrointestinal radiographic studies reveal that a loop of small intestine has passed through the epiploic foramen into the omental bursa and is constricted by the margins of the foramen as the intestine fills. The constriction should not be surgically relieved by opening the epiploic foramen because this procedure would risk cutting the

    (A) abdominal aorta

    (B) hepatic artery

    (C) hepatic vein

    (D) hypogastric plexus

    (E) pancreatic duct

17. A 26-year-old man is stabbed in the left chest during a bar brawl. Several days after he is treated, he returns to the physician complaining of decreased function in his left arm. Physical examination reveals a winged left scapula and an inability to raise his left arm above the horizontal. Osteopathic manipulation has failed to improve his condition. Which of the following nerves is most likely affected?

    (A) Axillary

    (B) Long thoracic

    (C) Lower subscapular

    (D) Suprascapular

    (E) Thoracodorsal

18. A patient is transported to the emergency department with a knife wound to the right fifth intercostal space at the midaxillary line. Which of the following structures is likely to have been damaged?

    (A) Liver

    (B) Right atrium

    (C) Right pulmonary artery

    (D) Superior vena cava

    (E) Upper lobe of right lung

19. A patient has chronic somatic dysfunction at T11-L1. An IVP is scheduled. You review your anatomy of the kidney. Which of the following renal structures is most medially located?

    (A) Major calyx

    (B) Minor calyx

    (C) Renal cortex

    (D) Renal pelvis

    (E) Renal pyramid

20. A 19-year-old woman comes to the emergency department after falling while on roller-blades. There is a 3-cm laceration over the lateral aspect of the knee penetrating so deep that the head of the fibula is apparent. A radiograph of the leg is negative for any fractures. A noticeable foot-drop occurs while the patient walks. Further examination reveals inability to dorsiflex or evert the foot. Which of the following best explains her injury?

(A) The common peroneal nerve was severed

(B) The peroneal muscles were detached from the head of the fibula

(C) The superficial peroneal nerve was severed

(D) The tibial nerve was severed

(E) The talus is in plantar flexion

21. A resident physician is performing a pelvic examination on a young woman. The fingers of one of her hands are in the patient's vagina, palpating the cervix. The other hand is pressing on the abdomen. With the palm of this hand, the physician feels a bony structure in the lower midline. She notes that there is no somatic dysfunction during her palpation of this structure. This structure is most likely the

(A) coccyx

(B) ilium

(C) ischium

(D) pubis

(E) sacrum

22. A 45-year-old man with a history of stable angina presents to the emergency department with an episode of chest pain that is not relieved by rest or nitroglycerin. After stabilization in the telemetry unit for 2 days, he undergoes a thallium stress test. The results show reduced perfusion of the lateral wall of the left ventricle. Which artery is most likely occluded?

(A) Left anterior descending

(B) Left circumflex

(C) Left main coronary

(D) Right coronary

(E) Anterior interventricular

23. Which of the labeled structures is responsible for the secretion of renin?

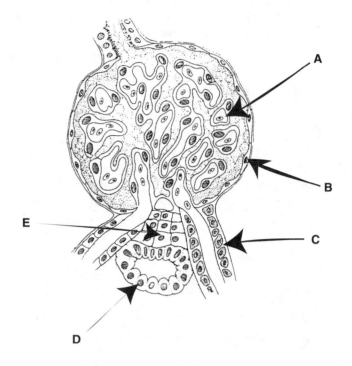

(A) A

(B) B

(C) C

(D) D

(E) E

24. A 4-day-old boy is brought to the pediatric clinic because of breathing difficulties and poor feeding. He coughs, chokes, and spits up milk very soon after beginning to suckle. Physical examination and radiographs reveal the presence of the most common type of tracheoesophageal fistula. The infant's defect likely resulted from

(A) failure of the buccopharyngeal membrane to rupture

(B) failure of the tracheoesophageal ridges to fuse

(C) incomplete formation of the septum secundum

(D) incomplete recanalization of the larynx

(E) patent thyroglossal duct

25. A 40-year-old man complains of loss of sensation over the right scrotum and on the medial right thigh. Structural examination reveals somatic dysfunction at T10-L2 on the right. Damage to which of the following nerves would result in such symptoms?

    (A) Genitofemoral
    (B) Iliohypogastric
    (C) Ilioinguinal
    (D) Lateral cutaneous
    (E) Pudendal

26. A neonate has a prominent defect at the base of his spine through which his meninges and spinal cord protrude. A failure of which of the following processes is the most common cause of this type of defect?

    (A) Development of the body
    (B) Development of the pedicle
    (C) Development of primary vertebral ossification centers
    (D) Development of the superior articular process
    (E) Fusion of the vertebral arches

27. A surgeon is first on the scene after a serious automobile accident. He finds a passenger bleeding profusely from the neck and correctly surmises that the bleeding is from the carotid artery. To control the bleeding, the surgeon can compress the carotid artery against the anterior tubercle of which of the following vertebrae?

    (A) Second cervical
    (B) Third cervical
    (C) Fourth cervical
    (D) Fifth cervical
    (E) Sixth cervical

28. MRI reveals that a 62-year-old man has a brain tumor growing in his interhemispheric fissure at the level of the central sulcus. The tumor produces neurologic dysfunction of the cerebral cortex on either side of the tumor. A neurologic examination of this patient would most likely reveal

    (A) ataxia
    (B) hemiplegia
    (C) paraplegia
    (D) quadriplegia
    (E) rigidity

29. Brunner's glands secrete an alkaline product that helps achieve optimal pH for the activity of pancreatic enzymes. Where are these glands located?

    (A) At the base of villi throughout the small intestine
    (B) In the epithelium of the ampulla of Vater
    (C) In the mucosa and submucosa of the jejunum
    (D) In the submucosa of the duodenum
    (E) In the submucosa of the ileum

30. A 24-year-old man presents with pain in his right wrist that resulted when he fell hard on his outstretched hand. Physical examination reveals pain, swelling, erythema, and decreased range of motion in the right wrist. Radiographic studies indicate an anterior dislocation of a proximal row carpal bone that articulates with the most lateral proximal row carpal bone. Which of the following bones was dislocated?

    (A) Capitate
    (B) Lunate
    (C) Scaphoid
    (D) Trapezoid
    (E) Triquetrum

31. A patient needs an arterial blood gas drawn from the femoral artery (in the femoral triangle, which is bounded superiorly by the inguinal ligament). Which of the following structures form the lateral borders of the femoral triangle?

    (A) Adductor longus and gracilis
    (B) Adductor longus and sartorius
    (C) Gracilis and pectineus
    (D) Gracilis and sartorius
    (E) Pectineus and sartorius

32. A 43-year-old woman is diagnosed with a condition that causes excruciating pain near her nose and mouth. The involved nerve is derived from which of the following branchial arches?

    (A) First
    (B) Second
    (C) Third
    (D) Fourth
    (E) Fifth

33. An infant is born with an abnormally developed falciform ligament. The hepatogastric and hepatoduodenal ligaments are also malformed. These developmental anomalies are most likely due to abnormal development of the

    (A) dorsal mesoduodenum

    (B) dorsal mesogastrium

    (C) pericardioperitoneal canal

    (D) pleuropericardial membranes

    (E) ventral mesentery

34. When removing an impacted mandibular third molar, the oral surgeon must warn the patient of possible lasting numbness of the tip of the tongue. This loss of general sensation is due to damage to the

    (A) auriculotemporal nerve

    (B) chorda tympani

    (C) lingual nerve

    (D) mental nerve

    (E) mylohyoid nerve

35. A resident physician is demonstrating the correct technique for inserting a subclavian central venous line. He has a medical student palpate the clavicle, then the chest wall below it. The first bony structure that can be palpated below the inferior margin of the medial portion of the clavicle is the

    (A) acromion

    (B) atlas

    (C) first rib

    (D) manubrium

    (E) second rib

36. The primordium of the respiratory system that forms the internal epithelial lining of the trachea, bronchi, and lungs is derived entirely from which of the following embryologic entities?

    (A) Foregut endoderm

    (B) Midgut endoderm

    (C) Splanchnic mesoderm

    (D) Stomodeum

    (E) Both endoderm and mesoderm

37. An infant born to an alcoholic mother had microcephaly and cardiac abnormalities and died despite resuscitative efforts. During which of the following periods of pregnancy is alcohol most teratogenic?

    (A) First 2 weeks

    (B) 3rd through 9th weeks

    (C) 9th through 12th weeks

    (D) 12th through 16th weeks

    (E) 16th through 20th weeks

38. A 15-year-old girl with a history of chronic rhinitis, allergy, asthma, and nasal polyposis presents with fever and dental pain. Physical examination reveals acute tissue-texture changes at T1-T4. She is diagnosed with maxillary sinusitis. Mucopurulent exudate would be most likely to drain through an ostium in the

    (A) bulla ethmoidalis

    (B) hiatus semilunaris

    (C) inferior nasal meatus

    (D) sphenoethmoidal recess

    (E) superior nasal meatus

39. A patient presents to the physician complaining of "something wrong with her foot" that causes her to trip and fall. Physical examination reveals an inability to dorsiflex (extend) the foot and a loss of sensation between the first and second toes. Osteopathic examination reveals somatic dysfunction at L4-L5. There is no other motor or sensory loss. Which of the following nerves was most likely injured?

    (A) Deep peroneal

    (B) Femoral

    (C) Superficial peroneal

    (D) Sural

    (E) Tibial

40. The endothelial lining of the aorta is composed of which of the following tissue types?

    (A) Pseudostratified epithelium

    (B) Simple columnar epithelium

    (C) Simple cuboidal epithelium

    (D) Simple squamous epithelium

    (E) Stratified columnar epithelium

41. One week following a sexual encounter at a ski resort in Colorado, a young woman develops a painful, swollen knee joint. The osteopathic structural examination found no somatic dysfunction in the spine at T10-L2; however, a decrease was found in the flexion and extension of the knee. The tests for ligamentous and meniscal changes are negative. The emergency department physician suspects gonococcal arthritis and wants to confirm this by sending joint fluid for bacterial culture. He uses the standard suprapatellar approach and passes a needle from the lateral aspect of the thigh into the region immediately proximal to the patella. Through which of the following muscles does the needle pass?

    (A) Adductor magnus

    (B) Gracilis

    (C) Iliacus

    (D) Sartorius

    (E) Vastus lateralis

42. A 67-year-old man has an abnormal neurologic exam. An electroencephalogram is subsequently performed and reveals delta waves over his left frontal lobe. Which of the following was the most likely abnormal finding on his neurologic exam?

    (A) Left hemiparesis

    (B) Left hemisensory loss

    (C) Left homonymous hemianopia

    (D) Right hemiparesis

    (E) Right hemisensory loss

43. A 23-year-old woman wearing high-heeled shoes inverts and sprains her ankle while running down a flight of stairs. There are multiple tender points, as well as ecchymosis, swelling, and decreased range of motion. Which of the following ligaments did she most likely injure?

    (A) Anterior talotibial

    (B) Calcaneofibular

    (C) Calcaneotibial

    (D) Deltoid

    (E) Medial collateral

Questions 44-50

<u>SET A</u>

Directions: For each numbered item (**patient presentation**), select the one lettered heading (**joint**) most closely associated with it. Each lettered heading may be selected once, more than once, or not at all.

   (A) hinge joint

   (B) pivot joint

   (C) condyloid joint

   (D) saddle joint

   (E) ball and socket joint

   (F) plane joint

   (G) immovable joint

   (H) slightly moveable joint

44. A patient diagnosed with osteoarthritis presents with hip pain.

45. A patient injured during a game of football complains of knee pain.

46. A 40-year-old woman slipped and fell on her wrist.

47. A 28-year-old woman comes in complaining of suprapubic tenderness; urinalysis and culture and sensitivity are negative.

48. A 19-year-old man sprains his thumb while catching a baseball.

49. A patient slipped on ice and complains of elbow pain.

50. A patient slipped and fell; x-ray reveals dislocation of the proximal radioulnar joint.

Anatomy (Gross Anatomy, Neuroanatomy, Embryology, and Histology)

ANSWERS AND EXPLANATIONS

1.	C		26.	E
2.	D		27.	E
3.	E		28.	C
4.	E		29.	D
5.	E		30.	B
6.	A		31.	B
7.	C		32.	A
8.	D		33.	E
9.	D		34.	C
10.	A		35.	E
11.	C		36.	A
12.	B		37.	B
13.	E		38.	B
14.	C		39.	A
15.	E		40.	D
16.	B		41.	E
17.	B		42.	D
18.	A		43.	B
19.	D		44.	E
20.	A		45.	F
21.	D		46.	C
22.	B		47.	H
23.	C		48.	D
24.	B		49.	A
25.	C		50.	B

1. **The correct answer is C.** The bladder is supplied by the vesicular branches of the internal iliac arteries. The internal iliacs arise from the common iliac artery. Note that this is a simple fact question (Which artery supplies the urinary bladder?) embedded in a clinical scenario.

   The external iliac (**choice A**) also arises from the common iliac artery. It makes no contribution to the blood supply of the bladder.

   The inferior epigastric (**choice B**) is a branch of the external iliac artery. It serves as a landmark in the inguinal region. Indirect inguinal hernias lie lateral to the inferior epigastric arteries, whereas direct inguinal hernias lie medial to these vessels. A good mnemonic is MDs don't LIe. (Medial-Direct, Lateral-Indirect).

   The internal pudendal (**choice D**) is a branch of the anterior division of the internal iliac artery. It gives rise to the inferior rectal artery, perineal artery, artery of the bulb in men, urethral artery, deep artery of the penis or clitoris, and dorsal artery of the penis or clitoris.

   The lateral sacral (**choice E**) is a branch of the posterior division of the internal iliac artery. It supplies sacral structures.

2. **The correct answer is D.** The right gastroepiploic artery, off the gastroduodenal artery, supplies the right half of the greater curvature of the stomach and could be directly affected by ulceration of the greater curvature of the stomach at a site this close (4 cm) to the pyloric sphincter.

   The left gastric artery (**choice A**), off the celiac trunk, supplies the left half of the lesser curvature of the stomach.

   The left gastroepiploic artery (**choice B**), off the splenic artery, supplies the left half of the greater curvature of the stomach. Although it anastomoses with the right gastroepiploic artery, it is unlikely that this artery would be directly damaged by ulceration of the stomach near the pyloric sphincter.

   The right gastric artery (**choice C**), off the proper hepatic artery, supplies the right half of the lesser curvature of the stomach.

   The short gastric artery (**choice E**), actually one of several (4-5) short gastric arteries, off the splenic artery (occasionally the left gastroepiploic), supplies the fundus of the stomach, which is most distant from the pylorus.

3. **The correct answer is E.** The anterior pituitary produces prolactin. The structure originates from Rathke's pouch, which is itself a diverticulum of the roof of the stomodeum.

   The cerebral vesicle (**choice A**) lies close to Rathke's pouch.

   The infundibulum (**choice B**) comes in contact with Rathke's pouch at the 5th week of development.

   The neurohypophysis (**choice C**) gives rise to the posterior pituitary.

   The proctodeum (**choice D**) is also known as the anal pit.

4. **The correct answer is E.** The trabeculae carneae are ridges of myocardium in the ventricular wall. Remember that the Latin root "carne-" means "flesh" and that the ventricles are "fleshier" than the atria.

   The auricle (**choice A**) is derived from the fetal atrium; it has rough myocardium known as musculi pectinati.

   The crista terminalis (**choice B**) is the vertical ridge that separates the smooth portion of the right atrium from the rough portion; it extends longitudinally from the superior vena cava to the inferior vena cava.

   The fossa ovalis (**choice C**) is the fetal foramen ovale, an opening in the interatrial septum that allows blood entering the right atrium from the inferior vena cava to pass directly to the left side of the heart.

   The sinus venarum (**choice D**) is the smooth-walled portion of the atrium that receives blood from the superior and inferior vena cava. It is derived from the fetal sinus venosus.

5. **The correct answer is E.** This is the classic presentation of a psoas abscess. This clinical entity was formerly a fairly common complication of vertebral tuberculosis, but is now rare in clinical practice in this country. The psoas muscle is covered by a fibrous sheath known as the psoas fascia. This sheath is open superiorly, permitting an infection involving the soft tissues around the spine to enter the sheath, then track down to the groin.

   The adductor longus (**choice A**) is a muscle of the anterior thigh and is not related to the lumbar portion of the back.

   The gluteus maximus (**choice B**), gluteus minimus (**choice C**), and piriformis (**choice D**) are muscles of the buttock with no relationship to the groin.

6. **The correct answer is A.** The uncus, which is the medial protrusion of the parahippocampal gyrus, is an external structure seen on the ventral surface of the temporal lobe. The amygdala is a collection of nuclei that lies directly beneath the uncus.

The caudate nucleus (**choice B**) is a deep nuclear structure that lies lateral to the lateral ventricles.

The claustrum (**choice C**) is a thin and elongated nucleus that lies just medial to the insular cortex.

The hippocampus (**choice D**) is a nuclear structure that lies in the interior of the parahippocampal gyrus.

The putamen (**choice E**) is a nuclear structure that resides lateral to the caudate and medial to the claustrum.

7. **The correct answer is C.** This child has a Meckel diverticulum, an ileal outpocketing typically located within 50-75 cm of the ileocecal valve. It is a congenital anomaly resulting from the persistence of the vitelline (omphalomesenteric) duct. Approximately half cause ulceration, inflammation, and gastrointestinal bleeding because of the presence of ectopic acid-secreting gastric epithelium. Pancreatic tissue may sometimes occur in these diverticula as well. Note that this is the most common type of congenital gastrointestinal anomaly.

    Something else to keep in mind: A favorite question attendings ask on the wards is the rule of 2's associated with Meckel diverticulum: it occurs in about 2% of children, occurs within approximately 2 feet of the ileocecal valve, contains 2 types of ectopic mucosa (gastric and pancreatic), and its symptoms usually occur by age 2.

    None of the other answer choices has a relationship to Meckel diverticulum.

8. **The correct answer is D.** The serratus anterior plays a major role in holding the scapula against the body wall. If paralyzed, the primary clinical sign is "winging" of the scapula, especially when raising the arm or pushing the body away from a wall. In addition, it aids in rotation of the scapula, raising the glenoid cavity when the arm is abducted beyond the horizontal. The serratus anterior is innervated by the long thoracic nerve, which runs very superficially on the superolateral thoracic wall, where it is especially prone to injury.

    The levator scapulae (**choice A**) elevates the scapula. It is not involved in holding the scapula against the body wall. Its innervation, derived from the cervical plexus (C3, 4), is not damaged by injury to the superolateral thoracic wall.

    Although the pectoralis minor (**choice B**) has a scapular attachment (to the coracoid process), it is not involved in holding the scapula against the body wall. Its innervation, the medial pectoral nerve, is not likely to be damaged by injury to the superolateral thoracic wall.

    The rhomboid major (**choice C**) primarily retracts the scapula. It does not have an important role in holding the scapula against the body wall. Its innervation, the

dorsal scapular nerve, is not easily damaged by injury to the superolateral thoracic wall.

Although the supraspinatus (**choice E**) plays a role in arm abduction, it is essential to the initiation of this movement (the first 20-30 degrees) before there is significant rotation of the scapula. It is not involved in holding the scapula against the body wall (although it is important in holding the head of the humerus against the glenoid fossa). Its innervation, the suprascapular nerve, would not be damaged by injury to the superolateral thoracic wall.

9. **The correct answer is D.** During the growth of the primary follicle, there is a proliferation of follicular cells, an increase in the size of the oocyte, and formation of a connective tissue capsule around the follicle by the follicular cells. Soon thereafter, small spaces begin to appear in the follicular mass. These spaces fuse to form the follicular cavity, or antrum. Once the antrum develops, the follicle is termed a secondary follicle.

    The Graafian follicle (**choice A**) is the mature follicle that extends through the entire cortex and bulges out at the ovarian surface.

    The primary follicles (**choice B**) are relatively small and spherical, with a central oocyte and one or more layers of cuboidal-like follicular cells.

    The primary oocytes, which are arrested in prophase of their first meiotic division, are contained within the primordial follicles (**choice C**) as inactive reserve follicles.

    Recall the sequence of oogenesis:

    Primordial follicle (contain primary oocytes) → Primary follicle → Secondary follicle → Graafian follicle

    There is no tertiary follicle (**choice E**) in the sequence of oogenesis; it would equate to a mature follicle.

10. **The correct answer is A.** The esophageal venous plexus, which drains into the azygos and hemiazygos veins within the thorax, has anastomoses with branches of the left gastric vein. Thus, following blockage of the portal vein, portal blood may enter the superior vena cava via the azygos system. Other important portacaval connections include the superior rectal vein with the middle and inferior rectal veins; paraumbilical veins with epigastric veins (engorgement of these vessels results in *caput medusae*); and the colic and splenic veins with renal veins and veins of the posterior body wall.

    The gonadal veins (**choice B**) exclusively drain the gonads (although in the female, the ovarian vein communicates with the uterovaginal plexus). These vessels have no anastomoses with portal vessels.

The internal iliac veins (**choice C**), which drain most of the pelvis and much of the inferior extremities, have no demonstrated portal anastomoses.

The splenic vein (**choice D**) is incorrect because it is itself a component of the portal venous system.

The vesical venous plexus (**choice E**), which is situated well within the pelvis and drains the bladder and the prostate (or uterus and vagina), has no association with portal vessels.

11. **The correct answer is C.** The patient has a cerebellar lesion. Cerebellar dysfunction can lead to a variety of motor dysfunctions, including truncal ataxia (appearing similar to the gait of an intoxicated individual), intention tremor (uncontrolled shaking of affected extremity present only with purposeful movement), dysdiadochokinesia (the inability to perform rapid and regular alternating movements), dysmetria (inability to stop movements at the desired point), dysarthria (ataxic speech), hypotonia, and nystagmus.

During the 4th week of embryonic development, the anterior end of the neural tube develops three vesicles: the prosencephalon (forebrain), the mesencephalon (midbrain), and the rhombencephalon (hindbrain). By the 6th week, five vesicles (listed in the answer options) have developed. The rhombencephalon has now developed into the metencephalon and myelencephalon. The cerebellum and pons derive from the metencephalon.

The diencephalon (**choice A**), which is derived from the prosencephalon, develops into the thalamus, hypothalamus, epithalamus, subthalamus (everything with the word "thalamus"), posterior lobe of the pituitary, and neural retina.

The mesencephalon (**choice B**), or midbrain, is the only brain vesicle that does not produce a secondary vesicle; it remains the mesencephalon.

The myelencephalon (**choice D**), which is derived from the rhombencephalon, develops into the medulla oblongata.

The telencephalon (**choice E**), which is derived from the prosencephalon, develops into the cerebral hemispheres (cerebral cortex, basal ganglia, and deep white matter).

12. **The correct answer is B.** Solid knowledge of cardiac anatomy and its clinical correlations are crucial for performing physical examinations (and answering COMLEX questions). This question tests two facts. First it requires that you recognize the patient has mitral stenosis. Classic clues to this diagnosis are "low-pitched, rumbling, diastolic murmur," "open-

ing snap," and "rheumatic fever." The mitral valve is the most commonly affected valve in rheumatic fever, followed by the aortic and tricuspid valves. The question then asks you where sounds generated by a faulty mitral valve will be best heard on physical exam. The mitral valve is most audible over the left fifth intercostal space at the midclavicular line.

The pulmonary valve is most audible over the left second intercostal space (**choice A**). Pulmonic stenosis is associated with tetralogy of Fallot, a common cyanotic congenital heart disease.

The tricuspid valve is most audible over the left lower sternal border (**choice C**). This valve is primarily affected in IV drug abusers with endocarditis.

The aortic valve is most audible over the right second intercostal space (**choice D**). Aortic stenosis is associated with angina, syncope, and congestive heart failure. A systolic murmur that radiates to the carotids is heard on exam, along with a systolic ejection click.

No particular structure is best heard over the right fifth intercostal space (**choice E**).

13. **The correct answer is E.** The optic cups derive from the optic vesicles, which are evaginations of the diencephalon. The anterior two layers of the optic cup (neurectoderm), in association with choroidal mesoderm, give rise to the ciliary body and the iris. The optic cup also gives rise to the neural and pigment layers of the retina.

Retinal ganglion cell axons (**choice A**), which run in the optic stalk, become the nerve fibers of the optic nerve.

Closure of the choroid fissure in the optic stalk (**choice B**) occurs during the 7th week of development. The former optic stalk is then called the optic nerve.

Mesoderm surrounding the optic cup (**choice C**) becomes the sclera and choroid of the eye.

Mesoderm surrounding the optic stalk (**choice D**) gives rise to the meninges surrounding the optic nerve.

14. **The correct answer is C.** The locus coeruleus is a dense collection of neuromelanin-containing cells in the rostral pons, near the lateral edge of the floor of the fourth ventricle. The fact that it appears blue-black in unstained brain tissue gave rise to its name, which means "blue spot" in Latin. These cells, which contain norepinephrine, provide the majority of noradrenergic innervation to the forebrain, including the cerebral cortex.

The basal nucleus of Meynert (**choice A**), a part of the substantia innominata, is a major collection of forebrain cholinergic neurons. These neurons (together with neurons in septal nuclei) innervate the neocortex, hippocampal formation, and the amygdala. The basal nucleus is one of the structures that degenerates in Alzheimer disease.

The caudate nucleus (**choice B**) is part of the basal ganglia, located immediately lateral to the lateral ventricles. There are at least two important cell types in the caudate. GABAergic projection neurons (the majority) innervate the globus pallidus and substantia nigra pars reticulata. The GABAergic neurons degenerate in Huntington disease, leading to enlarged lateral ventricles that are clearly visible on MRI. The caudate also contains cholinergic interneurons, which provide most of the acetylcholine to the striatum (caudate and putamen). The balance of striatal acetylcholine and dopamine is important for the treatment of patients with extrapyramidal symptoms, such as Parkinson disease or parkinsonism accompanying therapy with antipsychotic medications.

The raphe nuclei (**choice D**) are located in the midline at most levels of the brainstem. They contain serotonergic cell bodies that innervate virtually every part of the CNS.

The substantia nigra (**choice E**) is located in the midbrain and consists of the substantia nigra pars compacta and the substantia nigra pars reticulata. The substantia nigra pars compacta contains the nigrostriatal neurons that are the source of striatal dopamine. This cell group degenerates in Parkinson disease or in response to neurotoxic agents such as MPTP. The substantia nigra pars reticulata consists predominately of GABAergic neurons that innervate the thalamus.

15. **The correct answer is E.** The surgeon has asked the medical student to test for tetany, which can occur if the blood supply to the parathyroid glands (through the superior and inferior thyroid arteries) is disrupted during thyroid surgery. Specifically, the medical student is being asked to tap with his fingers the muscles of mastication, notably the masseter, which because of its strength is a sensitive indicator of tetany. Tetany will be seen as an abnormally strong jerk or contraction related to the hypocalcemia that can develop if secretion of parathyroid hormone is inadequate.

16. **The correct answer is B.** The hepatic artery is one component of the portal triad: the hepatic artery, common bile duct, and portal vein. These structures constitute the porta hepatis and lie in the free edge of the lesser omentum as it forms the epiploic foramen. Opening the epiploic foramen would therefore involve cutting the porta hepatis and, possibly, the hepatic artery and/or other components of the portal triad.

The abdominal aorta (**choice A**) is retroperitoneal, posterior to the omental bursa. It is not associated with the epiploic foramen and would not likely be damaged by surgery to open the foramen.

The hepatic vein (**choice C**) returns blood from the liver to the inferior vena cava and is not associated with the epiploic foramen. In contrast, the portal vein, part of the portal triad, brings venous blood to the liver.

The hypogastric plexus (**choice D**) is a plexus of autonomic nerves found in the superior pelvis and the posterior abdominal wall in the inferior abdomen. This plexus is not close to the epiploic foramen, so it is unlikely to be injured by surgery in that region.

The pancreatic duct (**choice E**) is not a boundary of the epiploic foramen.

17. **The correct answer is B.** The serratus anterior, innervated by the long thoracic nerve, is responsible for stabilization of the scapula during abduction of the arm from 90 to 180 degrees. When the long thoracic nerve is damaged, it is difficult to elevate the arm above the horizontal. This nerve arises from C5, 6, and 7. Remember: a "winged scapula" is a classic clue for long thoracic nerve injury.

Note that the supraspinatus muscle, innervated by the suprascapular nerve (**choice D**), is responsible for abducting the arm from 0 degrees to about 30 degrees. The rest of the motion to 180 degrees is performed by the deltoid muscle, which is innervated by the axillary nerve (**choice A**). However, the motion from 90 to 180 degrees also requires a stable scapula and therefore depends on the long thoracic nerve.

The axillary nerve (**choice A**) is a branch of the posterior cord of the brachial plexus (C5, C6). It is particularly susceptible to injury in shoulder dislocations that displace the humeral head or in fracture of the surgical neck of the humerus. A poorly placed crutch may also damage this nerve, causing paralysis of the teres minor and deltoid muscles. Arm abduction is impaired, and there is associated loss of sensation over the lower half of the deltoid.

The lower subscapular nerve (**choice C**) innervates the teres major, which is responsible for adducting and medially rotating the arm. It is a branch of the posterior cord (C5, C6) of the brachial plexus.

The suprascapular nerve (**choice D**) innervates the supraspinatus and infraspinatus muscles, which are responsible for abduction and lateral rotation of the arm. The nerve is derived from the C5 and C6 nerve roots.

The thoracodorsal nerve (**choice E**) innervates the latissimus dorsi muscle, which is responsible for adduction and extension of the arm. The nerve arises from the posterior cord (C7, C8) of the brachial plexus.

18. **The correct answer is A.** Any perforating wound occurring below the level of the fourth intercostal space on the right side may damage the liver, which is protected by the rib cage, although it is an abdominal organ lying inferior to the diaphragm.

    At its most lateral aspect, the right atrium (**choice B**) forms the right border of the heart, which extends from the third costal cartilage to the sixth costal cartilage just to the right of the sternum.

    The right pulmonary artery (**choice C**) enters the hilus of the lung at the level of the T5 vertebra. Since the ribs are angled downward as they pass forward, this entry occurs above the level of the fifth intercostal space at the midaxillary line.

    The superior vena cava (**choice D**) enters the right atrium at the level of the third costal cartilage.

    At the midaxillary line, the oblique fissure of the right lung (**choice E**) passes between the inferior and middle lobes.

19. **The correct answer is D.** This is a relatively simple question that requires you to visualize the relationship among the key parts of the kidney and to identify the one that lies most medially. Since the kidneys ultimately drain into the ureter at their medial poles, you are looking for the structure that is closest to the ureter. The correct answer is the renal pelvis. The renal pelvis is the dilated upper portion of the ureter that receives the major calyces.

    In terms of the other answer choices, the order from most lateral to most medial is as follows: renal cortex (**choice C**), renal pyramid (**choice E**), minor calyx (**choice B**), major calyx (**choice A**), and then renal pelvis (**choice D**).

20. **The correct answer is A.** The common peroneal nerve wraps around the lateral aspect of the head of the fibula and is highly susceptible to damage during lacerations or blunt injuries to the lateral knee. Foot-drop with loss of dorsiflexion or eversion is characteristic.

    Only the peroneus longus completely attaches to the fibular head (**choice B**). Other muscles that attach in other places along the tibia and fibula provide dorsiflexion and eversion for the foot (e.g., extensor digitorum longus, peroneus brevis, extensor hallucis longus, and tibialis anterior).

    The common peroneal nerve then branches into the superficial (**choice C**) and deep peroneal nerves, which

supply the muscles of the anterior compartment of the leg and cutaneous areas of the distal anterior leg, dorsum of the foot, and most of the digits.

The tibial nerve (**choice D**) supplies all the muscles in the posterior compartment of the leg (e.g., tibialis posterior, flexor digitorum longus, gastrocnemius, and soleus).

The talus being in plantar flexion (**choice E**) does not result in foot drop.

21. **The correct answer is D.** The resident is feeling the two pubic bones, which are joined at the midline by the symphysis pubis. Experienced obstetrician/gynecologists can often perceive the softening of the symphysis pubis that occurs during late pregnancy as a "springiness" of the pubic bones during palpation.

    The coccyx (**choice A**) is the caudal terminus of the vertebral column, generally formed by the fusion of four rudimentary vertebral bodies. It is also called the tailbone.

    The ilium (**choice B**) is one of the two "wings" that form the lateral sides of the pelvic cavity and support the abdominal contents.

    The ischium (**choice C**) is the portion of the pelvis on which a person sits.

    The sacrum (**choice E**) is the triangular bone situated just beneath the lumbar vertebrae.

22. **The correct answer is B.** In some patients with coronary artery disease, thallium stress tests may be performed instead of cardiac catheterization to determine the vessels involved and the extent of occlusion. The left circumflex (LCx) branch supplies the lateral wall of the left ventricle; in 10% of the population, it also supplies the posterior wall and AV node.

    The left anterior descending (LAD) branch of the left coronary artery (**choice A**) supplies the anterior wall of the left ventricle and the anterior portion of the interventricular septum (**choice E**).

    The left main coronary artery (**choice C**) gives rise to both the LCx and the LAD.

    The right coronary artery (RCA; **choice D**) supplies the right ventricle; in 90% of the population, it supplies the AV node and posterior and inferior walls of the left ventricle.

23. **The correct answer is C.** This question requires that you know two pieces of information: (1) renin is secreted from the juxtaglomerular (JG) cells; and (2) the location of the JG cells in a picture that includes both the glomerulus and the juxtaglomerular apparatus. Remember that renin is responsible for converting angiotensinogen to angiotensin I, which is subsequently converted

to angiotensin II in the lungs by an important enzyme appropriately called angiotensin-converting enzyme. Angiotensin II helps preserve blood pressure both by its potent vasoconstrictor properties and by its ability to stimulate aldosterone secretion from the adrenal cortex.

The label for **choice A** points to the glomerular basement membrane.

The label for **choice B** points to the epithelium of Bowman's capsule.

The label for **choice D** points to the macula densa cells, which are thought to sense sodium concentration in the distal convoluted tubule.

The label for **choice E** points to the Polkissen cells. Their function is unknown.

24. **The correct answer is B.** The tracheoesophageal ridges are two longitudinal ridges that separate the respiratory diverticulum from the foregut. Eventually, they fuse to form a septum separating the esophagus (dorsal) from the trachea (ventral) and lung buds, maintaining a communication only rostrally at the pharynx. Incomplete formation of the tracheoesophageal septum (by fusion of ridges) results in the most common type of tracheoesophageal fistula, whereby the proximal part of the esophagus ends as a blind sac (esophageal atresia), while the distal part is connected to the trachea by a narrow canal just above the bifurcation. This defect occurs in approximately 1 in 2,500 births.

The buccopharyngeal membrane is a bilaminar membrane (ectoderm externally, endoderm internally) separating the stomodeum (mouth) from the pharynx. The membrane ruptures at about 4 weeks. The buccopharyngeal membrane is not involved in formation of the esophagus and trachea; therefore, failure to rupture (**choice A**) would not lead to tracheoesophageal fistula.

The septum secundum is a membrane that forms on the right side of the developing interatrial wall of the heart. It is not associated with formation of the esophagus and trachea; therefore, failure to close would not lead to tracheoesophageal fistula. Failure of formation of the septum secundum (**choice C**) leads to a patent foramen ovale, a relatively common atrial septal defect.

Incomplete recanalization of the larynx (**choice D**) is relatively rare and results in a membrane (laryngeal web) that may partially obstruct the airway. Though there may be difficulty breathing, there should be little problem with swallowing and keeping milk down.

The thyroid gland forms from a primordium associated with development of the tongue that eventually descends into the neck. For a short time, it remains connected

to the tongue by a narrow canal called the thyroglossal duct. Although the duct normally closes, it occasionally remains patent (**choice E**) or develops cysts, which are usually asymptomatic unless they become infected. They do not interfere with breathing or feeding and do not involve the trachea or esophagus.

25. **The correct answer is C.** This question allows us to review the sensory innervation of the perineum and vicinity. The ilioinguinal nerve supplies the skin of the scrotum and the medial thigh with sensory fibers.

The genitofemoral nerve (**choice A**) supplies motor fibers to the cremaster muscle and a small area of skin on the thigh, giving rise to the cremasteric reflex.

The iliohypogastric nerve (**choice B**) supplies the skin of the anterior lower abdominal wall.

The lateral cutaneous nerve (**choice D**) of the thigh supplies the skin over the lateral surface of the thigh.

The pudendal nerve (**choice E**) gives off branches that supply the external anal sphincter, the lower half of the anal canal, perianal skin, and skin on the posterior surface of the scrotum.

26. **The correct answer is E.** The condition described is spina bifida with myelomeningocele. A failure of the posteriorly located vertebral arches to fuse posteriorly causes spina bifida, which can vary in severity from a completely asymptomatic minor abnormality to protrusion of the spinal cord and roots through an open skin defect, with a very real risk of minor trauma or infection causing paralysis.

The bodies of the vertebrae (**choice A**) are the stacking ovoid structures on the anterior aspect of the spinal canal.

The pedicles (**choice B**) attach the body ring that surrounds the spinal canal to the body of the vertebrae.

Failure of development of one of the paired primary ossification centers (**choice C**) of the body can produce very severe scoliosis.

The superior articular process (**choice D**) articulates with the inferior articular facet of the vertebra above it.

27. **The correct answer is E.** The sixth cervical vertebra is a critical boundary of the root of the neck. To enter the neck from the chest, the vascular structures pass through a ringlike opening bounded by the scalene muscles laterally, the sternum and first ribs anteriorly, and the vertebrae (notably C6).

28. **The correct answer is C.** Knowledge of the motor homunculus of the precentral gyrus (primary motor cortex) is necessary to answer this question. The parts of the cortex that control the legs are buried within the

interhemispheric fissure. Paraplegia indicates weakness of both legs.

Ataxia (**choice A**) is clumsiness or incoordination that is not caused by weakness or sensory loss. It is most commonly caused by a lesion of the cerebellum or of the dentatorubrothalamic tract.

Hemiplegia (**choice B**) is weakness of an arm and leg. This could be caused by a very large lesion on one-half of the motor strip. It would include the cortex inside the interhemispheric fissure (controlling the legs) and the area of cortex present on the medial and superior aspect of the motor strip (controlling the arms).

Quadriplegia (**choice D**) is weakness of all four extremities. If the lesion were present in the motor strip, it would have to extend from the interhemispheric portion of both motor strips to the medial and superior aspects of both motor strips.

Rigidity (**choice E**) is hypertonia that is uniform throughout passive movement. This type of dysfunction is caused by lesions of the basal ganglia, most commonly the nigrostriatal dopaminergic pathway.

29. **The correct answer is D.** Brunner's glands are located in the submucosa of the duodenum. These glands are connected to the intestinal lumen by ducts that open into certain crypts. They secrete an alkaline product that protects the duodenal mucosa from the acidic chyme and helps achieve optimal pH for pancreatic enzymes.

   Note that if you did not recall the location of Brunner's glands, the question's description of their function allowed you to deduce it, on the basis of your knowledge of the anatomy of the small intestine. You should have immediately ruled out **choices C and E** because they are too far from the pancreas. **Choices B and D** would therefore remain as the best possible answers because of their proximity to the pancreas. If you remembered the structure and function of the ampulla of Vater, you were left with the correct answer.

   Let's review some other key features of intestinal histology by way of the wrong answer choices.

   The small intestinal villi (**choice A**) are outgrowths of the mucosa into the lumen. Their epithelium contains columnar absorptive cells and goblet cells (which produce acid glycoproteins that protect and lubricate the lining of the intestine). Near the base of each villus are tubular glands called crypts, whose lining is continuous with the simple columnar epithelium of the villus. The crypts include Paneth cells, which produce acidophilic cytoplasmic granules containing bactericidal enzymes. The lamina propria of the small intestine penetrates

the core of the villi and is composed of blood vessels, lymphatics, fibroblasts, and smooth muscle cells.

The ampulla of Vater (**choice B**) receives bile from the common bile duct and the main pancreatic duct, delivering it to the duodenum through the major duodenal papilla.

The mucosa and submucosa of the jejunum (**choice C**) are both included in the permanent folds called the plica circulares.

The submucosa of the ileum (**choice E**) is the home of Peyer's patches, which are large aggregates of lymphoid nodules.

30. **The correct answer is B.** The lunate is in the proximal row and articulates with the scaphoid laterally (this being the most lateral of the proximal row). The lunate is the most commonly dislocated carpal bone. It is usually displaced anteriorly by rotation on its proximal, convex surface (where it articulates with the radius). The displaced bone may compress the median nerve in the carpal tunnel, leading to pain, sensory loss, and/or paralysis.

   The capitate (**choice A**) is a carpal bone in the distal row. It articulates with the hamate (the most medial of this row).

   The scaphoid (**choice C**), the most commonly fractured carpal bone, is the most lateral bone of the proximal row. Patients with scaphoid fractures have an increased risk for avascular necrosis.

   The trapezoid (**choice D**) is a carpal bone of the distal row and articulates with the most lateral of this row (trapezium).

   The triquetrum (**choice E**), although in the proximal row of carpal bones, is the most medial carpal bone of the proximal row.

31. **The correct answer is B.** You should know the boundaries of the femoral triangle: the inguinal ligament above, the medial border of the sartorius laterally, and the medial border of the adductor longus on the inner aspect of the thigh.

   The gracilis muscle (**choices A, C, and D**) runs roughly parallel to the adductor longus but is not usually considered part of the triangle.

   The pectineus muscle (**choices C and E**) is found on the floor of the femoral triangle.

32. **The correct answer is A.** The clinical history suggests trigeminal neuralgia, which is characterized by extreme pain along the distributions of the maxillary and mandibular subdivisions of the fifth cranial nerve. The trigeminal nerve is derived from the first branchial arch.

The second branchial arch (**choice B**) gives rise to the muscles of facial expression and is innervated by the facial nerve, cranial nerve VII.

The third branchial arch (**choice C**) is innervated by the ninth cranial nerve, the glossopharyngeal, which innervates the stylopharyngeus muscle.

The fourth branchial arch (**choice D**) gives rise to most pharyngeal constrictor muscles and is innervated by the tenth cranial nerve, the vagus nerve.

The fifth brachial arch (**choice E**) gives rise to certain laryngeal cartilages and muscles, along with the fourth brachial arch.

33. **The correct answer is E.** The ventral mesentery forms the falciform ligament, ligamentum teres, and lesser omentum, which can be divided into the hepatogastric and hepatoduodenal ligament.

The dorsal mesoduodenum (**choice A**) is the mesentery of the developing duodenum, which later disappears so that the duodenum and pancreas lie retroperitoneally.

Both omental bursa and the greater omentum are derived from the dorsal mesogastrium (**choice B**), which is the mesentery of the stomach region.

The pericardioperitoneal canal (**choice C**) embryologically connects the thoracic and peritoneal canals.

The pleuropericardial membranes (**choice D**) become the pericardium and contribute to the diaphragm.

34. **The correct answer is C.** The lingual nerve is a branch of the mandibular division of the trigeminal nerve that conveys general sensation from the anterior two-thirds of the tongue. It enters the oral cavity by passing just under the mandibular third molar between the medial pterygoid muscle and the mandibular ramus.

The auriculotemporal nerve (**choice A**) is a branch of V3 that passes from the infratemporal fossa to the parotid region. It contains sensory fibers from the region in front of the ear and the temporomandibular joint, and also conveys postganglionic parasympathetic fibers to the parotid salivary gland.

The chorda tympani (**choice B**) is a branch of CN VII that travels with the lingual nerve in the floor of the mouth. It carries taste fibers from the anterior two-thirds of the tongue and preganglionic parasympathetic fibers that synapse in the submandibular ganglion.

The mental nerve (**choice D**) is a sensory branch of the inferior alveolar nerve that supplies the skin of the chin and lower lip.

The mylohyoid nerve (**choice E**) is a motor branch of the inferior alveolar nerve that supplies the mylohyoid and anterior belly of the digastric muscles.

35. **The correct answer is E.** The palpable space immediately inferior to the clavicle is the first intercostal space, and the bone below it is the second rib.

The acromion (**choice A**) is the lateral extension of the scapular spine.

The atlas (**choice B**) is the first cervical vertebra, articulating with the occipital bone above and the axis below.

The first rib (**choice C**) is hidden under the clavicle.

The manubrium (**choice D**) is the most superior portion of the sternum.

36. **The correct answer is A.** The internal epithelial lining of the trachea, bronchi, and lungs form from a diverticulum of the ventral foregut wall (endoderm) called the respiratory diverticulum.

The midgut endoderm (**choice B**) gives rise to the internal epithelial lining of much of the gastrointestinal tract, duodenum, small intestine, ascending colon, and right two-thirds of transverse colon.

The splanchnic mesoderm (**choice C**) contributes only to the smooth muscle coat and cartilaginous skeleton of trachea and bronchi.

The stomodeum (**choice D**) is of ectodermal origin and gives rise to the mouth. The stomodeum eventually becomes continuous with the endodermal foregut of the larynx (and trachea) and the esophagus.

The internal epithelial lining of the trachea, bronchi, and lungs is derived entirely from ventral foregut endoderm, not from both endoderm and mesoderm (**not choice E**). Splanchnic mesoderm contributes only to the smooth muscle coat and cartilaginous skeleton.

37. **The correct answer is B.** Embryonic tissue is most susceptible to teratogens during the 3rd through 9th weeks of pregnancy. This is when organogenesis, as well as most major congenital anomalies, occurs. Since brain development occurs throughout pregnancy, however, it is wisest for a pregnant woman to avoid alcohol for all 9 months of gestation.

The first 2 weeks (**choice A**) of pregnancy are not generally associated with teratogenicity, unless so many of the cells of the conceptus are irreversibly damaged that death results. Otherwise, the abundance of undifferentiated cells present can compensate for the damage.

The 9th through 12th weeks (**choice C**) are associated with minor congenital anomalies, including those of the eyes, palate, teeth, and ears.

The 12th through 16th weeks (**choice D**) and 16th through 20th weeks (**choice E**) are associated with minor congenital anomalies, including those of the eyes, teeth, ears, and external genitalia. Minor CNS anomalies may occur during the 20th week.

38. **The correct answer is B.** This patient has two risk factors for sinusitis: chronic rhinitis and allergy. She probably also has aspirin allergy, which is associated with the triad of nasal polyps, asthma, and sinusitis. In maxillary sinusitis, exudate may drain into the middle meatus through an ostium in the hiatus semilunaris, which contains openings to the frontal and maxillary sinuses and anterior ethmoidal cells.

The bulla ethmoidalis (**choice A**), also part of the middle meatus, contains an opening to the middle ethmoidal air cells.

The inferior nasal meatus (**choice C**) receives fluid from the nasolacrimal duct, which drains tears from the medial aspect of the orbit to the nasal cavity.

The sphenoethmoidal recess (**choice D**) is located above the superior concha and contains an opening for the sphenoid sinus.

The superior nasal meatus (**choice E**) is located above the superior concha and contains an opening for the sphenoid sinus.

39. **The correct answer is A.** The deep peroneal nerve arises from the common peroneal nerve (L4-S2). It innervates the postaxial muscles of the anterior compartment of the leg, which dorsiflex (extend) the foot. Damage to the nerve therefore produces "foot-drop"—a classic clue to deep peroneal nerve pathology. The nerve gives rise to many branches, one of which innervates the skin between the first and second toes.

The femoral nerve (**choice B**) contains fibers from L2-L4. It supplies flexor muscles of the thigh, extensors at the knee joint, and cutaneous areas of the thigh. The saphenous nerve branches off it and supplies the knee joint and the skin on the medial aspect of the foot.

The superficial peroneal nerve (**choice C**) supplies the muscles of the lateral compartment of the leg and is responsible for foot eversion. It also conveys sensory information from most of the dorsal surface of the foot.

The sural nerve (**choice D**) also arises from the common peroneal nerve and innervates the skin of the lateral calf.

The tibial nerve (**choice E**) innervates the hamstrings as well as muscles of the calf and sole of the foot. "Clawing of the toes" is a classic clue to tibial nerve injury.

40. **The correct answer is D.** Endothelium lines the cardiovascular and lymphatic vessels and is composed of simple squamous epithelium. The mesothelium that lines the pleural, pericardial, and peritoneal cavities is also composed of a single layer of simple squamous epithelium.

Pseudostratified epithelium (**choice A**) is found in the epithelial lining of the respiratory tract, as well as in the transitional epithelium of the urinary system.

In simple columnar epithelium (**choice B**), the cells are taller than they are wide. This epithelium can be found in the intestinal absorptive surface.

Simple cuboidal epithelium (**choice C**) can be found in the ducts of many glands.

Stratified columnar epithelium (**choice E**) can be found in portions of the male urethra.

41. **The correct answer is E.** This route passes through the vastus lateralis to penetrate the knee joint via the suprapatellar bursa, allowing aspiration of joint fluid for culture. The vastus lateralis, together with the vastus medialis, vastus intermedius, and rectus femoris, forms the quadriceps muscle.

The adductor magnus (**choice A**) is on the inner and anterior aspect of the upper thigh.

The gracilis (**choice B**) is on the inner aspect of the thigh.

The iliacus (**choice C**) is on the lateral, proximal aspect of the thigh.

The sartorius (**choice D**) passes diagonally from the lateral hip to the medial knee.

42. **The correct answer is D.** A normal waking adult characteristically shows alpha activity over the posterior regions of the head, some beta activity in the fronto-central regions, and few (if any) theta waves over the temporal areas. Delta waves are not present in normal adults during wakefulness. The delta waves over his left frontal lobe indicate a lesion in this area. The left primary motor cortex resides in this region and would produce a right hemiparesis if damaged.

A left hemiparesis (**choice A**) could be caused by a lesion of the right primary motor cortex, located in the frontal lobe.

A left hemisensory loss (**choice B**) could be produced by a lesion of the right primary somatosensory cortex, located in the parietal lobe.

A left homonymous hemianopia (**choice C**) could be caused by a lesion in the visual pathway after the optic chiasm (right optic tract, right optic radiations, right visual cortex).

A right hemisensory loss (**choice E**) could be produced by a lesion of the left primary somatosensory cortex, located in the parietal lobe.

43. **The correct answer is B.** The most common type of ankle sprain is lateral, which occurs as a result of excessive inversion of the foot and dorsiflexion of the ankle. The calcaneofibular [not calcaneotibial (**choice C**)] and anterior talofibular [not talotibial (**choice A**)] ligaments may tear, producing marked swelling and

pain. These two ligaments combined with the posterior talofibular ligament constitute the lateral ligament of the ankle.

The deltoid ligament (**choice D**), also known as the medial ligament of the ankle, is a very strong, thick structure located at the medial malleolus. Excessive eversion would be the most likely mechanism of injury.

The medial collateral ligament (**choice E**) is damaged in lateral blows to the knee.

44. **The correct answer is E.** The hip is a ball and socket joint with polyaxial motion and spherical articular surfaces.

45. **The correct answer is F.** The knee is a plane joint with polyaxial motion and flat articular surfaces.

46. **The correct answer is C.** The wrist is a condyloid joint with movement in two axes. This is commonly referred to as an "egg and spoon" type of joint.

47. **The correct answer is H.** The patient has a pubic symphysis dysfunction. The pubic symphysis is a slightly moveable joint. This is a symphysis of two bones with fibrocartilage between them to create the joint.

48. **The correct answer is D.** The thumb is a saddle joint that has movement around two axes and movements that are similar to a condyloid joint.

49. **The correct answer is A.** The elbow is a hinge joint with movement around one axis (flexion and extension).

50. **The correct answer is B.** The proximal radioulnar joint is an example of a pivot joint with movement around one axis (i.e., rotation).

Anatomy (Gross Anatomy, Neuroanatomy, Embryology, and Histology)

1. On structural examination, you find somatic dysfunction at T10. Which of the following embryonic structures gives rise to the adrenal cortex?

   (A) Ectoderm

   (B) Endoderm

   (C) Mesoderm

   (D) Mesonephros

   (E) Neural crest cells

2. A 42-year-old man presents with chronic indigestion. Physical examination reveals somatic dysfunction at T5-T9. A gastric biopsy is performed on a 42-year-old man. As the pathologist inspects the specimen, he observes numerous, normal cuboidal-to-columnar cells with apical membrane-bound secretion granules in the gastric glands. From which area of the stomach was the biopsy specimen most likely taken?

   (A) Cardiac region

   (B) Columns of Morgagni

   (C) Fundic region

   (D) Greater omentum

   (E) Pyloric region

3. During a football game, a player sustains a powerful blow to the lateral side of his weight-bearing leg. Osteopathic examination reveals a positive anterior drawer test and multiple tender points along the medial joint space. He experiences excruciating knee pain and is unable to walk. The three structures most likely to be injured are the

   (A) anterior cruciate and lateral collateral ligaments and the lateral meniscus

   (B) anterior cruciate and medial collateral ligaments and the medial meniscus

   (C) posterior cruciate and lateral collateral ligaments and the lateral meniscus

   (D) posterior cruciate and medial collateral ligaments and the lateral meniscus

   (E) posterior cruciate and medial collateral ligaments and medial meniscus

4. A mother brings her 5-year-old daughter to the physician complaining that the child still seems to regularly wet herself despite having been toilet-trained. The physician orders an IV pyelogram, which demonstrates a complete duplication of the ureter on the right side. Although one ureter opens normally into the bladder, the other opens ectopically into the vagina. This congenital anomaly is caused by

   (A) duplication of the proximal mesonephric (Wolffian) duct

   (B) early division of the ureteric bud

   (C) ectopic growth of the pronephros

   (D) improper union of excretory tubules and collecting tubules

   (E) persistence of embryonic ureters as the kidney ascends from the pelvis to the superior abdomen

5. Which of the following is the embryologic precursor of the fibrous remnant that runs in a fissure on the visceral surface of the liver?

   (A) Ductus arteriosus

   (B) Ductus venosus

   (C) Hepatic portal vein

   (D) Lateral splanchnic artery

   (E) Left umbilical artery

6. Injury to the lower division of the facial nerve during parotid surgery will result in

   (A) inability to furrow the brow (to frown) on the same side

   (B) numbness over the angle and mental region of the jaw on the same side

   (C) ptosis of the eye on the same side

   (D) weakness in closing the eye on the same side

   (E) weakness of the lower lip on the same side

7. After finding chronic somatic dysfunction at T1-T4, an arteriogram is performed on a patient with atherosclerosis. Luminal narrowing of which of the following vessels would compromise blood flow through the renal arteries?

   (A) Abdominal aorta

   (B) Celiac trunk

   (C) Common iliac artery

   (D) Inferior mesenteric artery

   (E) Superior mesenteric artery

8. A patient has chronic somatic dysfunction at T1-T4, which has not resolved with treatment. A full workup is done, and the patient is diagnosed with thyroid cancer. Following thyroidectomy, hoarseness of the voice may occur. This condition is caused by damage to the

   (A) internal laryngeal nerve

   (B) recurrent laryngeal nerve

   (C) thyroarytenoid muscle

   (D) vestibular folds

   (E) vocal folds

9. During an automobile accident, a person sustains a "broken neck" and dies after a small bony fragment is driven into his spinal cord. From which of the following bones was this fragment most likely derived?

   (A) Atlas

   (B) Axis

   (C) Seventh cervical vertebrae

   (D) Sixth cervical vertebrae

   (E) Third cervical vertebrae

10. The pedal pump lymphatic technique moves lymph to a structure that receives lymph from the lumbar trunks and the intestinal trunks. What vertebra is the structure located near?

    (A) L1, L2

    (B) L3, L4

    (C) S2, S3

    (D) T9, T10

    (E) T11, T12

11. A nursing home patient who aspirates while lying on his back would be most likely to develop pneumonia involving which of the following sites?

    (A) Anterior segment of the right upper lobe

    (B) Apical segment of the right lower lobe

    (C) Inferior lingular segment of the left upper lobe

    (D) Lateral segment of the right middle lobe

    (E) Superior lingular segment of the left upper lobe

12. A patient has a tiny (0.2 cm), but exquisitely painful, tumor under the nail of her index finger. Local anesthetic block to a branch of which of the following nerves would be most likely to provide adequate anesthesia for the surgical removal of the mass?

    (A) Axillary

    (B) Median

    (C) Musculocutaneous

    (D) Radial

    (E) Ulnar

13. Which of the following pharyngeal pouches develops into the palatine tonsil?

    (A) First
    (B) Second
    (C) Third
    (D) Fourth
    (E) Fifth

14. A 35-year-old woman with severe dysmenorrhea, prolonged menstrual periods, and chronic somatic dysfunction at T10-L2 due to large uterine fibroids undergoes a hysterectomy. Which of the following structures is the gynecologist most likely to inadvertently ligate during surgery?

    (A) Internal iliac artery
    (B) Internal iliac vein
    (C) Ovarian artery
    (D) Ureter
    (E) Uterine vein

15. A prostate-specific antigen (PSA) level is drawn from a 54-year-old man as part of a routine health evaluation after finding chronic tissue changes at T10-L2. Which of the following embryonic structures gives rise to the organ being screened for carcinoma?

    (A) Genital tubercle
    (B) Processus vaginalis
    (C) Testis cords
    (D) Tunica albuginea
    (E) Urogenital sinus

16. A football player is examined by the team physician following a shoulder injury during a game. Preliminary x-ray films show an inferior dislocation of the humerus. On further examination, there is weakness in lateral rotation and abduction of the arm. The nerve most likely affected is the

    (A) axillary
    (B) dorsal scapular
    (C) radial
    (D) suprascapular
    (E) thoracodorsal

17. A 20-year-old man is stabbed immediately to the left of the body of the sternum at the fifth intercostal space. The knife most likely penetrated the

    (A) left atrium
    (B) left ventricle
    (C) right atrium
    (D) right ventricle
    (E) stomach

18. An elderly woman with osteoporosis is taken to the emergency department following a fall. One of her legs appears shortened and is externally rotated. A fracture of which part of the femur is suggested by these findings?

    (A) Greater trochanter
    (B) Lateral epicondyle
    (C) Medial epicondyle
    (D) Neck
    (E) Shaft

19. An otherwise healthy first-year medical student visits the student health office for a physical examination. He is taking no medications. He is concerned because he has noticed several painless uniform "large bumps" at the back of his tongue. These are most likely

    (A) aphthous ulcers
    (B) candidal colonies
    (C) circumvallate papillae
    (D) filiform papillae
    (E) fungiform papillae

20. An oblique x-ray view of a patient with right middle lobar pneumonia demonstrates an area of consolidation bounded by sharp, intersecting, relatively straight lines above and below. These lines correspond to which of the following?

    (A) Diaphragm above and oblique fissure below
    (B) Oblique fissure above and breast shadow below
    (C) Oblique fissure above and transverse fissure below
    (D) Transverse fissure above and diaphragm below
    (E) Transverse fissure above and oblique fissure below

21. Intramuscular injections should be given in the upper, outer quadrant of the buttocks to prevent damage to which of the following nerves?

    (A) Common peroneal
    (B) Lateral femoral cutaneous
    (C) Obturator
    (D) Sciatic
    (E) Superior gluteal

22. A sharp instrument passing through the superior orbital fissure would most likely sever which of the following structures?

    (A) Abducens nerve
    (B) Facial nerve
    (C) Mandibular nerve
    (D) Maxillary nerve
    (E) Middle meningeal artery

23. A patient presents to the emergency department after sustaining a laceration of the first web space of his hand in a rock-climbing accident. Which of the following structures is also likely to be injured?

    (A) Deep branch of radial nerve
    (B) Opponens pollicis
    (C) Radial artery
    (D) Recurrent branch of median nerve
    (E) Superficial palmar arch

24. A football player experiences an anterior dislocation of the shoulder. Cutaneous sensation over the lower half of the deltoid muscle is impaired. These findings suggest damage to which of the following nerves?

    (A) Axillary
    (B) Median
    (C) Musculocutaneous
    (D) Radial
    (E) Ulnar

25. A patient with a left adrenal mass is scheduled for surgery. The surgeon is planning to approach the suprarenal area by removing the 12th rib. With this approach, the surgeon should take particular care to avoid damaging which of the following structures?

    (A) Aorta
    (B) Diaphragm
    (C) Pancreas
    (D) Stomach
    (E) Vena cava

26. While performing an osteopathic structural examination of the knee, you get a positive posterior drawer test. Which of the following prevents hyperextension of the knee?

    (A) Anterior cruciate ligament
    (B) Lateral semilunar cartilage
    (C) Medial semilunar cartilage
    (D) Posterior cruciate ligament
    (E) Transverse ligament

27. During anatomy lab, a medical student notes a fibrous band that runs on the visceral surface of the liver. It is attached on one end to the inferior vena cava and on the other end to the left branch of the portal vein. In the embryo, this structure corresponds to the

    (A) ductus venosus
    (B) ligamentum teres
    (C) ligamentum venosum
    (D) umbilical arteries
    (E) umbilical vein

28. In a patient suspected of a pituitary abnormality, which of the following hormones is secreted by anterior pituitary cells that stain with acidic dyes?

    (A) ACTH
    (B) FSH
    (C) LH
    (D) Prolactin
    (E) TSH

29. A 4-year-old boy with recurrent urinary tract infections is evaluated for renal/urinary tract abnormalities with a voiding cystourethrogram (VCUG). Reflux is discovered, so an intravenous pyelogram (IVP) is performed. The renal anatomy appears normal. On the IVP, which of the following structures would have been seen emptying into the renal pelvis?

    (A) Major calyx
    (B) Minor calyx
    (C) Renal pyramid
    (D) Ureter
    (E) Cortex

30. A neonate is observed to have a cleft lip. Which of the following is the most likely etiology of this malformation?

    (A) Abnormal development of the third and fourth pharyngeal pouches
    (B) Bony defects of the malar bone and mandible
    (C) Failure of the maxillary processes and medial nasal swellings to fuse
    (D) Incomplete joining of the palatine shelves
    (E) Insufficient migration of neural crest cells

31. A patient's left hypoglossal nerve (CN XII) is injured during a carotid endarterectomy. Which of the following would most likely result from this injury?

    (A) Decreased gag reflex on the left
    (B) Decreased salivation from the left submandibular and sublingual salivary glands
    (C) Deviation of the tongue to the left on protrusion
    (D) Inability to elevate the pharynx on the left during swallowing
    (E) Inability to perceive sweet and salt taste sensation on the anterior part of the left side of the tongue

32. Incomplete fusion of the embryonic endocardial cushions can produce which of the following congenital defects?

    (A) Atrioventricular septal defect
    (B) Coarctation of the aorta
    (C) Pulmonary stenosis
    (D) Tetralogy of Fallot
    (E) Transposition of the great vessels

33. Following fracture of the humerus, an adult patient has a biopsy of the healing area. Which of the following types of bone will the biopsy most likely show?

    (A) Cancellous
    (B) Compact
    (C) Spongy
    (D) Trabecular
    (E) Woven

34. When tapping a pleural effusion, it is important to pass the needle immediately above the rib to prevent damage to which of the following structures in the subcostal groove?

    (A) Intercostal artery and vein
    (B) Intercostal nerve
    (C) Intercostal nerve and artery
    (D) Intercostal nerve and vein
    (E) Intercostal nerve, artery, and vein

35. A newborn boy does not pass meconium until 48 hours after his birth. Several weeks later his mother complains that he has not been passing stool regularly. Anorectal manometry reveals increased internal anal sphincter pressure on rectal distention with a balloon. The patient's disorder may be attributed to

    (A) defective recanalization of the colon
    (B) failure of neural crest cells to migrate into the colonic wall
    (C) herniation of abdominal contents into the umbilical cord
    (D) persistence of the proximal end of the yolk stalk
    (E) presence of a rectourinary fistula

36. A blockage of the cerebral aqueduct will produce an increase in pressure initially in the

    (A) foramen of Magendie
    (B) foramina of Luschka
    (C) fourth ventricle
    (D) interventricular foramen
    (E) third ventricle

37. A mother comes to the office for a cranial sacral evaluation of her infant. Which of the following anatomic landmarks is the site of the anterior fontanelle in an infant?

    (A) Bregma

    (B) Coronal suture

    (C) Lambda

    (D) Pterion

    (E) Sagittal suture

38. On physical examination, the upper body of a 7-year-old boy appears much more developed than his lower body. Blood pressure in the upper extremities exceeds that of the lower extremities. On cardiac examination, there is a midsystolic murmur over the anterior chest and back. The child's lower extremities are cold, and femoral pulses are absent. The part of the vascular system that is affected in this disorder is derived from which of the following embryologic structures?

    (A) Bulbus cordis

    (B) Ductus arteriosus

    (C) Right common cardinal vein

    (D) Right horn of sinus venosus

    (E) Third, fourth, and sixth aortic arches

39. A urologist performs a cystoscopy to examine the bladder and the openings of the ureters into the bladder. After distention of the bladder with air, the physician slowly passes the cystoscope up the urethra into the bladder. In which direction should she turn the head of the cystoscope to see the ureteric orifices and examine for blockage?

    (A) Anterior and inferior

    (B) Anterior and superior

    (C) Posterior and inferior

    (D) Posterior and superior

    (E) Anterior and medial

40. The extraocular muscles are derived from which of the following structures?

    (A) Branchial arches

    (B) Optic cup ectoderm

    (C) Somites

    (D) Somitomeres

    (E) Splanchnic mesoderm

41. A surgeon performing an appendectomy makes an incision through the ventrolateral abdominal wall. The layers of the abdominal wall are shown below.

    1. Internal oblique

    2. External oblique

    3. Peritoneum

    4. Transversus abdominis

    Which of the following corresponds to the order of penetration of the layers of the abdominal wall?

    (A) 1-3-4-2

    (B) 2-1-3-4

    (C) 2-1-4-3

    (D) 4-1-2-3

    (E) 4-2-1-3

42. A patient with acute cholecystitis experiences referred pain to the right shoulder and has somatic dysfunction at T5-T9 on the right side. Which of the following dermatomes is most likely involved?

    (A) C1-C2

    (B) C3-C5

    (C) C6-C8

    (D) T1-T3

    (E) T4-T6

43. Which of the following structures is lined with epithelium derived from mesoderm of the ureteric bud?

    (A) Bowman's capsule

    (B) Distal convoluted tubule

    (C) Loop of Henle

    (D) Proximal convoluted tubule

    (E) Ureter

Questions 44-50

SET A

Directions: For each numbered item (**patient presentation**), select the one lettered heading (**etiology**) most closely associated with it. Each lettered heading may be selected once, more than once, or not at all.

   (A) spondylosis

   (B) spondylolysis

   (C) spondylolisthesis

   (D) spondylitis

   (E) ankylosing spondylitis

   (F) spina bifida occulta

   (G) diskitis

   (H) spinal stenosis

44. Your patient is a migrant farm worker who complains of severe lower back pain that has been worsening over time. X-ray reveals that L1 and L2 lumbar vertebrae are destroyed and the disk space between them is narrowed by caseation. A lumber spine bone biopsy is positive for *Mycobacterium tuberculosis*.

45. A 24-year-old man complains of lower back pain after playing football. There is no numbness, tingling, or radiation. Lower extremity motor strength is 5/5. L-spine x-ray reveals an anterior displacement of L5 on S1.

46. An 81-year-old woman complains of chronic neck pain and denies any trauma. An x-ray of the cervical spine reveals degeneration of the C5-C6 intervertebral disk and some mild disk herniation.

47. An 11-year-old boy complains of lower back pain that started after he fell while playing soccer. An x-ray of the lumbar spine reveals a stress fracture of the pars interarticularis of L5.

48. The mother of a 4-year-old girl states that her child has had fevers of 37.8-40.0 C (100.0-104.0 F) for the past 10 days, associated with lumbar paravertebral muscle spasms and pain. On examination you note an exaggerated lumbar lordotic posture. Blood cultures are sterile; erythrocyte sedimentation rate is elevated. X-ray demonstrates a narrowed L4-L5 disk space, and a subsequent MRI demonstrates inflammatory swelling of the disk space.

49. A patient of yours is a professional football player about to be signed on to a new team. As part of his physical examination, an x-ray of his lumbar spine was required, which showed a failure of the L5 lamina to fuse.

50. A 66-year-old man complains of chronic lower back pain and stiffness. The pain has been intermittent, but the pain and stiffness are worsening. There is bilateral radiation down both legs. X-rays of the spine reveal fusion of L4, L5, and S1, and squaring and demineralization of the vertebrae with calcification of the anterior and lateral spinal ligaments.

Anatomy (Gross Anatomy, Neuroanatomy, Embryology, and Histology)

TEST 2

ANSWERS AND EXPLANATIONS

1. C
2. C
3. B
4. B
5. B
6. E
7. A
8. B
9. B
10. A
11. B
12. B
13. B
14. D
15. E
16. A
17. D
18. D
19. C
20. E
21. D
22. A
23. C
24. A
25. B

26. A
27. A
28. D
29. A
30. C
31. C
32. A
33. E
34. E
35. B
36. E
37. A
38. E
39. C
40. D
41. C
42. B
43. E
44. D
45. C
46. A
47. B
48. G
49. F
50. E

1. **The correct answer is C.** The mesoderm gives rise to the adrenal cortex. In addition, it also gives rise to connective tissue, cartilage, bone, muscle, blood and lymph vessels, kidneys, gonads, serous membranes lining body cavities, and the spleen.

   The ectoderm (**choice A**) gives rise to the CNS, peripheral nervous system, epidermis and its appendages, mammary glands, pituitary gland, tooth enamel, and the neural crest.

   The endoderm (**choice B**) gives rise to the parenchyma of the tonsils, thyroid and parathyroid glands, thymus, liver, pancreas, the epithelial lining of the gastrointestinal and respiratory tracts, urinary bladder, urethra, and auditory tube.

   The mesonephros (**choice D**) functions as an interim kidney in the embryo.

   The neural crest cells (**choice E**) give rise to cells of the spinal and cranial nerves, autonomic ganglia, melanocytes, leptomeninges, connective tissue and bone of branchial arch origin, and the adrenal medulla.

2. **The correct answer is C.** The pathologist saw normal chief cells, which are abundant in the body and fundus of the stomach. Chief cells secrete pepsinogen, which is stored in apical membrane-bound granules. The body and fundus of the stomach contain high concentrations of four other types of cells in the epithelium. The *parietal* (oxyntic) cells are large, pyramidal, and acidophilic with central nuclei (like a "fried egg"). They make and secrete HCl. The *mucous neck* cells secrete mucus and appear clear. The *enteroendocrine* cells have affinity for silver stains and exhibit a positive chromaffin reaction; these cells synthesize amines, polypeptides, or proteins.

   The cardiac region (**choice A**) is a narrow, circular band at the transition between the esophagus and stomach, consisting of shallow gastric pits and mucous glands. It does not normally contain an abundance of chief cells.

   The columns of Morgagni (**choice B**) are found in the rectum, not in the stomach. These are mucous membrane infoldings in the submucosa of the proximal anal canal. They would not contain chief cells.

   The greater omentum (**choice D**) is a four-layered fold of peritoneum that hangs from the greater curvature of the stomach and attaches to the transverse colon. It would not contain chief cells.

   The pyloric region (**choice E**) has deep gastric pits into which tubular glands open. The predominant secretion is mucus. It does not normally contain an abundance of chief cells.

   Note that in this question you could have automatically eliminated choices B and D, since they are not gastric structures. If nothing else, you would have improved your guessing odds to 33%.

3. **The correct answer is B.** The anterior cruciate and medial collateral ligaments and the medial meniscus are sometimes called the "unhappy triad," because they are commonly injured in lateral blows to the knee that forcefully abduct the tibia. A good mnemonic is "MAMM" (for Medial collateral, Anterior cruciate, and Medial Meniscus). Damage to the anterior cruciate ligament is characterized by the ability to push the tibia too far forward on the femur.

   Damage to the lateral collateral ligaments and lateral menisci are very uncommon (**choices A, C, and D**) and would be expected if the tibia were forcefully adducted.

   Damage to the posterior cruciate ligaments (**choices C, D, E**) is extremely rare and is characterized by the ability to push the tibia too far backward on the femur.

4. **The correct answer is B.** The collecting system of the kidney, including the ureters, develops from an outgrowth of the distal mesonephric duct called the ureteric bud. The ureteric bud grows into the metanephros and induces the formation of the excretory system (nephrons). Early splitting of the ureteric bud may result in partial or complete duplication of the ureter. One of the buds typically opens into the bladder. The lower, abnormal bud usually opens more inferiorly and may communicate with the vagina or urethra in females.

   The mesonephric duct (**choice A**) is the drainage system of the mesonephros (the second "incarnation" of the kidney). The mesonephros, like the pronephros, eventually degenerates and almost completely disappears (to be replaced by metanephros) by the 2nd month of gestation. With the mesonephros gone, the duct no longer functions in urine drainage. In females it also degenerates, whereas in males it persists to become the epididymis and ductus deferens.

   The pronephros (**choice C**) is the first "incarnation" of the kidney. It rapidly regresses so that by 4 weeks post-fertilization, all indications of it have completely disappeared.

   During normal kidney formation there is union of the excretory tubules derived from the metanephros and the collecting tubules derived from the mesonephric duct. However, when the union does not occur properly (**choice D**), the outcome is not incontinence but rather the formation of renal cysts.

Renal arterial branches of the abdominal aorta form and then degenerate as the kidney ascends from the pelvis to the superior abdomen; one or more supernumerary renal arteries may persist. The ureters do not undergo a similar process during development (**choice E**); once formed, the embryonic ureters persist and continue to develop into the adult ureters.

5. **The correct answer is B.** The structure described is the ligamentum venosum, which is derived from the ductus venosus.

    The ductus arteriosus (**choice A**) is derived from the sixth aortic arch. It obliterates to form the ligamentum arteriosum.

    The hepatic portal vein (**choice C**) is derived from the vitelline vein.

    The lateral splanchnic arteries (**choice D**) arise from each side of the dorsal aorta. They supply intermediate mesoderm and derivatives and give rise to renal, suprarenal, phrenic, and testicular or ovarian arteries.

    The umbilical arteries (**choice E**) give rise to the internal iliac arteries proximally and the medial umbilical ligaments distally.

6. **The correct answer is E.** The motor component (special visceral efferent) of the facial nerve (CN VII) exits the skull via the stylomastoid foramen, passes lateral to the styloid process, and then enters the parotid gland. Within the gland, two divisions can usually be identified (upper and lower), which in turn give off five named branches that innervate the muscles of the face. The upper division gives rise to the temporal and zygomatic branches, which collectively innervate the frontalis, corrugator, and orbicularis oculi muscles. The lower division gives off the buccal, mandibular, and cervical branches. The largest, the buccal, innervates the muscles attaching to the upper lip, including the orbicularis oris and the levators, as well as the buccinator and the muscles of the nose. The mandibular branches innervate the muscles of the lower lip and of the chin, whereas the cervical branch innervates the platysma muscle. There are usually communicating branches between the named terminal nerves so that overlapping innervation of the muscles occurs. If the lower division is injured, there will be weakness (not frank paralysis because of the innervation overlap) of the muscles that attach to the lower lip.

    An inability to furrow the brow (**choice A**) would be caused be denervation of the corrugator supercilii and frontalis muscles, which are innervated by the upper division of the facial nerve.

    Choice B is wrong because once the facial nerve emerges from the stylomastoid foramen, it is a pure motor nerve (special visceral efferent, or branchiomotor nerve). It carries no sensory nerve fibers.

    Ptosis (a drooping of the upper eyelid; **choice C**) is the result of a paralysis of the levator palpebrae muscle, which is innervated by the oculomotor (CN III) nerve.

    Choice D is not correct because the orbicularis oculi muscle is innervated by branches from the upper division of the facial nerve.

7. **The correct answer is A.** The renal arteries emerge from the abdominal aorta at about the level of the L1/L2 intervertebral disk and travel at nearly right angles to it (on the right, passing posterior to the inferior vena cava) to enter the hilum of the kidney.

    The celiac trunk (**choice B**) gives off the common hepatic, splenic, and left gastric arteries.

    The common iliac artery (**choice C**) gives off the internal and external iliac arteries. Occasionally, a persistent, supernumerary renal artery may be seen arising from the junction of the abdominal aorta and the common iliac artery. In addition, an unascended pelvic kidney may be supplied by the common iliac artery.

    The inferior mesenteric artery (**choice D**) gives off the superior rectal, sigmoid, and left colic arteries.

    The superior mesenteric artery (**choice E**) gives off the inferior pancreaticoduodenal, intestinal (ileal and jejunal), right colic, middle colic, and ileocolic arteries.

8. **The correct answer is B.** The recurrent laryngeal nerves are branches of the vagus (CN X), and supply all intrinsic muscles of the larynx except the cricothyroid. The right recurrent laryngeal nerve recurs around the right subclavian artery. The left recurrent laryngeal nerve recurs in the thorax around the arch of the aorta and ligamentum arteriosum. Both nerves ascend to the larynx by passing between the trachea and esophagus, close to the thyroid gland.

    The internal laryngeal (**choice A**) nerve is a purely sensory branch of the superior laryngeal nerve.

    The thyroarytenoid (**choice C**) is an intrinsic muscle of the larynx; its inner fibers are specialized as the vocalis muscle, which is related to the vocal ligament. It is not usually at risk during thyroid surgery.

    The vestibular folds (**choice D**), or false vocal folds, are located superior to the true vocal folds inside the larynx. They are not concerned with phonation.

    The vocal folds (**choice E**) form the boundaries of the rima glottidis inside the larynx and are not vulnerable during thyroidectomy.

9. **The correct answer is B.** The odontoid process is the part of the axis (second cervical vertebrae) that fits into and articulates with the atlas (first cervical vertebrae). It is susceptible to traumatic fracture, and bony fragments can injure the spinal cord. The scenario presented is unfortunately realistic, and a similar mechanism is thought to cause deaths by execution-style hanging.

    The atlas (**choice A**) is the first cervical vertebra; it receives the odontoid process of the axis.

    Fracture of the lower cervical vertebrae (**choices C, D, and E**) does not usually cause sudden death, but may cause paralysis of any or all limbs depending on the amount of damage done.

10. **The correct answer is A.** The cisterna chyli performs this function. It is the dilated initial portion of the thoracic duct, which lies near vertebrae L1 and L2.

11. **The correct answer is B.** Aspiration pneumonia is a common complication observed in nursing home patients. The most probable site of the pneumonia can be anticipated by knowing the anatomy of the bronchial tree, since the aspirated fluid usually flows downhill. In a supine or nearly supine patient, the fluid flows into the trachea and then into either of the (typically the right) main bronchi. The first posteriorly located branch is the one leading to the apical aspect of (either) lower lobe. The lateral and posterior segments of the lower lobes are also supplied by posteriorly branching segmental bronchi. In contrast, the posterior aspects of the upper lobes are somewhat protected by an initial anteriorly directed bifurcation before their segmental bronchi arise. All other segments of the bronchial tree and their corresponding portions of lung are more anterior.

12. **The correct answer is B.** The tumor in question is probably a benign glomus tumor, which is notorious for producing pain far out of proportion to its small size. The question is a little tricky (but important clinically for obvious reasons) because the most distal aspect of the dorsal skin of the fingers, including the nail beds, is innervated by the palmar digital nerves rather than the dorsal digital nerves. Specifically, the median nerve, through its palmar digital nerves, supplies the nail beds of the thumb, index finger, middle finger, and half the ring finger.

    The axillary nerve (**choice A**), musculocutaneous nerve (**choice C**), and radial nerve (**choice D**) do not supply the nail beds. The radial nerve does supply the more proximal skin of the back of the index finger.

    The ulnar nerve (**choice E**) supplies the nail beds of the small finger and half the ring finger.

13. **The correct answer is B.** The epithelial lining of the second pharyngeal pouch buds into the mesenchyme to form the palatine tonsil. Part of the pouch remains in the adult as the tonsillar fossa.

    It is important to review the other choices, since pharyngeal pouch derivatives are typically tested on the COMLEX Level 1:

    The first pharyngeal pouch (**choice A**) develops into the middle ear cavity and eustachian tube.

    The third pharyngeal pouch (**choice C**) develops into the thymus and the inferior parathyroid glands.

    The fourth pharyngeal pouch (**choice D**) gives rise to the superior parathyroid glands. Recall that abnormal development of the third and fourth pouches leads to DiGeorge syndrome and results in hypocalcemia, as well as abnormal cellular immunity and consequent susceptibility to viral and fungal illnesses.

    The fifth pharyngeal pouch (**choice E**) gives rise to the C cells of the thyroid gland. These cells secrete calcitonin—a hormone that lowers serum calcium.

14. **The correct answer is D.** The ureter passes directly inferior to the uterine artery, lateral to the body of the uterus near its junction with the cervix ("water flows under the bridge"). During a hysterectomy, therefore, the ureter (instead of the uterine artery) may be inadvertently ligated.

    The internal iliac artery (**choice A**) gives rise to the uterine artery, the primary blood supply of the uterus.

    The internal iliac vein (**choice B**) receives blood from the uterine vein (**choice E**), the primary venous drainage of the uterus.

    The ovarian artery (**choice C**) arises from the abdominal aorta and is the primary blood supply of the ovaries.

15. **The correct answer is E.** It is recommended that PSA (prostate-specific antigen) levels be measured annually in men older than 50 to screen for prostatic carcinoma (and to record a baseline level). The prostate is immediately derived from the prostatic urethra, which is derived from the urogenital sinus.

    The genital tubercle (**choice A**) gives rise to the glans penis.

    The processus vaginalis (**choice B**) is a coelomic extension into the scrotal swelling that carries with it extensions of the body wall to form the inguinal canal during the descent of the testes.

    The testis cords (**choice C**) are composed of primitive germ cells, which give rise to spermatogonia, and sex cord cells, which differentiate into Sertoli cells.

The tunica albuginea (**choice D**) is derived from mesenchyme and condenses to form the fibrous connective tissue capsule of the testis.

16. **The correct answer is A.** Because of the proximity of the axillary nerve to the glenohumeral joint, a fracture of the surgical neck of the humerus or an inferior dislocation of the humerus could damage the nerve. The axillary nerve innervates the deltoid muscle. The deltoid abducts, adducts, flexes, extends, and rotates the arm medially. The axillary nerve also innervates the teres minor, which rotates the arm laterally.

    The dorsal scapular nerve (**choice B**) innervates both the major and minor rhomboid muscles. These muscles raise the medial border of the scapula upward and laterally.

    The radial nerve (**choice C**) innervates muscles involved in the movement of the forearm and hand.

    The suprascapular nerve (**choice D**) innervates the supraspinatus and infraspinatus. The supraspinatus abducts the arm, whereas the infraspinatus rotates the arm laterally. This nerve travels along the posterior aspect of the scapula and would not easily be subjected to injury in a dislocation of the shoulder joint.

    The thoracodorsal nerve (**choice E**) innervates the latissimus dorsi, which adducts, extends, and rotates the arm medially.

17. **The correct answer is D.** The right ventricle comprises most of the anterior surface of the heart.

    The left atrium (**choice A**) and the left ventricle (**choice B**) are located more posteriorly.

    The right atrium (**choice C**) is located more superiorly and to the right.

    The stomach (**choice E**) is located more inferiorly and to the left.

18. **The correct answer is D.** This is the classic presentation of a fracture of the neck of the femur. This type of fracture typically occurs in postmenopausal women with significant bone resorption due to osteoporosis. Dislocation of the head of the femur can produce a similar effect. The change in the position of the leg is due to the action of the gluteal muscles, particularly the gluteus maximus.

    Fracture of the femur at the greater trochanter (**choice A**) produces a less dramatic effect, because only the gluteus medius and gluteus minimus attach to it, and the overall structure of the femur remains intact.

    Fractures occurring lower in the femur, involving the epicondyles (**choices B and C**) or shaft (**choice E**), would not produce outward rotation of the entire leg.

19. **The correct answer is C.** This medical student has apparently not yet studied the anatomy of the tongue. Otherwise, he would have recognized the large bumps at the back of his tongue as circumvallate papillae. These are large circular structures surrounded by moat-like depressions. The lateral surfaces of these papillae contain taste buds.

    Aphthous ulcers (**choice A**) are small, white or red mouth lesions.

    Candidal colonies (**choice B**) appear in thrush, which occurs more commonly in the immunocompromised host or in those taking antibacterial drugs. You are told that the patient is healthy and not taking medications, making this condition unlikely.

    Filiform papillae (**choice D**) are the most numerous papillae of the tongue. They are elongated cones that create the tongue's rough texture. They do not contain taste buds.

    Fungiform papillae (**choice E**) are mushroom-shaped structures scattered among the filiform papillae. They frequently contain taste buds.

20. **The correct answer is E.** The transverse fissure above (between the right upper and right middle lobes) and the oblique fissure below (between the right middle and right lower lobes) are often strikingly visible on the oblique view in patients with right middle lobar pneumonia. The diaphragm and the breast may also be seen but do not overlap the middle lobe on the oblique view.

21. **The correct answer is D.** Injections are given in the upper, outer quadrant of the buttocks to prevent damage to the sciatic nerve, which is present in the lower quadrant. The other nerves listed are not particularly vulnerable to injections into the buttocks.

    The common peroneal nerve (**choice A**) is a branch of the sciatic nerve that diverges from it in the popliteal fossa. It then divides into the superficial and deep peroneal nerves.

    The lateral femoral cutaneous nerve (**choice B**) derives from the lumbar plexus, emerges slightly below the anterior superior iliac spine, and supplies the skin of the anterior thigh down to the knee.

    The obturator nerve (**choice C**) derives from the lumbar plexus, diverges from the femoral nerve in the psoas muscle, and passes medially along the lateral pelvic wall to run in the obturator canal, where it divides into anterior and posterior divisions. The anterior division generally supplies the gracilis, adductor brevis, and adductor longus; the posterior division generally supplies the obturator externus and the adductor part of the adductor magnus.

The superior gluteal nerve (**choice E**) is a branch of the sacral plexus. It supplies the gluteus minimus and medius and the tensor fascia lata. Only small branches of this nerve are likely to be encountered in the upper outer quadrant of the buttock, making injection here relatively safe.

22. **The correct answer is A.** A good way to remember what goes through the superior orbital fissure is that everything that innervates the eye, other than the optic nerve, passes through this fissure. This includes the oculomotor nerve (CN III), the trochlear nerve (CN IV), the ophthalmic nerve (V1), and the abducens nerve (CN VI).

The facial nerve (CN VII; **choice B**) passes through the internal auditory meatus.

The mandibular nerve (V3; **choice C**) passes through the foramen ovale.

The maxillary nerve (V2; **choice D**) passes through the foramen rotundum.

The middle meningeal artery (**choice E**) passes through the foramen spinosum.

23. **The correct answer is C.** After crossing the floor of the anatomic snuff box, the radial artery passes deep to the tendon of extensor pollicis longus to enter the palm deeply in the space between the first and second metacarpals (first web space). Within this space, it contributes to the formation of the deep palmar arterial arch.

The deep branch of the radial nerve (**choice A**), or posterior interosseous nerve, supplies the deep muscles of the extensor forearm. It does not enter the palm. The superficial branch of the radial nerve conveys sensory information from the dorsum of the hand, particularly from the skin of the first web space.

The opponens pollicis (**choice B**) arises from the trapezium and the flexor retinaculum. It inserts on the lateral aspect of the first metacarpal and lies deep to abductor pollicis brevis and flexor pollicis brevis in the thenar eminence.

The recurrent branch of the median nerve (**choice D**) supplies the muscles of the thenar eminence. It leaves the median nerve following that nerve's passage through the carpal tunnel, and passes between abductor pollicis brevis and flexor pollicis brevis. It supplies both of these muscles and the opponens pollicis, which lies deep to them. The median nerve also supplies the first two lumbrical muscles.

The superficial palmar arch (**choice E**) is formed mainly by the ulnar artery, with a contribution from the radial artery. It lies more distally in the palm than the deep palmar arch.

24. **The correct answer is A.** The axillary nerve can be damaged during anterior dislocation of the shoulder, causing loss of sensation in the skin overlying the lower half of the deltoid muscle.

The median nerve (**choice B**) supplies sensation to the anterior arm, palm, and distal aspects of the lateral three-and-a-half fingers.

The musculocutaneous nerve (**choice C**) supplies sensation to the lateral surface of the arm and forearm.

The radial nerve (**choice D**) supplies sensation to the back of the arm, forearm, and hand.

The ulnar nerve (**choice E**) supplies sensation to the medial side of the arm, forearm, and hand.

25. **The correct answer is B.** The diaphragm is at particular risk because it is closely related to both the 12th rib and the suprarenal area. Surgeons sometimes call this the "perilous pleura" because of the care they must exercise with this approach. The close physical relationship also accounts for the pleural effusions seen in some patients with kidney infections. The other structures listed in the answers are not particularly vulnerable during the suggested surgical approach.

26. **The correct answer is A.** The anterior cruciate ligament passes from its anterior attachment on the anterior aspect of the intercondylar eminence upward and laterally and posteriorly to attach to the medial side of the lateral condyle of the femur. Thus, in normal movement, as the condyles of the femur rotate backward on the head of the tibia, the anterior cruciate ligament is put under stretch and comes to arrest rotation at full extension.

The lateral (**choice B**) and medial (**choice C**) semilunar cartilages (the menisci) function to aid in rotation of the condyles; they do so by moving on the tibia. The medial cartilage is attached to the tibial collateral ligament, and the lateral one has the meniscofemoral ligament and the popliteus muscle attached to it. During rotation of the condyles of the femur, these various attachments pull on the menisci, causing them to move in concert. By being thicker at their peripheral margins and conforming to the tibial surface of the associated condyles, these two cartilages also aid in joint stability.

The posterior cruciate ligament (**choice D**), which extends between the dorsal aspect of the posterior intercondylar fossa of the tibia and the lateral surface of the medial condyle, comes under full tension during flexion of the knee joint. Actually, both the anterior and posterior cruciate ligaments, in all joint positions, are under some degree of tension. This provides stability to the full range of movements of the knee.

The transverse ligament (transverse genicular ligament; **choice E**) is a fibrous band of connective tissue that connects the anterior end of the lateral meniscus to the anterior end of the medial meniscus of the knee. By the nature of its attachments, it would not contribute to the control of knee extension; in fact, this ligament is often absent.

27. **The correct answer is A.** This question could have tricked you if you didn't catch the key words, "in the embryo." If you read the question too quickly and thought you were going to be asked to identify the structure described, you probably chose **choice C** (ligamentum venosum), since that is indeed the structure in question. In the embryo, however, this fibrous band is actually the ductus venosus. The ductus venosus is an embryonic vessel that allows blood to bypass the fetal liver; this prevents the depletion of oxygen and nutrient-rich blood in the hepatic sinusoids.

    The embryonic umbilical arteries (**choice D**) become the medial umbilical ligaments.

    The embryonic umbilical vein (**choice E**) actually becomes the fibrous ligamentum teres (**choice B**). The ligamentum teres is located in the free margin of the falciform ligament.

28. **The correct answer is D.** The cells of the anterior pituitary can be classified as chromophils (stain with dyes) or chromophobes (do not stain with dyes). The chromophils can be further divided into acidophils (stain with acidic dyes) and basophils (stain with basic dyes). The acidophils include the somatotrophs, which secrete growth hormone, and the mammotrophs, which secrete prolactin.

    The basophils include the corticotrophs, which secrete ACTH (**choice A**), the gonadotrophs, which secrete FSH and LH (**choices B and C**), and the thyrotrophs, which secrete TSH (**choice E**).

29. **The correct answer is A.** Children with recurrent urinary tract infections should be further evaluated for renal/urinary tract abnormalities with a voiding cystourethrogram (VCUG). If the VCUG shows no urinary reflux, an ultrasound should be performed to evaluate the upper urinary tract and kidney. If reflux is present, an intravenous pyelogram (IVP) or radionuclide scan may be performed to detect renal scarring. (Note that the number one cause of urinary reflux in children is posterior urethral valves.) A normal IVP would be expected to display normal renal anatomy, in which two cup-shaped major calyces unite to form the renal pelvis.

    The minor calyces (**choice B**), of which there are usually 7-14, first unite into 2 (sometimes 3) major calyces before emptying into the renal pelvis.

The renal pyramids (**choice C**) represent the region where the collecting tubules of the kidney are located (separated from each other by renal columns in which glomeruli and convoluted tubules are located). At their apices (renal papilla), the collecting tubules constituting the renal pyramids discharge urine into the minor calyces. These collecting tubules are too small to be filled by contrast material in pyelograms; hence, the renal papilla are seen on the IVP as dark, unfilled indentations of the minor calyces.

The ureter (**choice D**) receives urine from the renal pelvis, not the other way around.

The renal cortex (**choice E**) contains all of the convoluted tubules, cortical collecting ducts, and glomeruli. These structures are too small to be filled by contrast material and would be seen as dark.

30. **The correct answer is C.** Cleft lip is caused by the failure of the maxillary processes to fuse with the medial nasal swellings.

    Abnormal development of the third and fourth pharyngeal pouches (**choice A**) can give rise to DiGeorge syndrome, which is characterized by underdevelopment or absence of several structures, including the thymus and parathyroids.

    Bony defects of the malar bone and mandible (**choice B**) are associated with mandibulofacial dysostosis, which is mainly due to abnormal development of derivatives of the first arch. This condition is characterized by downward sloping palpebral fissures; hypoplasia of the malar and mandibular bones; macrostomia; high or cleft palate; abnormally shaped, low-set ears; and unusual hair growth patterns. If pits or clefts appear between the mouth and ear, the condition is called Franceschetti syndrome. If the condition is limited to the orbit and malar region, it is termed Treacher-Collins syndrome. Insufficient migration of neural crest cells (**choice E**) is an important factor as well.

    When the palatine shelves fail to join together (**choice D**), cleft palate results. Cleft lip and cleft palate commonly co-occur.

31. **The correct answer is C.** The hypoglossal nerve is a pure motor nerve (general somatic efferent) to the intrinsic muscles of the tongue. If the nerve is damaged, denervation atrophy of the affected side will permit the intact musculature of the opposite side to operate unopposed, thereby protruding the tongue to the side of the injury.

    The gag reflex (**choice A**) is mediated by the glossopharyngeal nerve (CN IX; afferent limb) and the vagus nerve (CN X; efferent limb).

Choice B is incorrect because the preganglionic parasympathetic fibers that regulate these two salivary glands are carried by the chorda tympani (which joins with the lingual nerve) to the submandibular ganglion. Postganglionic fibers are then distributed to these glands.

The muscles responsible for elevation of the pharynx (**choice D**) are innervated primarily by the vagus nerve (CN X).

Choice E is incorrect because taste fibers for the anterior two-thirds of the tongue are carried via the chorda tympani to the facial nerve (CN VII) and hence to the brainstem.

32. **The correct answer is A.** The endocardial cushions form the fibrous tissue "skeleton" of the heart, which lies between the chambers of the heart. A failure of fusion of the cushions can cause an atrioventricular defect, which, in extreme cases, can make the heart behave as if it were a single chamber. Surgical correction of a large defect may be difficult and may not yield an effective heart, since other malformations, such as small ventricular size, may coexist.

The causes of coarctation of the aorta (**choice B**) are unclear but are not thought to be related to incomplete fusion of the endocardial cushions.

Pulmonary stenosis (**choice C**) can be caused by fusion of the cusps of the semilunar valve, or by unequal division of the truncus arteriosus.

Tetralogy of Fallot (**choice D**) is caused by failure of the pulmonary trunk and aorta to line up with the ventricular openings.

Transposition of the great vessels (**choice E**) results from abnormal migration of neural crest cells, leading to failure of spiral development of the aorticopulmonary septum.

33. **The correct answer is E.** Bone is formed by type I collagen fibers, ground substance, and hydroxyapatite crystals. The collagen is oriented in a layered or lamellar fashion. It can be parallel (trabecular bone and periosteum) or concentric (Haversian system). When bone is formed quickly, as in a healing fracture site, metabolic bone disease, or tumor, the collagen is randomly oriented and is called woven bone.

Compact bone (**choice B**) is the dense calcified external part of the bone. It is lamellar bone.

Cancellous (**choice A**), spongy (**choice C**), and trabecular (**choice D**) bone are all synonymous terms for the thinner network of bone within the cortex. These are also lamellar bone.

34. **The correct answer is E.** All three structures lie in the subcostal groove below a rib. Third- and fourth-year students are sometimes offered the chance to help tap a patient's pleural effusion, and can look a little foolish if the resident has to stop them because they have forgotten this basic anatomic point and have entered the intercostal space in the middle or upper region.

35. **The correct answer is B.** The infant has Hirschsprung disease (more common in males), a diagnosis that should spring to mind in an infant who fails to pass meconium soon after birth and presents with chronic constipation. Diagnosis is made most easily and most reliably by anal manometry and/or rectal biopsy. On manometry, internal anal sphincter pressure increases on rectal balloon distention in patients with Hirschsprung disease (normally, pressure decreases with distention). Rectal biopsy reveals an absence of ganglion cells (which are derived from neural crest cells) in a portion of the colonic wall. Barium enema would show a transition zone between the aganglionic area of bowel (narrow) and the region of normal bowel proximal to it (dilated).

Defective recanalization of the colon (**choice A**) results in rectal atresia. In this condition, there is no communication between the rectum and anal canal. Therefore, neither meconium nor stool can be passed.

Herniation of abdominal contents into the umbilical cord (**choice C**) describes a congenital omphalocele. This occurs because of the failure of all or part of the intestines to return into the abdominal cavity during the 10th week of gestation.

Persistence of the proximal end of the yolk stalk (**choice D**) results in Meckel diverticulum, an ileal outpouching that is more prevalent in males. It usually contains ectopic gastric mucosa, which can cause ulceration and bleeding. Inflammation of the diverticulum may produce symptoms and signs similar to appendicitis.

The presence of a rectourinary fistula (**choice E**) would result in the passage of meconium, stool, and gas into the urine.

36. **The correct answer is E.** The CSF circulates through the ventricular system as follows: from the lateral ventricles through the interventricular foramen (**choice D**) into the third ventricle (**choice E**) through the cerebral aqueduct (of Sylvius) to reach the fourth ventricle (**choice C**) and out the foramina of Luschka (**choice B**) and Magendie (**choice A**) into the subarachnoid space. Once the CSF is in the subarachnoid space, it is absorbed through arachnoid villi into dural sinuses, where it mixes with the venous blood. Therefore, a blockage of the cerebral aqueduct, which connects the third and fourth ventricles, will produce an increase in pressure initially in the third ventricle.

37. **The correct answer is A.** Bregma represents the point where the coronal and sagittal sutures intersect; it is the site of the anterior fontanelle.

The coronal suture (**choice B**) lies between the frontal and parietal bones.

Lambda (**choice C**) represents the point where the sagittal and lambdoid sutures intersect; it is the site of the posterior fontanelle in infants.

The pterion (**choice D**) is the point on the lateral aspect of the skull where the greater wing of the sphenoid, parietal, frontal, and temporal bones converge. Recall that the pterion is the landmark for the middle meningeal artery and that a blow to the temple (e.g., as could occur in boxing) can lead to a middle meningeal arterial bleed and an epidural hemorrhage.

The sagittal suture (**choice E**) is located between the two parietal bones.

38. **The correct answer is E.** This patient has coarctation of the aorta (constriction of the ascending aorta), which is suggested by a midsystolic murmur over the anterior part of the chest and back, hypertension in the upper extremities, and absent or delayed pulsations in the femoral arteries. The upper extremities and thorax may be more developed than the lower extremities. Patients with coarctation of the aorta may experience symptoms such as cold extremities as a result of tissue ischemia. The truncus arteriosus gives rise to the proximal portions of the ascending aorta and the pulmonary trunk. The third, fourth, and sixth aortic arches and the right and left dorsal aortae contribute to the remainder of the aorta.

The bulbus cordis (**choice A**) gives rise to the right ventricle and the aortic outflow tract.

In 98% of cases, coarctation of the aorta takes place immediately distal to the offshoot of the left subclavian artery, close to the junction of the ductus arteriosus (**choice B**) with the aorta.

The right common cardinal vein (**choice C**) gives rise to the superior vena cava.

The right horn of the sinus venosus (**choice D**) gives rise to the smooth part of the right atrium.

39. **The correct answer is C.** The submucosa and mucosa lining the inside of the bladder are highly folded when the bladder is empty, but are loosely adherent to the underlying muscle and move against each other, smoothing the folds of the bladder wall as it fills. The only site where the attachment of mucosa to muscle is tight is the triangularly shaped trigone of the bladder, located on the posterior bladder floor (i.e., posterior and inferior). The internal wall here is smooth even when the bladder is empty. All ducts that open into the bladder (including the internal ureteric orifices) do so at the angles of the trigone; hence, they are not stretched or pulled by the movement of the bladder wall as the bladder fills. In the distended bladder, the internal ureteric openings are approximately 5 cm apart.

40. **The correct answer is D.** The somitomeres are specialized masses of mesoderm found in the head region that give rise to the muscles of the head. The extraocular muscles are derived from somitomeres 1, 2, 3, and 5.

The branchial arches (**choice A**) give rise to muscles of mastication (arch 1), muscles of facial expression (arch 2), and muscles of the pharynx and larynx (arches 3-6), as well as additional small muscles.

The optic cup ectoderm (**choice B**) gives rise to the muscles of the iris (sphincter and dilator pupillae). These are the only muscles not formed from mesoderm.

Somites (**choice C**) give rise to the inferior muscles of the neck.

Splanchnic mesoderm (**choice E**) gives rise to smooth muscle of the viscera and the heart muscle.

41. **The correct answer is C.** Questions like these are particularly amenable to the use of test-taking strategies because even if you don't know 100% of the answer, you will be able to eliminate some answer choices on the basis of knowledge you do have. For example, you probably are aware that the peritoneum does not lie above the transversus abdominis muscle, enabling you to eliminate choice A and increase your chances of answering correctly by 20%. Note that this is a question surgeons love to ask students, so keep this information in mind in the OR!

42. **The correct answer is B.** Pain in the liver and gallbladder can be referred to C3-C5 dermatomes of the right shoulder. Many people are familiar with the projection of cardiac pain to the left shoulder, which is a similar phenomenon. Pancreatic disease can also produce left shoulder pain. On physical examination, referred pain can usually be distinguished from pain truly originating in the perceived area by palpation and manipulation of the area. Local physical manipulation does not usually alter the character or intensity of referred pain, but it does alter those features of skin, joint, or muscle pain truly localized to the region.

43. **The correct answer is E.** The transitional epithelium that lines the ureter, the renal pelvis, and the major and minor calyces is derived from mesoderm of the ureteric bud. Similarly, the cuboidal epithelium of the collecting tubules derives from ureteric bud mesoderm.

The simple squamous epithelium lining Bowman's capsule (**choice A**) is derived from mesoderm of the metanephric vesicle.

The simple cuboidal epithelium lining the distal convoluted tubule (**choice B**) is derived from mesoderm of the metanephric vesicle.

The simple squamous epithelium lining the loop of Henle (**choice C**) is derived from mesoderm of the metanephric vesicle.

The proximal convoluted tubule (**choice D**) is lined with simple columnar epithelium derived from mesoderm of the metanephric vesicle.

44. **The correct answer is D.** Spondylitis is defined as an inflammation of the vertebra. Here we have a case of Potts disease. This is an advanced stage of spondylitis.

45. **The correct answer is C.** Spondylolisthesis is an anterior displacement of one vertebral body relative to the one just below it.

46. **The correct answer is A.** Spondylosis is degeneration of the intervertebral disk. In the early stages it shows on x-ray as silhouette changes of the disk. In the final stages, one sees ankylosis of the involved vertebral bodies.

47. **The correct answer is B.** Spondylolysis can occur congenitally or traumatically. In this case, it was a fracture of the pars interarticularis.

48. **The correct answer is G.** Diskitis is an acute inflammation of the disk space. It is a benign self-limited inflammation that occurs at ages 2-7 years. Symptoms are mild fevers of 37.8 to 38.4 C (100.0 to 101.1 F) and back pain and stiffness, with no neurologic deficits. Treatment consists of rest, NSAIDs, and antibiotics for 4 to 6 weeks.

49. **The correct answer is F.** This hidden defect is one of the most common congenital anomalies of the lumbar spine. It is a failure of fusion of the lamina of the lumbar vertebrae. Physical findings may include hypertrichosis or a hyperpigmented area. It is most commonly found on x-ray.

50. **The correct answer is E.** Ankylosing spondylitis is an inflammatory disease that is possibly associated with antigen HLA-B27. It prefers men to women by 3:1 and starts to manifest at approximately 20-30 years of age. Its symptoms start as dull back pain, morning stiffness, loss of spinal mobility, and pain in the sacroiliac joint with motion or strong palpatory pressure. In the late stages of the disease, a bamboo spine is a radiographic finding.

Physiology

1. A 42-year-old woman complains of a burning pain in the upper middle region of her abdomen. The pain usually occurs about 2 hours after a meal and frequently awakens her at night. Antacids can usually relieve the pain within a few minutes. Physical examination reveals that T5–T9 has chronic tissue changes. An x-ray film reveals a typical duodenal ulcer identified as a discrete crater in the proximal portion of the duodenal bulb. Because the woman does not have a history of chronic use of aspirin or other nonsteroidal antiinflammatory drugs (NSAIDs), the bacterium *Helicobacter pylori* is assumed to be the major factor in the etiology of the ulcer. Which of the following is likely to be normal in this woman?

   (A) Basal acid output

   (B) Fasting serum gastrin

   (C) Gastrin response to a meal

   (D) Maximal acid output

   (E) Parietal cell mass

2. A series of photographs taken of a middle-aged man over a period of 2 decades demonstrates gradual coarsening of facial features and progressive protrusion of the brows. Upon questioning, the patient reports having to wear larger shoes than he did as a young man. Which of the following pair of hormones normally regulates the hormone responsible for these changes?

   (A) Dopamine and norepinephrine

   (B) LH and hCG

   (C) Prolactin and FSH

   (D) Somatostatin and GHRH

   (E) TSH and ACTH

3. Given these data below, what is the net filtration pressure at the glomerulus?

   > Glomerular hydrostatic pressure = 44 mm Hg
   > Bowman's capsule hydrostatic pressure = 9 mm Hg
   > Osmotic pressure of plasma = 28 mm Hg
   > Osmotic pressure of tubular fluid = 0

   (A) −5 mm Hg

   (B) 7 mm Hg

   (C) 25 mm Hg

   (D) 63 mm Hg

   (E) 81 mm Hg

4. A 50-year-old woman undergoes surgery to remove a large abdominal tumor. Histologic findings show that the mass contains a large number of blood vessels. Several metastases were found 2 months after surgery. A decrease in which of the following is the most likely cause for the development of metastases after the removal of the large tumor?

   (A) Basic fibroblast growth factor (bFGF)

   (B) Endostatin

   (C) Growth hormone

   (D) Platelet-derived growth factor (PDGF)

   (E) Transforming growth factor (TGFβ)

5. A 48-year-old man presents to the emergency department with chest pain that radiates to his jaw and left shoulder. Osteopathic examination reveals T4 FRS_L. Angina pectoris is suspected, and he is sent for an angiogram. The test reveals an atherosclerotic coronary artery that is 50% occluded. The blood flow through this artery is reduced by

   (A) 1/2

   (B) 1/4

   (C) 1/8

   (D) 1/16

   (E) 1/32

6. A 24-year-old man becomes paraplegic after he severs his spinal cord at T1 in an automobile accident. Chronic constipation is a problem, but he wants to be as independent as possible in its treatment. His physician advises him to distend the rectum digitally on a regular schedule to initiate the defecation reflex. Rectal distention causes which of the following in this patient?

   (A) Closure of the glottis

   (B) Contraction of the internal anal sphincter

   (C) Increased abdominal pressure

   (D) Increased peristaltic waves

   (E) Relaxation of the external anal sphincter

Questions 7-8

CASE A

A patient trapped in a house fire is injured by the inhalation of smoke. Carbon dioxide is transported in the blood by a variety of mechanisms.

7. Which of the following is quantitatively the most important method for transporting CO_2?

   (A) As carbaminohemoglobin

   (B) As CO_2 in gas bubbles

   (C) As CO_2 in physical solution

   (D) As sodium bicarbonate in red cells

   (E) As sodium bicarbonate in serum

8. What would cause the oxygen-hemoglobin dissociation curve to shift to the left?

   (A) Carbon monoxide poisoning

   (B) Decreased pH

   (C) Increased 2,3-diphosphoglycerate (2,3-DPG)

   (D) Increased P_{CO_2}

   (E) Increased temperature

9. A prisoner has gone on a hunger strike. Which of the following substances can be converted to glucose to supply the needs of the brain during starvation?

   (A) Acetoacetate

   (B) Acetone

   (C) Amino acids

   (D) Beta-hydroxybutyrate

   (E) Fatty acids

10. A 54-year-old man is seen in clinic with complaints of palpitations and light-headedness. Physical examination is remarkable for a heart rate of greater than 200 min and a blood pressure of 75/40 mm Hg. Which of the following adjustments have probably occurred in the cardiac cycle?

    (A) Diastolic time has decreased and systolic time has increased

    (B) Diastolic time has decreased but systolic time has decreased more

    (C) Systolic time has decreased and diastolic time has increased

    (D) Systolic time has decreased but diastolic time has decreased more

    (E) Systolic time has decreased but diastolic time has not changed

11. A 25-year-old man visits a friend living in a mountain cabin at an altitude of 5000 meters. After 5 days, he has an increase in ventilation rate and a decrease in arterial P_{CO_2}. Which of the following physiologic changes is also expected?

    (A) Decreased production of erythropoietin

    (B) Decreased 2,3-diphosphoglycerate (2,3-DPG)

    (C) Increased renal excretion of H^+ ions

    (D) Increased renal excretion of HCO_3-

    (E) Pulmonary vasodilation

12. As part of an experimental study, a volunteer agrees to have 10 g mannitol injected intravenously. After sufficient time for equilibration, blood is drawn, and the concentration of mannitol in the plasma is found to be 65 mg/100 mL. Urinalysis reveals that 10% of the mannitol had been excreted into the urine during this time period. What is the approximate extracellular fluid volume of this volunteer?

    (A) 10 L

    (B) 14 L

    (C) 22 L

    (D) 30 L

    (E) 42 L

13. In clinical trials, an experimental drug is found to cause impotence in a large percentage of male patients. Inhibition of which of the following could be responsible for this side effect?

    (A) Conversion of DHT to testosterone
    (B) Forward motility factor
    (C) Nitric oxide synthase (NOS)
    (D) Oxytocin
    (E) Prostaglandins

14. A healthy 22-year-old female medical student has an exercise stress test at a local health club. Which of the following is most likely to decrease in her skeletal muscles during exercise?

    (A) Arteriolar resistance
    (B) Carbon dioxide concentration
    (C) Lactic acid concentration
    (D) Sympathetic nervous activity
    (E) Vascular conductance

Questions 15-16

CASE B

15. A volume-pressure diagram of the left ventricle during one cardiac cycle of a normal heart is shown above. Which point on the diagram marks the beginning of systole?

    (A) A
    (B) B
    (C) C
    (D) D
    (E) E

16. Which of the following points on the left ventricular pressure-volume loop represents the mitral valve opening?

    (A) A
    (B) B
    (C) C
    (D) D
    (E) E

17. A 43-year-old man with a recurrent history of ulcer disease associated with diarrhea and a strong family history of duodenal ulcer disease is suspected of having Zollinger-Ellison syndrome (gastrinoma). Physical examination reveals chronic somatic dysfunction at T5-T9 bilaterally. Secretin (1 U/kg) is given as a rapid IV injection to test for gastrinoma. Which of the following results would support the existence of gastrinoma following secretin administration?

    (A) Gastrin release from antrum
    (B) Increased serum gastrin
    (C) Inhibition of gastric emptying
    (D) Inhibition of gastric secretion
    (E) Stimulation of pancreatic HCO_3- secretion

18. Blood is drawn from a 14-year-old boy with bacterial meningitis for a complete blood count. The leukocyte count is elevated. Which of the following is released by the predominant type of white blood cell present?

    (A) Histamine
    (B) Leukotrienes
    (C) Lysozyme
    (D) Peroxidase
    (E) Vasoactive amines

19. A 21-year-old man is competing in a weight-lifting competition. He lifts 325 lb over his head and holds it there for 5 seconds. Suddenly, his arms give way and he drops the weight to the floor. Which of the following receptors is responsible for this sudden muscle relaxation?

    (A) Free nerve ending
    (B) Golgi tendon organ
    (C) Merkel disk
    (D) Muscle spindle
    (E) Pacinian corpuscle

Questions 20-21

CASE C

A 16-year-old type 1 diabetic is noncompliant with his required insulin therapy and develops hyperglycemia after eating several pieces of hard candy.

20. The release of which of the following intestinal hormones would most likely be stimulated?

   (A) Gastric inhibitory peptide (GIP)

   (B) Gastrin

   (C) Motilin

   (D) Secretin

   (E) Somatostatin

21. In a normal patient, the primary metabolic effect of the principal hormone secreted by the alpha cells of the pancreas is

   (A) augmentation of calcium deposition in bone

   (B) increase of amino acid storage in the liver

   (C) promotion of lipogenesis in liver and adipose tissue

   (D) inhibition of gluconeogenesis

   (E) stimulation of glycogenolysis

22. A 57-year-old woman with a 30-year history of alcoholism and liver disease visits her physician complaining of abdominal swelling and shortness of breath. Physical examination reveals a shifting dullness, an abdominal fluid wave, and chronic somatic dysfunction of right paraspinal tissues at T5-T9. The physician determines that she has severe ascites. Which of the following factors contributes to the accumulation of fluid in the abdominal cavity?

   (A) Decreased plasma epinephrine and norepinephrine

   (B) Decreased plasma volume

   (C) Increased hepatic lymph flow

   (D) Increased hydrostatic pressure in splanchnic capillary beds

   (E) Increased natriuresis

23. A 33-year-old man complains that his chest hurts when he eats, especially when he eats meat. Physical examination shows somatic dysfunction on the left paraspinal tissues of T2-T8. An x-ray film shows a dilated esophagus, and achalasia is suspected. Esophageal manometry is used to confirm the diagnosis. Swallowing induced relaxation is reduced at which anatomic location in this man?

   (A) Lower esophageal sphincter

   (B) Lower esophagus

   (C) Middle esophagus

   (D) Pharynx

   (E) Upper esophageal sphincter

Questions 24-25

CASE D

A substance that is filtered, but not secreted or reabsorbed (substance X), is infused into a volunteer until a steady state plasma level of 0.1 mg/mL is achieved. The subject then empties his bladder and waits 1 hour, at which time he urinates again. The volume of urine in the second specimen is 60 mL, and the concentration of substance X is 10 mg/mL.

24. What is the glomerular filtration rate (GFR) in this individual?

   (A) 30 mL/min

   (B) 60 mL/min

   (C) 100 mL/min

   (D) 300 mL/min

   (E) 600 mL/min

25. Which of the following can be determined by calculating the clearance of para-aminohippuric acid (PAH)?

   (A) Extracellular fluid (ECF) volume

   (B) Effective renal plasma flow (ERPF)

   (C) Glomerular filtration rate (GFR)

   (D) Plasma volume

   (E) Total body water (TBW)

26. A 40-year-old man with sleep apnea participates in a sleep study. During his evaluation, normal sawtooth waves are observed on his EEG tracing. This pattern is associated with which period of sleep?

    (A) REM
    (B) Stage 1
    (C) Stage 2
    (D) Stage 3
    (E) Stage 4

27. A 48-year-old white female secretary presents with progressive difficulty typing over the past month. She also notes that her hands begin to feel numb and weak after typing for long periods of time. There is somatic dysfunction at T1-T4, as well as pain when the transverse carpal ligaments are struck. On testing, which of the following deficits would be predicted?

    (A) Difficulty in abducting the fifth finger
    (B) Difficulty in adducting the thumb
    (C) Difficulty in flexing digits two and three at the metacarpophalangeal joints
    (D) Loss of sensation over the lateral half of the dorsum of the hand
    (E) Loss of sensation over the lateral half of the palm

28. A 70-year-old woman undergoes a gastrectomy for Zollinger-Ellison syndrome. Her physician informs her that she will need to take intramuscular vitamin B_{12} shots for the rest of her life. Absence of which of the following cell types is responsible for this vitamin replacement requirement?

    (A) Chief cells
    (B) G cells
    (C) Goblet cells
    (D) Mucous neck cells
    (E) Parietal cells

29. In a person weighing 75 kg, the volumes of total body water (TBW), intracellular fluid, and extracellular fluid are, respectively

    (A) 40L, 30L, 10L
    (B) 45L, 30L, 15L
    (C) 45L, 35L, 10L
    (D) 50L, 25L, 25L
    (E) 50L, 35L, 15L

30. A 35-year-old, sexually active woman visits her gynecologist complaining of mild, right-sided, lower abdominal pain but no other symptoms. Physical examination reveals no guarding, bowel sounds are present, and there is no somatic dysfunction. There are also no peritoneal signs. Her surgical history is significant for an appendectomy at age 10. Her last period occurred 14 days ago. Which of the following endometrial changes corresponds to this stage of the patient's menstrual cycle?

    (A) Apical movement of secretions in the glandular cells
    (B) Degeneration of the glandular structures
    (C) Glandular glycogen accumulation in the functionalis
    (D) Growth of the spiral arteries
    (E) Tissue expansion by cellular hypertrophy

31. Which sequence of the numbered statements below correctly describes the pathway of lymphatic flow on the left side of the body?

    1) Junction of left internal jugular and left subclavian
    2) Lymph capillaries
    3) Thin lymph vessels
    4) Thoracic duct

    (A) 2-1-3-4
    (B) 2-3-1-4
    (C) 2-3-4-1
    (D) 2-4-1-3
    (E) 2-4-3-1

32. The following data were collected from a normal patient before and after an intervention. Assume that plasma osmolarity and glomerular filtration rate remain constant.

	Before	After
Urine osmolarity (mOsm/L)	900	250
Urine flow rate (mL/min)	0.65	2.3
Fractional clearance of sodium	1%	1%
Osmolar clearance (mL/min)	2.0	2.0

The intervention that would best account for the observed changes is

(A) administration of furosemide

(B) administration of hydrochlorothiazide

(C) administration of lithium

(D) a high dietary intake of potassium

(E) a transfusion of 2 L isotonic saline

33. An unlabeled container of blood product is left in a laboratory. The technician must determine whether the sample is serum or plasma. An elevated level of which of the following substances would identify the specimen as plasma?

(A) Albumin

(B) Erythrocytes

(C) Fibrinogen

(D) Granulocytes

(E) Serotonin

34. A Swan-Ganz catheter inserted into a patient with acute respiratory distress syndrome (ARDS) records a pulmonary artery wedge pressure of 6 mm Hg. The same pressure would be expected in which of the following structures?

(A) Aorta

(B) Left atrium

(C) Left ventricle

(D) Right atrium

(E) Systemic veins

35. A hysterical patient is hyperventilating and doubles his alveolar ventilation. If his initial alveolar PA_{CO_2} was 40 mm Hg, and his CO_2 production remains unchanged, what will his alveolar P_{CO_2} be on hyperventilation?

(A) 80 mm Hg

(B) 60 mm Hg

(C) 20 mm Hg

(D) 10 mm Hg

(E) 4 mm Hg

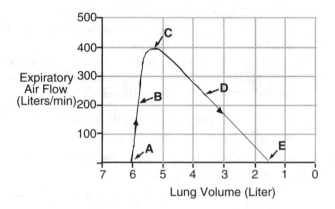

36. The maximum expiratory flow-volume curve shown above was obtained from a normal, healthy volunteer. Which point on the curve represents residual volume?

(A) A

(B) B

(C) C

(D) D

(E) E

37. A 42-year-old obese woman experiences episodic abdominal pain. She notes that the pain increases after the ingestion of a fatty meal. There is somatic dysfunction in the right paraspinal tissue at T5-T9. The action of which of the following hormones is responsible for the postprandial intensification of her symptoms?

(A) Cholecystokinin (CCK)

(B) Gastrin

(C) Pepsin

(D) Secretin

(E) Somatostatin

38. In a normal patient, if renal vascular resistance is decreased to 50% of its initial value, with no change in renal artery or renal vein pressure, which of the following combinations of changes will occur?

	Renal Blood Flow	Renal Artery (O_2)	Renal O_2 Use
(A)	double	increase	no change
(B)	double	no change	increase
(C)	increase 50%	decrease	increase
(D)	increase 50%	increase	no change
(E)	decrease 50%	no change	decrease

39. In a normal patient, adrenocorticotropic hormone (ACTH) promotes the production of cortisol by stimulating which of the following reactions?

    (A) 11-Deoxycortisol to cortisol

    (B) 17-Hydroxyprogesterone to 11-deoxycortisol

    (C) Cholesterol to pregnenolone

    (D) Pregnenolone to progesterone

    (E) Progesterone to 17-hydroxyprogesterone

40. A 69-year-old man presents with unilateral hearing loss. A lesion in which of the following structures could be responsible for this loss?

    (A) Inferior colliculus

    (B) Lateral lemniscus

    (C) Medial geniculate body

    (D) Medial lemniscus

    (E) Organ of Corti

41. A young boy presents with failure to thrive. Biochemical analysis of a duodenal aspirate after a meal reveals a deficiency of enteropeptidase (enterokinase). The levels of which the following digestive enzymes would be affected?

    (A) Amylase

    (B) Colipase

    (C) Lactase

    (D) Pepsin

    (E) Trypsin

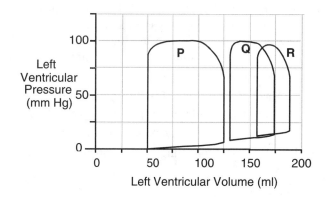

42. Above are volume-pressure diagrams (work diagrams) depicting changes in left ventricular volume and pressure during one cardiac cycle for a normal heart, a failing heart, and a failing heart after treatment with digitalis. Which of the following best describes the relationship of the volume-pressure diagrams with the stated conditions?

	Normal	Before Digitalis	After Digitalis
(A)	P	Q	R
(B)	P	R	Q
(C)	Q	R	P
(D)	R	P	Q
(E)	R	Q	P

43. A patient with congestive heart failure has been placed on salt and fluid restriction to improve his symptoms. Which of the following areas of the adrenal gland would be expected to increase in activity in a patient subjected to salt restriction?

    (A) Adrenal medulla

    (B) Zona fasciculata of the adrenal cortex

    (C) Zona glomerulosa of the adrenal cortex

    (D) Zona reticularis of the adrenal cortex

    (E) There is no area of increased activity

44. A medical student is studying the fluid exchange in skeletal muscle capillaries in a laboratory animal. He determines that fluid is being forced out of a capillary with a net filtration pressure of 8 mm Hg, and he obtains the following laboratory values:

    Capillary hydrostatic pressure = 24 mm Hg

    Capillary colloid osmotic pressure = 17 mm Hg

    Interstitial hydrostatic pressure = 7 mm Hg

    Which of the following is the interstitial osmotic pressure?

    (A) −9 mm Hg

    (B) −8 mm Hg

    (C) −6 mm Hg

    (D) 6 mm Hg

    (E) 8 mm Hg

45. A 32-year-old man and his wife have gone to a fertility clinic and had a successful implantation. By the time of implantation in the uterine endometrium, the typical fertilized ovum has divided into how many cells?

    (A) 2

    (B) 4

    (C) 8

    (D) 16

    (E) >50

46. In a patient diagnosed with von Willebrand disease, which of the following binds to von Willebrand factor at the platelet membrane?

    (A) Adenosine diphosphate (ADP)

    (B) Calcium

    (C) Glycoprotein GPIb

    (D) Platelet factor 3 (PF3)

    (E) Prostacyclin

47. A 25-year-old woman involved in an automobile accident is admitted as an emergency patient. A major artery severed in her leg caused an estimated 600 mL blood to be lost. Her blood pressure is 90/60 mm Hg. Which of the following would be expected to increase in response to hemorrhage?

    (A) Arteriolar diameter in skeletal muscle

    (B) Sodium excretion

    (C) Sympathetic nerve activity

    (D) Vagal nerve activity

    (E) Water excretion

48. Your patient has nephrotic syndrome. Which of the following Starling force changes is the primary cause of the edema seen?

    (A) Decreased capillary hydrostatic pressure (P_c)

    (B) Decreased capillary oncotic pressure (π_c)

    (C) Decreased interstitial hydrostatic pressure (P_i)

    (D) Decreased interstitial oncotic pressure (π_i)

    (E) Increased capillary hydrostatic pressure (P_c)

49. Which of the following would most likely be observed in the lungs during an autopsy of a 2-week-old infant who died of neonatal respiratory distress syndrome?

    (A) Alveoli filled with neutrophils

    (B) Dense fibrosis of the alveolar walls

    (C) Enlarged air spaces

    (D) Hyaline membranes and collapsed alveoli

    (E) Normal lung histology for age

50. An accidental, brief occlusion of the right femoral artery produces transient ischemia in the leg of a patient. The cellular edema seen in reversibly injured cells in a muscle biopsy taken from the patient is most closely related to an increase in which of the following?

    (A) Intracellular Ca^{2+}

    (B) Intracellular K^+

    (C) Intracellular Mg^{2+}

    (D) Intracellular Na^+

    (E) Na^+/K^+ ATPase pump activity

Physiology

ANSWERS AND EXPLANATIONS

1.	B		26.	A
2.	D		27.	C
3.	B		28.	E
4.	B		29.	B
5.	D		30.	D
6.	D		31.	C
7.	E		32.	C
8.	A		33.	C
9.	C		34.	B
10.	D		35.	C
11.	D		36.	E
12.	B		37.	A
13.	C		38.	B
14.	A		39.	C
15.	C		40.	E
16.	A		41.	E
17.	B		42.	B
18.	C		43.	C
19.	B		44.	E
20.	A		45.	E
21.	E		46.	C
22.	D		47.	C
23.	A		48.	B
24.	C		49.	D
25.	B		50.	D

1. **The correct answer is B.** The fasting serum gastrin is normal in patients with duodenal ulcer (DU); however, the gastrin response to a meal (**choice C**) is increased. The increase in serum gastrin following a meal occurs, in part, because acid suppresses gastrin release less effectively in DU patients compared with controls.

    DU patients have an increase in parietal cell mass (**choice E**), which may be caused by the trophic (growth promoting) effects of gastrin.

    Patients with DU have an increased basal acid output (**choice A**) that totally disappears following eradication of the *H. pylori* infection.

    However, the increase in maximal acid output (**choice D**), which occurs in response to IV gastrin, can remain following eradication of the *H. pylori* infection and is likely to result from the increased parietal cell mass.

2. **The correct answer is D.** The disease is acromegaly, which is typically produced by a growth hormone-secreting pituitary adenoma. Growth hormone synthesis is predominately regulated by hypothalamic GHRH (growth hormone releasing hormone), and its pulsatile secretion is predominately regulated by hypothalamic somatostatin.

    Choice A: Dopamine and norepinephrine are catecholamines that regulate smooth muscle tone and cardiac function.

    Choice B: Luteinizing hormone (LH) regulates sex steroid hormone production by both testes and ovaries. Human chorionic gonadotropin (hCG) is produced by the placenta and has actions similar to LH.

    Choice C: Prolactin regulates menstruation and lactation. Follicle stimulating hormone (FSH) regulates ovarian and testicular function.

    Choice E: Thyroid stimulating hormone (TSH) regulates secretion of thyroid hormones. Adrenocorticotropin (ACTH) regulates glucocorticoid secretion.

3. **The correct answer is B.** There is more than one way to think about this question. One way is to determine which of each of the descriptions corresponds to P_c, P_i, π_C, and π_i and then to use the Starling equation for net filtration pressure: $(P_c - P_i) - (\pi_c - \pi_i)$. Perhaps faster and more intuitive is to just envision that the filtration pressure will be the difference between the forces pushing fluid out and the forces pulling fluid back into the glomerulus. The pushing forces are the hydrostatic pressure of the glomerulus (44 mm Hg) and the osmotic pressure of the tubular fluid (0). So the total pressure forcing fluid from the glomerulus into the tubular fluid is 44 mm Hg. The forces pulling the fluid back are the hydrostatic pressure of the Bowman's capsule (9 mm Hg) and the osmotic

pressure of the plasma (28 mm Hg). The total pressure pushing the fluid back into the glomerulus is $9 + 28 = 37$ mm Hg. The difference between the forces favoring filtration and those opposing it is therefore $44 - 37 = 7$ mm Hg.

4. **The correct answer is B.** Tumors produce both angiogenic and anti-angiogenic factors (also called angiostatic factors). Angiogenic factors stimulate the growth of blood vessels (angiogenesis), whereas angiostatic factors inhibit blood vessel growth (anti-angiogenesis). Angiogenic factors such as VEGF and bFGF have relatively long half-lives in the blood compared with angiostatic factors such as endostatin or angiostatin. Large tumors often produce sufficient amounts of angiostatic factors to suppress the growth of blood vessels in small, undetectable tumors present elsewhere in the body. This suppression of angiogenesis in the smaller tumors also suppresses the overall growth of the tumors, because the small tumors cannot grow without an adequate blood supply, i.e., tumor growth is angiogenesis-dependent. When the large tumor is removed, the blood levels of angiostatic factor (endostatin) decrease, allowing angiogenesis to occur in the smaller tumors. The smaller tumors grow rapidly as a consequence of this angiogenesis and can be detected within a few weeks. Endostatin is a fragment of collagen XVIII, which inhibits angiogenesis and shrinks tumors. It shows promising behavior as an anticancer agent in early, preclinical trials.

    The astute student may wonder how angiogenesis can occur in large tumors in the presence of angiostatic factors. The answer is that angiogenesis occurs when the levels (or activities) of angiogenic factors become greater compared with the levels of angiostatic factors, i.e., both angiogenic and angiostatic factors may be present in a tumor, but angiogenesis occurs when the influence of angiogenic factors predominates. The student may also ask how a large tumor can suppress angiogenesis in small tumors when both angiostatic and angiogenic factors are released from the large tumor. The answer is that angiostatic factors have long half-lives in the blood compared with that of angiogenic factors, as discussed above. Thus, the smaller tumors "see" higher levels of angiostatic factors compared with angiogenic factors.

    Basic fibroblast growth factor (bFGF; **choice A**) is a powerful angiogenic agent, both in vitro and in vivo, and is produced by many different types of cells. bFGF is also a potent mitogen for cells of mesenchymal, neural, and epithelial origin. Overexpression of bFGF can result in tumor production.

Growth hormone (**choice C**) has a general effect to cause growth of all, or almost all, tissues of the body, but does not appear to stimulate angiogenesis to a significant extent in solid tumors.

Platelet-derived growth factor (PDGF; **choice D**) is actually three molecules, each of which is a dimeric combination of two distinct but structurally related peptide chains. PDGF isoforms are potent mitogens for connective tissue cells, smooth muscle cells, and some epithelial and endothelial cells. PDGF is thought to have a role in neoplastic transformation and tumor pathogenesis.

Transforming growth factor (TGFβ; **choice E**) is a polypeptide growth factor. It is generally stimulatory for cells of mesenchymal origin and inhibitory for cells of epithelial or neuroectodermal origin. It is an important mediator of the formation of extracellular matrix.

5. **The correct answer is D.** According to the equation, $R = 8\eta l / \pi r^4$, where R is resistance, η is viscosity of blood, l is the length of the blood vessel, and r^4 is the radius of the blood vessel wall to the fourth power, the resistance is inversely proportional to the fourth power of the radius. In other words, if the radius is reduced by one-half, the resistance is multiplied by 16. In addition, blood flow can be expressed as the following: $Q = \Delta P / R$, where Q is blood flow, DP is the pressure gradient at both ends of the vessel, and R is the resistance. Blood flow is inversely proportional to resistance. So when the resistance is increased by 16-fold, blood flow must decrease by 16-fold.

6. **The correct answer is D.** Defecation is initiated by defecation reflexes. An intrinsic reflex mediated entirely by the local enteric nervous system is stimulated when feces enters the rectum. Distention of the rectum initiates afferent signals that spread through the myenteric plexus to initiate peristaltic contractions in the descending colon, sigmoid, and rectum and force the feces toward the anus.

The internal anal sphincter is relaxed (compare with **choice B**), and, if the external anal sphincter (**choice E**) is *voluntarily* relaxed at the same time, defecation will occur. This intrinsic defecation reflex works together with a more powerful reflex that involves the sacral elements of the spinal cord. The cord reflex is also initiated by distention of the rectum, which transmits afferent signals to the sacral cord and then back to the descending colon, sigmoid, rectum, and anus by way of parasympathetic fibers in the pelvic nerves. These parasympathetic signals greatly intensify the peristaltic contractions, adding considerable power to the defecation process. The lower neurons of the second, third, and fourth sacral roots, which provide the sensory and motor fibers for the defecation reflex, are intact when the spinal cord is injured at a higher level.

However, the afferent signals entering the spinal cord initiate other effects that require an intact spinal cord. These include closing the glottis (**choice A**) and increasing abdominal pressure (**choice C**), both of which together move the fecal contents downward. Voluntary relaxation of the external anal sphincter then allows the feces to be expelled from the body. Loss of voluntary aid to the defecation process following spinal transection or injury can make defecation a difficult process; however, excitation of the cord defecation reflex (either digitally or with an enema) can usually produce adequate defecation.

7. **The correct answer is E.** Red blood cells (and many other blood cells) contain the enzyme carbonic anhydrase, which catalyzes the intracellular conversion of CO_2 to bicarbonate and H^+ ion. Most of the bicarbonate in the red cell is exchanged across the plasmalemma for chloride ion. This means that although the bulk of the production of bicarbonate occurs in the red cell (**choice D**), the bulk of the actual transport occurs in serum. Carbonic anhydrase is not present in serum. Bicarbonate can also be produced in serum by nonenzymatic means, but the process is slow.

CO_2 is also carried as carbaminohemoglobin (**choice A**), which forms when CO_2 binds to an NH_2 side group of the hemoglobin protein, rather than to the heme iron (Fe^{2+}), as with carbon monoxide and oxygen.

CO_2 is not transported in the form of bubbles (**choice B**), which is a good thing, because gas bubbles are effectively emboli, which can lead to considerable morbidity or death.

Some CO_2 is carried directly dissolved in blood (**choice C**). It is 20 times more soluble in blood than is O_2.

8. **The correct answer is A.** The loading of O_2 is facilitated when the oxygen dissociation curve shifts to the left, and the unloading of O_2 is facilitated when the oxygen dissociation curve shifts to the right. Carbon monoxide (CO) poisoning is extremely dangerous for several reasons. CO left-shifts the oxygen dissociation curve, which interferes with the unloading of O_2. Also, CO, which has approximately 240 times the affinity for hemoglobin than O_2 does, preferentially binds to available sites on hemoglobin.

The remaining answer choices all shift the oxygen-hemoglobin dissociation curve to the right. A good way to remember the conditions that promote dissociation of O_2 is to think of exercising muscle, which has decreased pH (**choice B**) from lactic acid build-up and increased P_{CO_2} (**choice D**), increased 2,3-DPG (2,3-diphosphoglycerate; **choice C**) because of increased glycolysis, and increased temperature (**choice E**).

9. **The correct answer is C.** During starvation, the diet is inadequate to provide sufficient glucose to maintain the brain, yet the brain requires glucose as an energy source. Glucose used in the brain during starvation is synthesized from amino acids, primarily derived from muscle protein. This use of amino acids in starvation leads to profound muscle wasting.

The ketone bodies (acetoacetate, **choice A**; acetone, **choice B**; and beta-hydroxybutyrate, **choice D**) produced during starvation and diabetic ketoacidosis are derived from adipose triacylglycerols. Although these compounds can be used in biochemical pathways in the brain, they cannot completely replace glucose in that organ. Furthermore, glucose cannot be synthesized from these precursors.

Fatty acid (**choice E**) degradation cannot be used to produce glucose. It can be used, however, to produce ketone bodies that can be used by the brain as a source of intermediates for some synthetic pathways.

10. **The correct answer is D.** Under normal conditions, one-third of the cardiac cycle is spent in systole and two-thirds spent in diastole. As heart rate increases dramatically, the time spent in diastole falls precipitously but the time spent in systole falls only slightly.

A large increase in heart rate must produce a decrease in both diastole and systole (compare with **choice A**).

The major change with increased heart rate is in diastole, not systole (compare with **choice B**).

Heart rate cannot increase if diastolic time increases (**choice C**).

An increase in heart rate must be accompanied by a decrease in diastolic time (compare with **choice E**).

11. **The correct answer is D.** Compensation for high altitude includes an increase in the renal excretion of bicarbonate. The diminished barometric pressure found at high altitude causes arterial hypoxia, which is sensed by peripheral chemoreceptors. The ventilation rate increases, thereby causing a respiratory alkalosis. The kidney then compensates by increasing the excretion of HCO_3-.

Erythropoietin is increased, not decreased, in chronic hypoxia and at high altitude (**choice A**). Increased erythropoietin leads to an increased hematocrit.

Another adaptation to high altitude is increased 2,3-DPG (compare with **choice B**), which shifts the oxygen dissociation curve to the right. This facilitates the release of O_2 in the tissues.

High altitude leads to respiratory alkalosis. The renal compensation is a metabolic acidosis characterized by decreased H^+ excretion and increased HCO_3- excretion. Respiratory acidosis is renally compensated with a metabolic alkalosis that would include increases in H^+ excretion (**choice C**).

Pulmonary vasoconstriction, not vasodilation (**choice E**), occurs in response to alveolar hypoxia, such as would occur at high altitudes.

12. **The correct answer is B.** Volume = amount/concentration.

The amount of mannitol in the volunteer is equal to the amount injected minus the amount excreted: $10 g - 1 g = 9 g = 9000$ mg. Therefore,

$$\text{Volume} = \frac{9000}{65 \text{ mg}/100 \text{ mL}} = 13.8 \text{ L}$$

13. **The correct answer is C.** Penile erection is mediated by the parasympathetic nervous system. The neurons involved are termed nonadrenergic, noncholinergic (NANC) autonomic neurons, and they release nitric oxide (NO). NO binds to the iron in the heme molecule of guanylate cyclase, activating it to form cGMP. This results in a decrease in intracellular calcium and subsequent smooth muscle relaxation and vasodilatation in the corpus cavernosa, producing erection. Nitric oxide synthase (NOS) is the enzyme required for the formation of NO from circulating arginine, and androgens are necessary to maintain normal amounts of this enzyme. Inhibition of this enzyme could result in impotence (although most currently used drugs that have impotence as a side effect do not affect NOS).

Inhibition of the conversion of testosterone to DHT, not DHT to testosterone (**choice A**), would be accomplished by a 5-alpha-reductase inhibitor. This could cause impotence by its anti-androgen effect. In fact, finasteride, a clinically used 5-alpha-reductase inhibitor, produces drastic decreases in libido in some men.

Inhibition of forward motility factor (**choice B**) would hamper sperm motility and result in infertility, not impotence.

Inhibition of oxytocin (**choice D**) or prostaglandins (**choice E**) would result in failure to ejaculate (ejaculatory incompetence), not impotence.

14. **The correct answer is A.** The increase in muscle blood flow that occurs during exercise is caused by dilation of the arterioles (i.e., decreased arteriolar resistance). In normal skeletal muscles, the blood flow can increase as much as 20-fold during strenuous exercise. Most of this increase in blood flow can be attributed to the dilatory actions of metabolic factors (e.g., adenosine, lactic acid, carbon dioxide) produced by the exercising muscles.

Exercise causes the concentration of carbon dioxide (**choice B**) and lactic acid (**choice C**) to increase in the muscles.

Mass discharge of the sympathetic nervous system (**choice D**) occurs throughout the body during exercise, causing arterioles to constrict in most tissues. The arterioles in the exercising muscles, however, are strongly dilated by vasodilator substances released from the muscles.

A decrease in vascular conductance (**choice E**) occurs when the vasculature is constricted. Resistance and conductance are inversely related, so that a decrease in arteriolar resistance is associated with an increase in arteriolar conductance.

15. **The correct answer is C.** The various points on the volume-pressure diagram correspond to specific events of the cardiac cycle as follows:

    Choice A: The mitral valve opens, and the *period of filling* begins.

    Choice B: This is the *period of filling*.

    Choice C: This marks the beginning of *systole*. The mitral valve closes, and S1 can be heard. The end-diastolic pressure (5 mm Hg) and end-diastolic volume (125 mL) can be determined on the Y-axis and X-axis from this point.

    Choice D: This is the period of *isovolumetric contraction*. Left ventricular pressure increases rapidly, but left ventricular volume remains constant. All heart valves are closed.

    Choice E: The aortic valve opens, which marks the beginning of the *period of ejection*. The pressure at this point is equal to the diastolic blood pressure, which is about 80 mm Hg on the diagram.

16. **The correct answer is A.** The mitral valve opens at the beginning of diastole, when the left ventricle is at its lowest pressure.

    Point B represents ventricular filling. Pressure in the left ventricle gradually increases as blood begins to enter it from the left atrium during diastolic ventricular filling.

    Point C represents the closing of the mitral valve.

    Point D represents isovolumetric contraction. It occurs when the left ventricle contracts in response to ventricular filling (**B**) but has not yet achieved enough pressure to force open the aortic valve (**E**).

17. **The correct answer is B.** Gastrinomas are gastrin-secreting tumors usually present in the pancreas. Patients with gastrinoma have high serum gastrin levels, which lead to hypersecretion of gastric acid and consequent duodenal and jejunal ulcers. Injection of secretin is the most specific and easiest test for gastrinoma.

Secretin inhibits antral release of gastrin (**choice A**), but it stimulates release of gastrin from gastrin tumors (gastrinoma) in almost all patients. A doubling of serum gastrin 5-10 minutes after administration of secretin (1 U/kg), coupled with acid hypersecretion and increased basal serum gastrin, strongly indicates the presence of gastrinoma. Secretin can inhibit gastric emptying (**choice C**), inhibit gastric secretion (**choice D**), and stimulate pancreatic HCO_3^- secretion (**choice E**), but these effects are not diagnostic for gastrinoma.

18. **The correct answer is C.** This question requires you to know that bacterial infections are associated with an elevated neutrophil count. These leukocytes have 3-5 nuclear lobes and are filled with granules that contain bactericidal products, including lysozyme. Note that neutrophils normally constitute 54% to 62% of leukocytes, so if you were unsure of the percentages occurring in response to bacterial infections, **choice C** would still have been a good guess. Had the infection been viral, there would have been an increase in lymphocytes instead.

Histamine (**choice A**) is released by basophils and mast cells, along with other vasoactive amines (**choice E**). Slow-reacting substance of anaphylaxis, which consists of leukotrienes LTC4, LTD4, and LTE4 (**choice B**), is also released by these cells, which possess large spheroidal granules. Basophils and mast cells are basophilic (thus their name) and metachromatic, because of the presence of heparin, a glycosaminoglycan.

Eosinophils contain peroxidase (**choice D**). These white blood cells have a bilobed nucleus and possess acidophilic granules in their cytoplasm. They also contain hydrolytic enzymes. Note that an increased eosinophil count is associated with parasitic infections, allergies, asthma, and some neoplasms.

19. **The correct answer is B.** Normally, stretching of muscle results in a reflex contraction: the harder the stretch, the stronger the contraction. At a certain point, when the tension becomes too great, the contracting muscle suddenly relaxes. The reflex that underlies this sudden muscle relaxation is called the Golgi tendon organ (GTO) reflex, also known as the inverse stretch reflex or autogenic inhibition. The GTO is an extensive arborization of nerve endings (encapsulated by a connective tissue sheath and located near the muscle attachment) that is connected in series with the extrafusal skeletal muscle fibers. As a result, GTOs respond to muscle tension rather than muscle length. Increased tension leads to stimulation of Ib afferents, which inhibit the homonymous muscle via spinal interneurons.

Free nerve endings (**choice A**) are unmyelinated, unencapsulated nerve endings that penetrate the epidermis. These types of receptors respond to pain and temperature.

Merkel disks (**choice C**) are composed of specialized tactile epidermal cells and their associated nerve endings. They are located in the basal layer of the epithelium and are slowly adapting receptors that respond to touch and pressure.

Muscle spindles (**choice D**) are spindle-shaped bundles of muscle fibers (intrafusal fibers) that are encapsulated by connective tissue. Muscle spindles are arranged in parallel with extrafusal skeletal muscle fibers, so they sense the length of the muscle. They are innervated by Group Ia and II sensory afferent neurons.

Pacinian corpuscles (**choice E**) are unmyelinated nerve endings surrounded by thin, concentric layers of epithelioid fibroblasts. In transverse section, this receptor resembles a sliced onion. They are found primarily in the deep layer of the dermis, loose connective tissue, male and female genitalia, mesentery, and visceral ligaments. They are rapidly adapting receptors that respond to touch and pressure.

20. **The correct answer is A.** Gastric inhibitory peptide (GIP) is produced in the duodenal and jejunal mucosa by K cells and is released in response to intraluminal glucose and fatty acids. GIP is sometimes called "glucose-dependent insulinotropic" peptide because it stimulates pancreatic insulin secretion in the presence of hyperglycemia. Note that although GIP release would be stimulated, the hormone would not have a pronounced effect in this type 1 diabetic, whose pancreatic islet cells do not produce adequate amounts of insulin.

Gastrin (**choice B**) is synthesized and stored primarily in the G cells of the stomach and TG cells of the stomach and small intestine. The stimuli for gastrin secretion include increased vagal discharge, digestive products, calcium salts, and gastric distention. Gastrin stimulates HCl secretion by parietal cells, histamine release from enterochromaffin cells, pepsinogen secretion by chief cells, gastric blood flow, and contraction of gastric circular smooth muscle. It has a trophic effect on gastric and small-intestinal mucosa and the pancreas, increases lower esophageal sphincter (LES) tone, and is a weak stimulus for the secretion of pancreatic enzymes and bicarbonate.

Motilin (**choice C**) is produced in the M and enterochromaffin cells of the duodenum and jejunum. Secretion occurs during fasting. Motilin acts to regulate the migrating myoelectric complex (MMC).

Secretin (**choice D**) is synthesized and stored in the S cells of the mucosa of the upper intestine. Acidification of the duodenal mucosa and the presence of fat and protein degradation products in the duodenum stimulate its secretion. The main role of secretin is to stimulate bicarbonate secretion from the pancreas and liver.

Somatostatin (**choice E**) is synthesized and stored in the D cells of the pancreatic islets, in the gastric antrum, and throughout the intestine. It is also present in the hypothalamus. It inhibits the release of gastrin, cholecystokinin (CCK), and most other gastrointestinal hormones. In brief, it "shuts off" the gut. Somatostatin inhibits the release of glucagon by pancreatic alpha cells, as well as the release of insulin by the pancreatic beta cells (of the islets of Langerhans).

21. **The correct answer is E.** Glucagon is released from the alpha cells of the pancreas in response to hypoglycemia and stimulates glycogenolysis to increase serum glucose.

Augmented calcium deposition in bone (**choice A**) is achieved by calcitonin, which is secreted by the C-cells in the thyroid gland. Glucagon plays no role in calcium metabolism.

Glucagon favors the conversion of amino acids to glucose (gluconeogenesis) rather than their storage in the liver (**choice B**).

Insulin (which generally has opposite effects of glucagon) promotes lipogenesis in the liver and in adipose tissue (**choice C**).

Glucagon stimulates gluconeogenesis (**choice D**).

22. **The correct answer is D.** Ascites often occurs in patients with cirrhosis and other forms of severe liver disease and is usually noticed by the patient because of abdominal swelling. Shortness of breath may occur because the diaphragm is elevated when the accumulation of fluid becomes more pronounced. A number of factors contribute to accumulation of fluid in the abdominal cavity. Portal hypertension plays an important role in the production of ascites by raising capillary hydrostatic pressure within the splanchnic bed.

Elevated serum levels of epinephrine and norepinephrine (compare with **choice A**), resulting from increased central sympathetic outflow, is found in patients with cirrhosis and ascites.

The increased sympathetic output leads to decreased natriuresis (compare with **choice E**) by activation of the renin-angiotensin system and diminished sensitivity to atrial natriuretic peptide.

Interstitial fluid often weeps freely from the surface of the cirrhotic liver because of distortion and obstruction of hepatic lymphatics (compare with **choice C**). This interstitial fluid has a high protein concentration because the endothelial lining of the hepatic sinusoids is discontinuous. The entry of protein-rich interstitial fluid into the peritoneal cavity may account for the high protein concentration present in the ascitic fluid of some patients.

23. **The correct answer is A.** Achalasia is a disorder of esophageal motility that affects the lower esophageal sphincter (LES) and lower two-thirds of the esophageal body. The LES remains tonically contracted and does not relax as food moves down the esophagus. Therefore, food cannot move easily from the esophagus into the stomach. The distal esophagus often becomes greatly dilated. Patients with achalasia most commonly complain of dysphagia (difficulty swallowing), chest pain, and regurgitation.

    During swallowing, the bolus of food is propelled through the pharynx (**choice D**) by peristaltic contractions.

    These contractions, along with relaxation of the upper esophageal sphincter (**choice E**), propel the bolus of food into the esophagus. Relaxation of the upper esophageal sphincter occurs normally in patients with achalasia.

    The middle and lower esophagus (**choices B and C**) propel the bolus toward the stomach by coordinated contractions of the muscle layers.

24. **The correct answer is C.** Because substance X is filtered, but not secreted or reabsorbed (like inulin), the clearance of substance X can be used to approximate GFR.

    GFR = $[U]_X \times V / [P]_X$, therefore,

    GFR = (10 mg/mL) × (60 mL/hour) / (0.1 mg/mL)

    = (10 mg/mL) × (1 mL/min) / (0.1 mg/mL)

    = 100 mL/min

    Note that you need to convert 60 mL/hour to 1 mL/min to get the correct answer in the correct units. Checking to make sure the units are correct will help make sure you are using the formula properly.

25. **The correct answer is B.** At less than saturating concentrations, PAH is completely secreted into the proximal tubule and excreted into the urine. Therefore, the volume of plasma cleared of PAH is approximately equal to the volume of plasma flowing through the peritubular capillaries, also called the effective renal plasma flow, or ERPF.

$$\text{ERPF} = \frac{U_{PAH} \times V}{P_{PAH}}$$

The ECF volume (**choice A**) can be calculated by measuring the volume of distribution of solutes that move freely across capillary walls but cannot permeate cell membranes (e.g., inulin and mannitol).

GFR (**choice C**) is best calculated using a substance that is freely filtered at the glomerulus, not reabsorbed, and only minimally secreted into the urine. Creatinine fits the bill and is used clinically to measure the GFR (inulin also works and is used experimentally). Whereas the creatinine excretion exceeds filtration by 10% to 20% (because of the secretion), creatinine clearance is still a good approximation for GFR because the error due to secretion is balanced by an overestimation of plasma creatinine inherent in the measurement technique.

$$\text{GRF} = \frac{U_{creatine} \times V}{P_{creatine}}$$

The plasma volume (**choice D**) can be measured by measuring the volume of distribution of radioactively labeled serum albumin or of Evans blue dye (binds to albumin).

Total body water (TBW; **choice E**) can be measured by measuring the volume of distribution of tritium, deuterium, or antipyrine.

26. **The correct answer is A.** Sawtooth waves appearing in bursts are associated with REM sleep.

    Stage 1 (**choice B**) is associated with 4-7-Hz theta waves.

    Stage 2 (**choice C**) is associated with 12-14-Hz sleep spindles and K-complexes.

    Stage 3 (**choice D**) is associated with <4-Hz, high-amplitude delta waves.

    Stage 4 (**choice E**) is characterized by an EEG composed of about 50% delta waves.

    Note that beta waves (15-18 Hz) occur during periods of more intense mental activity while awake. Alpha waves (8-12 Hz) occur during awake, relaxed states. REM is the stage of sleep that most resembles the awake state on the EEG.

27. **The correct answer is C.** This is a classic presentation of carpal tunnel syndrome, which typically affects women between the ages of 40 and 60 who chronically perform repetitive tasks that involve movement of the structures that pass through the carpal tunnel. One important structure that passes through the carpal tunnel is the median nerve. Patients often note tingling, loss of sensation, or diminished sensation in the digits. There is also often a loss of coordination and strength in the thumb, because the median nerve also sends fibers to the abductor pollicis brevis, flexor pollicis brevis, and

the opponens pollicis. A final function of the median nerve distal to the carpal tunnel is control of the first and second lumbricals, which function to flex digits two and three at the metacarpophalangeal joints and extend interphalangeal joints of the same digits.

Abduction of the fifth digit (**choice A**) is a function controlled by the ulnar nerve, which does not pass through the carpal tunnel.

Adduction of the thumb (**choice B**) is a function of the adductor pollicis, which is the only short thumb muscle that is not innervated by the median nerve, but rather by the deep branch of the ulnar nerve.

Sensation of the lateral half of the dorsum of the hand (**choice D**) is mediated by the radial nerve, which also does not pass through the carpal tunnel.

Sensation over the lateral aspect of the palm (**choice E**) is mediated by the median nerve; however, the branch innervating the palm (palmar cutaneous branch of the median nerve) passes superficially to the carpal tunnel.

28. **The correct answer is E.** The parietal cells of the stomach produce intrinsic factor, a glycoprotein that binds vitamin B_{12} in the lumen of the stomach and facilitates its absorption in the terminal ileum. Patients without a stomach and those with pernicious anemia (autoimmune destruction of parietal cells) require B_{12} replacement therapy. Recall that B_{12} deficiency will lead to megaloblastic anemia and the COMLEX-favorite picture of a blood smear with hypersegmented neutrophils. Note that parietal cells also synthesize and secrete HCl.

Chief cells (**choice A**) are responsible for secreting pepsinogen, the precursor to pepsin.

G cells (**choice B**) secrete gastrin, which stimulates secretion of acid by the parietal cells found in the body and fundus of the stomach. Zollinger-Ellison syndrome is caused by a pancreatic or duodenal tumor that secretes gastrin (a gastrinoma). It is characterized by the development of severe peptic ulcer disease.

Goblet cells (**choice C**) are part of the mucosa of the small intestine, not the stomach. They produce glycoproteins (mucins) that protect and lubricate the lining of the intestine.

Mucous neck cells (**choice D**) secrete mucus and are located in the necks of the gastric glands.

29. **The correct answer is B.** Total body water (TBW) in liters equals approximately 60% of body weight in kilograms and therefore equals 45 L in a 75-kg person. Intracellular volume = 2/3 of TBW and is therefore 30 L in this case. Extracellular volume = 1/3 of TBW and is therefore 15 L in this case.

Choices A, C, D, and E do not satisfy these conditions.

30. **The correct answer is D.** This patient appears to be experiencing *mittelschmerz*, abdominal pain occurring at the time of ovulation that can mimic acute appendicitis (which is ruled out because of the patient's surgical history). If this information did not clue you into the stage of the menstrual cycle, you are told explicitly that the patient's last menstrual period was 14 days ago. Therefore, she is at the conclusion of the proliferative (estrogenic) phase. This stage begins during the latter period of menstrual flow and continues through the 13th-14th day of a typical 28-day cycle; it is characterized by regrowth of the endometrium. The epithelial cells of the glandular structures remaining after menstruation migrate and proliferate to cover the new mucosal surface. Also, the spiral arteries grow into the regenerating endometrium (this process continues through the secretory stage as well). Significant edema develops by the end of the proliferative stage and continues to develop during the secretory phase.

Apical movement of secretions in the glandular cells (**choice A**) occurs during the secretory phase.

Degeneration of the glandular structures (**choice B**) occurs during the premenstrual stage of the cycle.

Glandular glycogen accumulation in the functionalis (**choice C**) occurs during the secretory phase.

Tissue expansion by cellular hypertrophy (**choice E**) occurs during the secretory phase since mitosis of the endometrial tissue has ceased at this point.

31. **The correct answer is C.** On the left side of the body, the lymphatic fluid flows from the lymphatic capillaries, to the thin lymphatic vessels, and then to the thoracic duct, which empties into the junction of the left internal jugular and left subclavian veins. On the right side, lymphatic fluid flows from the lymphatic capillaries to the thin lymphatic vessels, to the right thoracic duct, which empties into the junction of the right internal jugular and the right subclavian veins.

32. **The correct answer is C.** Lithium inhibits the action of antidiuretic hormone (ADH; vasopressin) on the V2 receptors in the collecting duct that regulate the permeability to water. Therefore, lithium administration will decrease water permeability in the collecting duct, which will increase urine flow rate and decrease urine osmolarity. Since ADH has minimal effects on sodium reabsorption in humans, the fractional clearance of sodium and the osmolar clearance are unaffected. (Osmolar clearance refers to the clearance of all particles, including sodium and anions, from the plasma per minute.)

Furosemide (**choice A**) inhibits the active reabsorption of sodium, potassium, and chloride in the thick ascending limb. This will deplete the medullary gradient, which could result in a slightly hypotonic urine, but furosemide will significantly increase the fractional clearance of sodium and hence the osmolar clearance.

Hydrochlorothiazide (**choice B**) inhibits the active reabsorption of sodium chloride from the distal convoluted tubule. Since the distal tubule is in the renal cortex, it will not inhibit the ability of the kidney to concentrate urine and therefore will not decrease the urine osmolarity so dramatically. It will also increase the fractional clearance of sodium, and hence the osmolar clearance, but not as much as with furosemide.

High dietary intake of potassium (**choice D**) will increase plasma potassium levels, which will increase aldosterone secretion by direct action on the adrenal cortical cells. The aldosterone will decrease fractional clearance of sodium and will not increase urine flow rate.

Increased isotonic plasma volume (**choice E**) will increase atrial natriuretic factor (ANF), which will inhibit sodium reabsorption in the nephron and thus increase the fractional clearance of sodium as well as osmolar clearance.

33. **The correct answer is C.** This is a really simple definition question: What is the difference between serum and plasma? Essentially, serum is derived from plasma by the extraction of fibrinogen and coagulation factors II, V, and VIII. This can be achieved by allowing whole blood to clot, then removing the clot.

Albumin (**choice A**) is present in both serum and plasma.

Neither erythrocytes (**choice B**) nor granulocytes (**choice D**) are present in either serum or plasma.

Serotonin (**choice E**) levels may be increased in serum because of the platelet breakdown that occurs during the extraction process. Serotonin is normally found in the highest concentration in platelets, as well as in the enterochromaffin cells and myenteric plexus of the gastrointestinal tract. The brain and the retina contain smaller amounts.

34. **The correct answer is B.** Pressure in the left atrium can be approximated by wedging an arterial catheter into a small branch of the pulmonary artery. Remember that the pulmonary vascular tree abuts the left atrium anatomically. The pulmonary artery carries deoxygenated blood from the right ventricle into the pulmonary circulation, where it is oxygenated and then returned to the left atrium via the pulmonary veins.

Aortic (**choice A**) pressure is usually five times greater than pulmonary artery pressure.

Left ventricular (**choice C**) pressure is usually about six times greater than right ventricular pressure.

Right atrial (**choice D**) and systemic venous (**choice E**) pressures can be estimated on the basis of central venous pressure (CVP), which is the pressure present in the great veins as they enter the right atrium. CVP is measured by placing a catheter into the thoracic great veins.

35. **The correct answer is C.** This question requires use of the alveolar ventilation equation:

$$PA_{CO_2} = \frac{\dot{V}CO_2}{\dot{V}_A}, \text{ where}$$

PA_{CO_2} = is the partial pressure of alveolar CO_2

$\dot{V}CO_2$ is CO_2 production

$\dot{V}A$ is alveolar ventilation

If $\dot{V}CO_2$ remains constant and alveolar ventilation doubles, PA_{CO_2} must decrease to half its original value. Therefore, PA_{CO_2} equals 20 mm Hg after hyperventilation.

Memorizing the formula is not necessary if you think about this intuitively: If CO_2 production remains constant and alveolar ventilation doubles, the partial pressure of alveolar CO_2 must decrease to half its original value and would therefore equal 20 mm Hg after hyperventilation.

36. **The correct answer is E.** The maximum expiratory flow-volume (MEFV) curve is created when the patient inhales as much air as possible and then expires with maximal effort until no more air can be expired. The amount of air that remains in the lungs after maximal expiration is the residual volume, and is depicted by point E. Note that the absolute value of the residual volume cannot be determined from a MEFV curve alone. Additional studies, such as helium dilution, are needed to determine the absolute value.

Choice A is the lung volume at the total lung capacity; however, absolute lung volumes cannot be determined from a MEFV curve without additional methods. The other points on the curve correspond to the following:

At **choice B**, the patient has just begun to exhale with a maximal effort at this point.

At **choice C**, the patient is exhaling with a maximal effort and the rate of air flow has reached its maximal value of nearly 400 L/minute at this high lung volume.

The descending portion of the curve (**choice D**) represents the maximum expiratory flow at each lung volume along the curve. This portion of the curve is sometimes referred to as the "effort-independent" portion of the curve because the patient cannot increase expiratory flow rate further by expending greater effort.

37. **The correct answer is A.** This woman has a risk profile (female, fat, forties) and symptomatology consistent with gallstones (cholelithiasis). As would be expected, contraction of the gallbladder following a fatty meal often exacerbates the pain caused by gallstones. Cholecystokinin (CCK) is the hormone responsible for stimulation of gallbladder contraction; the release of CCK is stimulated by dietary fat. It is produced in I cells of the duodenum and jejunum. In addition to gallbladder contraction, CCK also stimulates pancreatic enzyme secretion and decreases the rate of gastric emptying.

Gastrin (**choice B**) is produced by the G cells of the antrum and duodenum. Gastrin stimulates the secretion of HCl from the parietal cells and pepsinogen from the chief cells of the stomach. Gastrin secretion is stimulated by gastric distention, digestive products (e.g., amino acids), and vagal discharge.

Pepsin (**choice C**) is a protease produced by the chief cells of the stomach (as pepsinogen). It is involved in the digestion of proteins. Pepsinogen release is stimulated by vagal stimulation, gastrin, local acid production, secretin, CCK, and histamine.

Secretin (**choice D**) is produced by the S cells of the duodenum. It is secreted primarily in response to acidification of the duodenal mucosa. Secretin stimulates the secretion of bicarbonate-containing fluid from the pancreas and biliary ducts. This neutralization allows pancreatic enzymes to function. Secretin also inhibits gastric acid production and gastric emptying.

Somatostatin (**choice E**) is produced by the D cells of the pancreatic islets and in the gastric and intestinal mucosa. Somatostatin is an inhibitory hormone; it inhibits most gastrointestinal hormones, gallbladder contraction, gastric acid and pepsinogen secretion, pancreatic and small intestinal fluid secretion, and both glucagon and insulin release.

38. **The correct answer is B.** Renal blood flow = (renal artery pressure – renal vein pressure)/renal vascular resistance (RVR). Therefore, if RVR is decreased to half its original value, with no pressure changes, renal blood flow must double (not increase 50%). Increased blood flow to the kidney increases renal oxygen use by increasing glomerular filtration rate, which increases the filtered load of sodium and other solutes. Since active sodium reabsorption is load-dependent, increased tubular fluid sodium increases all active sodium reabsorption, which requires more ATP hydrolysis and synthesis (and hence more oxygen use). Renal artery oxygen concentration does not change, since it is dependent on normal lung function, not oxygen extraction by the kidney.

39. **The correct answer is C.** All of the choices listed are reactions that occur in the synthetic pathway from cholesterol to cortisol. ACTH stimulates the first reaction in the pathway: cholesterol to pregnenolone. This reaction is catalyzed by the enzyme cholesterol desmolase.

The next step in the pathway is pregnenolone to progesterone (**choice D**); progesterone is then converted to 17-hydroxyprogesterone (**choice E**); 17-hydroxyprogesterone is converted to 11-deoxycortisol (**choice B**) by the enzyme 21 beta-hydroxylase; and the 11-deoxycortisol is then converted to cortisol (**choice A**).

40. **The correct answer is E.** The sequence of the auditory pathway is as follows: Organ of Corti → spiral ganglion in the cochlea → vestibulocochlear nerve (CN VIII) → cochlear nuclei (dorsal and ventral) → superior olivary nuclei → lateral lemniscus → inferior colliculus → medial geniculate nucleus of the thalamus (MGN) → primary auditory cortex (Heschl's gyrus).

Each ear projects to both sides of the brainstem and cortex via multiple commissures, including the trapezoid body (which contains fibers crossing contralateral to the superior olivary nucleus), the commissure of the inferior colliculus (connecting the right and left inferior colliculi), and another commissure that connects the right and left nuclei of the lateral lemniscus. Therefore, a lesion of any structure up until the superior olivary nuclei will produce an ipsilateral deafness. The only structure listed that is proximal to the superior olivary nuclei is the organ of Corti (**choice E**).

The inferior colliculus (**choice A**), the lateral lemniscus (**choice B**), and the medial geniculate body (**choice C**) all receive information from both ears, and unilateral hearing loss could not result from a lesion of any of these structures.

The medial lemniscus (**choice D**) is not a part of the auditory system. It is part of the somatosensory system, which conveys proprioception, discriminative touch, and vibration information. More specifically, neurons of the gracile and cuneate nuclei send projections that decussate as the internal arcuate fibers and ascend as the medial lemniscus to synapse in the ventroposterolateral nucleus (VPL) of the thalamus.

41. **The correct answer is E.** Enteropeptidase, formerly called enterokinase, activates trypsinogen by limited proteolytic digestion to give trypsin. Trypsin is itself capable of activating trypsinogen, which produces a positive feedback effect. Trypsin also activates chymotrypsinogen (and several other proteolytic enzymes), so deficiency of enteropeptidase results in a severe deficiency of enzymes that digest protein.

Amylase (**choice A**) aids in the breakdown of starches to oligosaccharides, maltose, and maltotriose.

Colipase (**choice B**), along with other lipases, functions to digest fats.

Lactase (**choice C**) is a brush-border disaccharidase that hydrolyzes the bond between galactose and glucose in lactose.

Pepsin (**choice D**) is a proteolytic enzyme secreted in an inactive form (pepsinogen) by the chief cells of the stomach. Pepsinogen is activated by stomach acid, and so is not dependent on enteropeptidase. Pepsin alone will not replace the activities of other proteolytic enzymes, partly because food does not remain in the stomach for an extended period of time.

42. **The correct answer is B.** Diagram P shows a normal heart with an end-diastolic volume (EDV) of 125 mL and an end-systolic volume (ESV) of 50 mL. Stroke volume (SV) can be calculated as EDV − ESV = 75 mL, and ejection fraction can be calculated as SV/EDV = 0.6. The untreated failing heart (diagram R) has an EDV of ~188 mL, an ESV of ~156, an SV of ~32 mL, and an ejection fraction of only ~0.17. Note also that the peak systolic pressure of the failing heart (95 mm Hg) is lower than that of the control heart (100 mm Hg). Treatment with digitalis (diagram Q) has increased the contractility of the myocardium. This increase in contractility has increased stroke volume to 45 mm Hg and ejection fraction to 0.26. Note also on diagram Q that the peak systolic pressure has returned to a normal value of 100 mm Hg and is better maintained throughout systole.

43. **The correct answer is C.** This question requires you to equate salt restriction with an increased synthesis of aldosterone (aldosterone promotes sodium reabsorption) and then to remember that aldosterone is produced in the zona glomerulosa of the adrenal cortex. The zona glomerulosa is the outermost layer of the adrenal cortex.

The adrenal medulla (**choice A**) secretes catecholamines.

The zona fasciculata (**choice B**) is the middle layer of the adrenal cortex. It primarily secretes glucocorticoids.

The zona reticularis (**choice D**) is the innermost layer of the adrenal cortex. It primarily secretes androgens such as dehydroepiandrosterone (DHEA).

Salt restriction causes increased activity in the zona glomerulosa of the adrenal cortex because of the increased synthesis; therefore, **choice E** is incorrect.

44. **The correct answer is E.** To calculate the direction and driving force for fluid movement, use the Starling equation [net filtration pressure = $(P_c - P_i) - (\pi_c - \pi_i)$]. The net pressure in this case is positive because fluid is being forced out of the capillary.

P_c = capillary hydrostatic pressure = 18, π_c = capillary colloid osmotic pressure = 25, and π_i = interstitial osmotic pressure = 9. Substituting these values into the equation and solving for P_i, we get:

8 mm Hg = (24 − 7) − (17 − π_i) mm Hg

π_i = 8 mm Hg

45. **The correct answer is E.** By the time of implantation, approximately 7 days after ovulation, the fertilized ovum has developed to the blastocyst stage. At this stage, the blastocyst typically contains 100 or more cells, which have differentiated into an inner cell mass (designed to become the embryo) and trophoblast (which surrounds both the outer edge of the inner cell mass and a large fluid-filled cavity). The blastocyst is able to burrow into the endometrium in less than 24 hours after touching the endometrial surface. During the next several days, a primitive placenta begins to develop that penetrates the maternal capillary bed and begins circulating maternal blood by about day 11.

46. **The correct answer is C.** Glycoprotein GPIb on the platelet membrane binds von Willebrand factor, a plasma protein that circulates in a complex with factor VIII.

ADP (**choice A**) is a powerful inducer of platelet aggregation and strengthens the platelet plug by the addition of more activated platelets.

Calcium (**choice B**) is essential for increasing the degree of platelet aggregation and for strengthening the platelet plug. It is also a necessary cofactor in the coagulation cascade [required for the conversion of factors IX to IXa, X to Xa, V to Va, and prothrombin (factor II) to thrombin (factor IIa)].

Platelet factor 3 (PF3; **choice D**) is involved in platelet plug formation.

Prostacyclin (**choice E**) is synthesized by blood vessel endothelial cells and inhibits platelet aggregation.

47. **The correct answer is C.** The decrease in blood pressure caused by hemorrhage activates the baroreceptor reflex, which tends to increase sympathetic nerve activity and decrease parasympathetic (vagal) nerve activity (**choice D**). The increase in sympathetic nerve activity constricts arterioles in skeletal muscle (**choice A**) and elsewhere in the body. The fact that the patient has lost 600 mL blood and yet her blood pressure has decreased only slightly from a normal value of about 120/80 mm Hg may be

attributed to the following compensatory responses: baroreceptor reflex, chemoreceptor reflex, epinephrine and norepinephrine released from the adrenal medulla, formation of angiotensin II, formation of vasopressin, and the capillary fluid shift mechanism.

Activation of the renin-angiotensin system during hemorrhage also plays an important role in maintaining blood pressure. Angiotensin II increases blood pressure acutely by constricting arterioles throughout the body (**choice A**), and chronically by decreasing the renal excretion of both salt (**choice B**) and water (**choice E**). The decrease in salt and water excretion returns blood volume to a normal value.

48. **The correct answer is B.** This question illustrates an important strategy: knowing what you're looking for before you consider the answer choices. If you thought about the answer before considering the choices, this question was very straightforward and simple. If, on the other hand, you considered each answer choice in turn, you no doubt got pretty confused and wasted a lot of precious test time.

The first thing to remember is that nephrotic syndrome is defined as proteinuria (>3.5 g/day) with concurrent hypoalbuminemia and hyperlipidemia. The loss of protein in the urine results in a decreased oncotic pressure in the vascular space (decreased π_c). This decrease in capillary oncotic pressure promotes movement of fluid into the interstitium and the development of edema. This is also the cause of edema in patients with liver disease.

Decreased interstitial oncotic pressure (π_i; **choice D**) would actually promote the movement of fluid into the vasculature; it would not lead to edema. The same thing would occur with decreased capillary hydrostatic forces (P_c; **choice A**).

Although decreased interstitial hydrostatic pressure (P_i; **choice C**) would lead to edema, it is not the mechanism of action in nephrotic syndrome.

Although increased capillary hydrostatic pressure (**choice E**) does lead to edema, it is not the mechanism at work in nephrotic syndrome. It is, however, the mechanism of edema in the setting of both congestive heart failure (increased capillary hydrostatic pressure due to inefficient pumping of the heart, leading to pooling) and glomerulonephritis (increased intravascular volume due to inefficient excretion by the kidney).

49. **The correct answer is D.** Neonatal respiratory distress syndrome is a disease of immaturity. The immature lung is not able to produce sufficient surfactant to prevent collapse of many alveoli. Severe diffuse damage to alveoli causes precipitation of protein ("hyaline membranes") adjacent to many alveolar walls. In infants who survive, particularly if oxygen was used for therapy, the lungs eventually become heavily fibrotic (misnamed bronchopulmonary dysplasia).

Abundant neutrophils (**choice A**) would not be seen unless the patient had also developed pneumonia.

Fibrosis (**choice B**) is a late, not early, feature of respiratory distress syndrome.

The air spaces are collapsed, not enlarged (**choice C**), in this condition.

The histology in these patients is usually markedly abnormal (**not choice E**).

50. **The correct answer is D.** The cellular edema observed during reversible cell injury is usually due to decreased ATP levels. In the presence of lower ATP levels, there is less activity of the Na^+/K^+ ATPase on the plasmalemma. This, in turn, leads to a shift of Na^+ into the cell and K^+ out of it. The pump does not normally transport the same amount of Na^+ out of and K^+ into the cell, so when the pump fails, there is a new flow of solute in the form of Na^+ into the cell. When this solute adds to the higher intracellular osmotic pressure relative to the extracellular osmotic pressure (due to all of the proteins and small molecules trapped in the cell), water flows into the cell to "dilute" its counterpart.

Ca^{2+} (**choice A**) and Mg^{2+} (**choice C**) do not play a direct role in cellular edema.

Both the Na^+/K^+ ATPase activity (**choice E**) and intracellular K^+ (**choice B**) are usually decreased during cellular edema.

Physiology

TEST 2

1. In a controlled experiment, radiolabeled ATP is injected into an isolated muscle. The muscle is stimulated and allowed to contract for 10 seconds. An autoradiogram from a biopsy of the muscle will show radiolabeled ATP bound to

   (A) actin
   (B) myosin
   (C) sarcoplasmic reticulum
   (D) tropomyosin
   (E) troponin C

2. A physician decides to conduct a neurochemical experiment to measure extracellular neurotransmitter levels in the brain following electrical stimulation of the raphe nuclei. Which of the following neurotransmitter levels would be expected to rise?

   (A) Acetylcholine
   (B) Dopamine
   (C) Gamma-amino-butyric acid (GABA)
   (D) Norepinephrine
   (E) Serotonin

3. A 60-year-old man with heart disease is brought to the emergency department. Physical examination reveals chronic somatic dysfunction at T1-T4. Cardiovascular evaluation reveals a resting O_2 consumption of 200 mL/min, a peripheral arterial O_2 content of 0.20 mL O_2/mL of blood, and a mixed venous O_2 content of 0.15 mL O_2/mL of blood. What is his cardiac output?

   (A) 2.5 L/min
   (B) 4 L/min
   (C) 10 L/min
   (D) 25 L/min
   (E) 100 L/min

4. Administration of an experimental drug that acts on peripheral nervous system (PNS) myelin is shown to increase the space constant of an axon in a peripheral nerve. Action potentials traveling down the axon would be predicted to be

   (A) faster
   (B) larger
   (C) slower
   (D) smaller
   (E) unchanged

5. A patient undergoes a total gastrectomy because of a proximally located gastric cancer. After the surgery, which of the following digestive enzymes will be produced in inadequate amounts?

    (A) Amylase

    (B) Chymotrypsin

    (C) Lipase

    (D) Pepsin

    (E) Trypsin

6. A patient has a bone-marrow biopsy to determine if he has leukemia. What is the normal myeloid to erythroid ratio in bone marrow?

    (A) 1:1

    (B) 1:3

    (C) 1:10

    (D) 3:1

    (E) 10:1

7. Which of the following characteristics is similar for spermatogenesis and oogenesis?

    (A) Age at which meiosis begins

    (B) Amount of cytoplasm retained

    (C) DNA replication during meiosis

    (D) Length of prophase I

    (E) Transmission to fetus of mitochondrial DNA

8. In a normal patient, which of the following is found in the respiratory zone of the lung?

    (A) Goblet cells

    (B) Main bronchi

    (C) Mucous cells

    (D) Terminal bronchioles

    (E) Type I epithelial cells

9. A 28-year-old man decides to donate a kidney to his brother, who is in chronic renal failure, after HLA typing suggests that he would be a suitable donor. He is admitted to the hospital, and his right kidney is removed and transplanted into his brother. Which of the following indices would be expected to be decreased in the donor after full recovery from the operation?

    (A) Creatinine clearance

    (B) Creatinine production

    (C) Daily excretion of sodium

    (D) Plasma creatinine concentration

    (E) Renal excretion of creatinine

10. In a normal patient, release of which of the following peptides leads to an increase in the secretion of pancreatic enzymes into the small intestine?

    (A) Cholecystokinin

    (B) Gastrin

    (C) Motilin

    (D) Secretin

    (E) Somatostatin

11. In a normal patient, which of the following directly inhibits insulin secretion?

    (A) Alpha$_2$-adrenergic agonist

    (B) Beta$_2$-adrenergic agonist

    (C) Cholecystokinin

    (D) Glucagon

    (E) Ingestion of a high-sugar meal

12. A patient placed on a ventilator in the intensive care unit has an anatomic dead space of 150 mL. If the ventilator has a dead space of 350 mL and a rate of 20/min, which tidal volume should be selected for the ventilator to provide an alveolar ventilation of 6 L/min?

    (A) 1200 mL

    (B) 1000 mL

    (C) 800 mL

    (D) 600 mL

    (E) 400 mL

13. A 55-year-old woman stopped menstruating approximately 3 months ago. Worried that she may be pregnant, she decides to have a pregnancy test. The result is negative. Which of the following series of test results will confirm that the woman is postmenopausal?

    (A) Decreased LH, decreased FSH, increased estrogen
    (B) Decreased LH, increased FSH, decreased estrogen
    (C) Increased LH, decreased FSH, decreased estrogen
    (D) Increased LH, increased FSH, decreased estrogen
    (E) Increased LH, increased FSH, increased estrogen

14. A child falls and bumps her head on the floor. Tissue factor is exposed beneath the endothelium of traumatized blood vessels. Which of the following procoagulant proteins binds to tissue factor and initiates the clotting cascade?

    (A) Factor V
    (B) Factor VII
    (C) Factor X
    (D) Fibrinogen
    (E) Prothrombin

15. A 63-year-old man with essential hypertension has gone several weeks without taking his medications. He arrives at the emergency department after falling on his outstretched right hand. He has a heart rate of 90 min and a blood pressure of 170/115 mm Hg. His structural examination reveals chronic tissue changes at T1-T4 and some erythmatous, swollen tissue around his right wrist. Which of the following is most likely to be decreased in the skeletal muscles of his legs?

    (A) Adenosine levels
    (B) Arterial blood pressure
    (C) Arteriolar resistance
    (D) Blood flow
    (E) Venous oxygen concentration

16. A man with normal lungs overdoses on secobarbital, causing hypoventilation. He is brought to a hospital where the barometric pressure is 500 mm Hg. Alveolar PCO_2 rises to 80 mm Hg, and the respiratory exchange ratio is 1.0. Assuming that the patient's condition remains unchanged, what percentage of inspired O_2 will return his alveolar P_{O_2} to normal (100 mm Hg)?

    (A) 55
    (B) 40
    (C) 36
    (D) 28
    (E) 24

17. In the clotting process, as the hemostatic plug develops, fibrin polymerizes into monomeric threads that are held together by noncovalent bonds. Which clotting protein increases the strength of the clot by cross-linking the newly formed fibrin threads?

    (A) Factor XIII
    (B) High molecular weight kininogen (HMWK)
    (C) Plasminogen
    (D) Thrombin
    (E) von Willebrand Factor (vWF)

18. Under normal conditions, the main drive for respiration is the

    (A) arterial P_{CO_2} acting through central chemoreceptors
    (B) arterial P_{CO_2} acting through peripheral chemoreceptors
    (C) arterial pH acting through central chemoreceptors
    (D) arterial pH acting through peripheral chemoreceptors
    (E) arterial P_{O_2} acting through central chemoreceptors

19. A construction worker has a serious accident in which his rib cage and abdominal muscles become completely paralyzed. He is still able to breathe, however, because his diaphragm continues to contract. At which level might his spinal cord injury have occurred?

    (A) C2
    (B) C7
    (C) L3
    (D) T5
    (E) T12

20. A 49-year-old mildly obese man with no history of heart disease is prescribed a diet and aerobic exercise regimen. Which of the following is most important for maintaining adequate cardiac output during exercise?

    (A) Decreased cardiac index
    (B) Decreased diastolic blood pressure
    (C) Increased heart rate and stroke volume
    (D) Increased systemic vascular resistance
    (E) Increased somatic dysfunction

21. A woodworker operating a bandsaw accidently injures his wrist, severing his radial artery and producing severe hemorrhage. As he loses blood, his body tries to compensate for the developing hypotension by increasing sympathetic outflow. The postganglionic signals carrying the impulses to constrict his arterioles are transmitted along which of the following fiber types?

    (A) A-δ fibers
    (B) B fibers
    (C) C fibers
    (D) Ia fibers
    (E) Ib fibers

22. In a normal, relaxed patient, which of the following regulates the frequency of gastrointestinal slow waves?

    (A) Circadian rhythms
    (B) Dietary intake of fiber
    (C) Intrinsic pacemaker regions within the smooth muscle
    (D) Local levels of cholecystokinin secretion
    (E) Systemic levels of catecholamines and corticosteroids

23. A 1-week-old infant has a coarctation of the aorta just distal to the subclavian arteries. The blood pressure distal to the constriction is 50% lower than normal. Which of the following is increased in this infant?

    (A) Blood flow in the lower body
    (B) Glomerular filtration rate
    (C) Plasma levels of angiotensin II
    (D) Renal excretion of sodium
    (E) Renal excretion of water

24. A 65-year-old woman receives 3 liters of 0.9% saline following a minor surgical procedure. This results in increased right atrial filling and contraction, as well as activation of type B baroreceptors. Which of the following is most likely to be secreted in response?

    (A) Aldosterone
    (B) Antidiuretic hormone (ADH)
    (C) Atrial natriuretic factor (ANF)
    (D) Norepinephrine
    (E) Renin

25. In a patient with no history of kidney disease, which of the following regions of the nephron is capable of the greatest level of sodium reabsorption?

    (A) Collecting duct
    (B) Distal convoluted tubule
    (C) Proximal convoluted tubule
    (D) Thick ascending limb of the loop of Henle
    (E) Descending limb of the loop of Henle

26. The second heart sound corresponds to which of the following points on an atrial pressure tracing?

    (A) a wave
    (B) c wave
    (C) v wave
    (D) x descent
    (E) y descent

27. A 65-year-old woman with renal failure presents for hemodialysis. Her physical examination is significant for long-standing somatic dysfunction at T11-L1. She is found to be anemic and is given a dose of erythropoietin along with her usual vitamin and mineral supplements. Erythropoietin stimulates which of the following intermediates in hematopoiesis?

    (A) Basophilic erythroblasts

    (B) Colony forming units-erythroid (CFU-E)

    (C) Multipotential stem cells

    (D) Proerythroblasts

    (E) Reticulocytes

28. After an accident at work resulting in severe hemorrhage, a machinist is rushed to the emergency department. Which of the following sets of autonomic responses would be predicted in this patient?

	Heart rate	Bowel sounds	Pupil diameter
(A)	Decreased	Decreased	Dilated
(B)	Decreased	Increased	Constricted
(C)	Decreased	Increased	Dilated
(D)	Increased	Decreased	Constricted
(E)	Increased	Decreased	Dilated

29. In a tissue capillary, the interstitial hydrostatic pressure is 2 mm Hg, the capillary hydrostatic pressure is 25 mm Hg, and the interstitial oncotic pressure is 7 mm Hg. If the net driving force across the capillary wall is 3 mm Hg favoring filtration, what is the capillary oncotic pressure?

    (A) 21 mm Hg

    (B) 23 mm Hg

    (C) 24 mm Hg

    (D) 25 mm Hg

    (E) 27 mm Hg

30. A medical student volunteers to have his lung volumes and capacities measured for his organ physiology laboratory class. He is connected to a spirometer containing a known concentration of helium. He is instructed to breathe several times until the helium has equilibrated between the spirometer and his lungs. He is then instructed to inhale and then to passively exhale. Calculations are made to determine the amount of air remaining in his lungs, which is called the

    (A) expiratory reserve volume

    (B) functional residual capacity

    (C) inspiratory capacity

    (D) inspiratory reserve volume

    (E) residual volume

31. A 78-year-old woman has a mean arterial pressure of 120 mm Hg and a heart rate of 60/min. She has a stroke volume of 50 mL, cardiac output of 3000 mL/min, and a right atrial pressure of 0 mm Hg. What is the total peripheral resistance (in mm Hg/mL/min) in this woman?

    (A) 0.01

    (B) 0.02

    (C) 0.04

    (D) 0.08

    (E) 0.10

32. A 23-year-old man with diabetes mellitus has a glomerular filtration rate (GFR) significantly greater that normal, especially when he consumes excessive amounts of sweets. A decrease in which of the following parameters would tend to increase the glomerular capillary hydrostatic pressure?

    (A) Afferent arteriolar resistance

    (B) Bowman's capsular hydrostatic pressure

    (C) Capillary filtration coefficient

    (D) Efferent arteriolar resistance

    (E) Plasma colloid osmotic pressure

33. Which of the following gastrointestinal hormones is structurally related to secretin?

    (A) Cholecystokinin

    (B) Gastrin

    (C) Glucagon

    (D) Somatostatin

    (E) Substance P

34. With time, blood stored in a blood bank tends to become relatively depleted of 2,3-diphosphoglycerate (2,3-DPG). What effect does this have on the hemoglobin-oxygen dissociation curve?

    (A) Shifts the curve to the left, so that the hemoglobin has a decreased oxygen affinity

    (B) Shifts the curve to the left, so that the hemoglobin has an increased oxygen affinity

    (C) Shifts the curve to the right, so that the hemoglobin has a decreased oxygen affinity

    (D) Shifts the curve to the right, so that the hemoglobin has an increased oxygen affinity

    (E) Does not change the dissociation curve

35. During spermatogenesis, crossing over occurs during the meiotic division of which of the following cells?

    (A) Primary spermatocytes

    (B) Secondary spermatocytes

    (C) Spermatids

    (D) Spermatogonia

    (E) Spermatozoa

36. The cyclic secretion pattern of which of the following hormones is represented by the dotted line in the figure below?

    (A) Estrogen

    (B) Follicle-stimulating hormone (FSH)

    (C) Gonadotropin-releasing hormone (GnRH)

    (D) Luteinizing hormone (LH)

    (E) Progesterone

37. A 66-year-old woman complains of fatigue to her physician. Her pulse is 80/min and her hematocrit is 32%. Ultrasound shows an end-systolic volume of 65 mL and an end-diastolic volume of 115 mL. Which of the following is the ejection fraction in this woman?

    (A) 0.29

    (B) 0.32

    (C) 0.43

    (D) 0.51

    (E) 0.62

38. Under normal conditions virtually 100% of the filtered load of glucose is reabsorbed by the kidney tubules. Which part of the tubule shown below is expected to have the highest concentration of glucose under normal conditions (letters represent answer choices)?

39. Which of the following conditions is associated with a lifelong requirement for administration of parenteral vitamin B_{12}?

  I. Pernicious anemia
  II. Removal of colon
  III. Removal of gallbladder
  IV. Removal of ileum
  V. Removal of jejunum
  VI. Removal of stomach

 (A) I only
 (B) I and V
 (C) I, IV, and V
 (D) I, IV, and VI
 (E) I, V, and VI

40. A 42-year-old man develops acute renal failure. Physical examination is notable for warm, swollen tissue at T11-L1. Laboratory studies also reveal hypocalcemia. What is the most likely mechanism underlying this electrolyte disturbance?

 (A) Hyperphosphatemia
 (B) Hyponatremia
 (C) Increased sensitivity to 1,25-dihydroxyvitamin D
 (D) Increased sensitivity to parathyroid hormone (PTH)
 (E) Metabolic alkalosis

41. A patient with lung cancer has one lung removed. When he is at rest, his pulmonary artery pressure is within normal limits. However, when he tries to exercise, the pulmonary artery pressure rises rapidly. Which of the following best explains this finding?

 (A) The airway resistance of the lung is limiting during exercise
 (B) The compliance of the lung limits blood flow
 (C) Pulmonary vessels constrict during exercise
 (D) Recruitment of additional pulmonary vessels is not adequate during exercise
 (E) The volume of the single lung is inadequate during exercise

42. A heroin addict is found unconscious in an alley with an empty syringe beside him. When his blood gases are checked, which of the following would be expected?

 (A) Metabolic acidosis
 (B) Metabolic alkalosis
 (C) Normal pH balance
 (D) Respiratory acidosis
 (E) Respiratory alkalosis

43. A 55-year-old man develops a deep venous thrombosis that dislodges and travels to the left lung, completely blocking a branch of the left pulmonary artery. Physical examination reveals acute somatic dysfunction at T2-T8 on the left side. Which of the following is true about the partial pressure of oxygen in that area of the lung?

    (A) It is equal to arterial blood PO_2

    (B) It is equal to atmospheric pressure PO_2

    (C) It is equal to inspired PO_2

    (D) It is equal to mixed venous blood PO_2

    (E) It is less than mixed venous blood PO_2

44. A 19-year-old man is rushed to the emergency department after being shot in the chest. He has lost a great deal of blood and appears very pale. His skin is cool and clammy, and his mental status is altered. On exam he is tachycardic and tachypneic, and the jugular veins are collapsed. Urinary output is minimal. Which of the following is most consistent with the patient's condition?

	Preload	Cardiac Output	Vascular Resistance	Mixed Venous O_2
(A)	↑	↑	↑	↓
(B)	↑	↓	↓	↑
(C)	↓	↓	↑	↓
(D)	↓	↓	↓	↑
(E)	↓	↓	↓	↓

45. Which of the following clinical observations is directly related to the increase in compliance seen in patients with emphysema?

    (A) Barrel chest

    (B) Chronic cough

    (C) Excessive mucus production

    (D) Long, slow, deep breathing pattern

    (E) Pink face

46. Biopsy of the lung from a patient with chronic lung disease demonstrates a honeycomb appearance on gross inspection and fibrosis with inflammation of the alveolar walls on microscopic examination. The patient's blood gas studies are within normal limits. If spirometry were performed on this patient, which of the following would most likely be seen?

    (A) Decreased airway resistance

    (B) Decreased compliance

    (C) Increased functional residual capacity (FRC)

    (D) Increased lung volume

    (E) Increased tidal volume

47. In a patient who has a history of recurrent deep-vein thrombosis, deficiency of which of the following factors usually predisposes to thrombosis rather than bleeding?

    (A) V

    (B) VIII

    (C) IX

    (D) X

    (E) XII

48. The osmotic fragility test would be most useful for the diagnosis of which of the following disorders?

    (A) Alpha thalassemia minor

    (B) Beta thalassemia major

    (C) Hereditary spherocytosis

    (D) Sickle cell anemia

    (E) Sickle cell trait

49. In a healthy patient's heart ventricular depolarization is due to a sodium influx through which of the following?

    (A) Voltage-gated calcium channels

    (B) Slow channels

    (C) Slow calcium-sodium channels

    (D) Fast channels

    (E) Voltage-gated potassium channels

50. Carotid sinus massage is performed on a patient with a stable narrow-complex supraventricular tachycardia. Which of the following physiologic reflex changes is occurring as a result of this maneuver?

    (A) A decrease in afferent activity to the medulla

    (B) An increase in blood pressure

    (C) An increase in heart rate

    (D) An increase in sympathetic activity to the heart

    (E) An increase in parasympathetic activity to the heart

Physiology

ANSWERS AND EXPLANATIONS

1.	B	26.	C	
2.	E	27.	B	
3.	B	28.	E	
4.	A	29.	E	
5.	D	30.	B	
6.	D	31.	C	
7.	C	32.	A	
8.	E	33.	C	
9.	A	34.	B	
10.	A	35.	A	
11.	A	36.	A	
12.	C	37.	C	
13.	D	38.	A	
14.	B	39.	D	
15.	A	40.	A	
16.	B	41.	D	
17.	A	42.	D	
18.	A	43.	C	
19.	B	44.	C	
20.	C	45.	A	
21.	C	46.	B	
22.	C	47.	E	
23.	C	48.	C	
24.	C	49.	D	
25.	C	50.	E	

1. **The correct answer is B**. During the contraction cycle, ATP binds to myosin, causing the dissociation of myosin from actin.

   Actin (**choice A**) forms cross-bridges with myosin but does not bind to ATP.

   The sarcoplasmic reticulum (**choice C**) is involved in storing and releasing Ca^{2+} for muscle contraction.

   Tropomyosin (**choice D**) is a thin filament that runs alongside actin. In the absence of calcium, tropomyosin lies in the groove of the actin filament and blocks actin's myosin-binding sites.

   Troponin C (**choice E**) is the calcium-binding subunit of the troponin complex. When troponin C binds calcium, a conformational change causes tropomyosin to shift, thereby exposing the myosin-binding sites on actin.

2. **The correct answer is E.** Serotonin is the primary neurotransmitter of the raphe nuclei. Ascending serotonin projections from the dorsal and median raphe nuclei distribute diffusely throughout the brain. Other raphe nuclei provide descending serotonin projections to the spinal cord and brainstem.

   Cell bodies that contain acetylcholine (**choice A**) are found in the basal nucleus of Meynert (which degenerates in Alzheimer disease), in the medial septum and diagonal band complex, and in the striatum.

   Dopamine- (**choice B**) containing cell bodies are found in the midbrain (in the substantia nigra pars compacta and in the ventral tegmental area). The cell bodies in the hypothalamus contribute to the tuberoinfundibular pathway.

   GABA (**choice C**) is the primary inhibitory neurotransmitter of the brain and is therefore located throughout the brain. Such areas include the cerebellar cortex, striatum, globus pallidus, and substantia nigra pars reticulata.

   Norepinephrine- (**choice D**) containing neurons are found predominantly in the locus ceruleus of the pons and midbrain.

3. **The correct answer is B.** Cardiac output can be measured by way of O_2 consumption using the Fick principle:

   $$\text{Cardiac output} = \frac{O_2 \text{ consumption}}{([O_2] \text{ arterial} - [O_2] \text{ venous})}$$

   In this case, oxygen consumption was 200 mL/min, $[O_2]$ arterial was 0.20 mL O_2/mL of blood, and $[O_2]$ venous was 0.15 mL O_2/mL of blood:

   $$\text{Cardiac output} = \frac{200 \text{ mL/min}}{0.20 \text{ mL } O_2/\text{mL blood} - 0.15 \text{ mL } O_2/\text{mL blood}}$$
   $$= 4000 \text{ mL/min}$$
   $$= 4.0 \text{ L/min}$$

   Choice A corresponds to a very low cardiac output, as average cardiac output is approximately 5 L/min.

   Choices C, D, and E are illogical since the heart is virtually incapable of pumping so much blood in 1 minute, especially in a patient with heart disease.

4. **The correct answer is A.** The space constant of an axon reflects the amount of passive or electrotonic spread of current within the axon. The larger the space constant, the further the current can spread, allowing action potentials to propagate faster. This is why myelin increases the conduction velocity of action potentials down an axon. Conversely, demyelination decreases the space constant and slows action potential conduction.

5. **The correct answer is D**. Pepsin is secreted (in an inactive or zymogen form as pepsinogen) by the chief cells of the stomach. Pepsinogen is activated by contact with stomach acid. Although protein digestion usually begins with the actions of hydrochloric acid and pepsin, pancreatic enzymes complete the job as the food passes into the small intestine.

   Amylases (**choice A**) hydrolyze $1 \rightarrow 4$ glycosidic linkages of starches to produce oligosaccharides, maltose, maltotriose, and limit dextrins. These enzymes are produced by the pancreas and salivary glands.

   Chymotrypsin (**choice B**) is a proteolytic enzyme released by the pancreas as the inactive proenzyme, chymotrypsinogen.

   Lipases (**choice C**) are mostly released by the pancreas and serve to digest various lipids, including triacylglycerols.

   Trypsin (**choice E**) is a proteolytic enzyme released by the pancreas as the inactive proenzyme trypsinogen.

6. **The correct answer is D.** The ratio of cells in bone marrow developing along myeloid lines to cells developing along erythroid lines is 3:1. An alternative way to remember the normal marrow composition is that it typically contains about 60% granulocytes and their precursors; 20% erythroid precursors; 10% lymphocytes, monocytes, and their precursors; and 10% unidentified or disintegrating cells. These numbers are worth remembering, because shifts away from normal values may be a subtle clue to marrow abnormalities.

7. **The correct answer is C.** The actual process of manipulation of DNA and chromosomes during meiosis is very similar in spermatogenesis and oogenesis. However, the processes also differ in many other respects:

    In oogenesis, the process of meiosis begins before birth and arrests between birth and puberty in prophase I. In contrast, spermatogenesis does not begin until puberty (**see choice A**).

    The egg retains a large volume of cytoplasm (**choice B**), whereas nearly all the cytoplasm is stripped during formation of a sperm.

    As noted above, in oogenesis, meiosis is arrested in prophase I, which is consequently very prolonged in the female. In spermatogenesis, meiosis is completed in a much shorter time (**choice D**).

    Both the egg and the sperm have mitochondria, but those of the sperm are left outside when the sperm nucleus enters the egg and consequently do not contribute to the mitochondrial genome of the fetus. Instead, the mitochondria are transmitted from the egg to the fetus (**choice E**). Traits coded for by mitochondrial DNA are therefore inherited in a matrilineal fashion.

8. **The correct answer is E.** There are two zones in the lung: the conducting zone (where there is no gas exchange) and the respiratory zone (where there is gas exchange). Of all of the structures listed, only type I epithelial cells are located in the respiratory zone. Type I epithelial cells are the primary structural cells of the alveolar wall. Type II epithelial cells, also located in the alveoli, produce surfactant.

    Goblet cells (**choice A**), which are mucus-secreting cells, are present in the conducting airways.

    The main bronchi (**choice B**) are part of the conducting airways.

    Mucous cells (**choice C**), which are mucus-secreting cells, are present in the conducting airways.

    Terminal bronchioles (**choice D**) are the most distal part of the conducting airways. Respiratory bronchioles, which are just distal to the terminal bronchioles, are part of the respiratory zone. These two types of bronchioles can be differentiated from each other by whether they have alveoli budding from their walls. Respiratory bronchioles have alveoli, terminal bronchioles do not.

9. **The correct answer is A.** Because creatinine is freely filtered by the glomerulus, but not secreted or reabsorbed to a significant extent, the renal clearance of creatinine is approximately equal to the glomerular filtration rate. In fact, creatinine clearance is commonly used to assess renal function in the clinical setting. When a kidney is removed, the total glomerular filtration rate decreases because 50% of the nephrons have been removed,

which causes the creatinine clearance to decrease. In turn, the plasma creatinine concentration (**choice D**) increases until the rate of creatinine excretion by the kidneys (**choice E**) is equal to the rate of creatinine production by the body. Recall that creatinine excretion = GFR $\times$ plasma creatinine concentration. Therefore, creatinine excretion is normal when GFR is decreased following removal of a kidney because the plasma concentration of creatinine is elevated.

Creatinine is a waste product of metabolism. Creatinine production (**choice B**) is directly related to the muscle mass of an individual, but is independent of renal function.

The daily excretion of sodium (**choice C**) is unaffected by the removal of a kidney. The amount of sodium excreted each day by the remaining kidney exactly matches the amount of sodium entering the body in the diet.

10. **The correct answer A.** Release of cholecystokinin is stimulated by the presence of peptides, amino acids, or fatty acids in the small intestine. Cholecystokinin acts on the pancreas to stimulate secretion of pancreatic enzymes that aid in the digestion of these compounds.

    Gastrin (**choice B**) secretion, which is stimulated by the presence of peptides or amino acids in the lumen of the stomach, produces an increase in gastric H^+ secretion.

    Motilin (**choice C**) is a hormone that regulates the migrating myoelectric complex, a series of contractions that occur during fasting, clearing the stomach and small intestine of any residual food.

    Secretin (**choice D**) secretion, which is stimulated by the presence of H^+ and fatty acids in the duodenum, causes an increase in pancreatic and biliary HCO_3^- release and a decrease in gastric H^+ release.

    Somatostatin (**choice E**) secretion, which is stimulated by the presence of H^+ in the lumen, results in decreased release of all gastrointestinal hormones and decreased H^+ secretion in the stomach.

11. **The correct answer is A.** Alpha$_2$-receptor agonists directly inhibit pancreatic insulin secretion.

    Beta$_2$-adrenergic agonists (**choice B**) stimulate insulin secretion.

    Cholecystokinin (**choice C**) is a hormone that causes not only gallbladder contraction, but also insulin secretion from the pancreas.

    Pancreatic glucagon release (**choice D**) acts as a paracrine stimulus for insulin secretion.

    Ingestion of high-sugar meals (**choice E**) is a stimulus for the secretion of insulin from the pancreas.

12. **The correct answer is C.** Recall that total ventilation is equal to alveolar ventilation plus dead space ventilation. This can be expressed mathematically as:

$$V_T \times n = V_A \times n + V_D \times n, \text{ where}$$

V_T = tidal volume

V_A = the volume of alveolar gas in the tidal volume

V_D = dead space

n = respiratory frequency

To calculate the answer, just plug the given values into this equation and solve for V_T. Realize also that the dead space is the combined dead space of the patient and the ventilator: 150 mL + 350 mL = 500 mL. Do not forget to check your units: you need to convert 6 L/min to 6000 mL/min.

$$(V_T \times 20/\text{min}) = (6000 \text{ mL/min}) + (500 \text{ mL } 20/\text{min})$$

$$(V_T \times 20/\text{min}) = 16,000 \text{ mL/min}$$

$$V_T = 800 \text{ mL}$$

13. **The correct answer is D.** During menopause, there is a loss of functioning follicles in the ovaries such that GnRH-stimulated LH and FSH secretion do not result in normal estrogen secretion. The low estrogen levels cannot inhibit gonadotropin secretion in a negative-feedback fashion, resulting in very high levels of LH and FSH.

    Choices A, B, C, and E do not accurately describe normal hormonal levels in menopause.

14. **The correct answer is B.** The extrinsic pathway of clotting begins with tissue factor binding to Factor VII or Factor VIIa. All other clotting proteins require proteolytic cleavage to become active; however, Factor VII has a low level of activity in its inactive form and can act with tissue factor and phospholipids to initiate the clotting cascade. In the extrinsic pathway, Factor VII cleaves Factor X to Xa (**choice C**), which acts in concert with Factor V (**choice A**) to cleave prothrombin to thrombin (**choice E**). The final step in the coagulation pathway is the cleavage of fibrinogen to fibrin by thrombin (**choice D**). Fibrin polymerizes and cross-links, thereby forming a hemostatic net of insoluble protein.

15. **The correct answer is A.** The skeletal muscles of the body have a normal blood flow even when blood pressure is chronically elevated. Organs and tissues in which the vasculature has primarily a nutritive function (e.g., brain, heart, and skeletal muscle) regulate their blood flow in accordance with the metabolic needs of the tissues. These tissues exhibit short-term autoregulation of blood flow such that the increase in flow caused by an elevated arterial pressure is minimized by constriction of the arterioles. The constriction is caused in part by decreased levels of adenosine (an endogenous vasodila-

tor) in the tissues. The rate of adenosine production in a tissue is a function of its metabolic rate, which is not affected significantly by an increase in systemic pressure. When blood flow to the muscle increases, the adenosine is literally washed from the muscle, lowering the tissue levels of adenosine. The decrease in adenosine concentration causes small arteries and arterioles in the muscle to constrict, and this increase in resistance (**choice C**) maintains blood flow (**choice D**) at a normal rate in the face of increased arterial pressure (**choice B**). The overall process is called autoregulation of blood flow.

Venous oxygen concentration (**choice E**) does not decrease in the skeletal muscles of hypertensives because blood flow is maintained at an adequate level to meet the nutritional demands of the muscles.

16. **The correct answer is B.** The patient is hypoventilating because of the effects of barbiturates on respiration. This question requires use of the alveolar gas equation:

$$P_{A_{O_2}} = P_{I_{O_2}} - P_{A_{CO_2}}/R, \text{ where}$$

$P_{A_{O_2}}$ = the partial pressure of alveolar O_2

$P_{I_{O_2}}$ = the partial pressure of inspired O_2

$P_{A_{CO_2}}$ = the partial pressure of alveolar CO_2

R = respiratory exchange ratio

We know that $P_{A_{O_2}}$ = 100 mm Hg, $P_{A_{CO_2}}$ = 80 mm Hg, and $R = 1$, so we can solve for $P_{I_{O_2}}$:

$$100 \text{ mm Hg} = P_{I_{O_2}} - 80 \text{ mm Hg}/1$$

$$P_{I_{O_2}} = 180 \text{ mm Hg}$$

$P_{I_{O_2}} = F_{O_2} \times (P_B - P_{H_2O})$, where F_{O_2} is the fraction of inspired O_2 and P_B is the barometric pressure. P_{H_2O} is the water vapor pressure in the airways and always remains constant at 47 mm Hg. Solving for F_{O_2}:

$$180 \text{ mm Hg} = F_{O_2} \times (500 \text{ mm Hg} - 47 \text{ mm Hg})$$

$$F_{O_2} \approx 0.40$$

For this patient to re-establish a normal value for alveolar P_{O_2}, a 40% oxygen mixture must be inhaled. (The percent of oxygen present in the atmosphere is 21%.)

17. **The correct answer is A.** Fibrinogen is cleaved by thrombin twice as it is activated to form fibrin. The initial cleavage causes it to polymerize, and the second causes it to branch. Thrombin also activates Factor XIII to XIIIa, which cross-links the fibrin strands and strengthens the clot.

High molecular weight kininogen (HMWK; **choice B**) is a cofactor in the intrinsic pathway that converts Factor XI to XIa.

Plasminogen (**choice C**) is a central proenzyme in clot lysis. When plasminogen is converted to plasmin, it digests fibrin threads, as well as a number of protein factors including Factors V, VIII, XII, and prothrombin.

Thrombin (**choice D**) is an enzyme derived from prothrombin. It converts fibrinogen to fibrin and activates factor XIII.

von Willebrand Factor (vWF; **choice E**) is a tissue-bound protein that is exposed with vascular trauma and helps in the process of platelet adhesion.

18. **The correct answer is A.** The most important factor in the control of minute-to-minute ventilation is arterial P_{CO_2}, which influences chemoreceptors located near the ventral surface of the medulla. As arterial P_{CO_2} rises, CO_2 diffuses from cerebral blood vessels into the CSF. Carbonic acid is formed and dissociates into bicarbonate and protons. Protons directly stimulate these central chemoreceptors, resulting in hyperventilation. Hyperventilating reduces the P_{CO_2} in the arterial blood and subsequently in the CSF.

Peripheral chemoreceptors located in the carotid and aortic bodies respond to increases in P_{CO_2} (**choice B**), but are less important than the central chemoreceptors. It is estimated that when a normal subject hyperventilates in response to inhalation of CO_2, less than 20% of the response can be attributed to the peripheral receptors. However, they respond more quickly than their central counterparts and are thought to play a role in regulating ventilation after abrupt changes in P_{CO_2}.

There are no known central chemoreceptors that respond to either arterial pH (**choice C**) or arterial P_{O_2} (**choice E**).

Carotid chemoreceptors (**choice D**) cause hyperventilation in response to decreases in arterial pH; however, CO_2 acting through central chemoreceptors is the most important regulator of ventilation under normal conditions.

19. **The correct answer is B.** Trauma to the lower cervical cord (at C7, for example) can cause the pattern described in the question stem, since the lesion is below the origin of the phrenic nerve, but above the origin of the nerves innervating the muscles of the rib cage and abdomen.

Trauma high in the neck at C2 (**choice A**), above the origin of the phrenic nerve (C3-C5 nerve roots), would cause diaphragmatic paralysis as well.

A lesion at L3 (**choice C**) would spare all of the accessory respiratory muscles, as well as the diaphragm.

A lesion at T5 (**choice D**) would spare part of the accessory muscles of the rib cage.

A lesion at T12 (**choice E**) would spare the accessory muscles of the rib cage.

20. **The correct answer is C.** Both increased stroke volume and heart rate are important for maintaining an adequate cardiac output during exercise.

There is an increased, not decreased, cardiac index (**choice A**) during isotonic exercise.

Diastolic blood pressure usually remains unchanged during isotonic exercise; it is not decreased (**choice B**). In contrast, systolic blood pressure usually rises during isotonic exercise.

There is decreased, not increased, systemic vascular resistance (**choice D**) during isotonic exercise.

Increased somatic dysfunction (**choice E**) would not help maintain adequate cardiac output; it could impair it.

21. **The correct answer is C.** There are two systems currently used for classifying nerve fibers. The first system groups both sensory and motor fibers together, describing A-α, A-β, A-γ, A-δ, B, and C fibers. Another system relates only to sensory fibers, describing Ia, Ib, II, III, IV categories. Both classification schemes begin with large, myelinated fibers, progressing to finer, unmyelinated fibers.

The C fiber (or IV fibers) is the only type of fiber that is unmyelinated. Remember that preganglionic neurons are myelinated, but postganglionic neurons are unmyelinated. Neurons that carry slow pain and temperature information are also classified as C fibers. See the table below for more information.

Sensory and Motor Fibers	Sensory Fibers	Function
A-α	Ia (**choice D**)	Alpha motor neurons, primary afferents of muscle spindles
A-α	Ib (**choice E**)	Golgi tendon organ afferents, touch and pressure
A-β	II	Secondary afferents of muscle spindles, touch and pressure
A-γ		Gamma motor neurons
A-δ (**choice A**)	III	Touch, pressure; pain and temperature (fast)
B (**choice B**)		Preganglionic autonomic, visceral afferents
C (**choice C**)	IV	Postganglionic autonomic; pain and temperature (slow)

22. **The correct answer is C.** Slow waves are oscillating membrane potentials that are generated locally within the gastrointestinal smooth muscle. In each region of the gastrointestinal tract, intrinsic pacemaker cells within the smooth muscle independently generate slow waves. Slow-wave frequencies are relatively constant and are characteristic of each region of the gut, ranging from 3 slow waves/min in the stomach to 12 slow waves/min in the duodenum. The slow-wave frequency represents the maximal rate of contraction within a gut segment. When an action potential occurs at the peak of a slow wave (a spike burst), sufficient depolarization to initiate muscle contraction results. Therefore, increasing the amplitude of the slow waves makes a contraction more likely to occur, or makes the contraction more forceful.

There is no evidence that either circadian rhythms (**choice A**) or dietary fiber intake levels (**choice B**) have any effect on gastrointestinal slow wave frequencies.

Cholecystokinin (**choice D**), corticosteroids (**choice E**), and sympathetic stimulation may modify the frequency of action potentials and contractions by affecting the amplitude, rather than the frequency, of the slow waves.

23. **The correct answer is C.** The aorta is constricted at a point beyond the arterial branches to the head and arms but proximal to the kidneys. Collateral vessels in the body wall carry much of the blood flow to the lower body, and the arterial pressure in the lower body is about 50% lower compared with the pressure in the upper body. The lower-than-normal pressure at the level of the kidneys causes renin to be secreted and angiotensin to be formed. The angiotensin causes salt and water retention so that within a few days to weeks the arterial pressure in the lower body (at the level of the kidneys) increases to normal, but in doing so, the blood pressure in the upper body has increased to hypertensive levels. The kidneys are no longer ischemic when the blood pressure has increased; therefore, renin secretion

decreases and the formation of angiotensin returns to normal levels.

Blood flow in the lower body (**choice A**) is lower than normal at this early stage of aortic coarctation. However, blood flow can be normal above and below the constriction if the body is able to compensate fully.

The decrease in blood pressure at the level of the kidneys causes the glomerular filtration rate (**choice B**) to decrease.

Increase plasma levels of angiotensin II causes salt and water retention; thus, salt and water excretion (**choices D and E**) are decreased.

24. **The correct answer is C.** Activation of type B baroreceptors (atrial stretch receptors) results in secretion of atrial natriuretic factor (ANF), a polypeptide hormone that increases urinary sodium excretion and therefore decreases intravascular volume to maintain homeostasis. None of the remaining answer choices are appropriate physiologic responses to increased atrial filling.

Aldosterone (**choice A**) causes sodium retention by increasing sodium and water reabsorption in the distal convoluted tubule. This leads to an increased intravascular volume.

Activation of atrial baroreceptors results in increased secretion of ADH (**choice B**), a polypeptide hormone that decreases urine concentration and increases intravascular volume.

Norepinephrine (**choice D**) causes vasoconstriction and increased blood pressure, which can produce a reflex decrease in heart rate.

Renin (**choice E**) converts angiotensin I to angiotensin II, a potent vasoconstrictor that stimulates aldosterone secretion from the adrenal cortex, resulting in increased intravascular volume.

25. **The correct answer is C.** About 70% of the sodium entering the proximal convoluted tubule is actively reabsorbed. Chloride and water follow passively.

The collecting duct (**choice A**) reabsorbs about 3% to 5% of the entering sodium, via aldosterone-regulated, electrogenic Na^+-channel pumps. Antidiuretic hormone (ADH) increases H_2O permeability and reabsorption in this region.

The distal convoluted tubule (**choice B**) reabsorbs about 5% of the entering sodium, also via $Na^+/K^+/2Cl^-$ cotransport. This region is relatively impermeable to water.

The ascending limb of the loop of Henle (**choice D**) reabsorbs about 20% of the entering sodium via $Na^+/K^+/2Cl^-$ cotransport. This region is relatively impermeable to water.

The descending limb of the loop of Henle (**choice E**) is water-permeable. Hence, this area has a dilute sodium concentration.

26. **The correct answer is C.** The second heart sound and the v wave both occur during isovolumetric relaxation.

The onset of the a wave (**choice A**) occurs during atrial systole and coincides with the fourth heart sound, if present.

The onset of the c wave (**choice B**) coincides with the first heart sound and evolves into the x descent (**choice D**) during rapid ejection. It does not correspond to any heart sounds.

The y descent (**choice E**) occurs during rapid filling and does not correspond to any heart sounds.

27. **The correct answer is B.** The colony forming unit-erythroid (CFU-E) is a unipotential stem cell that develops from a burst forming unit-erythroid (BFU-E), which develops eventually from the multipotential stem cell. The BFU-E is somewhat responsive to erythropoietin, but the CFU-E is completely dependent on erythropoietin. Erythropoietin is normally released from the kidney in response to hypoxic or anemic conditions. Its half-life is about 3-6 hours. Clinically, it takes 5 days to see reticulocyte formation in the peripheral blood following erythropoietin administration.

The basophilic erythroblast (**choice A**) differentiates from the proerythroblast. It is recognizable by light microscopy and has a dark basophilic staining due to hemoglobin synthesis. It is not directly affected by erythropoietin, but is instead indirectly increased by the increase in precursor cells from the increase in CFU-E earlier in development.

The multipotential stem cell (**choice C**) appears earlier in development than CFU-E and does not increase with erythropoietin. The development of all major components of blood (RBC, WBC, and platelets) begins with the multipotential stem cell (CFU-S). This cell is non-committed and can self-renew. It is located in the bone marrow and is not recognizable by light microscopy.

The proerythroblast (**choice D**), which is the first recognizable cell in the red cell lineage, develops from the CFU-E cell. It is not affected directly by erythropoietin, but instead increases in number from the increased CFU-E cells.

The reticulocyte (**choice E**) is the enucleated cell just before the mature red blood cell. Reticulocytes enter the peripheral circulation but continue to synthesize hemoglobin. This cell is not directly stimulated by erythropoietin, but increases in number as a result of the increase in precursors.

28. **The correct answer is E.** This is simply a question about baroreceptor reflexes. The reflex response that would be anticipated after a decrease in blood pressure (e.g., after a hemorrhage) would be an increase in sympathetic outflow and a decrease in parasympathetic outflow. As a result, heart rate would increase, gastrointestinal motility would decrease, and the pupils would dilate.

29. **The correct answer is E.** The net driving force for fluid across a capillary wall is given by the following equation:

driving force =
(hydrostatic$_c$ – hydrostatic$_i$) – (oncotic$_c$ – oncotic$_i$)

where:

hydrostatic$_i$ = interstitial hydrostatic pressure

hydrostatic$_c$ = capillary hydrostatic pressure

oncotic$_i$ = interstitial oncotic pressure

oncotic$_c$ = capillary oncotic pressure

Substituting the values in the question stem: $3 = (25 - 2) - (x - 7)$. Simplifying, $3 = 23 - x + 7$, therefore $x = 27$.

30. **The correct answer is B.** There are two ways to arrive at the correct answer to this question. The first is to simply remember the definition of functional residual capacity (FRC): the amount of air remaining in the lungs after a passive expiration. The second way is to recall that the helium dilution technique described above is used to measure FRC and residual volume (RV), which narrows the reasonable option choices to B and E only. All of the other volumes and capacities can be directly measured with spirometry because they are blown into the spirometer. Only FRC and RV represent amounts of air that remain in the lungs.

Expiratory reserve volume (**choice A**) is the volume expelled by an active expiratory effort after passive expiration.

Inspiratory capacity (**choice C**) is the maximal amount of air inspired after a passive expiration.

Inspiratory reserve volume (**choice D**) is the amount of air inspired with a maximal inspiratory effort over and above the tidal volume.

Residual volume (**choice E**) is the amount of air remaining in the lungs after maximal expiration.

31. **The correct answer is C.** Total peripheral resistance (TPR) is equal to the pressure gradient across the circulation (mean arterial pressure – right atrial pressure) divided by the cardiac output. Thus, TPR = 120/3000 = 0.04 mm Hg/mL/min. The "ABC rule" is useful in remembering the relation between pressure (P), flow (Q), and resistance (R) because P = QR (note the alphabetical order). Note that knowledge of heart rate and stroke volume is not required to solve this problem because cardiac output is provided.

32. **The correct answer is A.** A decrease in the resistance of the afferent arteriole (i.e., arteriolar dilation) directly increases glomerular capillary hydrostatic pressure by lessening the drop in blood pressure that normally occurs along the vasculature proximal to the glomerulus. [Recall that the afferent arteriole is upstream from the glomerulus; the efferent arteriole is downstream from the glomerulus.] The glomerular capillary hydrostatic pressure is the determinant of glomerular filtration rate most subject to physiologic control.

Bowman's capsular hydrostatic pressure (**choice B**), capillary filtration coefficient (**choice C**), and plasma colloid osmotic pressure (**choice E**) are important determinants of GFR, but they do not have any direct effect to increase or decrease the glomerular capillary hydrostatic pressure.

A decrease in efferent arteriolar resistance (**choice D**) would tend to decrease the glomerular capillary hydrostatic pressure because the efferent arteriole is downstream from the glomerular capillaries.

33. **The correct answer is C.** Glucagon, secretin, and vasoactive intestinal polypeptide (VIP) are all structurally related.

Cholecystokinin (**choice A**) and gastrin (**choice B**) form another family of related hormones.

Neither somatostatin (**choice D**) nor substance P (**choice E**) are structurally related to secretin. In addition to their role in the gastrointestinal system, both hormones are also present in the brain.

34. **The correct answer is B.** 2,3-Diphosphoglycerate (2,3-DPG) is produced in red cells by a variation on the glycolytic pathway, and levels diminish when glycolysis by the red cells slows. The depletion of 2,3-DPG in stored blood causes the hemoglobin dissociation curve to shift to the left, leading to an increase in oxygen affin-

ity. This increase is helpful in the picking up of oxygen by hemoglobin in the lungs, but it can be very problematic in the release of oxygen from the blood in tissues. This is not just a theoretical point: considerable effort has been expended in developing improved solutions for storing packed red cells and methods for "restoring" older stored cells so that the 2,3-DPG levels are adequate. In practice, in otherwise reasonably healthy patients, older transfused blood will quickly regenerate 2,3-DPG when placed in the glucose-containing environment of the serum; however, even transiently decreased 2,3-DPG levels in a severely compromised patient can be dangerous.

35. **The correct answer is A.** Crossing over, a transposition of genetic information, occurs during the first meiotic (reduction) division, when the primary spermatocyte divides to form two secondary spermatocytes. This division does not consist of separation of sister chromatids after DNA replication, but rather involves the separation of previously paired, homologous chromosomes. Crossing over occurs during prophase of meiosis I.

The secondary spermatocyte (**choice B**) undergoes the second meiotic division, which results in four spermatids (**choice C**), each with the haploid number of chromosomes. The spermatids are located adjacent to the lumen of the seminiferous tubules and are distinguished by their small size. These cells undergo no further division, but become transformed into mature spermatozoa (**choice E**) through the process of spermiogenesis.

The spermatogonia (**choice D**) are the primitive germ cells. These cells give rise to the primary spermatocytes through repeated mitotic divisions.

Remember the sequence of spermatogenesis:

Spermatogonia (2n) → REPEATED MITOSES → Primary spermatocytes (2n) → FIRST MEIOTIC DIVISION → Secondary spermatocytes (n) → SECOND MEIOTIC DIVISION → Spermatids (n) → SPERMIOGENESIS → Spermatozoa (n)

36. **The correct answer is A.** Estrogen levels peak at the end of the follicular phase of the menstrual cycle, creating positive feedback to the hypothalamus and pituitary gland. This increases the number of GnRH spikes per 24 hours, causing a surge of both follicle-stimulating hormone (FSH) and luteinizing hormone (LH). It is the surge of LH, in combination with the high estrogen levels, that induces ovulation.

FSH levels (**choice B**) peak at ovulation.

Gonadotropin-releasing hormone (**choice C**) is released in pulses, not in a continuous pattern as is estrogen.

LH levels (**choice D**) peak at ovulation.

Progesterone (**choice E**) peaks during the premenstrual phase of the cycle. It is represented by the solid line on the graph.

37. **The correct answer is C.** Ejection fraction is a sensitive index of cardiac function equal to the ratio of stroke volume to end-diastolic volume. The stroke volume is equal to the difference between the amount of blood in the ventricle prior to systole (end-diastolic volume) and the amount of blood in the ventricle at the end of systole (end-systolic volume). Because the end-diastolic volume is 115 mL and the end-systolic volume is 65 mL, the stroke volume is $115 - 65 = 50$ mL. The ejection fraction is calculated as 50 mL / 115 mL = 0.43. Ejection fraction (normal value = 0.65) can be estimated by radionuclide angiography or echocardiography and is frequently depressed in systolic heart failure, even when the stroke volume itself is normal.

38. **The correct answer is A.** Glucose is freely filtered by the glomerular capillary membrane and totally reabsorbed in the proximal tubule under normal conditions. Therefore, the concentration of glucose is highest in the proximal portion of the proximal tubule. The concentration of glucose is essentially zero in the thin descending limb of loop of Henle (**choice B**), distal convoluted tubule (**choice C**), cortical collecting tubule (**choice D**), and medullary collecting tubule (**choice E**).

39. **The correct answer is D.** This question tests your knowledge of how vitamin B_{12} is normally absorbed. In summary, parietal cells in the gastric lining secrete a glycoprotein called intrinsic factor into the gastric lumen. This protein binds to vitamin B_{12}, protecting it from degradation and allowing for its eventual absorption. At the level of the ileum, B_{12} bound to intrinsic factor is actively reabsorbed. Therefore, a loss of intrinsic factor or of its reabsorption site, the ileum, would lead to the need for lifelong injection of vitamin B_{12}. Removal of the stomach would obviously lead to loss of intrinsic factor. Pernicious anemia is actually an autoimmune disease that targets the gastric epithelium. In many cases, patients have autoantibodies against intrinsic factor, preventing the absorption of ingested vitamin B_{12}.

Removal of the colon, jejunum, or gallbladder would not affect reabsorption of intrinsic factor or B_{12}. A total absence of bile (which occurs with bile duct blockage, but not with cholecystectomy) may lead to malabsorption of fat-soluble vitamins such as A, D, E, and K, but not of B_{12}.

40. **The correct answer is A.** Hyperphosphatemia associated with renal failure is the likely cause for this patient's hypocalcemic state. Phosphate excretion is impaired, and metabolic phosphate production is often increased. High serum levels of phosphate can lead to the deposition of calcium phosphate in tissues, decreasing the plasma calcium concentration.

Hyponatremia (**choice B**) in acute renal failure (ARF) is generally due to ingestion of water or inappropriate administration of hypotonic IV solutions. It does not directly affect the levels of calcium in the plasma.

Decreased, rather than increased, sensitivity to 1,25-dihydroxyvitamin D (**choice C**) is typical of ARF. Again, increased sensitivity to 1,25-dihydroxyvitamin D could result in hypercalcemia, not in hypocalcemia.

Decreased, rather than increased, sensitivity to parathyroid hormone (**choice D**) is typical of ARF. Regardless, since parathyroid hormone acts to increase serum calcium, increased sensitivity to parathyroid hormone (PTH) could result in hypercalcemia, not in hypocalcemia.

Metabolic alkalosis (**choice E**) is rare in ARF, but may accompany vomiting or may be due to therapeutic administration of bicarbonate. Metabolic acidosis, which is much more common, results from the failure of the kidneys to excrete the organic acids derived from the metabolism of dietary protein.

41. **The correct answer is D.** Removal of a lung, typically for treatment of lung cancer, has many physiologic consequences. The most obvious change is that the remaining lung fills the chest cavity (and typically displaces the heart across the midline). The volume of air that can be maximally inspired by the single lung is less than that inspired by two lungs. Another subtle change is that the pulmonary vascular bed is sufficiently large that it can accommodate the doubled blood flow at rest (by recruiting more alveolar wall capillaries), but there is not a sufficient reserve vascular bed to accommodate the larger blood flow produced during exercise.

Airway resistance (**choice A**) is decreased during exercise because of bronchodilation; this helps ventilate the lung.

Lung compliance (**choice B**) changes do not adversely affect blood flow during exercise.

Pulmonary vessels typically dilate, rather than constrict (**choice C**), during exercise.

Although the volume of the single lung (**choice E**) is less than that of two lungs, this would not account for an increase in pulmonary artery pressure.

42. **The correct answer is D.** Opioids, such as heroin, depress respiration centrally by reducing the responsiveness of brainstem respiratory centers to CO_2. The resulting hypoventilation leads to CO_2 retention because of the inability of the patient to "blow off" the CO_2. This increases the production of carbonic acid (H_2CO_3) by carbonic anhydrase present in red blood cells (which converts CO_2 to carbonic acid). Dissociation of carbonic acid to bicarbonate (HCO_3^-) and protons produces a respiratory acidosis.

Metabolic acidosis (**choice A**) is caused by a primary decrease in HCO_3^-, which can occur after tissue hypoxia (which increases levels of lactic acid) or in uncontrolled diabetes mellitus.

Metabolic alkalosis (**choice B**) is caused by an increase in HCO_3^-, which can occur subsequent to ingestion of alkali or a loss of gastric acid (vomiting).

Normal pH balance (**choice C**) might be anticipated if the respiratory acidosis persists, allowing time for the kidneys to compensate for the altered pH by conserving HCO_3^-. However, renal compensation takes several days (this patient had an acute heroin overdose) and is rarely complete.

Respiratory alkalosis (**choice E**) is caused by a decrease in P_{CO_2}, which can occur with hyperventilation.

43. **The correct answer is C.** Even though blood flow is interrupted to a portion of the lung, the lung will still continue to ventilate. There will be no gas exchange, and the PO_2 and PCO_2 of alveolar gas will approach that of inspired air ($PO_2 = 150$ mm Hg, and $PCO_2 = 0$ mm Hg).

Choice A indicates the normal situation.

The PO_2 of the lung will always be less than the PO_2 of the atmosphere (**choice B**) because air is warmed and moistened in the airways, so water vapor pressure must be accounted for. PO_2 in the atmosphere is approximately 160 mm Hg (0.21×760 mm Hg); PO_2 in the lung is approximately 150 mm Hg (760 mm Hg − 47 mm Hg) × 0.21 = 150 mm Hg (atmospheric pressure = 760 mm Hg; water vapor pressure = 47 mm Hg).

PO_2 of the lung would approximate mixed venous blood (**choice D**) if ventilation were blocked.

PO_2 of the lung cannot be less than that of mixed venous blood (**choice E**).

44. **The correct answer is C.** This case depicts a classic picture of hypovolemic shock due to hemorrhage. When blood volume is low, less blood fills the ventricles during diastole, corresponding to reduced preload.

Consequently, cardiac output is decreased because of the diminished stroke volume. Vascular resistance is increased to compensate for volume loss. Mixed venous oxygen levels are reduced because of the increased tissue demand of oxygen and the loss of hemoglobin.

The remaining choices are inconsistent with hemorrhagic shock.

45. **The correct answer is A.** A barrel chest with increased anterior/posterior diameter is commonly observed in patients with long-standing, severe emphysema. This change in chest shape occurs because these patients, who have high compliance of the lung proper, tend to function with their lungs to some degree "over-inflated" compared with people who have normal lung compliance. This over-inflation limits their ability to take further deep breaths. (The "balloon" of emphysematous lung remains compliant, but the "box" of the chest wall is not very compliant and limits the volume of air that can be inhaled.) Patients with moderately severe emphysema are able to maintain an adequate lung ventilation by taking many short breaths (compare with **choice D**); this physiology is sometimes expressed by describing these patients as "pink puffers" (**choice E**).

Chronic cough (**choice B**) in emphysema patients is not directly related to the change in compliance.

46. **The correct answer is B.** This patient has pulmonary fibrosis, which markedly decreases the compliance of the lung, thereby producing a small lung that is difficult to inflate (restrictive lung disease).

The airway resistance (**choice A**) would not be expected to change.

The functional residual capacity (FRC; **choice C**) would be expected to decrease, rather than increase.

The lung volume (**choice D**) is generally smaller than normal in patients with this disorder.

The tidal volume (**choice E**) would be expected to decrease, rather than increase.

47. **The correct answer is E.** Factor XII is unusual among coagulation factors in that its deficiency is associated with thrombosis rather than hemorrhage. The mechanism appears to be a deficient activation of fibrinolysis, and both thrombophlebitis and myocardial infarction have occurred in severely affected patients. The condition is inherited in an autosomal recessive manner. Many patients with mild-to-moderate factor XII deficiency are never detected; others are identified when a routine preoperative clotting screen demonstrates a greatly prolonged partial thromboplastin time.

Deficiency of each of the other factors (**choices A, B, C, and D**) is associated with hemorrhage.

48. **The correct answer is C.** Hereditary spherocytosis is due to an intrinsic abnormality in the membrane support structure of the red cell. A distinctive feature of this disorder is marked susceptibility of the red cells to lysis in hypotonic solutions. This feature is the basis of the osmotic fragility test, which is quite specific for spherocytosis.

Neither thalassemias (**choices A and B**) nor sickle cell disease (**choices D and E**) are characterized by a positive osmotic fragility test.

49. **The correct answer is D.** Membrane depolarization of the heart is due to a sodium influx through fast channels. Depolarization is the signal that causes these channels to quickly open and close. They are also called voltage-gated sodium channels.

Voltage-gated calcium channels (**choice A**) are channels that open more slowly after depolarization, allowing sodium as well as calcium to flow through. These calcium channels are also known by two other names: slow channels (**choice B**) because they open more slowly and slow calcium-sodium channels (**choice C**) because they allow both ions to pass through.

Voltage-gated potassium channels (**choice E**) close during depolarization and most of the plateau phase.

50. **The correct answer is E.** Carotid massage causes an increase in afferent activity to the medulla (not a decrease [**choice A**]) that causes stimulation of the vagus nerve, which results in an increase in the parasympathetic activity of the heart. This increase will lower the blood pressure (**choice B**) and lower the heart rate (**choice C**).

As a result of the pressure on the carotid sinus, the medulla interprets the rise in afferent activity as an increase in blood pressure, and there is a decrease in the sympathetic activity to the heart (**choice D**).

Biochemistry

1. A newborn presents with severe acidosis, vomiting, hypotonia, and neurologic deficits. Laboratory analysis reveals elevated levels of lactate and alanine. These observations suggest a deficiency of which of the following enzymes?

   (A) Alanine aminotransferase

   (B) Glutamate dehydrogenase

   (C) Lactate dehydrogenase

   (D) Phenylethanolamine N-methyltransferase

   (E) Pyruvate dehydrogenase

2. Several members of a family have an autosomal recessive disease characterized by intellectual deterioration, weakness, ataxia, seizures, and death at a young age. Special studies demonstrate a deficiency of cytochrome C oxidase activity. Which of the following subcellular organelles is defective in affected members of this family?

   (A) Golgi apparatus

   (B) Lysosomes

   (C) Mitochondria

   (D) Ribosomes

   (E) Smooth endoplasmic reticulum

Questions 3-4

SET A

Directions: For each numbered item (**test result**), select the one lettered heading (**disease/condition**) most closely associated with it. Each lettered heading may be selected once, more than once, or not at all.

   (A) G6PD deficiency

   (B) chronic tobacco abuse

   (C) asbestosis

   (D) COPD

   (E) asthma

   (F) pulmonary edema

   (G) Wilson disease

3. Peripheral blood smear reveals clumps of hemoglobin-degraded product found in RBCs stained with methylene blue.

4. A liver biopsy reveals a hyaline endoplasmic reticulum within the hepatocytes.

5. Which of the following citric acid cycle intermediates is required for heme synthesis?

   (A) α-Ketoglutarate

   (B) Fumarate

   (C) Isocitrate

   (D) Oxaloacetate

   (E) Succinyl-CoA

6. A 22-year-old woman presents with a fusiform swelling of the Achilles tendon, which, when biopsied, shows cholesterol-laden macrophages (foam cells) dispersed among the collagen fibers. She had been troubled with joint pains for several years. Both her mother and father developed arthritis associated with production of xanthomas, but their first symptoms occurred in middle age. She was referred to a nutritionist and treated with an enzyme inhibitor. Which of the following is most likely elevated in the blood of this woman?

(A) Chylomicron remnants

(B) Chylomicrons

(C) High density lipoproteins (HDL)

(D) Low density lipoproteins (LDL)

(E) Very low density lipoproteins (VLDL)

7. An infant has deficiency of a vitamin that acts as a co-enzyme for glutamate carboxylase would most likely present as which of the following syndromes?

(A) Hemolytic anemia in newborns

(B) Hypoprothrombinemia

(C) Megaloblastic anemia

(D) Neural tube defects in newborns

(E) Osteomalacia in adults

Questions 8-9

CASE A

8. A 26-year-old pregnant woman complains of persistent, dry, ulcerated skin over her knees and elbows. Examination of her eyes reveals small, gray plaques on the conjunctiva. This patient probably will develop which of the following conditions if she does not seek treatment?

(A) Diarrhea

(B) Beriberi

(C) Hypercarotenosis

(D) Blindness

(E) Scurvy

9. The earliest symptom of the above condition is

(A) keratomalacia

(B) night blindness

(C) xerosis

(D) endophthalmitis

(E) corneal ulceration

10. The pregnant mother of a 6-year-old son with glucose-6-phosphate dehydrogenase deficiency is very worried that her female fetus will have the disease. The father and mother are clinically normal. Which of the following is true about her baby?

(A) The baby has a 25% chance of clinical disease

(B) The baby has a 50% chance of being a carrier

(C) The baby has a 50% chance of clinical disease

(D) The baby will be a carrier

(E) The baby will have clinical disease

11. Which of the following is an example of a glycosylated integral membrane protein with seven transmembrane segments?

(A) Adenylate cyclase

(B) Beta-adrenergic receptor for epinephrine

(C) Cystic fibrosis transmembrane conductance regulator channel

(D) Glucose transporter

(E) Na^+/K^+ ATPase

12. A previously normal child begins deteriorating developmentally at about 6 months of age. She is seen by an ophthalmologist because she no longer responds to visual stimuli. A cherry-red spot on the macula is noted on ophthalmologic examination. The enzyme that is deficient in this child normally carries out which of the following functions?

(A) Degradation of glycogen in muscle

(B) Degradation of glycolipids in the brain

(C) Degradation of mucopolysaccharides in bone marrow

(D) Synthesis of glycoproteins in the liver

(E) Synthesis of peptides in the spleen

13. A 30-year-old vegetarian presents to his physician complaining of diminished sensation in his lower extremities. He has not eaten meat for the past 15 years. A complete blood count reveals hypersegmented neutrophils and elevated mean corpuscular volume. Which of the following findings would be expected on urinalysis?

(A) Argininosuccinic aciduria

(B) Cystinuria

(C) Hemoglobinuria

(D) Methylmalonic aciduria

(E) Propionic aciduria

14. Which of the following diseases has an X-linked recessive inheritance pattern?

    (A) Alpha$_1$-antitrypsin deficiency
    (B) Cystic fibrosis
    (C) Duchenne muscular dystrophy
    (D) Phenylketonuria
    (E) Tay-Sachs disease

15. A newborn vomits after each feeding of milk-based formula and does not gain weight. Biochemical testing reveals a severe deficiency of galactose-1-phosphate uridyltransferase, consistent with homozygosity. If this condition goes untreated, which of the following is the likely outcome for this patient?

    (A) Benign disease except for cataract formation
    (B) Chronic emphysema appearing in early adulthood
    (C) Chronic renal failure appearing in adolescence
    (D) Death in infancy
    (E) Gastrointestinal symptoms that remit with puberty

16. Following the ingestion of glyburide, a type 2 diabetic patient begins to experience anxiety, diaphoresis, and hunger. The patient subsequently ingests a health food bar containing glucose. The glycolytic degradation of the ingested glucose commences with the action of which of the following enzymes?

    (A) Aldolase
    (B) Hexokinase
    (C) Phosphofructokinase
    (D) Phosphoglucose isomerase
    (E) Pyruvate kinase

17. A 24-year-old woman with phenylketonuria (PKU) gives birth to her first child. Although there is no history of PKU in the father's family, the couple could not afford genetic testing of the father or consistent prenatal care. At birth, the child is small, microcephalic, and has elevated blood phenylalanine. What is the most likely explanation for this neonate's symptoms?

    (A) Father is a carrier of PKU
    (B) Maternal translocation with unbalanced segregation in meiosis I
    (C) Maternal translocation with unbalanced segregation in meiosis II
    (D) Maternal uniparental disomy
    (E) Phenylalanine was not adequately restricted from the mother's diet during pregnancy

18. A Guatemalan child with a history of meconium ileus is brought to a clinic because of a chronic cough. The mother notes a history of respiratory tract infections and bulky, foul-smelling stools. On physical examination, there is chronic bilateral tissue texture changes at T2-T7. After assessment of the respiratory tract illness, the physician should also look for signs of

    (A) cystinuria
    (B) hypoglycemia
    (C) iron deficiency anemia
    (D) sphingomyelin accumulation
    (E) vitamin A deficiency

19. A 30-year-old man has been fasting for religious reasons for several days. His blood glucose level is now about 60% of its normal value, but he does not feel lightheaded because his brain has reduced its need for serum glucose by using which of the following substances as an alternate energy source?

    (A) Apoprotein B
    (B) Beta-carotene
    (C) Beta-hydroxybutyrate
    (D) C-reactive protein
    (E) Coenzyme A

20. A patient with severe arthritis and urine that turns black on standing most likely has a deficiency of which of the following enzymes?

    (A) Arylsulfatase A
    (B) Glucose-6-phosphatase
    (C) Hexosaminidase A
    (D) Homogentisic oxidase
    (E) Muscle phosphorylase

21. A 2-year-old boy has a past medical history significant for mental retardation, hepatosplenomegaly, foam cells in the bone marrow, and neurologic deficits. The boy dies by the age of 3. Which of the following enzymes was most likely deficient in this child?

    (A) Alpha-galactosidase
    (B) Beta-glucocerebrosidase
    (C) Ceramidase
    (D) HMG-CoA reductase
    (E) Sphingomyelinase

22. A 58-year-old woman is admitted to the hospital with fever, abdominal cramps, and severe watery diarrhea. The symptoms began one day after attending a banquet. The structural examination reveals acute tissue-texture changes at T5-L2 bilaterally. She was treated with ciprofloxacin, but her condition did not improve. PCR amplification and analysis of a gene region in the bacteria isolated from the patient revealed a missense mutation that conferred resistance to ciprofloxacin. The missense mutation is most likely in the gene encoding an enzyme essential for which of the following functions?

    (A) DNA replication

    (B) Folate synthesis

    (C) mRNA translocation on a ribosome

    (D) Peptide bond formation

    (E) Reduction of folate to tetrahydrofolate

23. A 62-year-old man is prescribed a pharmaceutical agent that inhibits the activity of the enzyme HMG-CoA reductase. This patient most likely has which of the following conditions?

    (A) Chronic inflammation

    (B) Familial hypercholesterolemia

    (C) Hypertension

    (D) Hyperuricemia

    (E) Type 2 diabetes

24. A 5-year-old, mentally retarded boy is brought to the city from a rural community for evaluation. A careful history reveals mental retardation in a number of other family members, especially the males. Physical examination is remarkable for a long face with large ears, a large jaw, and bilateral enlargement of the testes. This presentation is suggestive of

    (A) Down syndrome

    (B) Edwards syndrome

    (C) Fragile X syndrome

    (D) Klinefelter syndrome

    (E) Turner syndrome

25. A patient had a liver biopsy. Liver cells in the culture were kept at 0 C (32 F) and treated with trypsin to digest the receptors on the cell surface. The temperature was then raised to 37 C (98.6 F), and radioactive LDL was added to the culture media. Several hours later, the labeled LDL was found to be inside the cells. This specific process of LDL uptake is

    (A) active transport

    (B) facilitated diffusion

    (C) phagocytosis

    (D) pinocytosis

    (E) receptor-mediated endocytosis

26. On physical examination, a newborn is found to have micrognathia, a prominent occiput, low-set ears, and rocker-bottom feet. There is very little mental development during the first months of life, and the infant dies of cardiac complications after 8 months. A complete karyotype of this child would show which of the following?

    (A) XO

    (B) XXY

    (C) Trisomy 13

    (D) Trisomy 18

    (E) Trisomy 21

27. A college student goes to a fraternity party and consumes large quantities of beer. The alcohol in the beer is metabolized by the liver, with almost half the alcohol being oxidized to acetaldehyde. In which of the following sites does this reaction occur?

    (A) Golgi bodies

    (B) Lysosomes

    (C) Mitochondrial matrix

    (D) Peroxisomes

    (E) Ribosomes

28. A genetic deficiency of glucose-6-phosphatase would be expected to produce which of the following sets of laboratory values?

	Serum glucose	Serum lactate	Serum pyruvate
(A)	High	High	High
(B)	High	High	Low
(C)	High	Low	Low
(D)	Low	High	High
(E)	Low	Low	Low

29. A neonate with ambiguous genitalia and microcephaly is suspected of having a genetic disease characterized by failure to metabolize 7-dehydrocholesterol to cholesterol. Which of the following is the most likely diagnosis?

    (A) Down syndrome

    (B) Edwards syndrome

    (C) Patau syndrome

    (D) Smith-Lemli-Opitz syndrome

    (E) WAGR syndrome

30. Poor oxygenation of tissues decreases the production of ATP necessary for many cellular functions. Which of the following processes is most immediately compromised in a typical cell when ATP production is inadequate?

    (A) Complex carbohydrate synthesis

    (B) Lipid synthesis

    (C) Na^+/K^+ ATPase function

    (D) Nucleic acid synthesis

    (E) Protein synthesis

31. A 23-year-old African American woman presents to the emergency department with severe abdominal pain and evidence of dehydration. Her past medical history is significant for numerous pulmonary infections and effusions of the knees. Her physical examination reveals stiff, fibrotic tissues paraspinally at T2-T7 and T10-L2. This patient's erythrocytes would be expected to exhibit

    (A) an absence of central pallor

    (B) deletion of all four alpha Hb genes

    (C) denaturation during deoxygenation

    (D) Heinz bodies on RBC staining

    (E) Increased osmotic fragility

32. When a cloned DNA fragment is used as a probe, a restriction fragment length polymorphism (RFLP) is revealed in the region adjacent to the centromere of chromosome 21. Four haplotypes exist: A, B, C, and D. An AB woman and a CD man have an ACC child with trisomy 21. Nondisjunction occurred in

    (A) the child during the first mitotic division

    (B) the father during meiosis I

    (C) the father during meiosis II

    (D) the mother during meiosis I

    (E) the mother during meiosis II

33. Absence of which of the following enzymes would impair the rate-limiting step of glycogenolysis?

    (A) α-1,4-Glucan transferase

    (B) Glycogen phosphorylase

    (C) Glycogen synthase

    (D) Phosphoglucomutase

    (E) UDP-glucose pyrophosphorylase

34. A patient with acute lymphocytic leukemia is treated appropriately with antineoplastic therapy. Inhibition of which of the following enzymes will help prevent side effects of this therapy?

    (A) Alpha-glucosidase

    (B) Angiotensin-converting enzyme

    (C) Beta-lactamase

    (D) Cyclooxygenase

    (E) Xanthine oxidase

35. A 4-year-old retarded child hurls himself into walls and bites his fingertips so severely that they must be heavily bandaged. This child most likely has a deficiency of which of the following enzymes?

   (A) Cystathionine synthase

   (B) Hexosaminidase A

   (C) Homogentisic acid oxidase

   (D) Hypoxanthine-guanine phosphoribosyltransferase

   (E) Phenylalanine hydroxylase

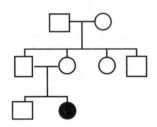

36. The patient shown in the pedigree above did poorly in school, then became increasingly forgetful and irrational. Over a period of years, he developed ataxia and began posturing. Eventually, he was demented and unable to care for himself. At autopsy, extensive cortical demyelination is observed. Microscopic examination of the areas of demyelination reveals numerous macrophages containing crystals that stain light brown with toluidine blue. This presentation is probably due to a deficiency of which of the following enzymes?

   (A) Arylsulfatase A

   (B) Galactocerebroside β-galactosidase

   (C) Glucocerebrosidase

   (D) Hexosaminidase A

   (E) Sphingomyelinase

37. A 28-year-old woman and a 25-year-old man present for genetic counseling. Both are white and have one sibling affected with cystic fibrosis. The most appropriate method to assess the risk of transmitting cystic fibrosis to a potential child would be

   (A) biochemical testing

   (B) fluorescence *in situ* hybridization (FISH)

   (C) karyotype analysis

   (D) polymerase chain reaction (PCR)

   (E) Western blot analysis

38. A 7-year-old girl is brought to the emergency department by her parents with a complaint of severe polyuria and polydipsia. The osteopathic structural examination is significant for T6-T11 somatic dysfunction. Laboratory examination reveals ketones in her urine. Which of the following is the most likely source of the ketones?

   (A) Free fatty acid breakdown

   (B) Gluconeogenesis

   (C) Glycogenolysis

   (D) Protein breakdown

   (E) Triglyceride breakdown

39. An infant receives an exchange blood transfusion due to severe neonatal jaundice. Red blood cell transfusion is required monthly, and at 6 months of age, a splenectomy is performed. Histologic examination of the spleen reveals marked hemosiderosis. Laboratory studies show:

	Patient	Normal
RBC	$2.54 \times 10^6/mm^3$	$3.5\text{-}5.5 \times 10^6/mm^3$
Hemoglobin	8.3 g/dL	12-16 g/dL
Hematocrit	23.4%	34-46%
Reticulocytes	27%	0.5-1.5%
Indirect bilirubin (conjugated)	6.1 mg/dL	0.4-3.4 mg/dL

Analysis of red cell glycolytic intermediates indicates markedly elevated concentrations of 2,3-bisphosphoglycerate, 3-phosphoglycerate, 2-phosphoglycerate, and phosphoenolpyruvate. Which of the following is the most likely diagnosis?

   (A) Glucose 6-phosphate dehydrogenase (G6PD) deficiency

   (B) Lead poisoning

   (C) Pyruvate kinase (PK) deficiency

   (D) Sickle cell anemia

   (E) β-Thalassemia

40. A concerned mother brings her 6-year-old child to the pediatric clinic for severe abdominal pain. The mother reports having found the child chewing on paint chips. Blood tests reveal microcytic hypochromic erythrocytes with basophilic stippling. Exposure to which of the following agents is the most likely cause of this child's presentation?

    (A) Arsenic
    (B) Cyanide
    (C) Gold
    (D) Lead
    (E) Mercury

41. Methotrexate is used as therapy for rheumatoid arthritis, but has many side effects related to competitive inhibition of the enzyme dihydrofolate reductase. These side effects can be decreased without interfering with the efficacy of methotrexate by ingestion of additional folate. If patients treated with methotrexate are given sufficient folate, which of the following would most likely occur?

    (A) Dihydrofolate reductase will have a higher apparent K_m for dihydrofolate
    (B) Dihydrofolate reductase will have a higher V_{max} than it would in the absence of methotrexate
    (C) Dihydrofolate reductase will have a lower apparent K_m for dihydrofolate
    (D) Dihydrofolate reductase will increase its affinity for methotrexate
    (E) Dihydrofolate reductase will reach the same V_{max} as it would in the absence of methotrexate

Questions 42–43

CASE B

A 69-year-old edentulous alcoholic man, who lives alone, is admitted to the hospital for evaluation of a shoulder wound that is not healing well. On physical examination, numerous ecchymoses are noted on the posterior aspect of his legs and thighs. Careful examination of the man's skin reveals minute hemorrhages around hair follicles and splinter hemorrhages in the nail beds. Laboratory examination is remarkable for a hemoglobin of 10 g/dL; no other hematologic abnormalities are noted.

42. The most likely diagnosis of this condition would be

    (A) hemophilia A
    (B) microcytic anemia
    (C) megaloblastic anemia
    (D) scurvy
    (E) vitamin E toxicity

43. Which of the following is the most appropriate therapy for this disorder?

    (A) Factor VIII
    (B) Iron
    (C) Vitamin B_{12}
    (D) Vitamin C
    (E) Vitamin K

44. A 45-year-old man is diagnosed with cancer of the proximal portion of the colon. The structural examination reveals chronic somatic dysfunction at T9–T12. His father died of colon cancer at the age of 52. He has three siblings. His 55-year-old brother has not been diagnosed with cancer, but his 57-year-old sister has an endometrial carcinoma, and his other sister died of ovarian cancer. A diagnosis of hereditary nonpolyposis colorectal cancer (HNPCC) is made. Which of the following types of mutations most likely occurred in this family?

    (A) A mutation causing defects in the mismatch repair system
    (B) A point mutation in the gene coding for an excision exonuclease
    (C) A reciprocal translocation between chromosomes 8 and 14, associated with the Epstein-Barr virus
    (D) Loss of the retinoblastoma (RB) tumor suppressor gene
    (E) Mutation causing defects in the match repair system

45. A 2-year-old boy is diagnosed with a biochemical defect involving hexosaminidase A. The patient's condition would be most appropriately categorized as belonging to which of the following general classes of defects?

    (A) Aminoacidopathy

    (B) Gangliosidosis

    (C) Lipid metabolism

    (D) Mucopolysaccharidosis

    (E) Porphyria

46. A 4-year-old boy is brought to the pediatrician because of gastroenteritis for three days, followed by a brief generalized seizure that left him semicómatose. The blood glucose level at admission is 18 mg/dL (0.10 mM) and urine is negative for glucose and ketones, but positive for a variety of organic dicarboxylic acids. Intravenous administration of glucose improves his condition within 10 minutes. Following diagnosis of an enzyme deficiency, his parents are cautioned to make sure he eats frequently. Which of the following is the most likely diagnosis?

    (A) Glucose-6-phosphatase deficiency

    (B) Hepatic glycogen phosphorylase deficiency

    (C) Medium chain acyl CoA dehydrogenase deficiency

    (D) Mitochondrial carbamoyl phosphate synthetase deficiency

    (E) Ornithine transcarbamoylase deficiency

47. A patient with short stature presents with hypoglycemia, hepatomegaly, bleeding diathesis, hepatic adenomas, and enlarged kidneys. Laboratory evaluation reveals the presence of increased lactate, cholesterol, triglyceride, and uric acid. This patient most likely has a deficiency of which of the following enzymes?

    (A) Brancher enzyme

    (B) Debrancher enzyme

    (C) Glucose-6-phosphatase

    (D) Hepatic phosphorylase

    (E) Muscle phosphorylase

48. A 50-year-old chronic alcoholic presents with dementia, paralysis of lateral gaze, and difficulty walking. Physical examination reveals chronic somatic dysfunction at T5-T9 in the right paraspinal area. The vitamin deficient in this patient is required as a cofactor for which of the following enzymes?

    (A) Aspartate aminotransferase

    (B) Methylmalonyl-CoA mutase

    (C) Prolyl hydroxylase

    (D) Pyruvate carboxylase

    (E) Pyruvate dehydrogenase

49. A 27-year-old medical student is unable to eat lunch and dinner during her clinical rotation. Which of the following enzymes is responsible for helping to maintain blood glucose levels by releasing glucose from its storage form in the liver?

    (A) Acetyl-CoA carboxylase

    (B) Glucose-6-phosphate dehydrogenase

    (C) Glycogen phosphorylase

    (D) Glycogen synthase

    (E) Thiolase

50. In the family shown below, individuals affected with profound deafness are represented by a shaded symbol.

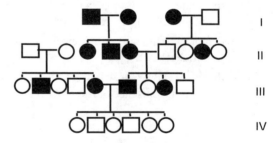

    The phenotypes of individuals in the fourth generation can best be explained by

    (A) autosomal dominant inheritance

    (B) locus heterogeneity

    (C) mitochondrial inheritance

    (D) multifactorial inheritance

    (E) X-linked dominant inheritance

Biochemistry

ANSWERS AND EXPLANATIONS

1.	E	26.	D
2.	C	27.	D
3.	A	28.	D
4.	G	29.	D
5.	E	30.	C
6.	D	31.	C
7.	B	32.	C
8.	D	33.	B
9.	B	34.	E
10.	B	35.	D
11.	B	36.	A
12.	B	37.	D
13.	D	38.	A
14.	C	39.	C
15.	D	40.	D
16.	B	41.	E
17.	E	42.	D
18.	E	43.	D
19.	C	44.	A
20.	D	45.	B
21.	E	46.	C
22.	A	47.	C
23.	B	48.	E
24.	C	49.	C
25.	E	50.	B

1. **The correct answer is E.** Pyruvate dehydrogenase (PDH) catalyzes the irreversible conversion of pyruvate to acetyl-CoA. If PDH is absent, pyruvate will be used in other pathways instead. Pyruvate will be converted to alanine via alanine aminotransferase (**choice A**) and to lactate via lactate dehydrogenase (**choice C**).

   Glutamate dehydrogenase (**choice B**) is involved in oxidative deamination, releasing ammonium ion for urea synthesis. Deficiency of this enzyme would not cause the symptoms described.

   Phenylethanolamine N-methyltransferase (**choice D**) is an enzyme involved in the synthesis of epinephrine. Deficiency of this enzyme would not cause the symptoms described.

2. **The correct answer is C.** This is Leigh's disease, a rare condition also known as subacute necrotizing encephalomyelopathy. The underlying problem is a defective form of cytochrome C oxidase, an electron transport chain component, in the mitochondria of muscle and brain. Clinically, the features described in the question stem are seen. Pathologically, there is a symmetric necrosis that affects central areas of the nervous system from the thalamus to the spinal cord. No effective treatment exists at this time.

   The Golgi apparatus (**choice A**) is involved in packaging materials for secretion outside the cell. You should associate the mucolipidosis I-cell disease with Golgi apparatus problems.

   Lysosomes (**choice B**) are the organelles that degrade many cellular products. Defects can produce a wide variety of lysosomal storage diseases, including Hurler and Hunter syndromes.

   Ribosomes (**choice D**) are the organelles that translate mRNA into proteins. There are no known diseases of ribosomes, probably because their function is so crucial that any problems produce death in utero.

   Hypertrophy of the smooth endoplasmic reticulum (**choice E**) in the liver is associated with conditions that stimulate the cytochrome P450 detoxification systems (e.g., barbiturate use and alcoholism).

3. **The correct answer is A.** These clumps are known as Heinz bodies, which are believed to be denatured hemoglobin caused by oxidative injury associated with a G6PD deficiency.

4. **The correct answer is G.** The correct name for these structures is Mallory bodies, and they are associated with Wilson disease or nutritional cirrhosis.

5. **The correct answer is E.** The porphyrin ring of heme is derived from the citric acid cycle intermediate succinyl-CoA and the amino acid glycine. The initial synthetic step, which is rate-limiting, is catalyzed by aminolevulinic acid synthase (ALA synthase).

   The other answer choices do not play a role in heme synthesis.

6. **The correct answer is D.** Deposition of xanthomas around the Achilles tendon is characteristic of familial type IIa hyperlipidemia, an autosomal dominant deficiency of the LDL receptor. The resultant reduced rate of LDL clearance leads to elevated LDL levels and hypercholesterolemia. For some poorly understood reason, arthritic pain in various joints, often prior to any appearance of xanthomas, is a characteristic of familial type IIa hyperlipidemia manifestation. Although Achilles tendonitis with associated xanthomas is common, other tendons may be involved. Symptoms in the heterozygous patient usually do not occur until the third or fourth decade, but homozygotes are affected much earlier, often in childhood. The patient was most likely treated with an HMG CoA reductase inhibitor such as simvastatin. Her condition carries a strong risk for cardiovascular disease. Although xanthomas are common in other familial hyperlipemias, such as type III and hepatic lipase deficiency, these are not associated with Achilles tendonitis.

   Chylomicron remnants (**choice A**) accumulate in familial type III hyperlipidemia (also known as familial dysbetalipoproteinemia) due to a lack of functional apolipoprotein E.

   Chylomicronemia (**choice B**) is associated with familial lipoprotein lipase deficiency (type I hyperlipoproteinemia). This rare autosomal recessive disease inhibits the clearance of the chylomicrons.

   HDLs (**choice C**) are the "good" lipoproteins; they have a protective effect against atherosclerosis. Their role is to take up free cholesterol from cell surfaces and circulating apolipoproteins.

   There is a tendency of VLDL (**choice E**) to be increased in several of the hyperlipoproteinemias, none of which produce the symptoms described. Familial type IV hyperlipidemia is probably the most significant, as it is associated with the hyperinsulinemia commonly observed in insulin-resistant, type 2 diabetes. The resultant concomitant increase in cholesterol and decrease in HDL lead to vascular disease, a critically important part of the insulin resistance syndrome.

7. **The correct answer is B.** Vitamin K acts as a coenzyme for glutamate carboxylase, which is an enzyme that catalyzes the carboxylation of glutamic acid side chains in several clotting factors (II, VII, IX, and X). Vitamin K deficiency can result in an accumulation of preprothrombin, a deficiency of prothrombin (hypoprothrombinemia), and an increase in clotting times.

Hemolytic anemia in newborns (**choice A**) can occur as a result of vitamin E, or tocopherol, deficiency. Vitamin E primarily acts as an antioxidant, protecting against peroxidation of polyunsaturated fatty acids in cellular membranes.

Vitamin B_{12}, or cobalamin, deficiency can lead to megaloblastic anemia (**choice C**), with or without associated nervous system neuropathy. This vitamin is required for two reactions in the human body: the methylation of homocysteine to methionine and the conversion of methylmalonyl-CoA to succinyl-CoA.

Folic acid deficiency is associated with megaloblastic anemia and neural tube defects in newborns (**choice D**). The coenzyme form of this vitamin is tetrahydrofolic acid, which acts as a carrier of one-carbon fragments in metabolism. A deficiency of folic acid is most commonly seen in pregnancy and alcoholism.

Vitamin D deficiency, which can occur either because of a lack of sunshine or with renal failure, can lead to osteomalacia in adults (**choice E**) and rickets in children. Vitamin D increases the intestinal absorption of calcium and phosphorus.

8. **The correct answer is D.** The patient has acute vitamin A deficiency, and the most serious complications are blindness and deafness.

    Choices A, B, and E are all conditions caused by deficiencies of other vitamins.

    Hypercarotenosis (**choice C**), caused by a large ingestion of vitamin A-containing foods, is the opposite of what the patient is suffering from.

9. **The correct answer is B.** The earliest symptom of vitamin A deficiency is night blindness.

    Choices A, D, and E are the late manifestations of this disease.

    Choice C is an early manifestation, but not the earliest.

10. **The correct answer is B.** Glucose-6-phosphate dehydrogenase disease is an X-linked condition. The father has a normal X chromosome since he does not have clinical disease. The mother has one normal X chromosome and one defective X chromosome, since her 6-year-old son has the disease and she does not. Therefore, the baby has a 50% chance of having two normal X chromosomes and a 50% chance of having one normal and one abnormal X chromosome, making her a carrier.

    Glucose-6-phosphate dehydrogenase deficiency is a defect in the pentose phosphate pathway of glucose metabolism, leading to defective production of reduced NADPH. Reduced NADPH is used in many biochemi-

cal pathways and is specifically used to regenerate the reduced form of glutathione that protects the body against oxidant drugs.

11. **The correct answer is B.** This question requires that you recognize the family of receptors that interact with G proteins to initiate a signal transduction cascade. These receptors are all glycosylated integral membrane proteins that have seven transmembrane segments. Beta-adrenergic receptors for epinephrine are an example.

    Adenylate cyclase (**choice A**) is an intracellular effector protein involved in signal transduction. It is not an integral membrane protein.

    The cystic fibrosis transmembrane conductance regulator channel (**choice C**) is a cyclic AMP-activated chloride channel.

    Glucose transporters (**choice D**) are integral membrane proteins with 12 membrane-spanning domains.

    Na^+/K^+ ATPase (**choice E**) pumps sodium into and potassium out of the cell. It provides energy for active transport by hydrolyzing ATP.

12. **The correct answer is B.** Tay-Sachs disease is a severe autosomal recessive disease characterized clinically by mental retardation, blindness, muscular weakness, and death by 3 years of age. The cherry-red spot is a classic clue for Tay-Sachs disease. The disease is prevalent in Ashkenazi (East European) Jews. Hexosaminidase A normally functions to hydrolyze a bond between N-acetylglucosamine and galactose in the polar head of the ganglioside GM_2, an N-acetylneuraminic acid-containing glycolipid found in high concentration in the brain. Without hexosaminidase A activity, this ganglioside accumulates, leading to degenerative CNS changes.

13. **The correct answer is D.** This patient has vitamin B_{12} deficiency (a COMLEX favorite). Absence of vitamin B_{12} as a cofactor in the conversion of methylmalonyl-CoA to succinyl-CoA results in the accumulation of methylmalonyl-CoA, which is subsequently excreted in the urine. Methylmalonyl-CoA mutase deficiency can also cause this type of aciduria.

    Vitamin B_{12}

    Methylmalonyl-CoA $\longrightarrow$ Succinyl-CoA

    Methylmalonyl-CoA mutase

    Argininosuccinic aciduria (**choice A**) can result from argininosuccinate lyase deficiency.

    Cystinuria (**choice B**) is the most common amino aciduria. It is an autosomal recessive disease, caused by a defect in the transport protein for lysine, arginine, cystine, and ornithine, that results in the excretion of these amino acids in the urine.

Hemoglobinuria (**choice C**) occurs with hemolytic anemias, not with megaloblastic anemia caused by vitamin B_{12} deficiency.

Propionic aciduria (**choice E**) can result from deficiency of biotin, propionyl-CoA carboxylase, or the enzyme that covalently attaches biotin to all carboxylases. In the latter case, additional organic acids accumulate as well.

14. **The correct answer is C.** Duchenne-type muscular dystrophy is the only disease listed that is X-linked; the other diseases are autosomal recessive. Remembering the genetics of myriad diseases is very problematic, but here are some imperfect rules of thumb that can help you out if you encounter an unfamiliar disease on an examination. Deficiencies of most enzymes are recessive (either autosomal or X-linked), since each person has at least two copies (from each of the parents) of each enzyme, and one working gene is usually enough (although careful evaluation of heterozygotes often shows mildly altered physiology). In contrast, alterations in structural proteins are often autosomal dominant, since having any amount of abnormal protein in structures such as basement membranes or in collagen tends to perturb their function. The number of common X-linked diseases (almost all recessive) is small and can be memorized: Duchenne muscular dystrophy, hemophilia A and B, chronic granulomatous disease, glucose-6-phosphate dehydrogenase deficiency, agammaglobulinemia, Wiskott-Aldrich syndrome, diabetes insipidus, Lesch-Nyhan syndrome, fragile X-syndrome, and color blindness.

Alpha$_1$-antitrypsin deficiency (**choice A**) is a deficiency of an enzyme (alpha$_1$-antitrypsin) that inhibits the action of various proteolytic enzymes. The two autosomal alleles for alpha$_1$-antitrypsin are codominantly expressed, such that they both contribute to the levels of circulating alpha$_1$-antitrypsin.

Cystic fibrosis (**choice B**) is an autosomal recessive disorder. The gene for cystic fibrosis has been localized to chromosome 7.

Phenylketonuria (**choice D**), in its classic form, is an autosomal recessive deficiency of phenylalanine hydroxylase.

Tay-Sachs disease (**choice E**) is caused by an autosomal recessive deficiency of the enzyme hexosaminidase A.

15. **The correct answer is D.** Galactosemia occurs in two very different clinical forms. Deficiency of galactokinase produces very mild disease; the only significant complication is cataract formation. In contrast, homozygous deficiency of galactose-1-phosphate uridyltransferase produces severe disease, culminating in death in infancy. In addition to galactosemia and galactosuria, these patients have impaired renal tubular resorption leading to aminoaciduria, gastrointestinal symptoms, hepa-

tosplenomegaly, cataracts, bleeding diatheses, hypoglycemia, and mental retardation. Pathologically, the CNS shows neuronal loss and gliosis, and the liver shows fatty change progressing to cirrhosis.

Benign disease with cataract formation (**choice A**) is characteristic of galactokinase deficiency.

Chronic emphysema (**choice B**) is not associated with homozygous galactose-1-phosphate uridyltransferase deficiency, but rather with alpha$_1$-antitrypsin deficiency.

Impaired tubular reabsorption (producing amino-aciduria) is seen within a few days or weeks of feeding milk to an infant with severe galactosemia, as opposed to chronic renal failure appearing in adolescence (**choice C**).

Gastrointestinal symptoms (**choice E**) certainly occur in homozygous galactose-1-phosphate uridyltransferase deficiency, but they would not be expected to remit with puberty. Instead, most untreated infants with this disorder show failure to thrive and die in infancy from wasting and inanition.

16. **The correct answer is B.** The process of glycolysis is defined as the sequence of reactions that converts glucose into pyruvate with the concomitant production of ATP.

Glycolysis begins when glucose is converted by hexokinase to glucose-6-phosphate. When this compound interacts with the enzyme phosphoglucose isomerase (**choice D**), fructose-6-phosphate is formed. Fructose-6-phosphate is then converted by phosphofructokinase (**choice C**) to form fructose 1,6-bisphosphate, which is subsequently converted to glyceraldehyde 3-phosphate by aldolase (**choice A**). After a number of enzymatic reactions, phosphoenolpyruvate is formed.

Phosphoenolpyruvate is converted to pyruvate by pyruvate kinase (**choice E**), and the glycolytic pathway is then completed.

17. **The correct answer is E.** The child is affected at birth, indicating in utero exposure to high levels of maternally derived phenylalanine. Women with PKU must strictly adhere to their special diet during pregnancy to avoid adversely affecting the fetus.

Even if the father is a carrier of PKU (**choice A**) and the child is homozygous for the PKU allele (phenylalanine hydroxylase gene), there would have been no symptoms in the infant until 4-5 days after birth, providing the maternal blood phenylalanine level was in the normal range throughout pregnancy.

Maternal translocation with unbalanced segregation in meiosis I (**choice B**) and maternal translocation with unbalanced segregation in meiosis II (**choice C**) would likely have no effect on phenylalanine levels but might lead to trisomy.

Maternal uniparental disomy (**choice D**) simply means that two copies of a chromosome are derived from the mother and implies paternal nullisomy. Although there are rare occurrences of uniparental disomy, this mechanism is not known to be involved in any case of PKU. If maternal uniparental disomy occurred, the child would be expected to have PKU, and as in **choice A**, symptoms would not occur until 4-5 days after birth.

18. **The correct answer is E.** This child probably has cystic fibrosis. In this disorder, an abnormality of chloride channels causes all exocrine secretions to be much thicker and more viscous than normal. Pancreatic secretion of digestive enzymes is often severely impaired, with consequent steatorrhea and deficiency of fat-soluble vitamins, including vitamin A.

Cystinuria (**choice A**) is a relatively common disorder in which a defective transporter for dibasic amino acids (cystine, ornithine, lysine, arginine; *COLA*) leads to saturation of the urine with cystine, which is not very soluble in urine, and precipitates out to form stones.

Hypoglycemia (**choice B**) is not a prominent feature in children with cystic fibrosis who are on a normal diet. Hyperglycemia may occur late in the course of the disease.

Iron deficiency anemia (**choice C**) is not regularly found in children with cystic fibrosis.

Sphingomyelin accumulation (**choice D**) is generally associated with deficiency of sphingomyelinase, as seen in Niemann-Pick disease.

19. **The correct answer is C.** Ketone bodies, which include acetoacetate, beta-hydroxybutyrate, and acetone, are produced by the liver in the fasting state by beta-oxidation of fatty acids. They are then released into the blood stream, where they can be used as alternative energy sources for other organs, such as muscle, kidney, and brain. The brain specifically still requires a small amount of circulating glucose to function, but the amount required is reduced when ketone bodies are available.

Apoprotein B (**choice A**) is one of the proteins that hold lipoproteins together.

Beta-carotene (**choice B**) is a vitamin with antioxidant properties.

C-reactive protein (**choice D**) is a serum protein produced by the liver that rises during infections and in inflammatory states.

Coenzyme A (**choice E**) is found in mitochondria and carries acetyl groups into the citric acid, or tricarboxylic acid, cycle.

20. **The correct answer is D.** The patient has alkaptonuria (ochronosis), a deficiency in the phenylalanine-tyrosine pathway that specifically blocks the metabolic degradation of homogentisic acid. The disease is hereditary (autosomal recessive) but does not typically become clinically evident until about the 4th decade of life, when the degenerative arthropathy becomes a problem.

Arylsulfatase A (**choice A**) is deficient in metachromatic leukodystrophy, one of the lysosomal storage diseases.

Glucose-6-phosphatase (**choice B**) is deficient in von Gierke disease, one of the glycogenoses.

Hexosaminidase A (**choice C**) is deficient in Tay-Sachs disease, one of the lysosomal storage diseases.

Muscle phosphorylase (**choice E**) is deficient in McArdle disease, one of the glycogenoses.

21. **The correct answer is E.** The patient has characteristics of Niemann-Pick disease, an autosomal-recessive condition caused by a deficiency of the enzyme sphingomyelinase. This condition is associated with mental retardation, hepatosplenomegaly, foam cells in the bone marrow, cherry red spots on the maculae in 40% of cases, and neurologic deficits. Furthermore, death by 3 years of age is common.

A deficiency of alpha-galactosidase (**choice A**) is associated with the X-linked disorder known as Fabry disease. This condition is characterized by renal failure, telangiectasia, skin rash, and pain in the lower extremities.

A deficiency of beta-glucocerebrosidase (**choice B**) is associated with the autosomal recessive disorder known as Gaucher disease. This condition is characterized by hepatosplenomegaly, neurologic deficits, and mental retardation.

Individuals with a deficiency of ceramidase (**choice C**) have Farber disease, which is associated with hoarseness, dermatitis, skeletal deformations, mental retardation, and hepatomegaly.

HMG-CoA reductase (**choice D**) is the enzyme that carries out the rate limiting step of cholesterol synthesis. Several agents used in the treatment of hyperlipidemia block the activity of this enzyme, resulting in a decrease in LDL and total cholesterol.

22. **The correct answer is A.** Ciprofloxacin, a quinolone derivative, inhibits DNA gyrase (prokaryotic topoisomerase II) essential for DNA replication. A mutation in the gene for DNA gyrase has made the enzyme insensitive to the effects of ciprofloxacin.

Folate synthesis (**choice B**) is inhibited by sulfamethoxazole, not ciprofloxacin.

mRNA translocation on a ribosome (**choice C**) is inhibited by erythromycin, not ciprofloxacin.

Peptide bond formation (**choice D**) is inhibited by chloramphenicol, not ciprofloxacin.

Reduction of folate to tetrahydrofolate (**choice E**) is inhibited by trimethoprim, not ciprofloxacin.

23. **The correct answer is B.** The "statins" are a class of medications that inhibit the activity of the enzyme HMG-CoA reductase. Medications such as pravastatin and simvastatin produce a reversible inhibition of this enzyme, which subsequently leads to a reduction in LDL, total cholesterol, and triglycerides in patients with familial hypercholesterolemia.

Chronic inflammation (**choice A**) can be effectively treated with cyclooxygenase inhibitors, including non-steroidal antiinflammatory drugs (NSAIDs), such as naproxen and ibuprofen, and cyclooxygenase-2 (COX-2) inhibitors, such as rofecoxib and celecoxib.

Essential hypertension (**choice C**) can be treated with angiotensin-converting enzyme (ACE) inhibitors, such as captopril. These agents decrease angiotensin production and reduce systolic and diastolic blood pressure.

Hyperuricemia (**choice D**) can be treated with allopurinol, which inhibits the activity of xanthine oxidase, leading to decreased production of uric acid.

One of the treatment measures for type 2 diabetes (**choice E**) is to inhibit the activity of the enzyme alpha-glucosidase. Acarbose, an alpha-glucosidase inhibitor, helps prevent postprandial surges in blood glucose levels.

24. **The correct answer is C.** Enlarged testes are the most specific phenotypic feature to suggest Fragile X syndrome in an individual who appears to have a hereditary mental retardation. The condition has unusual genetics, as it is related to expansion of a CGG repeat sequence located on the X chromosome. The larger the number of repeats, the higher the probability of significant retardation; hence, the retardation tends to become more severe in successive generations, as more CGG repeats accumulate. Sisters of affected males tend to show milder retardation than their brothers.

Features of Down syndrome (**choice A**), or trisomy 21, include mental retardation, epicanthal folds, dysplastic ears, hypotonia, a horizontal palmar crease (simian crease), redundant neck skin, and a short trunk.

Edwards syndrome (**choice B**), or trisomy 18, causes death in infancy. Characteristics include rocker-bottom feet, low-set ears, micrognathia, congenital heart disease, and mental retardation.

Klinefelter syndrome (47, XXY; **choice D**) is associated with testicular atrophy, a eunuchoid body shape, long extremities, and a small penis.

Turner syndrome (45, X; **choice E**) produces a female phenotype with short stature, ovarian dysgenesis, and webbing of the neck.

25. **The correct answer is E.** Even though the surface LDL receptors were digested by the trypsin, the recycling of unoccupied receptors to the cell surface provides a continual supply of new receptors to bind the labeled LDL. The LDL-receptor complex is internalized by receptor-mediated endocytosis.

Active transport (**choice A**) is the energy-dependent movement of molecules across a membrane and against a concentration gradient.

Facilitated diffusion (**choice B**) is the transport of low-permeability molecules with the aid of a carrier protein.

Phagocytosis (**choice C**) is the process by which cells such as macrophages and neutrophils engulf large particles.

Pinocytosis (**choice D**), which is the uptake of small molecules in solution, is receptor-independent.

26. **The correct choice is D.** This chromosomal aberration is known as Edwards syndrome, or trisomy 18. It is characterized by mental deficiency, growth retardation, prominent occiput, micrognathia, low-set ears, rocker-bottom feet, and ventricular septal defect.

XO (**choice A**) is the karyotype of Turner syndrome. It is characterized by short stature, webbed neck, and hypogonadism.

XXY (**choice B**) represents Klinefelter syndrome. It is usually undetected at birth but is characterized by tall stature, male hypogonadism, and sometimes mental retardation.

Trisomy 13 (Patau syndrome; **choice C**) is characterized by mental retardation, nervous system malformations, rocker-bottom feet, polydactyly, and cleft lip and palate.

Trisomy 21 (Down syndrome; **choice E**) is characterized by mental retardation, protruding tongue, simian crease, congenital heart defects, and a flat nasal bridge.

27. **The correct answer is D.** Peroxisomes are interesting cell organelles that were historically neglected because they are present in only small numbers in most mammalian cells. In the liver, however, these single membrane-bound organelles are present in large numbers and are important in detoxification and long chain fatty acid metabolism. The clinically important degradation of ethanol to (potentially toxic) acetaldehyde occurs in

humans in both peroxisomes and the smooth endoplasmic reticulum (P450 system). Disulfiram (Antabuse), used to discourage alcoholics from drinking, blocks the next reaction, in which acetaldehyde is oxidized to (nontoxic) acetate. This reaction, catalyzed by aldehyde dehydrogenase, occurs in the mitochondria.

Golgi bodies (**choice A**) are involved with packaging substances that are transported out of the cell.

Lysosomes (**choice B**) are sites of degradation of intracellular waste products.

The mitochondria (**choice C**) are involved with ATP production and contain both the electron transport chain and the citric acid (Krebs) cycle.

Ribosomes (**choice E**) are the sites of protein synthesis.

28. **The correct answer is D.** This is von Gierke disease, one of the glycogen storage diseases. The defect in glucose-6-phosphatase prevents release of glucose from glycogen across the liver cell membrane. The glucose-6-phosphate trapped in the liver cell is degraded to lactate and pyruvate, which are then released into the serum.

29. **The correct answer is D.** Smith-Lemli-Opitz syndrome is a recently described recessive genetic disease. It is the first single-gene (as opposed to trisomy or other gross chromosomal alterations) disease to be associated with multiple malformations. It presents with combinations of the following: microcephaly, mental retardation, hypotonia, incomplete development of the genitalia, high forehead, pyloric stenosis, and syndactyly of the second and third toes. The disease appears to have a carrier rate comparable to sickle cell disease or cystic fibrosis in selected populations (which are not yet well defined). Experiments reveal that nutritional therapies (such as the administration of vegetable oil supplemented by large amounts of cholesterol) begun within the first few weeks of life may markedly alter the course of this disease (unlike other devastating neurologic diseases that lack effective treatments).

Down syndrome (**choice A**), or trisomy 21, is a common cause of mental retardation, congenital heart disease, and premature aging.

Edwards syndrome (**choice B**), or trisomy 18, is a genetic defect that results in severely retarded infants who typically die within the first year of life. Characteristic features include micrognathia, a prominent occiput, congenital heart and kidney malformations, and low-set ears.

Patau syndrome (**choice C**), or trisomy 13, is characterized by severe mental retardation, microcephaly, microphthalmia, polydactyly, cleft lip and palate, renal defects, and cardiac abnormalities. Affected infants typically die before 1 year of age.

WAGR syndrome (**choice E**; for Wilms tumor, Aniridia, Genital anomalies, and mental Retardation) is associated with defects in several closely linked genes on chromosome 11.

30. **The correct answer is C.** Although ATP is important in cellular synthetic functions, its role in maintaining the Na^+/K^+ exchange across the plasmalemma is actually the most immediately important function for most cells. The direct effect of this is the energy (ATP) driven exchange of 3 Na^+ ions (which go from inside the cell to outside) for 2 K^+ ions (which go from outside to inside). This process requires considerable energy (1 ATP per $3Na^+/2K^+$ exchange), since both the Na^+ and K^+ are traveling against a concentration gradient. This direct effect of the Na^+/K^+ ATPase may seem trivial, but the secondary consequences are dramatic. The Na^+/K^+ ATPase helps establish the transmembrane potential of the cell (because the quantitatively uneven exchange of Na^+/K^+ drives more positive ions out of the cell than in), as well as both the Na^+ and K^+ gradients. All of these facilitate a wide variety of exchanges and transmembrane transport systems that allow entry into the cell of the large variety of small molecules and ions that it needs. The first microscopically visible effect of significant hypoxia is cellular edema, which is a consequence of distorted water balance, also an indirect function of the Na^+/K^+ ATPase.

31. **The correct answer is C.** Whenever the Step 1 exam specifies a patient's ethnic background, there is a good chance that it provides an important clue to the question. The patient described is an African American woman with symptoms and history suggestive of sickle cell anemia. The woman is experiencing the most frequent type of vaso-occlusive crisis seen in patients with this disease (infarctive). Crises may be precipitated by dehydration or infection. Hb electrophoresis is used to diagnose the illness, which is caused by an amino acid substitution of valine for glutamate in position 6 of the beta Hb chain. The resulting abnormal hemoglobin (HbS) tends to polymerize during low oxygen states, causing the red blood cells to assume a sickle shape.

Absence of central pallor (**choice A**) may be observed in patients with hereditary spherocytosis (usually autosomal dominant) resulting from abnormal red cell membrane proteins (e.g., spectrin, ankyrin). Spherocytes will exhibit increased osmotic fragility (**choice E**) because they have decreased surface area per unit volume.

Deletion of all four alpha genes (**choice B**) occurs in the most severe form of alpha thalassemia and is incompatible with life. It can result in hydrops fetalis and intrauterine death.

Heinz bodies (**choice D**) are clumps of Hb-degradation products seen when RBCs are stained with methylene blue. They are found in the peripheral blood smears of people with G6PD deficiency, especially common in males of Mediterranean or West African descent. Hemolysis occurs in response to oxidant stress that may be caused by drugs (e.g., antimalarials, sulfonamides, or nitrofurantoin) or the ingestion of fava beans.

32. **The correct answer is C.** The RFLP detects a region near the centromere of chromosome 21. The region around the centromere exhibits a phenomenon called crossover suppression. Since genetic exchange cannot happen in this area, the probe is a reliable marker for the individual chromosomes. During meiosis II, sister chromatids, which are two identical copies of the same chromosome, should separate. If a nondisjunction event occurs in this division, two copies of the same chromosome are passed to the progeny. In this case, both parents are heterozygous for the RFLP. The child received an A from the mother and two Cs from the father, leading us to conclude that the problem occurred in the father during meiosis II.

If a nondisjunction event of chromosome 21 occurs early in development, the result is a child who is a mosaic for trisomy 21 (**choice A**). This accounts for approximately 1% of children with trisomy 21. Since some of their cells are normal, these individuals show only a mild expression of the trisomy 21 phenotype.

During meiosis I, homologues that carry similar, but not identical, information separate. If a failure occurred in this division, we would expect the man to pass CD (**choice B**), and the woman to pass A or B, producing a child that was ACD or BCD.

If an AB woman had a failure in meiosis I (**choice D**), an AB gamete would be produced. When fertilized by the man's C or D sperm, a child that was ABC or ABD would result.

If an AB woman's sister chromatids failed to disjoin during meiosis II (**choice E**), AA or BB gametes would result. When fertilized by the CD male's sperm, a child that was AAC, AAD, BBC, or BBD would result.

33. **The correct answer is B.** The key to excelling in biochemistry on the COMLEX is to master the most clinically important elements of metabolic pathways, e.g., rate-limiting steps, irreversible steps, and steps involving enzymes affected by genetic diseases. In this case, glycogen phosphorylase is the enzyme involved in the rate-limiting step of glycogenolysis:

Glycogen phosphorylase

$$(Glucose)_n + P_i \longrightarrow (Glucose)_{n-1} + Glucose\text{-}1\text{-}P$$

Note that this enzyme is activated in response to the binding of glucagon to liver cell receptors or the binding of epinephrine to muscle receptors, via signal transduction.

α-1,4-Glucan transferase (**choice A**) is a debranching enzyme that removes three or four glucose units from a branch point and transfers them to the end of another chain. In this reaction, one α-1,4 bond is cleaved and another is formed. The elongated chain then becomes a substrate for glycogen phosphorylase.

Glycogen synthase (**choice C**) is the enzyme involved in the rate-limiting step of glycogen synthesis:

Glycogen synthase

$$(Glucose)_n + UDP\text{-}glucose \rightarrow (Glucose)_{n+1} + UDP$$

Note that this enzyme is inactivated in response to the binding of glucagon to liver cell receptors or the binding of epinephrine to muscle receptors.

Phosphoglucomutase (**choice D**) is a key enzyme in glycogen synthesis that reversibly converts glucose-6-phosphate to glucose-1-phosphate.

UDP-glucose pyrophosphorylase (**choice E**) is another key enzyme in glycogen synthesis:

UDP-glucose pyrophosphorylase

$$Glu\text{-}1\text{-}P + Uridine\text{-}P\text{-}P\text{-}P \longrightarrow UDP\text{-}Glu + PP_i$$

Note that the linkage formed between UDP and glucose is a high-energy bond that can provide energy to many biosynthetic reactions.

34. **The correct answer is E.** Following antineoplastic therapy for treatment of acute lymphocytic leukemia, patients often have a high level of urate secondary to the breakdown of nucleic acids. Therefore, patients are often given allopurinol to decrease plasma urate levels. Allopurinol prevents uric acid formation by inhibiting the enzyme xanthine oxidase. Decreasing uric acid levels will help prevent the formation of kidney stones as well as block the appearance of other deleterious effects of hyperuricemia.

Acarbose is an agent used in the treatment of type 2 diabetes. It inhibits the activity of alpha-glucosidase (**choice A**) in the intestinal tract, thereby helping to prevent postprandial hyperglycemia.

Inhibition of angiotensin-converting enzyme (**choice B**) will lower blood pressure and help prevent the "ventricular remodeling" that occurs secondary to congestive heart failure.

Beta-lactamase (**choice C**) inhibitors are combined with penicillin antibiotics to help improve their activity against bacteria that produce the enzyme beta-lactamase.

Nonsteroidal antiinflammatory drugs (NSAIDs) inhibit the activity of the enzyme cyclooxygenase (**choice D**), thereby decreasing the production of prostaglandins.

35. **The correct answer is D.** The combination of retardation and self-mutilation should lead you immediately to the diagnosis of Lesch-Nyhan disease. The hard part is remembering which enzyme is deficient in this disease. Hypoxanthine-guanine phosphoribosyltransferase (HGPRT) is part of the purine salvage pathway. A deficiency of this enzyme results in the inability to recycle purines and an overproduction of uric acid. Affected children are mentally retarded, have hyperuricemia and gout, and engage in compulsive self-destructive behaviors.

Deficiency of cystathionine synthase (**choice A**) results in homocystinuria, a disease characterized by elevated urinary homocystine. Afflicted children typically present with failure to thrive and visual problems due to lens displacement. In addition to cystathionine synthase deficiency, other causes of homocystinuria include methionine synthase deficiency and deficiency of pyridoxine, folate, or vitamin B_{12}.

Deficiency of hexosaminidase A (**choice B**) causes Tay-Sachs disease. This enzymatic deficiency results in the accumulation of GM_2 ganglioside. Clinical characteristics include mental retardation, blindness, and muscular weakness. A characteristic feature is the presence of a cherry-red spot on the macula. Remember that this disease is more common in Ashkenazi Jews and typically results in death by 3 years of age.

Deficiency of homogentisic acid oxidase (**choice C**), an enzyme involved in the degradation of tyrosine, results in a condition known as alkaptonuria. The classic finding of this typically benign disease is dark urine. There can also be darkening of connective tissue (e.g., ear cartilage may appear bluish).

Deficiency of phenylalanine hydroxylase (**choice E**) is one cause of phenylketonuria (PKU). Phenylalanine hydroxylase catalyzes the conversion of phenylalanine to tyrosine. In patients with PKU, tyrosine becomes an essential amino acid. Children with PKU have mental retardation, fair skin, and a characteristically musty body odor. (Note: if you see the adjective "musty" on the COMLEX, the answer is usually PKU.)

36. **The correct answer is A.** The presentation and autopsy findings are consistent with metachromatic leukodystrophy. The crystals in the macrophages that stained brown with toluidine blue are sulfatides, which accumulate in this disorder. The color shift seen in the toluidine blue stain is termed *metachromasia* (hence the term metachromatic leukodystrophy). The cause of metachromatic leukodystrophy is deficiency of arylsulfatase A.

Galactocerebroside β-galactosidase (**choice B**) deficiency produces Krabbe disease. In this disorder, multinucleated cells derived from macrophages (globoid cells) are seen around blood vessels. Electron microscopy of the macrophages reveals the presence of linear inclusions.

Glucocerebrosidase (**choice C**) deficiency results in Gaucher disease, characterized by accumulation of glucocerebrosides. Gaucher cells are distended with material that resembles crumpled tissue paper.

Hexosaminidase A (**choice D**) deficiency is associated with Tay Sachs disease, characterized by accumulation of GM_2 ganglioside in the central and autonomic nervous systems.

Sphingomyelinase deficiency (**choice E**) produces Niemann-Pick disease, in which sphingomyelin accumulates, especially in cells of the mononuclear phagocytic system.

37. **The correct answer is D.** Cystic fibrosis is an autosomal recessive disease caused by point mutations or small deletions in the gene encoding an integral membrane protein that functions as a chloride transporter. Although many mutations within the gene cause the phenotype, it is not practical or cost-effective to sequence the entire region to screen for a carrier. In the white population, however, the most frequent mutant allele causing cystic fibrosis is due to a small deletion at phenylalanine 508 in exon 10 on chromosome 7. This mutation accounts for greater than 50% of mutant cystic fibrosis alleles in white populations. An amplification of this region using the polymerase chain reaction (PCR) can be done, and the PCR products are sequenced and compared against the normal sequence for this region. If comparison reveals the deletion, the donor of that template DNA would be classified as a carrier. If the mutation is not present, the probability that the DNA donor is a carrier of cystic fibrosis is greatly reduced, but still exists. Most diagnostic laboratories will use this method to screen for between 4 and 10 of the most common mutations. Note that if a person belongs to a different ethnic group, PCR must be used to amplify the exons that contain the majority of cystic fibrosis mutations within that particular ethnic group.

Biochemical testing (**choice A**) is usually used to detect a defective enzyme or a reduced amount of the normal enzyme. It is more economical than DNA testing for detecting carriers or affected individuals. It is used in the detection of carriers of autosomal recessive diseases, such as Tay-Sachs disease, sickle cell anemia, and the thalassemias.

Fluorescence *in situ* hybridization (FISH; **choice B**) uses a DNA probe that has been labeled with a fluorescent compound to visualize locations on the chromosomes that have homology to the probe. It can be used to detect microdeletions in a gene of interest.

Karyotype analysis (**choice C**) is used to determine whether an individual's chromosomes are grossly normal in their number and structure. It can be used to detect trisomies, monosomies, and translocations, as well as large inversions and deletions.

Western blot analysis (**choice E**) is a technique commonly used to detect the presence of antibody against specific proteins in serum. It is primarily used as a confirmatory test for HIV infection.

38. **The correct answer is A.** The patient is presenting with signs and symptoms highly suggestive of type 1 diabetes. The primary source of ketones in the urine is free fatty acid breakdown. Ketone body formation occurs as follows: insulin deficiency → activated lipolysis → increased plasma free fatty acids → increased hepatic fatty acids → accelerated ketogenesis. In summary, as fatty acids break down, acetyl-CoA is generated. As acetyl-CoA levels increase, ketone bodies begin to form. When excessive amounts of ketone bodies are formed, the pathologic state known as ketosis can occur.

Gluconeogenesis (**choice B**) and glycogenolysis (**choice C**) occur when glucose is needed for the production of ATP in various cells in the body.

Protein breakdown (**choice D**) results in the formation of amino acids.

Triglyceride breakdown (**choice E**) results in the release of free fatty acids.

39. **The correct answer is C.** Taken together, severe neonatal jaundice, elevated indirect bilirubin, and exchange blood transfusion strongly suggest hemolysis. The hemoglobin and hematocrit values are low and reticulocytosis is present, indicating an anemia. Thus, this infant has a hemolytic anemia. Increased levels of 2,3-BPG, 3-PG, 2-PG, and PEP (all distal glycolysis intermediates) are consistent with a block in glycolysis below phosphoenolpyruvate. Only a hemolytic anemia induced by a PK deficiency meets all these criteria. Hemolytic anemias have been reported in association with deficiencies of most of the enzymes of glycolysis. Most are quite rare, but PK deficiency is the most common. There are many variant forms of PK deficiency, some affecting K_m, some V_{max}, and some allosteric regulation. Most have a relatively mild clinical symptomology limited to the red cell. The tissue specificity is a consequence of the fact that there is a red-cell–specific PK isozyme. The relative lack of severe symptoms is a consequence of the fact that many of the aberrations affect kinetic parameters rather than total

activity and because the body compensates with accelerated RBC production and the high 2,3 DPG level. The latter causes the hemoglobin to dump oxygen at a lower partial oxygen pressure.

G6PD deficiency (**choice A**) is the most common enzymatic effect causing hemolytic anemia. Over 300 different mutant forms of G6PD have been described, but only the "African" and the "Mediterranean" are common. Patients with either of these have few symptoms under normal conditions but can go into a hemolytic crisis when stressed by certain oxidizing drugs and infections, and in the case of the Mediterranean variant, by fava beans. In none of these variants do glycolytic intermediates accumulate.

Lead is a heavy metal that tends to bind to enzymes with multiple sulfhydryl groups, for example, pyruvate dehydrogenase and α-ketoglutarate dehydrogenase. Because of the key role these enzymes have in energy metabolism, lead poisoning (**choice B**) has multiple organ effects. The brain in particular is vulnerable because of its dependency on glucose. In this organ, lead poisoning causes delayed or inhibited development, permanent learning disabilities, and in acute cases, seizures, coma, and even death. Lead also lowers the hemoglobin level by interfering with the dehydration of aminolevulinic acid and the incorporation of iron into the protoporphyrin molecule. Thus, chronic lead poisoning will cause an anemia, but it will not be a hemolytic one.

Sickle cell anemia (**choice D**) is the most common hemoglobinopathy. It, like the common forms of glucose 6-phosphate dehydrogenase deficiency, provides a partial protection against malaria. The molecular defect is a substitution of glutamate by valine on position six of the beta-chain. The resultant product can form a tetramer with the alpha chains and is called hemoglobin-S (HbS). HbS has a low solubility in the deoxy form, and it precipitates when subjected to a low oxygen partial pressure. This causes red cells to sickle. These sickled cells can then block small vessels and cause a myriad of problems. Glycolytic intermediates do not accumulate.

β-Thalassemia (**choice E**) results from reduced synthesis of the hemoglobin β-chain. This leads to an excess of α-globin chains, which precipitate and prevent nascent red cells from maturing. Since there are two copies of the β-globin gene, some individuals only have one affected gene (β-thalassemia minor), whereas others have defects in both genes (β-thalassemia major). Individuals with β-thalassemia minor are essentially asymptomatic while those with β-thalassemia major require transfusions on a regular basis after their first or second year. Symptoms of anemia are delayed because the β-globin gene is not expressed until shortly before birth and fetal hemoglobin continues to be produced in the neonate. There is no accumulation of glycolytic intermediates.

40. **The correct answer is D.** This is a classic case of lead poisoning: chewing on paint chips, abdominal pain, and red blood cells with basophilic stippling. A related physical finding you would expect is lead lines at the gingival margins. X-ray films of the long bones would reveal increased radiodensity at the epiphyses.

Arsenic poisoning (**choice A**) acutely causes hemorrhagic gastroenteritis, fluid loss, and hypotension. Nausea, vomiting, abdominal pain, seizures, or coma may occur. The breath may exhibit a garlicky odor.

Cyanide poisoning (**choice B**) causes death within minutes. Generalized petechiae and a bitter almond smell are characteristic.

Gold toxicity (**choice C**) causes erythema and pruritus, as well as damage to hematopoietic organs.

Mercury toxicity (**choice E**) acutely causes lassitude, anorexia, and gastrointestinal symptoms. Chronic exposure produces emotional lability, memory loss and excitability (Mad Hatter disease), and polyneuropathies.

41. **The correct answer is E.** Folate (as 7,8-dihydrofolate) is converted to tetrahydrofolate by dihydrofolate reductase. Methotrexate is a competitive inhibitor of dihydrofolate reductase. Therefore, providing sufficiently high concentrations of folate will allow the enzyme to reach the same V_{max} as obtained in the absence of inhibitor.

Increasing substrate concentration would not increase (**choice A**) or decrease (**choice C**) the affinity (K_m) for the substrate dihydrofolate.

The V_{max} would not increase above the uninhibited V_{max} (compare with **choice B**) in the absence of methotrexate.

Increasing substrate concentration would not increase the affinity for methotrexate (**choice D**).

42. **The correct answer is D.** The patient is suffering from scurvy. Because he is edentulous, the classic picture (bleeding gums) is not seen. Instead, the description given is a good characterization of scurvy in this patient.

The fact there were no other hematologic abnormalities rules out **choice A**.

Although **choices B and C** also could result in ecchymosis and bleeding, it is unlikely that as an alcoholic he would be suffering from a condition other than a vitamin C or thiamine deficiency. It is highly unlikely that he would be suffering from iron or vitamin B_{12} deficiency.

Choice E presents with diarrhea and irritability.

43. **The correct answer is D.** The patient described has scurvy, resulting from a deficiency of dietary vitamin C. Absence of vitamin C leads to impaired hydroxylation of proline residues in the nascent procollagen chains, leading to weakness of blood vessel walls. Clinically, the deficiency syndrome is characterized by perifollicular hemorrhages, fragmentation of hairs, purpura, ecchymoses, splinter hemorrhages, and hemorrhages into muscle. In patients with normal dentition, gum changes (swelling, bleeding, loosening of teeth) are also noted. Without vitamin C supplementation, death may eventually occur.

Administration of factor VIII (**choice A**) would be indicated for factor VIII deficiency. This deficiency would also lead to a prolonged partial thromboplastin time (PTT), which was not noted.

Administration of iron (**choice B**) would be of benefit in iron-deficiency anemia, but there is no indication of a hypochromic, microcytic anemia in this patient. The anemia of scurvy is typically normochromic and normocytic because of bleeding.

Administration of vitamin B_{12} (**choice C**) would be indicated for a megaloblastic anemia. Although a macrocytic anemia may be observed in scurvy (because of concomitant dietary folate deficiency or perturbations in the folate pool), this patient did not show macrocytosis.

Administration of vitamin K (**choice E**) would be appropriate in the setting of vitamin K deficiency, which would produce a prolonged prothrombin time (PT), followed eventually by a prolonged PTT as the vitamin K-dependent factors (II, VII, IX, X, protein C, and protein S) are depleted.

44. **The correct answer is A.** Hereditary nonpolyposis colorectal cancer (HNPCC) is an autosomal dominant condition causing early colorectal cancer, often before the age of 50. Female relatives are also at high risk for endometrial and ovarian cancer. Nearly 90% of cases of HNPCC are linked to mutations in mismatch repair genes such as hMLH1 and hMSH2. The proteins encoded by these genes function during G2 of the cell cycle to repair areas of DNA with mismatched bases introduced during DNA replication. Dinucleotide (microsatellite) repeat instability is characteristic of tumor cells in HNPCC.

A point mutation in the gene coding for an excision exonuclease (**choice B**) is characteristic of xeroderma pigmentosum.

A reciprocal translocation between chromosomes 8 and 14 (**choice C**) is characteristic of Burkitt lymphoma. This translocation occurs near the *myc* gene and results in transcriptional activation of *myc*. There is a strong association between Burkitt lymphoma and infection with the Epstein-Barr virus.

Loss of the RB tumor suppressor gene (**choice D**) causes retinoblastoma. The RB gene products normally regulate the G1 to S transition, thereby promoting differentiation and inhibiting unrestricted cellular division. Mutations causing loss of RB gene function are usually inherited as a dominant trait. This also is true of tumor suppressor genes in general. The sequence of events follows: A defective allele is inherited, and then the second allele becomes mutated as an early somatic event. This leads to a high incidence of that cancer at an early age. Sporadic nonfamilial retinoblastomas are also reported. These usually occur at a later age and only affect one eye.

Mutations do not come from the match repair system (**choice E**) because this is a normal system.

45. **The correct answer is B.** Deficiencies of the enzyme hexosaminidase A result in Tay-Sachs disease, an autosomal-recessive disorder characterized by mental retardation, blindness, muscular weakness, and the appearance of a cherry red spot on the macula. Death by 3 years of age is common. This condition is most commonly seen in Ashkenazi Jews. Tay-Sachs can best be described as a gangliosidosis, since ganglioside GM_2 accumulates.

An example of an aminoacidopathy (**choice A**) would be the autosomal recessive phenylalanine hydroxylase deficiency associated with phenylketonuria.

Lipid metabolism (**choice C**) disorders often involve a defect at the LDL receptor. These types of disorders can be seen in patients with the autosomal dominant disorder familial hypercholesterolemia.

An example of a mucopolysaccharidosis (**choice D**) is an X-linked recessive deficiency of iduronate sulfatase, or Hunter syndrome.

Acute intermittent porphyria (**choice E**) is an autosomal dominant disorder involving a biochemical defect of porphobilinogen deaminase.

46. **The correct answer is C.** Hypoglycemia with hypoketosis after fasting suggests a block in fatty acid oxidation. Accumulation of organic dicarboxylic acids further indicates a fatty acyl-CoA dehydrogenase deficiency; most commonly this will be a medium chain acyl CoA dehydrogenase (MCAD) deficiency. MCAD deficiency is an autosomal recessive disease expressed with high frequency among people of Northern European descent. Homozygous individuals are unable to break down fatty acids, and so cannot use fat for energy production when glucose supplies are limited. This blockage may also lead to a secondary carnitine deficiency because the accumulated acyl-CoA is transesterified to produce acyl carnitine.

Because carnitine is required to transport fatty acids into mitochondria for oxidation, this also will increase tissue dependence on glucose metabolism. Because ketogenesis also depends on fatty acid catabolism, the brain has no source of ketones to use as an alternative fuel. Whether due to the primary block, the induced carnitine deficiency, or a combination of the two, the net result is acute hypoglycemia whenever glucose is not readily available. Symptoms most commonly appear between two months and two years, but they may be noted as early as two days or as late as six years, and on occasion, asymptomatic parents have first been diagnosed after one of their children have an episode. Generally, symptoms appear after a period of dietary carbohydrate deficiency; presumably, this is what happened in this boy due to his gastroenteritis. It has been estimated that MCAD accounts for about 1% of deaths due to sudden infant death syndrome (SIDS), and about 20% of children with MCAD die after the first episode. The hypoglycemia can occur quickly, and CNS symptoms become marked when venous blood glucose levels drop to about 20 mg/dL (0.11 mM). The mainstay of treatment is to remain well fed on a high carbohydrate diet. Some physicians also prescribe L-carnitine, which is claimed to help maintain blood glucose levels during sickness or other forms of stress.

Glucose 6-phosphatase deficiency (**choice A**) is a glycogen storage disease that will also lead to a fasting hypoglycemia, but ketone bodies would accumulate, and there would be no accumulation of organic dicarboxylic acids.

Hepatic glycogen phosphorylase deficiency (**choice B**) is a glycogen storage disease that will also lead to a mild fasting hypoglycemia with formation of ketone bodies, but without accumulation of organic dicarboxylic acids.

Mitochondrial carbamoyl phosphate synthetase deficiency (**choice D**) is a urea cycle enzyme deficiency disease that will cause hyperammonemia, not hypoglycemia, and accumulation of organic dicarboxylic acids.

Ornithine transcarbamoylase deficiency (**choice E**) is also a urea cycle enzyme deficiency disease that will cause hyperammonemia, rather than hypoglycemia, and accumulation of organic dicarboxylic acids.

47. **The correct answer is C.** The patient is presenting with the classic signs and symptoms of von Gierke disease, which is an autosomal recessive genetic disorder that usually manifests in the first 12 months of life. Laboratory evaluation often reveals the presence of increased lactate, cholesterol, triglyceride, and uric acid levels. This condition is caused by a basic enzyme defect involving glucose-6-phosphatase deficiency.

Brancher enzyme deficiency (**choice A**), otherwise known as Anderson disease, is associated with infantile failure to thrive, cirrhosis, liver failure, and extreme hypotonia.

Debrancher enzyme deficiency **(choice B),** also known as Cori disease, is characterized by hypoglycemia, hepatomegaly, short-stature, and myopathy. Laboratory evaluation often reveals the presence of normal lactate and uric acid and increased cholesterol and triglyceride levels.

Hepatic phosphorylase deficiency **(choice D)**, otherwise known as Hers disease, is associated with hepatomegaly and variable hypoglycemia.

Muscle phosphorylase deficiency **(choice E),** or McArdle disease, causes pain, cramps, and myoglobinuria on strenuous exercise. It is associated with episodes of increased creatine kinase and deficient lactate production.

48. **The correct answer is E.** This question is a "two-step" item, which is common on the COMLEX. First, you need to figure out from the clinical clues which vitamin deficiency you are dealing with. Next, you need to remember which enzymes utilize the deficient vitamin as a cofactor.

This patient has all the signs of Wernicke encephalopathy—a favorite Step 1 disease characterized by dementia, ataxia, and ophthalmoplegia. This disease typically occurs in alcoholics and is the result of thiamine deficiency. Thiamine pyrophosphate (TPP), the activated form of thiamine, is a cofactor in the oxidative decarboxylation of α-ketoacids. The four major enzymes requiring TPP are pyruvate dehydrogenase (pyruvate to acetyl-CoA; links glycolysis to TCA cycle), α-ketoglutarate dehydrogenase (TCA cycle), branched-chain ketoacid dehydrogenase (involved in metabolism of branched-chain amino acids; deficiency results in maple syrup urine disease), and transketolase (hexose monophosphate shunt).

Aspartate aminotransferase **(choice A)** is a transaminase involved in the transfer of the α-amino group from aspartate. The transaminases are a family of enzymes involved in amino acid degradation; they transfer the α-amino group from an amino acid to an α-ketoacid receptor (usually α-ketoglutarate). The transaminases require pyridoxal phosphate, a derivative of pyridoxine (vitamin B_6), as a cofactor.

Methylmalonyl-CoA mutase **(choice B)** catalyzes the conversion of methylmalonyl-CoA (a product of fatty acid oxidation and branched-chain amino acid catabolism) to succinyl-CoA, which can then enter the TCA cycle. This enzyme is one of two reactions in humans that requires deoxyadenosylcobalamin, the activated form of vitamin B_{12}, as a cofactor. The other is methionine synthase, which converts homocysteine to methi-

onine. Recall that vitamin B_{12} is absorbed in the stomach and that absorption requires intrinsic factor produced by gastric parietal cells. The classic finding of B_{12} deficiency is megaloblastic anemia. Peripheral neuropathy may also occur.

Prolyl hydroxylase **(choice C)** catalyzes the hydroxylation of prolyl residues in collagen biosynthesis. Along with lysyl hydroxylase, it requires vitamin C as a cofactor. Deficiency of vitamin C inhibits the cross-linking of collagen fibers, resulting in a condition known as scurvy. Scurvy is characterized by poor wound healing, fragile blood vessels, bleeding gums, and loose teeth.

Pyruvate carboxylase **(choice D)** catalyzes the first step in gluconeogenesis—the carboxylation of pyruvate to oxaloacetate. Biotin serves as the carrier of the "activated carboxyl" group in this reaction, as well as in the carboxylation reactions catalyzed by acetyl-CoA carboxylase (fatty acid synthesis) and propionyl-CoA carboxylase (branched-chain amino acid catabolism and odd-chain fatty acid oxidation).

49. **The correct answer is C.** Glycogen is the storage form of glucose and a readily mobilizable fuel store. When individuals do not consume adequate quantities of carbohydrates, the body responds by breaking down glycogen stores in the liver to maintain normal blood glucose levels. The two enzymes involved in the degradation and synthesis of glycogen are glycogen phosphorylase **(choice C)** and glycogen synthase **(choice D)**, respectively. The processes of glycogen synthesis and degradation are coordinated by a hormone-triggered cascade that ensures that when one enzyme is active, the other enzyme is inactive.

Acetyl-CoA carboxylase **(choice A)** is the key enzyme involved in fatty acid synthesis.

Glucose-6-phosphate dehydrogenase **(choice B)** is involved in the pentose phosphate pathway.

Thiolase **(choice E)** converts acetoacetyl-CoA into acetyl-CoA.

50. **The correct answer is B.** Locus heterogeneity refers to the situation in which the same phenotype is caused by defects in different genes. It is commonly seen in syndromes resulting from failures in a complex pathway, such as hearing. In this example, locus heterogeneity is indicated because of complementation. In generations I through III, deafness appears to be due to a single autosomal recessive trait. In generation IV, deaf parents produce normal hearing children, suggesting that the parents have defects in different genes. The children are heterozygous at both loci and so have normal hearing (complementation).

Autosomal dominant inheritance (**choice A**) would require multiple assumptions. In generation IV, the parents produce six normal children, although at best they are both heterozygous for the trait. The probability of that event, given that they are both heterozygous, is $(1/4)^6$. Even more troublesome is the mating between II-1 and II-2, in which normal parents produce affected children. Although it is possible that the gene is an autosomal dominant with incomplete penetrance, no data about this frequency are given, and this hypothesis still requires many more assumptions than the correct answer. Penetrance is the frequency at which the phenotype is expressed in a person who carries a particular genotype. It can complicate pedigree analysis.

Mitochondrial inheritance (**choice C**) would show a completely different pattern. Genetic information is transmitted to progeny on nuclear chromosomes, as well as on mitochondrial chromosomes. Since mitochondria are inherited only from the mother, if affected, she will give the trait to all of her progeny. A male with the trait will never transmit it to his progeny.

Multifactorial inheritance (**choice D**) is a nonmendelian inheritance pattern that depends on the incremental contributions of multiple loci to a single phenotype, as well as on contributions from environmental factors. Characteristics that exhibit a broad range of values, like height or eye color, are inherited in this manner.

X-linked dominant inheritance (**choice E**) affects either sex, but which of the children are affected depends on the sex of the affected parent. If the male parent is affected, he will produce only affected daughters and normal sons, because he gives his X chromosome to all of his daughters and none of his sons. If the female parent is affected, she contributes an X chromosome to both daughters and sons; hence, both can be affected. However, since she is almost always heterozygous for the trait, the probability is 50% that her children will receive a normal X chromosome. Remember that human females randomly inactivate one of their X chromosomes (Lyon hypothesis). Because of this inactivation, a female who is heterozygous for an X-linked dominant trait will tend to be both more mildly and more variably affected then a male with the same trait.

Biochemistry

1. A 3-year-old girl who is small for her age has had multiple hypoglycemic episodes associated with moderate fasting during periods of illness. In her most recent episode associated with influenza, her parents slept late, and at 10 AM were unable to rouse the child from sleep. Blood and urine samples collected at the emergency department reveal marked hypoglycemia, ketonuria, and ketonemia along with an appropriately low insulin level. The blood alanine level is abnormally low; however, infusion of alanine produces a rapid rise in blood glucose. The defect most likely responsible for these symptoms is found in which of the following pathways?

   (A) Gluconeogenesis

   (B) Glycogenolysis

   (C) Protein catabolism in muscle

   (D) Triglyceride hydrolysis in adipose tissue

   (E) β-Oxidation of fatty acids

2. A 60-year-old man complains of difficulty arising from a chair and initiating new movements. On examination, the physician notices a resting hand tremor and cogwheel rigidity. Osteopathic structural examination reveals no hip joint abnormalities. There are tissue-texture changes throughout the body. Which of the following amino acids is the precursor for the neurotransmitter that is deficient in the brain of this patient?

   (A) Glutamate

   (B) Glycine

   (C) Histidine

   (D) Tryptophan

   (E) Tyrosine

3. A patient has a pyruvate kinase deficiency. Which of the following diseases is clinically similar?

   (A) α-Thalassemia

   (B) β-Thalassemia

   (C) Glucose-6-phosphate dehydrogenase deficiency

   (D) Hereditary spherocytosis

   (E) Iron deficiency anemia

4. Your patient has recently developed an acid-base imbalance. Which of the following pairs of chemicals plays the most important role in extracellular and intracellular buffering?

	Extracellular fluid	Intracellular fluid
(A)	Bicarbonate	Calcium
(B)	Bicarbonate	Phosphate
(C)	Calcium	Phosphate
(D)	Phosphate	Bicarbonate
(E)	Phosphate	Calcium

5. A 40-year-old, formerly obese woman presents to her physician. She was very proud of having lost 80 lb during the previous 2 years, but has now noticed that her "hair is falling out." On questioning, she reports having followed a strict, fat-free diet. Her alopecia is probably related to a deficiency of which of the following vitamins?

   (A) A

   (B) C

   (C) D

   (D) E

   (E) K

6. Your patient has a genetic defect that doesn't allow the pentose phosphate pathway to shunt properly. Which of the following intermediates would be directly affected?

   (A) Fructose-1,6-bisphosphate
   (B) Fructose-6-phosphate
   (C) Glucose-6-phosphate
   (D) Phosphoenolpyruvate
   (E) Pyruvate

7. Uncontrollable bleeding from the umbilical stump of a neonate specifically suggests deficiency of which of the following coagulation factors?

   (A) Factor VIII
   (B) Factor IX
   (C) Factor XII
   (D) Factor XIII
   (E) Von Willebrand factor

8. A 25-year old woman with type 1 diabetes mellitus has maintained good glycemic control for several years. Recently she has gained 10 pounds and joined a group exercise program. By the end of her first 1-hour aerobics session, she is dizzy, nauseated, and feels faint. Physical examination reveals that T1-T9 have chronic paraspinal tissue texture changes. Which underlying mechanism is the most likely explanation for this episode?

   (A) Inadequate delivery of oxygen to the muscle
   (B) Stimulation of gluconeogenesis in the liver
   (C) Stimulation of glycogenolysis in liver
   (D) Stimulation of glycogenolysis in muscle
   (E) Translocation of GLUT4 to the cell membranes of myocytes

9. After a routine lab test, albumin is found to be lower than the normal value. Which of the following mechanisms does albumin reach the plasma through?

   (A) Clathrin-coated pits
   (B) Constitutive exocytosis
   (C) Pinocytosis
   (D) Receptor-mediated endocytosis
   (E) Regulated exocytosis

10. An infant diagnosed with phenylketonuria would be expected to be deficient in which of the following non-essential amino acids, assuming that it is not obtained from dietary sources?

    (A) Asparagine
    (B) Cysteine
    (C) Glutamine
    (D) Proline
    (E) Tyrosine

11. A patient has been diagnosed with an increased risk for myocardial infarction. Which of the following enzymes is most closely related to the role of folate in lowering the risk of cardiovascular disease?

    (A) Dihydrofolate reductase
    (B) Glycinamide ribonucleotide transformylase
    (C) Homocysteine methyltransferase
    (D) Ribonucleotide reductase
    (E) Thymidylate synthase

12. A 9-year-old girl with mild mental retardation was healthy at birth but presented during the first week of life with vomiting, lethargy, seizures, and hypertonia. An amino acid screen revealed elevated levels of leucine, isoleucine, and valine, so the child was put on a special diet restricted in these amino acids. She has had no medical problems related to her disease since that time. Which of the following enzymes is most likely deficient in this child?

    (A) Branched chain ketoacid dehydrogenase
    (B) Cystathionine synthase
    (C) Methylmalonyl CoA mutase
    (D) Ornithine transcarbamoylase
    (E) Propionyl CoA carboxylase

13. A 2-month-old boy is evaluated for failure to thrive. As the pediatrician is examining the patient, she witnesses a seizure. Structural examination reveals somatic dysfunction at T5-T8 and T11-L1. Physical examination is remarkable for hepatomegaly, a finding later confirmed by CT scan, which also reveals renomegaly. Serum chemistries demonstrate severe hypoglycemia, hyperlipidemia, lactic acidosis, and ketosis. Which of the following diagnoses best accounts for this presentation?

    (A) Gaucher disease
    (B) McArdle disease
    (C) Niemann-Pick disease
    (D) Pompe disease
    (E) Von Gierke disease

14. A patient with cancer asks about the toxic effects of the unconventional anticancer agent Laetrile, which is metabolized to cyanide. These toxic effects are probably due to an inhibition of which of the following enzymes?

    (A) 2,3-Bisphosphoglycerate mutase
    (B) Cytochrome oxidase
    (C) Guanylate cyclase
    (D) Na$^+$/K$^+$-ATPase
    (E) Phosphofructokinase-2

15. A 2-year-old child is brought to the pediatrician because of hematuria. Examination reveals hypertension and an abdominal mass. An osteopathic structural examination reveals T12 FRS$_R$. A tumor is localized to the right kidney, and biopsy reveals a stroma containing smooth and striated muscle, bone, cartilage, and fat, with areas of necrosis. The gene for this disorder has been localized to which of the following chromosomes?

    (A) 5
    (B) 11
    (C) 13
    (D) 17
    (E) 22

16. A jealous husband is concerned that his wife had an affair with her best friend's husband and that he is not the biologic father of their 7-month-old child. Restriction fragment length polymorphism (RFLP) analysis is performed on DNA samples from the two couples and from their two children (each couple has one child). The ethidium bromide-stained agarose gel used to separate the fragments is shown below. Which conclusion can be drawn from these results?

W$_1$ = wife 1; H$_1$ = husband 1; C$_1$ = child 1
W$_2$ = wife 2; H$_2$ = husband 2; C$_2$ = child 2

    (A) Husband 1 is the father of child 1
    (B) Husband 1 is the father of child 2
    (C) Husband 2 is the father of both children
    (D) Husband 2 is the father of child 1
    (E) Husband 2 is the father of child 2

17. The enzyme hypoxanthine guanine phosphoribosyl transferase (HGPRT) isolated from a child with Lesch-Nyhan syndrome is compared with HGPRT isolated from a healthy control individual. The results are shown in the graph below. Which of the following is the best conclusion about the HGPRT from the child with Lesch-Nyhan disease?

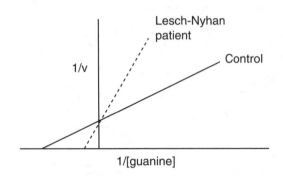

(A) A competitive inhibitor was added to the enzyme from the Lesch-Nyhan patient.

(B) The enzyme has a lower affinity for guanine than the control enzyme.

(C) The gene for HGPRT is repressed in the Lesch-Nyhan patient.

(D) There is an activating mutation in the HGPRT from the Lesch-Nyhan patient.

(E) There is more HGPRT in the Lesch-Nyhan cells.

18. A 25-year-old man and his wife go to a fertility clinic for evaluation. His wife has no significant past medical history and is given a "clean bill of health." He has had bronchiectasis and a history of recurrent sinusitis, and was diagnosed with situs inversus as a child. He is found to be sterile. What is the most likely cause of his infertility?

(A) Abnormal levels of sphingomyelinase

(B) Abnormal structure of cilia

(C) Fibrillin deficiency

(D) 47,XXY karyotype

(E) Hexosaminidase A deficiency

19. A child with cystic fibrosis presents with signs of a bleeding diathesis. Deficiency in which of the following factors is the most likely cause of this child's coagulo-pathy?

(A) Factor V

(B) Factor VIII

(C) Factor XII

(D) Protein C

(E) Prothrombin

20. A 57-year-old alcoholic man is brought to the emergency department in a state of global confusion, psychosis, and ataxia. On examination, ophthalmoplegia and polyneuropathy are also noted. The structural examination reveals chronic somatic dysfunction at T5-T9. Administration of which of the following would be the most appropriate treatment for this patient?

(A) Biotin

(B) Niacin

(C) Pyridoxine

(D) Riboflavin

(E) Thiamine

21. A pathologist is examining microscope slides of a skin biopsy from a patient with malignant melanoma. The pathologist notes in the microscopic description of the report that almost all of the melanoma cells have very large, visible nucleoli. This finding specifically suggests that these cells are making large amounts of which of the following?

(A) Cell surface markers

(B) Golgi apparatus

(C) Immunoglobulins

(D) New DNA

(E) Ribosomes

22. A 57-year-old sales representative for a biotechnology firm has a history of alcohol abuse and hyperuricemia. He attends an out-of-town conference and gorges himself on appetizers, including liver pâté, caviar, and sweetbreads before dinner. Early the following morning he develops a painful swelling in his big toe. The structural examination reveals that the right paraspinal area of T5-T9 has cool, ropy, and fibrotic tissue. In addition to the alcohol consumed with his meals, which other component may have contributed to this episode?

    (A) Carbohydrate

    (B) Cholesterol

    (C) Nucleic acid

    (D) Protein

    (E) Triglyceride

23. A significant difference between the pathways of glycogen synthesis and glycogen degradation is that the glucose molecules used in glycogen synthesis only are bound to which of the following nucleotides?

    (A) ADP

    (B) ATP

    (C) GDP

    (D) GTP

    (E) UDP

24. A neonate who initially appears healthy develops vomiting, diarrhea, abdominal pain, and hypoglycemia when weaning is attempted. There are acute tissue changes at T5-L2 associated with the symptoms. Other features include a generalized metabolic disturbance with lactic acidosis, hyperuricemia, and hyperphosphatemia. Hereditary fructose intolerance is confirmed with an IV fructose tolerance test, and strict dietary restriction of fructose is ordered to prevent the long-term complications of the condition. In addition to fructose, dietary intake of which of the following substances should also be restricted?

    (A) Galactitol

    (B) Galactose

    (C) Glucose

    (D) Lactose

    (E) Sucrose

25. A 10-year-old girl is admitted to the hospital because of a recurrent neurologic disorder. Her right arm and leg have become limp, and she is found to have lactic acidosis. Two months earlier, the girl had a grand mal seizure followed by cortical blindness with slow resolution. Muscle biopsy revealed ragged red muscle fibers and abnormal mitochondria. Which of the following pedigrees is most likely related to her disease?

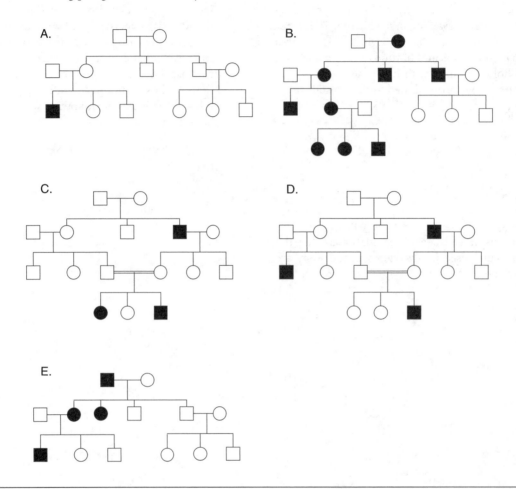

26. In the citric acid cycle, succinate thiokinase (succinyl-CoA synthetase) catalyzes the cleavage of the succinyl-CoA thioester bond with formation of a high-energy compound. This compound can then be used by the body in which of the following biochemical pathways?

    (A) Cysteine degradation
    (B) Elongation of the polypeptide chain
    (C) Epinephrine synthesis from tyrosine
    (D) Isopentyl pyrophosphate synthesis
    (E) Oxidative phosphorylation

27. An obese 76-year-old woman complains of chronic constipation, poor wound healing, and the inability to see well in the dark. The physical examination reveals small white patches on her conjunctiva. You suspect that this woman has a vitamin deficiency caused by which of the following?

    (A) Alcohol abuse
    (B) Malnutrition
    (C) Laxative abuse
    (D) Pellagra
    (E) Beriberi

28. A 72-year-old man presents to the hospital with a several week history of fatigue. Physical examination is remarkable for severe pallor. Neurologic examination reveals poor short-term memory and decreased vibration sense in his legs. Structural examination reveals acute paraspinal tissue changes at T1-T4. An ECG shows changes consistent with the presence of cardiac ischemia. The hemoglobin level is 4.1 g/dL, with a mean corpuscular volume of 105 μm^3, a white-cell count of 3100 per mm^3, and a platelet count of 55,000 per mm^3. The peripheral blood smear shows hypersegmentation of neutrophils, marked anisocytosis, poikilocytosis with some large oval erythrocytes, and basophilic stippling. Which of the following metabolic responses is most specific for the vitamin deficiency affecting this patient?

    (A) Decreased blood δ-aminolevulinic acid (ALA)

    (B) Decreased transketolase activity in erythrocytes

    (C) Decreased urinary homocysteine

    (D) Increased urinary methylmalonate (MMA)

    (E) Lactic acidosis

29. A 22-year-old woman with anorexia nervosa is seen in a specialty clinic that deals with eating disorders. A nutritional nurse estimates the content of the woman's regular diet. She is consuming about 125 g carbohydrate, 15 g protein, and 10 g fat daily. Her daily caloric intake is roughly equal to which of the following values?

    (A) 450 kcal/day

    (B) 650 kcal/day

    (C) 850 kcal/day

    (D) 1050 kcal/day

    (E) 1250 kcal/day

30. A scientist exposes a culture of a bacterium with minimal nutritional requirements to a chemical mutagen, then streaks out the bacteria on plates filled with a complex medium supplemented with all necessary nutrients. When the bacteria begin growing, she isolates individual colonies and tests each one for the ability to grow on a minimal medium. Cells derived from colonies unable to grow on a minimal medium are considered mutants, and their genome is sequenced. In one case, she finds that a two-nucleotide segment of DNA has been deleted. This event would most likely give rise to a

    (A) conservative mutation

    (B) frameshift mutation

    (C) missense mutation

    (D) nonsense mutation

    (E) silent mutation

31. A patient has a niacin deficiency. Dietary intake of which of the following amino acids can substitute for a portion of the daily requirement of niacin?

    (A) Alanine

    (B) Asparagine

    (C) Methionine

    (D) Proline

    (E) Tryptophan

32. Examination of a late aborted fetus reveals a small head, small eyes, prominent cleft lip and palate, six fingers on each hand, and dextrocardia. The developmental abnormalities noted in this fetus were probably due to

    (A) 5p-

    (B) 45,XO

    (C) trisomy 13

    (D) trisomy 18

    (E) trisomy 21

33. A patient has a past medical history significant for multiple infections involving the lungs, liver, and bones, as well as excessive inflammation with granulomas, gingivitis, aphthous ulcers, and seborrheic dermatitis. Osteopathic structural examination shows that T2-T8 has chronic paraspinal tissue changes and T7 FRS$_R$. This patient most likely has a deficiency of which of the following enzymes?

    (A) Muscle glycogen phosphorylase

    (B) Myeloperoxidase

    (C) NADPH oxidase

    (D) Transketolase

    (E) Xanthine oxidase

34. A 50-year-old man was admitted into the hospital of a leading research university with a diagnosis of hepatitis and early cirrhosis of the liver. His past medical history is significant for heavy smoking and only occasional consumption of alcohol. He did not use any drugs, and he had no viral infections. Physical examination reveals chronic paraspinal tissue-texture changes at T2-T8 with a Chapman reflex tender point at the interspace of ribs 5 and 6 just lateral to the costal margin. DNA studies showed that he was homozygous for the Z allele of α_1-antitrypsin, produced by a missense mutation that prevents the proper folding of the protein. A liver biopsy would most likely show accumulation of a proteinaceous substance in which of the following subcellular sites?

    (A) Endoplasmic reticulum

    (B) Extracellular matrix

    (C) Golgi apparatus

    (D) Inclusion bodies

    (E) Lysosomes

35. A 20-year-old develops weakness accompanied by difficulty in relaxation that is most pronounced in the hands and feet. Physical examination reveals somatic dysfunction at T2-T4 and T10-L2. Muscle biopsy demonstrates prominent ring fibers, centrally located nuclei, chains of nuclei, and disorganized sarcoplasmic masses. This condition has been associated with a mutation on which of the following chromosomes?

    (A) X

    (B) Y

    (C) 4

    (D) 5

    (E) 19

36. In a certain population, the frequency of color-blind males is 1 in 100. Assuming that the population is in Hardy-Weinberg equilibrium at this locus, the frequency of color-blind females is approximately

    (A) 0.0001

    (B) 0.0005

    (C) 0.01

    (D) 0.02

    (E) 0.025

37. A young woman is doing intense aerobic exercise. Aerobic glycolysis is being used for the source of energy for the muscle activity. In which of the following forms will the carbons derived from glucose enter the citric acid cycle?

    (A) Acetyl-CoA

    (B) Citrate

    (C) Oxaloacetate

    (D) Pyruvate

    (E) Succinate

38. An X-linked genetic disease affects a cation-transporting P-type ATPase, resulting in accumulation of copper in the intestinal epithelium because of failure to transport it normally into the blood. Infants with this disease have only 10% of normal blood copper levels. Arteriograms show elongation and tortuosity of major arteries. Bladder diverticula and subdural hematomas are also characteristic findings. These symptoms would most likely be caused by decreased activity of which of the following enzymes?

    (A) Cytochrome aa_3

    (B) Lysyl oxidase

    (C) Prolyl hydroxylase

    (D) Tyrosinase

    (E) γ-Glutamyl carboxylase

39. An Olympic runner participates in a 100-meter race. During this race, it is estimated that only ½ L oxygen will be consumed by the runner. However, more than 10 L oxygen would be consumed if the metabolism in this interval were entirely aerobic. The majority of ATP generated during this 100-meter race is derived from which of the following?

    (A) ATP stores

    (B) Creatine phosphate

    (C) Gluconeogenesis

    (D) Glycolysis

    (E) Lipolysis

40. A 57-year-old man with type 1 diabetes mellitus has progressive retinopathy. Physical examination reveals chronic somatic dysfunction at T1-T4. Ophthalmoscopic examination macular edema and retinal thickening with hard exudates of yellow-white lipid deposits. Which of the following contributes to hyperlipidemia in type 1 diabetes, and thus the risk for lipid deposition in the retina?

    (A) Glucose conversion to sorbitol in the lens

    (B) Overactive GLUT-2 in liver

    (C) Overactive GLUT-4 in adipose

    (D) Overactive hormone-sensitive lipase

    (E) Overactive lipoprotein lipase

41. A 34-year old woman presents to her physician complaining of oral ulcers. A careful history reveals that she is a strict vegetarian and does not eat meat, fish, poultry, eggs, or dairy products. She is found to have a severe riboflavin deficiency. The function of which of the following enzymes in the citric acid cycle would be most directly affected by the riboflavin deficiency?

    (A) Aconitase

    (B) Citrate synthase

    (C) Isocitrate dehydrogenase

    (D) Malate dehydrogenase

    (E) Succinate dehydrogenase

42. The pedigree below illustrates the mode of inheritance for which of the following diseases?

    (A) Glucose-6-phosphate dehydrogenase deficiency

    (B) Leber hereditary optic neuropathy

    (C) Neurofibromatosis

    (D) Sickle cell anemia

    (E) Tay-Sachs disease

43. A mother is informed that her daughter has an inherited disorder in which the administration of a "sugar-free" product that contains aspartame could be detrimental to her health. This patient most likely has which of the following genetic disorders?

    (A) Hyperornithinemia

    (B) Hyperuricemia

    (C) Hypervalinemia

    (D) Phenylketonuria

    (E) Wilson disease

44. A 2-year-old patient is diagnosed with retinoblastoma, which is associated with an abnormality in which of the following chromosomes?

    (A) 5

    (B) 8

    (C) 13

    (D) 21

    (E) X

Questions 45-50

<u>SET A</u>

For each numbered item (**patient presentation**), select the one heading (**enzyme**) most closely associated with it. Each lettered heading maybe used once, more than once, or not at all.

(A) Hexosaminidase A

(B) Beta-glucocerebrosidase

(C) Cystathionine synthase

(D) Homogentisic acid oxidase

(E) Phenylalanine hydroxylase

(F) Fumarylacetoacetate hydrolyase

(G) Alpha-L-iduronidase

(H) Glucose-6-phosphatase

(I) Sphingomyelinase

45. A 6-month-old child presents with mousy-smelling urine.

46. A 30-year-old patient presents with ochronosis, arthritis, and a history of passing black-colored urine.

47. A severely retarded infant presents with a cherry-red spot of the macula. Physical examination reveals no hepatosplenomegaly.

48. A 4-month-old infant presents with failure to thrive and has a cabbage-like body odor.

49. A 1-year-old presents with bilateral inguinal hernias. Physical examination reveals hepatosplenomegaly, exaggerated kyphosis, persistent nasal discharge, noisy breaths, and clouding of the corneas.

50. A couple presents for prenatal genetic testing because they are of Ashkenazi Jewish descent.

Biochemistry

ANSWERS AND EXPLANATIONS

1.	C		26.	B
2.	E		27.	C
3.	C		28.	D
4.	B		29.	B
5.	A		30.	B
6.	C		31.	E
7.	D		32.	C
8.	E		33.	C
9.	B		34.	A
10.	E		35.	E
11.	C		36.	A
12.	A		37.	A
13.	E		38.	B
14.	B		39.	D
15.	B		40.	D
16.	A		41.	E
17.	B		42.	B
18.	B		43.	D
19.	E		44.	C
20.	E		45.	E
21.	E		46.	D
22.	C		47.	A
23.	E		48.	F
24.	E		49.	G
25.	B		50.	A

1. **The correct answer is C.** A child with ketotic hypoglycemia following a period of fasting most likely has a defect in gluconeogenesis or in a pathway providing substrates for gluconeogenesis. Under fasting conditions, the primary substrate for gluconeogenesis is alanine derived from muscle protein. As muscle proteins are catabolized, the amino acid skeletons are used as fuel in the muscle, while the amino groups are transaminated to pyruvate, forming alanine, which is then transported to the liver and kidney cortex to be used in gluconeogenesis (Cahill cycle). In this child, alanine levels are abnormally low and infusion of alanine rapidly increases blood glucose. These findings rule out a defect in gluconeogenesis and are most consistent with a defect in protein catabolism in muscle.

Gluconeogenesis (**choice A**) was shown to be intact by the response to alanine infusion.

Glycogenolysis (**choice B**) is not involved, since liver glycogen stores would have been exhausted by this time. Moreover, defects in glycogenolysis should not produce such a severe hypoglycemia because they would be mitigated by gluconeogenesis and ketone body formation.

The ketosis indicates that triglyceride hydrolysis in adipose tissue (**choice D**) and β-oxidation of fatty acids (**choice E**) are functional, i.e., acetate is being formed and is being converted to ketones. However, the acetyl-CoA formed cannot contribute to net production of glucose because it cannot be converted to pyruvate.

2. **The correct answer is E.** This question requires three steps of logic. First, figure out the diagnosis (a classic case of Parkinson disease), then remember which neurotransmitter is involved in the disease (dopamine), and, finally, recall which amino acid serves as the precursor for that neurotransmitter (tyrosine). The hydroxylation of tyrosine by tyrosine hydroxylase results in DOPA, which is then decarboxylated to dopamine. Note that norepinephrine and epinephrine are also tyrosine derivatives, as are the melanins and the thyroid hormones thyroxine and triiodothyronine.

Glutamate (**choice A**) can be converted to the inhibitory neurotransmitter GABA by the action of glutamate decarboxylase.

Glycine (**choice B**) is involved in the synthesis of both creatine(alongwitharginineandS-adenosylmethionine) and heme (along with succinyl-CoA).

Histidine (**choice C**) can be decarboxylated to histamine, an important inflammatory mediator.

Tryptophan (**choice D**) can be converted to serotonin by a hydroxylation reaction (tryptophan hydroxylase) followed by a decarboxylation reaction.

3. **The correct answer is C.** Both pyruvate kinase deficiency and glucose-6-phosphate dehydrogenase deficiency are red cell enzyme deficiencies characterized clinically by long "normal" periods interspersed with episodes of hemolytic anemia triggered by infections and oxidant drug injury (antimalarial drugs, sulfonamides, nitrofurans). In both of these conditions, the cell morphology between hemolytic episodes is usually normal or close to normal.

The α (**choice A**) and β (**choice B**) thalassemias, in their major forms, are characterized by persistent severe anemia. In the trait forms, they are characterized by mild anemia.

Hereditary spherocytosis (**choice D**) is characterized by intermittent hemolysis. Unlike pyruvate kinase deficiency and glucose-6-phosphate dehydrogenase deficiency, however, oxidant drugs are not a specific trigger for hemolysis.

Iron deficiency anemia (**choice E**) is characterized by chronic anemia with hypochromic, microcytic erythrocytes.

4. **The correct answer is B.** Buffer systems usually work by having a molecule that can easily convert between two states by giving up or accepting a proton (H^+). If some of both forms of the molecule are present in the solution at the same time, the pH can be maintained at a relatively stable level. Within cells, the phosphate buffer system is the most important. This system uses HPO_4^{2-} and $H_2PO_4^{1-}$ as the two species, with the former capable of picking up H^+, and the latter capable of releasing it. In contrast, the most important inorganic buffer in extracellular fluid, including plasma, is the bicarbonate buffer system. This uses interconversions between HCO_3^- and H_2CO_3 and is unusual because any H_2CO_3 produced can be enzymatically split to CO_2 (carbon dioxide) and H_2O (water). The carbon dioxide can be "blown off" by increasing the depth or frequency of breathing, which allows the body to stretch the buffering ability of the bicarbonate. In contrast to the phosphate and bicarbonate systems, calcium does not bind H^+ and thus does not serve as a pH buffer. It is, however, tightly regulated (particularly intracellularly) because of its important roles as a second messenger and a trigger for muscle contraction.

5. **The correct answer is A.** This question is based on a real case. Although it is hard to develop a deficiency in oil-soluble vitamins (A, D, E, K) because the liver stores these substances, deficiency states can be seen in chronic malnutrition (specifically chronic fat deprivation) and chronic malabsorption. Vitamin A is necessary for formation of retinal pigments (deficiency can cause

night blindness) and for appropriate differentiation of epithelial tissues (including hair follicles, mucous membranes, skin, bone, and adrenal cortex).

Vitamin C (**choice B**), which is water soluble rather than oil soluble, is necessary for collagen synthesis.

Vitamin D (**choice C**) is important in calcium absorption and metabolism.

Vitamin E (**choice D**) is a lipid antioxidant that is important in the stabilization of cell membranes.

Vitamin K (**choice E**) is necessary for normal blood coagulation.

6. **The correct answer is C.** The hexose monophosphate shunt is an alternative route for the oxidation of glucose; it supplies the cell with NADPH and pentose sugars. The NADPH is used in many biosynthetic processes (e.g., fatty acid and cholesterol synthesis), whereas the pentoses are involved in the synthesis of nucleotides and some coenzymes. The pathway "shunts" from glucose-6-phosphate, which is oxidized in a series of NADPH-generating reactions, to ribulose-5-phosphate. The nonoxidative phase, which involves the transfer of C2 and C3 units from one sugar to another, follows. One resulting intermediate is fructose-6-phosphate (**choice B**), which can serve as a re-entry point to glycolysis, thereby closing the "shunt" loop.

Although all the other choices are glycolytic intermediates, they are not involved in the hexose monophosphate shunt.

7. **The correct answer is D.** Hereditary factor XIII deficiency is an autosomal recessive condition that is unusual among the factor deficiencies in that the presentation is often at birth, when the umbilical stump bleeds excessively, sometimes leading to the neonate's death. Factor XIII is necessary to stabilize clot formation; in its absence, clots will rapidly lyse. Cutaneous and muscular hematomas are common in affected patients. Bleeding after surgery and trauma can occur, including bleeding into the CNS. Spontaneous abortion in affected women is common. A factor XIII concentrate is available for treatment.

8. **The correct answer is E.** The woman is having an exercise-induced hypoglycemic episode. Exercise stimulates the uptake of glucose from the blood, thus lowering blood glucose levels. The normal response to this is to decrease blood insulin levels and increase glucagon levels, thereby stimulating glycogenolysis and restoring blood glucose. However, this person has type 1 diabetes mellitus and her insulin levels are determined largely by injection. Therefore, the insulin/glucagon ratio remained high, glycogenolysis could not be stimulated, and hypoglycemia resulted. It is time for her to ingest glucose in some readily absorbed form that should be carried by all type 1 diabetics.

This question requires you to associate translocation of GLUT4 with increased glucose uptake by muscle. Because glucose is a water-soluble molecule and cell membranes are lipid bilayers, specific transport proteins are required to get glucose into cells. This family of transporters is called GLUT, and there are five members, plus a sodium-dependent glucose transporter (SGLT1). Their properties are summarized in the following table.

Transporter	Location	Characteristics	Function
GLUT1	Brain, red cells, kidney, placenta, colon	Facilitative, bidirectional Insulin-independent	Uptake of glucose
GLUT2	Liver, pancreatic β cells Small intestine, kidney	Facilitative, bidirectional Insulin-independent	Rapid uptake and release of glucose Glucose sensor in pancreatic β cells
GLUT3	Brain, kidney, placenta	Facilitative, bidirectional Insulin-independent	Uptake of glucose
GLUT4	Cardiac and skeletal muscle, adipocytes	Facilitative, bidirectional **Insulin-dependent in adipose and muscle** **Exercise (AMP)–dependent in skeletal muscle**	Uptake of glucose by muscle and by adipocytes when glucose and insulin levels are high Uptake of glucose in skeletal muscle during exercise
GLUT5	Small intestine	Facilitative, bidirectional Insulin-independent	Lowers Km for fructose but also transports glucose
SGLT1	Small intestine and kidney	Na^+ cotransport system driven by the Na/K ATPase Only one that works against a concentration gradient	Uptake of glucose from the intestinal lumen and in the kidney proximal tubule

During fasting, much of the GLUT4 in skeletal muscle and adipose resides in the membranes of cytoplasmic vesicles. Increased insulin following a meal induces the translocation of these vesicles to the cell membrane, thus increasing glucose uptake (and lowering the peripheral blood glucose). In skeletal muscle, GLUT4 translocation is also stimulated by increased AMP associated with exercising muscle. This AMP-stimulated increase in GLUT4 and glucose uptake is independent of insulin. In this patient, the insulin dose has been adequate to maintain glycemic control. When she began the new exercise program, the additional AMP-stimulated glucose uptake was sufficient to cause hypoglycemia and the symptoms described. If the woman continues this exercise program, her physician should consider lowering the amount of insulin she takes.

Inadequate delivery of oxygen to the muscle (**choice A**) would produce different symptoms, such as pain and/or cramping.

Stimulation of gluconeogenesis in the liver (**choice B**) would increase blood glucose levels. However, gluconeogenesis would not be relevant even in a normal individual who had eaten recently (as long as hepatic glycogen levels were adequate).

Stimulation of glycogenolysis in liver (**choice C**) would increase blood glucose levels.

Stimulation of glycogenolysis in muscle (**choice D**) would occur in response to the lowering of intracellular glucose levels due to the exercise, but to the extent it maintained glucose levels near normal, this would prevent, not induce, symptoms of hypoglycemia

9. **The correct answer is B.** Constitutive (unregulated) exocytosis is the mechanism by which cells secrete plasma proteins. The vesicles involved are not coated with clathrin. This constitutive secretory pathway is also called the default secretory pathway, because vesicles not specifically tagged to go to a particular destination (e.g., lysosomes) will automatically go through this pathway. Constitutive exocytosis, which occurs in all cells, is also responsible for supplying the plasma membrane with newly synthesized lipids and proteins.

Receptor-mediated endocytosis (**choice D**) refers to the internalization of molecules (e.g., LDL) bound to a receptor on a cell, typically in the vicinity of a clathrin-coated pit (**choice A**).

Pinocytosis (**choice C**) ("cellular drinking" of fluids) is the endocytotic uptake of molecules in solution and does not involve receptors.

The secretion of hormones requires a signal before the clathrin-coated vesicle will fuse with the plasma membrane. This is known as regulated exocytosis (**choice E**).

10. **The correct answer is E.** The human body is able to synthesize roughly half the amino acids necessary to build protein. These amino acids, termed nonessential, include alanine, arginine, asparagine, aspartate, cysteine, glutamate, glutamine, glycine, proline, serine, and tyrosine. The amino acids that must be supplied in the diet are termed essential; these include histidine, isoleucine, leucine, lysine, methionine, phenylalanine, threonine, tryptophan, and valine. Phenylalanine undergoes hydroxylation to tyrosine, catalyzed by the enzyme phenylalanine hydroxylase. It is noteworthy that tyrosine becomes an essential amino acid in individuals lacking this enzyme. The hyperphenylalaninemias, which include phenylketonuria, result from impaired conversion of phenylalanine to tyrosine, and are also associated with mental retardation. This condition is associated with increased phenylalanine in blood and increased phenylalanine and its by-products (e.g., phenylpyruvate, phenylacetate, and phenyllactate) in urine.

Asparagine (**choice A**) is a member of the "oxaloacetate family"; its immediate precursor is aspartate.

The immediate precursor of cysteine (**choice B**) is serine. Serine is also the precursor of the nonessential amino acid glycine.

Glutamine (**choice C**), proline (**choice D**), and arginine are produced from glutamate. The synthesis of glutamate occurs by the reductive amination of alpha-ketoglutarate.

11. **The correct answer is C.** The conversion of homocysteine to methionine is catalyzed by homocysteine methyltransferase. An essential cofactor is the methylated form of vitamin B_{12} (methylcobalamin); the methyl group is obtained from N^5-methylenetetrahydrofolate. Thus, a deficiency of either vitamin increases the homocysteine concentration in the blood. Several different inborn errors of metabolism affecting this reaction cause homocystinuria, characterized by a marked increase in homocysteine levels. However, recent clinical studies have shown that a modest increase in homocysteine levels in "normal" individuals is a significant risk factor for cardiovascular disease and deep vein thrombosis. Moreover, these increased levels can be lowered by appropriate vitamin therapy.

Dihydrofolate reductase (**choice A**) is required to convert the folate to its active form, but it is not as closely related to the role of folate in lowering the risk of cardiovascular disease as is the cofactor for homocysteine methyltransferase.

Glycinamide ribonucleotide transformylase (**choice B**) catalyzes the transfer of a formyl group from N^{10}-formyltetrahydrofolate to the amino group of glycinamide ribonucleotide. Although it requires folate, it has no known role in lowering the risk of cardiovascular disease.

Ribonucleotide reductase (**choice D**) catalyzes the reduction of nucleoside diphosphates to their deoxy forms. Neither vitamin influences its activity, nor is its activity linked to cardiovascular disease

Thymidylate synthase (**choice E**) converts dUMP to dTMP. Although folate is required for its activity, it is not related to the role of folate in lowering the risk of cardiovascular disease.

12. **The correct answer is A.** Valine, leucine, and isoleucine are the branched chain amino acids. Deficiency of the branched chain ketoacid dehydrogenase causes maple syrup urine disease, in which branched chain ketoacids build up in blood, urine, and tissues. The urine has the odor of maple syrup and a metabolic acidosis is produced. Early diagnosis is essential to limit an irreversible mental retardation. Treatment consists of a special diet with limited amounts of these amino acids. If untreated, death occurs within a year.

Cystathionine synthase (**choice B**) converts homocysteine to cystathionine. A deficiency of this enzyme causes a form of homocystinuria (homocystinuria I).

Methylmalonyl CoA mutase (**choice C**) catalyzes a vitamin B_{12}–requiring step in the conversion of propionate from the amino acids threonine, valine, isoleucine, and methionine, and from odd numbered fatty acids to succinyl-CoA. Note that these are not the same set of amino acids involved in maple syrup urine disease, although the symptoms of the condition are somewhat similar. Deficiency of the methylmalonyl CoA mutase results most commonly in neonatal ketosis and metabolic acidosis with lethargy, vomiting, diarrhea, muscle hypotonia, and if not treated, coma and death. Some cases can be treated by restricting protein and supplementing with extra cobalamin.

Ornithine transcarbamoylase deficiency (**choice D**) is a urea cycle enzyme deficiency disease associated with hyperammonemia.

Propionyl CoA carboxylase (**choice E**) catalyzes a reaction analogous to that of acetyl-CoA carboxylase. Both form a malonyl derivative and require biotin as a cofactor. The carboxylation is a step in the conversion of propionate and odd numbered fatty acids to succinyl-CoA.

13. **The correct answer is E.** Von Gierke disease is a glycogen storage disease caused by a deficiency of glucose-6-phosphatase. It typically presents with neonatal hypoglycemia, hyperlipidemia, lactic acidosis, and ketosis. Failure to thrive is common in early life; convulsions

may occur because of profound hypoglycemia. The glycogen accumulation in von Gierke disease occurs primarily in the liver and kidneys, accounting for the enlargement of these organs. Gout may develop later because of the derangement of glucose metabolism.

Even if you do not remember all of the details of the presentation of these genetic diseases, you should be able to narrow the choices:

Gaucher (**choice A**) and Niemann-Pick (**choice C**) diseases are lipid storage diseases and would not be expected to produce hypoglycemia.

The other diseases are glycogen storage diseases, but McArdle (**choice B**) and Pompe (**choice D**) diseases affect muscle, rather than liver, and would not be expected to produce profound hypoglycemia, since the liver is the major source for blood glucose.

14. **The correct answer is B.** The byproduct cyanide strongly inhibits cytochrome oxidase (complex IV of the electron transport chain), causing loss of all ATP production associated with oxidative phosphorylation. Therefore, in a manner similar to the effects of hypoxia, cyanide poisoning causes rapid cell death. Highly aerobic tissues (nerves, muscle) are affected first.

2,3-Bisphosphoglycerate mutase (**choice A**) catalyzes the formation of 2,3-bisphosphoglycerate from 1,3-bisphosphoglycerate and is not inhibited by cyanide.

2,3-Bisphosphoglycerate is found in all cells in small quantities and is found in high concentrations in red cells.

Guanylate cyclase (**choice C**) catalyzes the formation of cGMP from GTP and is not inhibited by cyanide.

Na$^+$/K$^+$-ATPase (**choice D**) is coupled to the transport of various substances across cell membranes and accounts for the majority of the basal metabolic energy (BMR) utilization. It is not inhibited by cyanide.

Phosphofructokinase-2 (**choice E**) catalyzes the formation of fructose 2,6-bisphosphate from ATP and fructose 6-phosphate and is not inhibited by cyanide.

15. **The correct answer is B.** This is a two-step question. You first need to make the diagnosis, and you then need to recall the localization of this particular disease to a specific chromosome. In this case, everything in the vignette leads you to a diagnosis of Wilms tumor. Wilms tumor occurs in children and typically presents with an abdominal mass, as well as with hypertension, hematuria, nausea, and intestinal obstruction. Because the tumor is derived from mesonephric mesoderm, it can include mesodermal derivatives such as bone, cartilage, and muscle. The Wilms tumor suppressor gene (WT-1) has been localized to chromosome 11 (11p).

The remaining answer choices provide us the opportunity to discuss some other known relationships between genes and disease. This is a topic of intense research that is likely to be increasingly emphasized on the COMLEX examinations.

Chromosome 5 (**choice A**) is the site of the tumor suppressor gene APC, which is involved in the pathogenesis of colon cancer and familial adenomatous polyposis.

Chromosome 13 (**choice C**) is the site of the tumor suppressor gene for retinoblastoma and osteosarcoma (Rb), as well as the BRCA-2 gene for breast cancer.

Chromosome 17 (**choice D**) is the site of p53 (involved in most human cancers), NF-1 (neurofibromatosis type I), and BRCA-1 (breast and ovarian cancer).

Chromosome 22 (**choice E**) is home to the NF-2 gene, which is involved in neurofibromatosis type II.

16. **The correct answer is A.** Restriction length fragment polymorphism (RFLP) is a powerful tool that is used to compare DNA samples from several different sources. This technique has been used to convict or acquit criminals and has utility in the determination of paternity. Basically, total DNA is extracted (usually from a blood sample) and then digested with restriction enzymes. Restriction enzymes cut DNA at specific points (often palindromic sequences) called restriction sites. Differences in the DNA between two individuals will, with a very high probability, produce differences in the number and position of restriction sites, and so will produce differences in the length of the fragments made by digestion with restriction enzymes. The digested samples are then subjected to electrophoresis, and the fragments separated according to size. In the pattern shown, child 1 has a fragment approximately 7 kilobases (kb) in length that matches a similar fragment in the DNA of husband 1, verifying that he is the biologic father. No 7-kb fragment is found in husband 2, implying that he could not be the father. Interestingly, child 2 shows a 6-kb fragment that neither wife 2 nor husband 2 (nor husband 1) exhibit. An unexpected conclusion of this RFLP is that child 2 may not be the child of husband 2.

17. **The correct answer is B.** The graph shows that the patient's HGPRT has a higher K_m value than the HGPRT from the control cells; a higher K_m value means a lower affinity.

Although the resultant pattern would look like competitive inhibition (**choice A**), it would be a comparison between two different enzymes, not one enzyme with and without an inhibitor as described.

Since the V_{max} is the same, there is no evidence that there is less HGPRT (i.e., repression of the HGPRT gene; **choice C**) in the child's cells.

If a mutation activated the Lesch-Nyhan enzyme (**choice D**), either the V_{max} value would be higher or the K_m value lower. Neither is true.

Since the V_{max} is the same, there is no evidence that there is more HGPRT in the Lesch-Nyhan child's cells (**choice E**).

18. **The correct answer is B.** Kartagener syndrome, an autosomal recessive disorder characterized by bronchiectasis, sinusitis, and situs inversus, is classified as an "immotile cilia syndrome." It is associated with the absence of inner or outer dynein arms in the cilia. This leads to abnormal ciliary mobility of the sperm, producing infertility. Ciliary abnormalities in the respiratory tract lead to sinusitis and bronchiectasis.

Sphingomyelinase deficiency (**choice A**) occurs in Niemann-Pick disease (autosomal recessive transmission). Sphingomyelin accumulates in the phagocytes. "Foamy histiocytes" appear in the liver, spleen, lymph nodes, and skin. Clinical manifestations include hepatosplenomegaly and, in some cases, neurologic deterioration. Patients usually do not survive beyond 3 years of age.

Fibrillin deficiency (**choice C**) occurs in Marfan syndrome (autosomal dominant). Patients are characteristically tall and thin, and their fingers are spider-like (arachnodactyly). Anatomic abnormalities include ectopia lentis (displaced lens of the eye) and aortic dilatation predisposing to aortic aneurysm.

47,XXY karyotype (**choice D**), also known as Klinefelter syndrome, is characterized by male hypogonadism. It can cause male infertility, but nothing else in the question suggests this is the case. One would expect to see atrophic testes, tall stature, and gynecomastia. Mental retardation is sometimes present.

Hexosaminidase A deficiency (**choice E**) causes Tay-Sachs disease (autosomal recessive), which occurs most commonly in Ashkenazi Jews. The disease causes CNS degeneration and blindness, and patients exhibit motor and mental deterioration (e.g., loss of developmental milestones). A classic clue is a macular "cherry-red spot" on ophthalmoscopic examination. Patients usually do not survive beyond 3 years of age.

19. **The correct answer is E.** This question first requires you to make the connection between cystic fibrosis (CF) and bleeding. The connection is that CF patients have problems with pancreatic exocrine secretions and therefore have fat malabsorption, which, in turn, results in malabsorption of the fat-soluble vitamins A, D, E, and K. Vitamin K is essential in the post-translational modification of factors II (prothrombin), VII, IX, X, and proteins C and S.

Factors V (**choice A**), VIII (**choice B**), and XII (**choice C**) are not vitamin K dependent.

Although protein C (**choice D**) and protein S are vitamin K dependent, these proteins are endogenous anticoagulants involved in clot lysis, not clot formation. Therefore, deficiency of protein C would cause thrombosis, not bleeding.

20. **The correct answer is E.** The patient is presenting with the signs and symptoms of Wernicke encephalopathy, which consists of the classic triad of ophthalmoplegia, ataxia, and global confusion. This syndrome is considered a medical emergency and necessitates immediate administration of thiamine, or vitamin B_1.

Biotin (**choice A**) acts as a carrier of "activated carboxyl" groups for three key enzymes that catalyze carboxylation reactions. Symptoms of biotin deficiency include alopecia, skin and bowel inflammation, and muscle pain.

Niacin (**choice B**), or vitamin B_3, is converted to nicotinamide, which is then incorporated into the coenzymes NAD^+ and $NADP^+$. Pellagra, a condition associated with niacin deficiency, leads to diarrhea, dermatitis, and dementia.

Pyridoxine (**choice C**), or vitamin B_6, is utilized as the coenzyme pyridoxal phosphate. A deficiency in pyridoxine can lead to peripheral neuropathy and dermatitis.

Riboflavin (**choice D**), or vitamin B_2, is responsible for maintaining proper levels of both FMN and FAD. Individuals with riboflavin deficiency are likely to present with lesions of the lips, mouth, skin, and genitalia.

21. **The correct answer is E.** The nucleolus is the site of manufacture of ribosomal RNA with its subsequent packaging into ribosomes. Consequently, very large nucleoli indicate an increased rate of ribosome production, which, in turn, suggests an increased rate of production of proteins. Large nucleoli are seen in many active cancers but can also be prominent in benign conditions characterized by high metabolic rate, such as tissue repair after trauma.

Depending on the cells involved, the increased protein production associated with more ribosomes might produce more cell surface markers (**choice A**), but it is impossible to predict this simply from the presence of a large nucleolus.

You should associate a large Golgi apparatus (**choice B**) with transport of material to the cell surface.

Plasma cells that produce large amounts of immunoglobulins (**choice C**) may have large nucleoli, but more specifically have a very large endoplasmic reticulum and Golgi apparatus.

The nucleolus is not involved with new DNA (**choice D**) synthesis; this is done elsewhere in the nucleus.

22. **The correct answer is C.** Purines from ingested nucleic acids are converted to uric acid by intestinal epithelial cells and released into the blood for potential excretion by the kidney. Foods rich in DNA (caviar) or RNA (liver pâté and sweetbreads [pancreas], derived from organs with active protein synthesis) are particularly rich sources of purines, and their ingestion coupled with excess alcohol consumption presumably increased his plasma urate levels to the point at which uric acid crystallized in a susceptible joint. The resultant painful swelling is gout. The pain is caused by precipitation of uric acid crystals in the joints with attendant inflammation.

Carbohydrate (**choice A**), cholesterol (**choice B**), protein (**choice D**), and triglyceride (**choice E**) by themselves do not contain purines, and their metabolism does not contribute to the uric acid pool. To the extent that protein-rich foods are cellular, they will, however, contain nucleic acids that will be catabolized to uric acid.

23. **The correct answer is E.** In glycogen synthesis, one of the high-energy phosphate bonds of uridine triphosphate is used by the enzyme UDP-glucose pyrophosphorylase to form uridine diphosphate glucose:

Glucose-1-phosphate + UDP → UDP-glucose + PPi

This UDP-glucose can then bind to glycogen primers for formation of glycogen.

ADP (**choice A**) is produced when ATP transfers a high-energy phosphate group to another species. Intracellular ADP level is an important regulator of many energy-related pathways.

ATP (**choice B**) is the usual form of high-energy chemical storage used by the cell in a variety of reactions. One or, less commonly, two high phosphate groups from the ATP are transferred to molecules to drive otherwise chemically unfavored reactions. Binding of these molecules to ATP is usually transient.

GDP (**choice C**) is used in the citric acid cycle to form GTP as succinyl-CoA is converted to succinate.

GTP (**choice D**) is made in the citric acid cycle as succinyl-CoA is converted to succinate.

24. **The correct answer is E.** Several forms of genetic abnormalities of fructose can occur. The mildest, virtually asymptomatic, condition is essential (benign) fructosuria, due to a lack of fructokinase, which phosphorylates fructose. In marked contrast, the genetic abnormality of fructose metabolism described in the question stem is hereditary fructose intolerance (fructosemia), the most severe of these conditions. It is due to a deficiency of the enzyme aldolase B, which is found in liver, small intestine, and kidney. Aldolase B normally cleaves fructose-1-phosphate, and the severe abnormalities seen are related

to a disastrous depletion of intracellular phosphate, which is needed for making ATP and other phosphorylated compounds. Hereditary fructose intolerance requires very strict dietary control of fructose, which in practice means that not only fructose (fruit sugar) itself must be controlled, but the much more prevalent sucrose (table sugar) must also be controlled, since it is a disaccharide composed of fructose and glucose. The sugar alcohol sorbitol (an artificial sweetener) is also restricted, since this compound can also be converted to fructose.

Galactitol (**choice A**) is a sugar alcohol related to galactose, which need not be restricted in this condition.

Galactose (**choice B**) is a monosaccharide that is metabolized normally in this condition. Metabolic disorders associated with galactose metabolism, analogous to those of fructose, occur because of genetic defects in the kinase enzyme (galactokinase deficiency) and a transfer enzyme (galactose-1-phosphate uridyl transferase deficiency).

Glucose (**choice C**) is metabolized normally in this condition.

Lactose (**choice D**), a disaccharide composed of galactose and glucose, should be restricted in severe genetic diseases of galactose, as well as in lactose intolerance.

25. **The correct answer is B.** The condition described is MELAS (mitochondrial encephalomyopathy, lactic acidosis, and stroke-like episodes). Ragged red muscle fibers and disrupted mitochondria are seen on muscle biopsy. Two major features characterize mitochondrial patterns of transmission: no inheritance from an affected male, and usually all children of an affected female are affected. However, expression among siblings can vary to a considerable extent because there are so many mitochondria, each with their own set of genes, which are distributed into the eggs in a random fashion.

The pedigree in **choice A** is most likely a new mutation, but could be a recessive trait that has skipped several generations.

The pedigree in **choice C** is most likely autosomal recessive.

The pedigree in **choice D** is most likely X-linked recessive.

The pedigree in **choice E** is most likely X-linked dominant.

26. **The correct answer is B.** In this question, you need to know that GTP is synthesized when CoASH is cleaved from succinyl-CoA to form succinate in the citric acid cycle. You also need to know that GTP, rather than ATP, is used as the energy source in protein synthesis, specifically in the formation of the activated elongation factor to which tRNA binds, and in the transfer of the elongating chain from the P to the A site in the ribosome.

Cysteine degradation (**choice A**) requires O_2 and produces sulfite and then sulfate, which is secreted in urine.

Epinephrine synthesis from tyrosine (**choice C**) requires tetrahydrobiopterin, pyridoxal phosphate, oxygen, copper, and S-adenosylmethionine.

Isopentyl pyrophosphate synthesis from HMG CoA (**choice D**) requires NADPH and ATP, and releases CO_2.

Oxidative phosphorylation (**choice E**) uses NADH, $FADH_2$, coenzyme Q, oxygen, and a variety of cytochromes to produce ATP.

27. **The correct answer is C.** This patient is suffering from vitamin A deficiency. The earliest symptom is night blindness. The spots in the eyes are known as Bitot spots and are one of the earliest signs of vitamin A deficiency. In the United States, vitamin A deficiency is usually caused by fat malabsorption syndromes or mineral oil laxative abuse and occurs most commonly in elderly and urban, poor patients.

    Choices A and E are associated with a thiamin deficiency.

    Choice B is incorrect because the patient is obese.

    Choice D is associated with a niacin deficiency and is commonly due to alcoholism.

28. **The correct answer is D.** The combination of neurologic symptoms and megaloblastic anemia is characteristic of a vitamin B_{12} (cyanocobalamin) deficiency, which will also cause an increase in urinary methylmalonate (MMA) due to low activity of methylmalonyl CoA mutase. Megaloblastic anemia is caused by impaired DNA synthesis, which slows cell division, thus decreasing the count for cells with a rapid turnover. In the surviving cells, synthesis of cytoplasmic components proceeds unabated, while cellular division is slowed. Thus, these cells tend to be oversized, misshapen, and have various cytoplasmic inclusions. The direct cause of the decreased rate of DNA synthesis is the unavailability of folate, needed most acutely for conversion of dUMP to dTMP. Therefore, supplementation with folate will cause a rapid reversal of these symptoms. In the case described, there are also symptoms of neuropathy, a characteristic of vitamin B_{12} deficiency not associated with folate deficiency. In addition to causing neuropathy, a vitamin B_{12} deficiency will produce a secondary folate deficiency by preventing the regeneration of tetrahydrofolate.

    Cofactors derived from vitamin B_{12} carry out only two functions. One is in the conversion of homocysteine to methionine. N^5-methyltetrahydrofolate is a cosubstrate in this reaction and simultaneously loses its methyl moiety and is converted to tetrahydrofolate. N^5-methyltetrahydrofolate has no other function, and unless it is converted to a form that can be recycled,

it serves as a folate sink, making tetrahydrofolate unavailable for any other reaction. The other reaction requiring a vitamin B_{12} cofactor is catalyzed by methylmalonyl CoA mutase, in which methylmalonyl CoA is converted to succinyl CoA. This is the last step in the breakdown of odd carbon fatty acids, and inhibition of this reaction leads to odd carbon fatty acid accumulation in neuronal sheaths and, as a result, neuropathy.

Decreased blood δ-aminolevulinic acid (ALA; **choice A**) would occur with pyridoxine deficiency.

Decreased transketolase activity in erythrocytes (**choice B**) would occur with thiamine deficiency.

Because both cofactors are required to convert homocysteine to methionine, homocysteine levels would increase (compare with **choice C**) in the urine of either a folate- or vitamin B_{12}–deficient person.

Lactic acidosis (**choice E**) would occur in any condition in which lactate accumulates. These could involve many of the reactions in carbohydrate or oxidative metabolism, none of which are relevant to this question.

29. **The correct answer is B.** You may be asked to make this type of calculation on the COMLEX. You should know that 1 g of either protein or carbohydrate produces about 4 kcal = 4 calories (kcal) of energy, and 1 g of fat produces 9 kcal = 9 calories of energy. The calculation is then straightforward. The calories from carbohydrates are $125 \times 4 = 500$; from protein are $15 \times 4 = 60$; and from fat are $10 \times 9 = 90$. The total is $500 + 60 + 90 = 650$ kcal/day.

30. **The correct answer is B.** Deletion of two nucleotides will lead to a reading frame shift. The genetic code will be read differently from that point on until the end of the genome, or until another alteration in the DNA (e.g., the addition of two base pairs or the deletion of another base pair) restores the original reading frame. Often, this results in a truncated protein.

    A conservative mutation (**choice A**) is a missense mutation (see below) that leads to the substitution of a given amino acid with a chemically similar amino acid. For example, one codon for leucine is CUC. Replacement of the 5′ cytosine with an adenosine produces AUC, which codes for isoleucine.

    A missense mutation (**choice C**) is one that leads to the replacement of a given amino acid with a different amino acid.

    A nonsense mutation (**choice D**) introduces a stop codon instead of a codon specifying an amino acid, leading to premature chain termination.

    A silent mutation (**choice E**) is a mutation to a codon that specifies the same amino acid as the original codon, e.g., if ACU is mutated to ACC, threonine is still the amino acid specified by the code, and the protein is unchanged. Mutations in the third position (the wobble position) are generally the cause of silent mutations because of the degeneracy of the genetic code.

31. **The correct answer is E.** Tryptophan is an aromatic amino acid that contains an indole group. By a very complex series of minor enzymatic reactions, a small amount (~2%) of the tryptophan can be converted to quinolinate, which can then be used in place of niacin (nicotinic acid) in NAD (nicotinamide adenine dinucleotide) synthesis. Very high tryptophan levels can replace a portion of the dietary requirements for niacin. The nutritional disease pellagra (characterized by swollen tongue, dermatitis, neurologic dysfunction, and gastrointestinal dysfunction) usually occurs in the setting of combined tryptophan and niacin deficiency.

Alanine (**choice A**), the amino acid with a methyl R group, is a substrate of the liver enzyme alanine amino transferase (ALT, formerly called SGPT).

Asparagine (**choice B**) is one of the sources of ammonia for the urea cycle.

Methionine (**choice C**) is a sulfur-containing amino acid that is associated with associate with methyl group transfers.

Proline (**choice D**) is technically an imino acid, rather than an amino acid, with a ring structure. You should remember collagen has high proline concentration.

32. **The correct answer is C.** Chromosomal aberrations are common in spontaneously aborted fetuses. This fetus has Patau syndrome (trisomy 13). A convenient way to remember trisomy 13 is to think of polydactyly (remembered as 13 fingers) and midline defects, including microphthalmia (just one central "eye"); cleft lip, palate, or face; arrhinencephaly (failure of development of olfactory nerves and related brain); and dextrocardia or ventricular septal defect. The head is usually small, with profound mental retardation. In fetuses that survive until birth, death usually occurs in the neonatal period. Patau syndrome has an incidence of 1 in 6,000 births.

Features of *cri du chat* syndrome (5p-; **choice A**) include a catlike cry, severe mental retardation, microcephaly, and epicanthal folds.

Features of Turner syndrome (45, XO; **choice B**) include webbed neck, short stature, broad chest, low hairline, primary amenorrhea, coarctation of aorta, and streak ovaries.

Features of Edwards syndrome, or trisomy 18 (**choice D**), include severe mental retardation, ventricular septal defect, micrognathia, rocker-bottom feet, low-set ears, prominent occiput, and hypotonia.

Features of Down syndrome, or trisomy 21 (**choice E**), include mental retardation, flat nasal bridge, epicanthal folds, oblique palpebral fissures, dysplastic ears, horizontal palmar crease, redundant neck skin, short trunk, ventricular septal defect, acute lymphoblastic leukemia, and neurologic changes similar to those of Alzheimer disease.

33. **The correct answer is C.** The patient is presenting with signs and symptoms of chronic granulomatous disease of childhood. Patients with this condition usually present with a past medical history as described in the question stem. This pathologic condition is caused by a defect in the NADPH oxidase complex, resulting in neutrophils and other phagocytic cells that do not produce superoxides. Affected individuals therefore present with an inability to kill invading microbes that are engulfed by these phagocytic cells.

Muscle glycogen phosphorylase (**choice A**) deficiency is seen in patients with McArdle disease. These patients often experience muscle cramps and weakness on exercise.

Myeloperoxidase (**choice B**) deficiency usually is not associated with clinical abnormalities, except in patients with an underlying disease, such as diabetes. These patients may experience an increased frequency of fungal infections.

Transketolase (**choice D**) is an enzyme used to diagnose thiamine deficiency by measuring erythrocyte transketolase activity on addition of thiamine pyrophosphate.

Xanthine oxidase (**choice E**) is an enzyme responsible for the production of uric acid. Deficiency of this enzyme would result in the development of hypouricemia.

34. **The correct answer is A.** The patient has liver disease secondary to homozygosity for the Z allele of α_1-antitrypsin. α_1-Antitrypsin, more properly α_1-antiproteinase, is synthesized and secreted into the blood by the liver and macrophages. It is the principle serine protease of the human plasma, and it inhibits trypsin, elastin, and other proteases. It exists in several isoforms. Proteins such as α_1-antitrypsin that are normally secreted must fold properly in the endoplasmic reticulum in order to be transferred to the Golgi apparatus. Sporadic misfolded proteins will be escorted into the cytoplasm for degradation in proteasomes, but if the cell is accumulating large quantities, they accumulate in the endoplasmic reticulum. ZZ individuals produce large amounts of misfolded protein, which accumulates in the cisternae of the endoplasmic reticulum and causes hepatitis and cirrhosis.

Extracellular matrix (**choice B**) could not be a possibility because these misfolded proteins could not get into the Golgi apparatus, which is a necessary step on their way to being excreted.

The misfolded proteins would be unable to proceed to the Golgi apparatus (**choice C**).

"Inclusion bodies" (**choice D**) is a nonspecific term describing aggregate material accumulating in cells. The lysosomal storage diseases, including I-cell disease itself, result in inclusion bodies of material from endocytosis, phagocytosis, or autophagy that cannot be digested due to a lysosomal enzyme deficiency.

Misfolded proteins would accumulate in the ER, not in lysosomes (**choice E**).

35. **The correct answer is E.** The disease is myotonic dystrophy, which is an autosomal dominant disease; the affected gene has been localized to chromosome 19. Myotonic dystrophy is relatively common and is best thought of as a systemic disease, since it causes cataracts, testicular atrophy, heart disease, dementia, and baldness, in addition to muscular weakness.

A mutation on the X chromosome (**choice A**) causes Duchenne muscular dystrophy.

None of the muscle diseases are known to be related to defects on the Y chromosome (**choice B**).

Facioscapulohumeral dystrophy is associated with a defective gene on chromosome 4 (**choice C**).

Infantile hypotonia has been related to defective genes on chromosome 5 (**choice D**).

36. **The correct answer is A.** Color-blindness is an X-linked recessive trait. A male is hemizygous for the X chromosome and thus has only one copy of each trait. The frequency of an X-linked recessive in males is thus equal to the frequency of the allele in the population. From this, we know that q = 0.01 and p = 0.99. A female has two copies of each gene on the X chromosome, so the equation for Hardy-Weinberg equilibrium is the same as for the autosomal traits. In this case, a homozygous recessive female would occur at a frequency of q^2 or 0.0001.

Choice B, 0.0005, is incorrect. If you remembered that color-blindness was more frequent in males, but did not know how to use the equations to get the true estimate, you might have guessed this answer.

Choice C, 0.01, makes the assumption that the trait is autosomal, and so the frequencies of affected males and affected females are equal.

Choice D, 0.02, assumes that q = 0.01, and then calculates the frequency of carrier females (2pq).

Choice E, 0.025 is also incorrect; it is a distracter.

37. **The correct answer is A.** In aerobic glycolysis, glucose is degraded to pyruvate, which is then converted to acetyl-CoA, the form in which it actually enters the citric acid cycle. Two acetyl-CoAs, each containing two of the glucose's carbons, are produced from each glucose molecule. In addition, a total of two carbons from glucose are released as CO_2 when each of the two pyruvates are converted to acetyl-CoA.

Citrate (**choice B**) is the product formed in the citric acid cycle when acetyl-CoA condenses with oxaloacetate.

Oxaloacetate (**choice C**) is the citric acid cycle intermediate that condenses with acetyl-CoA to form citrate.

Two pyruvates (**choice D**) are produced from degradation of glucose. These are then converted to the two acetyl-CoAs that enter the citric acid cycle.

Succinate (**choice E**) is another citric acid cycle intermediate that forms when coenzyme A is removed from succinyl-CoA.

38. **The correct answer is B.** This infant has Menkes syndrome, also known as Ehlers-Danlos syndrome type IX or "kinky hair" disease. It is due to a defect in a copper transporting P-type ATPase, and in common with all of the Ehlers-Danlos diseases, it has a symptomology caused primarily by weak collagen. Most, if not all, copper-requiring enzymes are adversely affected by the associated copper deficiency. However, lysyl oxidase both requires copper and plays a direct role in collagen formation by catalyzing the cross-linking of collagen fibrils. A deficiency of this enzyme would thus be directly responsible for the described symptoms.

Cytochrome aa_3 (**choice A**) does require copper, but has no direct role in collagen formation. Deficient cytochrome aa_3 activity would principally affect muscles and nerves. The fact that these tissues appear to not be significantly affected may be a reflection of the fact that there is much more cytochrome aa_3 present than required for normal function. Thus, a loss of some activity would only reduce reserve capacity and have a minimal effect.

Prolyl hydroxylase (**choice C**) catalyzes the hydroxylation of proline on the nascent collagen fiber. Although clearly important for collagen synthesis, it does not require copper.

Tyrosinase (**choice D**) also is a copper-requiring enzyme. It plays an important role in the production of melanin, and the hypopigmentation associated with Menkes syndrome is undoubtedly due to hypoactivity of this enzyme. However, this is a relatively minor symptom and is not one of the ones described in the vignette.

γ-Glutamyl carboxylase (**choice E**) is a vitamin K–dependent enzyme that catalyzes the formation of γ-carboxyglutamate required for chelation of calcium ion by the clotting factors. It does not require copper, and it does not have a role in collagen formation.

39. **The correct answer is D.** The key to this question is understanding how and when the body utilizes fuel stores. The stores of ATP (**choice A**) will be used up in less than 1 second once the race has started. Creatine phosphate (**choice B**) will be the primary source of energy for the next 3 or 4 seconds. After the creatine phosphate stores are depleted, the majority of ATP needed to complete the race will be derived from glycolysis. If the race were to last for an extended period of time, then the processes of gluconeogenesis (**choice C**) and lipolysis (**choice E**) might be utilized. Gluconeogenesis is the process of synthesizing glucose in the liver from non-carbohydrate sources, such as amino and fatty acids. Lipolysis is the splitting up or decomposition of fat in the body.

40. **The correct answer is D.** In the absence of sufficient insulin or if there is decreased sensitivity to insulin, hormone-sensitive lipase in adipose tissue will be overactive. This will degrade stored triacylglycerols and release fatty acids into the blood.

Glucose conversion to sorbitol in the lens (**choice A**) will be enhanced due to the hyperglycemia of diabetes. This sorbitol will tend to accumulate in the lens, causing cataracts and probably contributing to other degenerative changes associated with diabetes. The reaction does not contribute to hyperlipidemia.

The GLUT-2 of liver (**choice B**) is insulin-independent and would not be affected.

The adipose and muscle glucose transporter, GLUT-4, will not be recruited maximally and will thus be underactive rather than overactive (**choice C**).

Lipoprotein lipase will be underactive rather than overactive (**choice E**). Underactive lipoprotein lipase will produce an increase in circulating triacylglycerol-rich lipoproteins by inhibiting their uptake into cells and will contribute to the hyperlipidemia.

41. **The correct answer is E.** To answer this question, you need two separate pieces of information. First, riboflavin (one of the B vitamins) is used to make the flavin part of FAD (flavin adenine dinucleotide). Second, of the citric acid cycle enzymes listed, only succinate dehydrogenase (which catalyzes the conversion of succinate to fumarate) uses FAD (which is converted to $FADH_2$) as a cofactor.

Aconitase (**choice A**) converts citrate to isocitrate and does not require a cofactor.

Citrate synthetase (**choice B**) combines acetyl-CoA and oxaloacetate to make citrate with the release of coenzyme A (which requires pantothenic acid for synthesis).

Isocitrate dehydrogenase (**choice C**) converts isocitrate to alpha-ketoglutarate and uses NAD^+ (which is con-

verted to $NADH + H^+$). The NAD^+ requires the vitamin niacin for synthesis.

Malate dehydrogenase (**choice D**) converts malate to oxaloacetate and uses NAD^+ (which is converted to $NADH + H^+$). The NAD^+ requires the vitamin niacin for synthesis.

42. **The correct answer is B.** Leber hereditary optic neuropathy is a relatively common cause of acute or subacute vision loss, especially in young men. It exhibits a mitochondrial inheritance pattern. The hallmark of this pattern is matrilineal inheritance. All the children of an affected woman will be affected since they receive mitochondrial genes only from the female parent. Affected males do not contribute mitochondria to progeny, so their children will not receive the trait.

Glucose-6-phosphate dehydrogenase (G6PD) deficiency (**choice A**) is an X-linked recessive disorder that affects the pentose phosphate pathway. The hallmark of X-linked recessive inheritance is an abundance of affected males and an absence of affected females. Males are hemi-zygous for the X chromosome, so the phenotype is expressed with only one dose of the gene. Females have two copies of the X chromosome, so they appear phenotypically normal although they may carry the recessive allele. Since a male inherits his X chromosome from his mother, if he is affected, she must carry the trait. Other X-linked recessive disorders include Lesch-Nyhan disease, hemophilia A, and Duchenne muscular dystrophy.

Neurofibromatosis (**choice C**) shows an autosomal dominant inheritance pattern, so the phenotype will be expressed if the allele is present in one dose. Deleterious autosomal dominants occur at very low frequencies, so affected individuals are almost always heterozygous for the trait. Since the gene is located on an autosome, both male and female progeny can be affected. Other autosomal dominant disorders include Ehlers-Danlos syndrome, Huntington disease, and osteogenesis imperfecta.

Sickle cell anemia (**choice D**) and Tay-Sachs disease (**choice E**) are both inherited in an autosomal recessive pattern. For the phenotype of the autosomal recessive to be expressed, the recessive allele must be present in two doses. Both male and female children can be affected. The hallmark feature is that unaffected parents have affected children of both sexes.

43. **The correct answer is D.** The administration of any product that contains phenylalanine, such as aspartame, to an individual with any of the hyperphenylalaninemias could be detrimental to his or her general health. The hyperphenylalaninemias result from an impaired conversion of phenylalanine to tyrosine. The

most common and clinically important of these is phenylketonuria, which is characterized by an increased concentration of phenylalanine in blood, increased concentration of phenylalanine and its by-products (such as phenylpyruvate, phenylacetate, and phenyllactate) in urine, and mental retardation. Phenylketonuria is caused by a deficiency of phenylalanine hydrolase.

Hyperornithinemia (**choice A**) is an inherited disorder of amino acid metabolism that results from a defect of the enzyme ornithine decarboxylase. This condition is associated with mental retardation, neuropsychiatric dysfunction, and protein intolerance.

Hyperuricemia (**choice B**) is a condition associated with higher than normal blood levels of uric acid. Gout may be produced if the hyperuricemia persists.

Hypervalinemia (**choice C**) is an inherited disorder of amino acid metabolism that results from a defect of the enzyme valine aminotransferase. This condition is associated with mental retardation, neuropsychiatric dysfunction, and protein intolerance.

Wilson disease (**choice E**) is an autosomal recessive disorder associated with an abnormality of the hepatic excretion of copper, resulting in toxic accumulations of the metal in the brain, liver, and other organs.

44. **The correct answer is C.** About 20% of patients with a chromosome 13 abnormality (13q-syndrome) develop retinoblastoma. There is also a genetic dominant form of retinoblastoma that has an 80% penetrance rate. Retinoblastomas that have a genetic basis are more likely to be bilateral than the spontaneous lesions. Microscopically, retinoblastomas are composed of masses of small hyperchromatic cells that may form small rosettes composed of radially arranged cells surrounding a central lumen.

45. **The correct answer is E.** This patient has phenylketonuria, which is caused by a complete or near complete deficiency of phenylalanine hydroxylase. The excess phenylalanine disrupts normal metabolism and causes brain damage. Urine odor is described as mousy, musty, or wolf-like.

46. **The correct answer is D.** This patient has alcaptonuria, which is caused by a deficiency of homogentisic acid oxidase. Physical manifestations consist of ochronosis (darkening of skin) and arthritis, usually occurring in the third to fourth decade of life. The only sign of this disorder as a child is black-colored urine when it is left standing.

47. **The correct answer is A.** This patient has Tay-Sach disease, which is caused by a deficiency of beta-hexosaminidase A. Tay-Sach is a lipid storage disease that manifests as a severely retarded infant with cherry-red spots of the macula. There are several sphingolipidoses that are associated with cherry red spots, but only Tay-Sach patients will have no hepatosplenomegaly.

48. **The correct answer is F.** This patient has tyrosinemia type I, which is caused by a deficiency of fumarylacetoacetate. Some of the clinical manifestations of an acute case are failure to thrive, developmental delay, irritability, vomiting, diarrhea, and fever usually occurring within the first six months of life. A cabbage-like odor of the urine and body is characteristic of the disease.

49. **The correct answer is G.** This patient has Hurler disease, which is caused by a deficiency of alpha-L-iduronidase. This deficiency causes a build up of dermatan and heparin sulfates in tissues and urine. Physical manifestations are hepatosplenomegaly, exaggerated kyphosis, persistent nasal discharge, and noisy breathing. The head is large and dolichocephalic, with frontal bossing and prominent sagittal and metopic sutures. Clouding of the corneas becomes evident by 12 months of age. Umbilical and inguinal hernias are common.

50. **The correct answer is A.** Tay-Sach disease is a lysosomal storage disease that is inherited as an autosomal recessive trait with a carrier rate of 1 in 30 among Ashkenazi Jews. The disease is caused by a deficiency of the lysosomal enzyme beta-hexosaminidase A.

Microbiology/Immunology

1. A 19-year-old man presents to the emergency department with pneumonia. Since the age of 6 months, he has had recurrent pneumonia and sinusitis due to *Streptococcus pneumoniae* and *Haemophilus influenzae*. Physical examination reveals chronic somatic dysfunction bilaterally at T2-T7. Careful assessment of his immune function would likely reveal abnormal function of the

   (A) B-lymphocytes

   (B) macrophages

   (C) natural killer cells

   (D) platelets

   (E) T-lymphocytes

2. A 20-year-old woman presents with a 2-day history of dysuria and increased urinary frequency. She states that she was recently married and was not sexually active prior to the marriage. Physical examination reveals a temperature of 100.7 F with normal vital signs. Gynecologic examination reveals no evidence of discharge, vaginitis, or cervicitis. Structural examination is significant for acute tissue changes paraspinally at T11-L2. Urinalysis reveals 14 white blood cells per high-powered field with many gram-negative rods. Which of the following is the most appropriate pharmacotherapy?

   (A) Ampicillin

   (B) Ceftriaxone

   (C) Fluconazole

   (D) Gentamicin

   (E) Metronidazole

3. A 35-year-old, sexually active man presents to his internist with a painless penile vesicle. Physical examination reveals inguinal lymphadenopathy. Structural examination reveals somatic dysfunction at T10-T11. The infecting organism is definitively diagnosed and is known to exist in distinct extracellular and intracellular forms. Which of the following is the most likely pathogen?

   (A) *Calymmatobacterium granulomatis*

   (B) *Chlamydia trachomatis*

   (C) *Haemophilus ducreyi*

   (D) *Neisseria gonorrhoeae*

   (E) *Treponema pallidum*

4. A neonate acquires meningitis during delivery. Which of the following organisms should be suspected?

   (A) *Escherichia coli* and *Streptococcus agalactiae*

   (B) *Haemophilus influenzae* and *Neisseria meningitidis*

   (C) *Haemophilus influenzae* and *Streptococcus pneumoniae*

   (D) *Listeria monocytogenes* and *Neisseria meningitidis*

   (E) *Staphylococcus aureus* and *Staphylococcus epidermidis*

5. A 24-year-old woman with a history of allergic rhinitis is involved in an automobile accident and sustains a splenic laceration. She undergoes abdominal surgery and is then transfused with four units of blood of the appropriate ABO and Rh type. As the transfusion progresses, she becomes rapidly hypotensive and develops airway edema, consistent with anaphylaxis. Which of the following pre-existing conditions best accounts for these symptoms?

   (A) AIDS

   (B) C1 esterase inhibitor deficiency

   (C) DiGeorge syndrome

   (D) Selective IgA deficiency

   (E) Wiskott-Aldrich syndrome

6. A 24-year-old woman in her third trimester of pregnancy presents with urinary frequency and burning for the past few days. She denies fever, nausea, vomiting, or chills. She takes no medications besides prenatal vitamins and is generally in good health. Physical examination is remarkable for mild suprapubic tenderness, and a urine dipstick is positive for white blood cells, protein, and a small amount of blood. Osteopathic examination reveals no pubic dysfunction and there are acute tissue changes at T11-L2. Culture produces greater than 100,000 colonies of gram-negative bacilli. Which of the following attributes of this uropathogenic organism is most strongly associated with its virulence?

(A) Bundle-forming pili
(B) GVVPQ fimbriae
(C) Heat labile toxins
(D) Heat stable toxins
(E) P pili

7. A 47-year-old grocer complains of diarrhea and painful arthritis. Physical examination is remarkable for lymphadenopathy and weight loss. Biopsy of his small bowel reveals PAS-positive macrophages within the lamina propria. Electron microscopic examination of the macrophages reveals small, rod-shaped structures. Which of the following is the most likely pathogen?

(A) *Clostridium difficile*
(B) *Enterotoxigenic Escherichia coli*
(C) *Isospora belli*
(D) *Salmonella* sp.
(E) *Tropheryma whippelii*

8. A 35-year-old man presents to the emergency department with intense back pain. Physical examination reveals acute tissue-texture changes in the right paraspinal area at T11-L1. He is hydrated and given pain medication. After several hours he passes a kidney stone. Laboratory analysis of the stone reveals that it is composed of struvite (magnesium ammonium phosphate). Infection with which of the following organisms promotes the production of such stones?

(A) *Escherichia coli*
(B) *Proteus mirabilis*
(C) *Pseudomonas aeruginosa*
(D) *Staphylococcus saprophyticus*
(E) *Ureaplasma urealyticum*

9. A 21-year-old man presents with cough, fever, and hemoptysis. Blood tests show significantly elevated BUN and creatinine. Immunofluorescent microscopy reveals a diffuse linear pattern of fluorescence along the basement membranes of alveolar septa and glomerular capillaries. Which type of hypersensitivity is associated with this disease?

(A) I
(B) II
(C) III
(D) IV
(E) Not discernible from the information given

10. A 47-year-old man with a history of sickle cell disease has had numerous hospitalizations requiring the placement of IV lines. The patient has poor peripheral venous access, and a catheter is placed in right subclavian vein. The patient subsequently develops right arm discomfort and swelling and a temperature of 40.1 C with chills. Multiple blood cultures are taken, and gram-positive cocci are isolated. The organism is catalase positive and produces whitish colonies on mannitol salt agar. The colonies are gamma-hemolytic on sheep blood agar. Which of the following organisms is the most likely cause of this patient's symptoms?

(A) *Enterococcus faecalis*
(B) *Staphylococcus aureus*
(C) *Staphylococcus epidermidis*
(D) *Streptococcus agalactiae*
(E) *Streptococcus pyogenes*

11. A 58-year-old alcoholic man with multiple dental caries develops a pulmonary abscess and is treated with antibiotics. Several days later, he develops nausea, vomiting, abdominal pain, and voluminous green diarrhea. Physical examination shows Chapman reflex tenderpoints bilaterally on the anterolateral aspect of the thighs. Which of the following antibiotics is most likely responsible for this patient's symptoms?

(A) Chloramphenicol
(B) Clindamycin
(C) Gentamicin
(D) Metronidazole
(E) Vancomycin

12. A 54-year-old man with chronic renal failure receives a kidney transplant and is given immunosuppressive therapy with cyclosporine. Over the next 6 months, the patient's creatinine levels progressively rise, and a needle biopsy of the kidney is performed. His physical examination reveals warm, boggy tissues paraspinally at T11-L1. What is the biopsy most likely to show?

(A) Intimal fibrosis, interstitial fibrosis, and tubular atrophy

(B) Linear deposition of immunoglobulin and complement in glomeruli

(C) Neutrophils, immunoglobulin, and complement in vessel walls

(D) T-cell interstitial infiltrate and edema

(E) Thickening of the blood vessel intima due to cellular proliferation

13. A 7-year-old boy presents to the pediatrician because his mother noticed a "smoky" color to his urine. On questioning the mother, it is revealed that the child had a sore throat several weeks ago that was left untreated. Physical examination reveals hypertension and mild generalized edema. Structural examination reveals acute somatic dysfunction at T1-T4. Urinalysis is significant for red blood cell casts. Which of the following accurately describes the microorganism responsible for this child's illness?

(A) It causes alpha-hemolysis on blood agar

(B) It is catalase positive

(C) It is coagulase positive

(D) It is sensitive to bacitracin

(E) It is sensitive to optochin

14. A baby born at 32 weeks' gestation with Apgar scores of 2 and 7 was placed in the neonatal intensive care unit. She developed a fever and leukocytosis; lumbar puncture revealed pleocytosis with increased protein, decreased glucose, and gram-positive rods. Which of the following organisms was most likely isolated from the CSF?

(A) *Escherichia coli*

(B) *Listeria monocytogenes*

(C) *Neisseria meningitidis*

(D) *Streptococcus agalactiae*

(E) *Streptococcus pneumoniae*

15. A young mother takes her infant to the pediatrician for the first time. The pediatrician notices the infant's teeth are yellow. The antibiotic this mother most likely took during pregnancy

(A) inhibits aminoacyl-tRNA binding

(B) inhibits peptidyl transferase

(C) interferes with cell wall synthesis

(D) is a large, cyclic, lactone-ring structure

(E) inhibits the synthesis of membrane lipids

16. A 32-year-old, blood type A positive man receives a kidney transplant from a blood type B positive female donor with whom he had a 6-antigen HLA match. Once the kidney is anastomosed to the man's vasculature, the transplant team immediately begins to observe swelling and interstitial hemorrhage. After the surgery, the patient developed fever and leukocytosis and produced no urine. Which of the following is the most likely explanation?

(A) Acute rejection due to antibody-mediated immunity

(B) Acute rejection due to cell-mediated immunity

(C) Chronic rejection due to cell-mediated immunity to minor HLA antigens

(D) Hyperacute rejection due to lymphocyte and macrophage infiltration

(E) Hyperacute rejection due to preformed ABO blood group antibodies

17. A 5-year-old child who has not had routine pediatric care develops a febrile disease with cough and a blotchy rash, and is brought to the emergency department. Structural examination reveals acute somatic dysfunction at T2-T7. On physical examination, there is cervical and axillary lymphadenopathy. Also noted is an erythematous, maculopapular rash behind the ears and along the hairline, involving the neck and, to a lesser extent, the trunk. Examination of this patient's oropharynx would likely reveal which of the following lesions?

(A) Adherent thin, whitish patch on gingiva

(B) Cold sores on the lips

(C) Curdy white material overlying an erythematous base on the oral mucosa

(D) Large shallow ulcers on the oral mucosa

(E) Multiple small white spots on the buccal mucosa

18. A 35-year-old man undergoes an appendectomy. Several days later, an abscess has formed at the surgical site. At that time, physical examination reveals acute somatic dysfunction at T9-T12. It does not improve with administration of a cephalosporin but does respond to nafcillin. The infecting organism most likely produced an enzyme that would hydrolyze which bond in the following molecule?

(A) A
(B) B
(C) C
(D) D
(E) E

19. After eating a dinner of leftovers that included rewarmed vegetable fried rice, a 17-year-old boy develops diarrhea and stomach pain. Physical examination reveals acute tissue changes at T5-L2 paraspinally. Which of the following is the most likely pathogen?

(A) *Bacillus cereus*
(B) *Campylobacter jejuni*
(C) *Clostridium botulinum*
(D) *Clostridium difficile*
(E) *Escherichia coli*

20. A 23-year-old woman with a history of sickle cell disease presents with fever and severe bone pain localized to her left tibia. An x-ray film reveals a lytic lesion, and blood cultures reveal infection. A bone culture grows gram-negative rods. Which of the following best describes the infecting organism?

(A) It is comma-shaped and sensitive to acidic pH
(B) It is an obligate intracellular parasite
(C) It is motile and does not ferment lactose
(D) It is motile and oxidase positive
(E) It is a nonmotile facultative anaerobe

21. A 33-year-old HIV-positive man complains of headache and blurred vision. Structural examination showed no somatic dysfunction in the cervical or thoracic region. Physical examination reveals papilledema and ataxia. Head CT is normal but CSF obtained by lumbar puncture reveals encapsulated organisms observable with India ink. Which of the following is true concerning this organism?

(A) It can also be identified with methenamine silver stain
(B) It consists of branching septate hyphae
(C) It exists as a mycelial form at room temperature and as yeast at 37 C
(D) It is an encapsulated nondimorphic yeast found worldwide
(E) It is a nonencapsulated dimorphic yeast that reproduces by budding

22. A French exchange student in a town near the Ohio River presents to the local hospital with headache, fever, malaise, and nonproductive cough. He became ill several days after cleaning and moving a chicken coop where hundreds of chickens had roosted for many years. Which of the following microorganisms is most likely responsible for his illness?

(A) *Actinomyces israelii*
(B) *Aspergillus fumigatus*
(C) *Candida albicans*
(D) *Coccidioides immitis*
(E) *Histoplasma capsulatum*

23. A 3-year-old girl presents with recurrent subcutaneous abscesses and furuncles. She has a history of pneumonia due to *Serratia marcescens*. There is chronic somatic dysfunction at T2-T7. Which of the following enzymes is most likely deficient in her neutrophils?

(A) Aldolase B
(B) Galactokinase
(C) Glucokinase
(D) Glucose-6-phosphate dehydrogenase
(E) NADPH oxidase

24. An otherwise healthy patient who has just received a prosthetic aortic valve develops postoperative fever. Blood cultures are done, and she is given broad-spectrum antibiotics. Two days later she is still febrile and clinically deteriorating. Which of the following is the most likely pathogen?

    (A) *Actinomyces israelii*

    (B) *Candida albicans*

    (C) *Histoplasma capsulatum*

    (D) *Nocardia asteroides*

    (E) *Trichophyton rubrum*

25. After high-dose chemotherapy and irradiation, a 35-year-old woman with acute myeloid leukemia in remission receives a bone marrow transplant from her HLA-matched brother. One week after the graft, the patient develops a fever and a maculopapular rash over her upper extremities and back. She also notes abdominal pain and diarrhea. Laboratory examination is remarkable for elevation of alkaline phosphatase and bilirubin. Which of the following is the most likely cause of this patient's symptoms?

    (A) Bacterial infection from the graft

    (B) Blast crisis

    (C) Graft-versus-host disease

    (D) Hyperacute graft rejection

    (E) Radiation toxicity

26. A 16-year-old boy with sickle cell disease is hospitalized for a severe infection. His spleen has autosplenectomized, and he has had other minor infections in the past. His symptoms include fever, chills, cough, and chest pain. Bacteria from the patient's sputum yield optochin-sensitive organisms with a positive Quellung reaction. Which of the following is the most likely pathogen?

    (A) *Escherichia coli*

    (B) *Haemophilus influenzae*

    (C) *Klebsiella pneumoniae*

    (D) *Neisseria gonorrhoeae*

    (E) *Streptococcus pneumoniae*

27. A 38-year-old AIDS patient presents to the clinic complaining of nausea, occasional vomiting, and "bumps" on his groin. On physical exam, the bumps are nontender, pedunculated, reddish-purple nodules in the inguinal and perirectal areas. His liver is palpable 8 cm below the right costal margin. Routine laboratory tests are remarkable only for slightly elevated aminotransferases and alkaline phosphatase levels. He has two pet cats and denies any foreign travel. Which of the following agents is the most likely cause of this patient's infection?

    (A) *Bartonella henselae*

    (B) Human papillomavirus

    (C) Molluscum contagiosum

    (D) *Rickettsia prowazekii*

    (E) *Treponema pallidum*

28. A 3-year-old boy presents with a 1-day history of loose stools, fever, abdominal cramping, headache, myalgia, and Chapman reflex tender points along the anterior lateral surface of his thighs. He has no blood in the stool. A careful history reveals that he has several pet turtles. Which of the following is the most likely pathogen?

    (A) *Chlamydia psittaci*

    (B) *Entamoeba histolytica*

    (C) *Salmonella* spp.

    (D) *Staphylococcus aureus*

    (E) *Yersinia enterocolitica*

29. A 52-year-old male with carcinoma complains of back pain. Physical examination reveals chronic somatic dysfunction at T5-T9 on the right side, which he states he has had since childhood. Which of the following viruses produces disease that is more severe if the infection occurs at a very young age?

    (A) Epstein-Barr virus

    (B) Hepatitis B virus

    (C) Measles virus

    (D) Poliovirus

    (E) Varicella zoster virus

30. A 20-year-old man with stridor is brought to the emergency department by his girlfriend. He had been complaining of abdominal pain earlier in the day. Physical examination is significant for well-demarcated regions of subcutaneous edema. Structural examination reveals acute tissue changes at T2-T8. He has had similar episodes before, and his mother and sister have the same condition. Which of the following substances is most likely deficient in this patient?

    (A) C1 esterase inhibitor

    (B) C3b inactivator

    (C) Factor H

    (D) Carboxypeptidase

    (E) Properdin

31. About a month after being bitten by a bat, a man develops an influenza-like illness. He subsequently develops striking mood changes, pharyngeal spasms with drooling, and seizures, and he falls into a coma. He eventually dies of his illness. This patient's deterioration was most likely caused by a virus from which of the following groups?

    (A) Bunyaviruses

    (B) Caliciviruses

    (C) Flaviviruses

    (D) Rhabdoviruses

    (E) Togaviruses

32. A diabetic patient has chronic sinusitis, which is eventually treated by evacuation of the contents of the maxillary and ethmoid sinuses. *Mucor* species are found when the material is examined histologically. The pathologist should notify the clinician immediately because *Mucor* can cause a virulent

    (A) meningitis

    (B) pneumonia

    (C) septicemia

    (D) skin infection

    (E) urinary tract infection

33. A 24-year-old woman has fever, malaise, and a dry, nonproductive cough. She also complains of headache, muscle aches, and leg pain. There is acute somatic dysfunction at T2-T7 bilaterally. Laboratory values are significant for elevated cold agglutinins. Which of the following microorganisms is responsible for her symptoms?

    (A) *Haemophilus influenzae*

    (B) *Klebsiella pneumoniae*

    (C) *Legionella pneumophila*

    (D) *Mycoplasma pneumoniae*

    (E) *Streptococcus pneumoniae*

34. A 25-year-old woman presents with a confluent maculopapular rash that began on her face then spread downward over her trunk. She states that 3 days ago she started having a fever and headache, with bilateral pain associated with the front and back of her neck. She also complains of joint pain. Which of the following diseases does she most likely have?

    (A) Infectious mononucleosis

    (B) Lyme disease

    (C) Roseola

    (D) Rubella

    (E) Rubeola

35. An 18-year-old, previously healthy woman presents to the student health service with fever, vomiting, and diarrhea. On physical examination, she is hypotensive, has an erythematous, red, sunburn-like skin rash, and multiple areas of acute somatic dysfunction. She is currently menstruating and has been using super-absorbent tampons. Which of the following findings from a positive blood culture would confirm the suspected diagnosis?

    (A) Organisms are acid-fast

    (B) Organisms are coagulase positive

    (C) Organisms grow on EMB (eosin-methylene blue) agar

    (D) Organisms grow on Thayer-Martin media

    (E) Organisms have positive Quellung reaction

36. Following a citywide outbreak of an exanthematous disease, three children at an urban elementary school develop a rash that begins on the face and neck and spreads to the rest of the body. Posterior auricular and posterior cervical lymphadenopathy is present. Distinct, rose-colored spots are seen on the palate, and the pharynx appears red. Which of the following procedures would be recommended for the rest of the students at the school?

    (A) A live, attenuated virus vaccine

    (B) A live, attenuated virus vaccine plus specific immunoglobulin

    (C) An inactivated (killed) virus vaccine

    (D) An inactivated (killed) virus vaccine plus specific immunoglobulin

    (E) Specific immunoglobulin only

37. A 7-month-old child presents with a 4-day history of fever, deepening cough, and dyspnea. Physical examination reveals acute somatic dysfunction at T2-T7 bilaterally. A chest x-ray film shows multiple interstitial infiltrates and hyperinflation of the lungs. Multinucleated giant cells with cytoplasmic inclusion bodies are seen when a nasal wash is inoculated into tissue culture. The most appropriate therapy includes administration of which of the following drugs?

    (A) Acyclovir

    (B) Ganciclovir

    (C) Ribavirin

    (D) Trifluorothymidine

    (E) Zidovudine

38. A formula-fed, 1-month-old boy is exposed to his sister, who has chickenpox. He does not develop signs of varicella. His mother had the infection 5 years ago. Which class of immunoglobulins did he acquire from his mother in utero that protected him from this virus?

    (A) IgA

    (B) IgD

    (C) IgE

    (D) IgG

    (E) IgM

39. After a normal physical examination, an osteopathic structural examination reveals chronic tissue changes at T5-T9 on the right. The 19-year-old army recruit then gives urine and blood samples for further testing. Serum analysis yields elevated ALT, HBsAg, Anti-HBc, HBeAg, and bilirubin. All other values are normal. What is the hepatitis B status of this recruit?

    (A) Asymptomatic carrier

    (B) Chronic active hepatitis

    (C) Fulminant hepatitis B

    (D) Recovered from acute self-limited HBV

    (E) Vaccinated against HBV

40. A 65-year-old man undergoes coronary artery bypass surgery that entails grafting the left internal mammary artery to the left main coronary artery to form an alternative conduit for blood flow. This patient received a(n)

    (A) allograft

    (B) autograft

    (C) homograft

    (D) isograft

    (E) xenograft

41. Following a barbecue hosted by a hunter who served "bear hamburgers," several guests develop abdominal pain and diarrhea; their condition progresses about a week later to fever, myalgia, periorbital edema, and petechial hemorrhages in the conjunctiva. A peripheral blood smear shows an increased eosinophil count. Which of the following is the most likely cause of these symptoms?

    (A) Anthrax

    (B) *Bacillus cereus* food poisoning

    (C) Botulism

    (D) *Escherichia coli* gastroenteritis

    (E) Trichinosis

42. A patient presents with right lower-quadrant pain, fever, and diarrhea. Physical examination reveals diffuse abdominal tenderness; laboratory examination shows a moderate leukocytosis, leading to a presumptive diagnosis of acute appendicitis. An osteopathic examination reveals no tenderness at the tip of the 12th rib. Surgical exploration of the abdomen reveals mesenteric adenitis, but the appendix is normal. Which of the following organisms is most likely responsible for these signs and symptoms?

    (A) Enteroinvasive *E. coli*
    (B) *Salmonella*
    (C) *Shigella*
    (D) *Vibrio cholerae*
    (E) *Yersinia enterocolitica*

43. A 68-year-old patient with alcoholic cirrhosis is hospitalized with ascites and esophageal varices. The patient's temperature is 38.3 C (101 F). Physical examination is significant for chronic and acute changes at T2-T9 bilaterally. Paracentesis reveals a polymorphonuclear cell count of 300/mm3. Which of the following is the most likely infecting organism?

    (A) *Bacillus cereus*
    (B) *Clostridium difficile*
    (C) *Escherichia coli*
    (D) *Entamoeba histolytica*
    (E) *Giardia lamblia*

44. A 4-year-old child who has had repeated infections with staphylococci and streptococci has normal phagocytic function and delayed hypersensitivity responses. Lymph node biopsy would most likely reveal

    (A) absence of postcapillary venules
    (B) absence of germinal centers
    (C) defective chemotactic response of neutrophils
    (D) depletion of paracortical areas
    (E) depletion of thymus-dependent areas

45. A 47-year-old man presents with a nonproductive cough and rales on his chest examination. Osteopathic structural examination reveals acute somatic dysfunction at T2-T8. A chest x-ray film suggests atypical pneumonia. The pneumonia resolves after treatment with azithromycin. A diagnosis of psittacosis is established by the presence of complement fixing antibodies against *Chlamydia psittaci* in the convalescent serum. Which of the following is the most likely occupation of this patient?

    (A) Cat breeder
    (B) Florist
    (C) Homeless shelter worker
    (D) Poultry farmer
    (E) Slaughterhouse worker

46. A 20-year-old college student presents to the university health clinic with sore throat, fever, and fatigue. Physical exam is significant for cervical lymphadenopathy and mild hepatomegaly. Structural examination reveals acutely edematous tissue on the right paraspinal area of T5-T9. Heterophile antibody tests are negative. Microscopic examination of an epithelial cell would be expected to reveal

    (A) an enlarged nucleus with peripherally displaced chromatin
    (B) conidia and septate hyphae
    (C) a giant nucleus surrounded by a clear zone
    (D) a multinucleated giant cell
    (E) staining with India ink

Questions 47-50

<u>CASE A</u>

A 21-year-old man complains of a tender papule on his penis that turns into an ulcer after 1 day. On examination the ulcer is 3 mm in diameter with irregular borders. There is bilateral painful inguinal adenopathy with draining abscesses.

47. The most likely diagnosis is

   (A) granuloma inguinale

   (B) chancroid

   (C) syphilis

   (D) lymphogranuloma venereum

   (E) herpes simplex virus 2

48. The causative etiology of this diagnosis is

   (A) a double-stranded DNA virus

   (B) *Calymmatobacterium granulomatis*

   (C) *Chlamydia trachomatis*

   (D) *Treponema pallidum*

   (E) *Haemophilus ducreyi*

49. The patient states he often forgets to take his medication properly. What would be the most appropriate treatment?

   (A) Tetracycline

   (B) Acyclovir

   (C) Doxycycline

   (D) Benzathine penicillin

   (E) Ceftriaxone

50. Which of the following is an associated condition?

   (A) Granuloma inguinale

   (B) Chancroid

   (C) Syphilis

   (D) Lymphogranuloma venereum

   (E) Gonorrhea

Microbiology/Immunology

ANSWERS AND EXPLANATIONS

1.	A	26.	E
2.	A	27.	A
3.	B	28.	C
4.	A	29.	B
5.	D	30.	A
6.	E	31.	D
7.	E	32.	A
8.	B	33.	D
9.	B	34.	D
10.	C	35.	B
11.	B	36.	A
12.	A	37.	C
13.	D	38.	D
14.	B	39.	B
15.	A	40.	B
16.	E	41.	E
17.	E	42.	E
18.	D	43.	C
19.	A	44.	B
20.	C	45.	D
21.	D	46.	C
22.	E	47.	B
23.	E	48.	E
24.	B	49.	E
25.	C	50.	C

1. **The correct answer is A.** The symptoms in the question suggest a deficiency known as common variable hypogammaglobulinemia, characterized by very low serum levels of IgG. In this congenital disease, the number of B cells is normal, but their ability to synthesize IgG and the other immunoglobulins is severely compromised, leading to recurrent streptococcal and *Haemophilus* infections. The onset of the recurrent infections usually begins between 6 and 12 months of age—concurrent with the decreasing levels of maternal IgG in the newborn. Treatment often involves giving IV gamma globulin to reduce the number of infections.

   Abnormal function of macrophages (**choice B**) such as that seen in chronic granulomatous disease results in recurrent infections with catalase-positive organisms. *Streptococcus* is a catalase-negative genus. Abnormal function of NK cells (**choice C**) is unlikely to present as recurrent bacterial infections, because these cells are primarily involved in cellular, rather than humoral, immunity.

   Platelets (**choice D**) are not directly involved in the immune response. Deficiencies in platelets lead to problems in clotting and produce bleeding disorders.

   T-cell deficiencies (**choice E**) result in severe viral, fungal, and protozoal infections, rather than recurrent bacterial infections.

2. **The correct answer is A.** The patient's presentation is consistent with a simple urinary tract infection; there is a short history of dysuria, increased urinary frequency, and the appearance of white blood cells and gram-negative rods in the urine. Urinary tract infections are common in women after they become sexually active. The infection is likely caused by urethral trauma during intercourse, which leads to bacterial contamination of the bladder. Since most of these infections are caused by *Escherichia coli* (a gram-negative rod), the most appropriate therapy would be ampicillin for around 10 days.

   Ceftriaxone (**choice B**) is the treatment of choice for uncomplicated infections with *Neisseria gonorrhoeae*, now that most strains are resistant to penicillin. IV ceftriaxone is a regimen reserved for the treatment of life-threatening infections.

   Fluconazole (**choice C**) is indicated for the treatment of vaginal candidiasis. Since there is no vaginal discharge and the patient has gram-negative rods in the urine, a diagnosis of vaginal candidiasis can be excluded.

   Gentamicin (**choice D**) would be an inappropriate choice. Most urinary tract infections caused by gram-negative rods are sensitive to ampicillin, and the potential for toxicity secondary to gentamicin is great.

   Metronidazole (**choice E**) is an antibiotic typically used in the treatment of vaginal *Trichomonas* and *Gardnerella* infections, as well as serious infections believed to be caused by anaerobic bacteria. Since there is no vaginal discharge and the patient has gram-negative rods in the urine, this is not the best choice for treatment.

3. **The correct answer is B.** This patient has lymphogranuloma venereum caused by *Chlamydia trachomatis* (type L1, 2, or 3). *Chlamydia* exhibit distinct infectious and reproductive forms. The extracellular infectious form is known as the elementary body (EB), which cannot reproduce. It attaches to the host cell and enters through endocytosis. Once inside the cell, the EB is transformed into the reticulate body (RB) within the endosome. The RB is capable of binary fission and divides within the endosome; fusion with other endosomes occurs to form a single large inclusion. Eventually, the RBs undergo DNA condensation and disulfide bond bridgings of the major outer membrane protein, forming EBs. The EBs are then released. Note that *C. trachomatis* is responsible for several sexually or perinatally transmitted diseases, including ocular trachoma (types A, B, and C), neonatal conjunctivitis, nongonococcal urethritis, cervicitis, and pelvic inflammatory disease (types D-K).

   Calymmatobacterium granulomatis (**choice A**) is a gram-negative rod that causes superficially ulcerated genital or inguinal papules that coalesce to form substantial lesions. The appearance of Donovan bodies in histiocytes is diagnostic of this infection.

   Haemophilus ducreyi (**choice C**) is a gram-negative rod that causes a soft, painful penile chancre, unlike that of a chlamydial or syphilitic lesion. This infection is common in the tropics.

   Neisseria gonorrhoeae (**choice D**) is a gram-negative diplococcus responsible for gonorrhea. Patients typically present with purulent penile discharge, not genital lesions.

   Treponema pallidum (**choice E**) is the spirochete responsible for syphilis. It may cause a firm, painless ulcer as a manifestation of primary syphilis, but the organism does not exist in distinct extracellular and intracellular forms as does *Chlamydia*. Secondary syphilis is associated with the appearance of condyloma lata—flat, gray, wart-like lesions.

4. **The correct answer is A.** The pattern of microbial causes of meningitis varies with the patient's age and clinical setting. The most common organisms encountered in neonatal meningitis are *Streptococcus agalactiae* (a group B *Streptococcus*) and *Escherichia coli*.

   Choice B: *Haemophilus influenzae* type B was the most common agent isolated in children aged 1–5 years (before 1990), but is much less common today because of the introduction of an effective vaccine. It is uncommon in neonates. *Neisseria meningitidis* is the most common agent isolated in patients aged 5–40 years (35% of children aged 5–15 years, and 20% of adults).

Choice C: *Haemophilus influenzae* type B was the most common agent isolated in children aged 1–5 years (before 1990), but is much less common today because of the introduction of an effective vaccine. *Streptococcus pneumoniae* occurs in all ages (40% of adult cases, 15% of childhood cases) but is uncommon in neonates (only 5% of cases).

Choice D: *Neisseria meningitidis* is the most common agent isolated in patients aged 5–40 years (35% of children aged 5–15 years, and 20% of adults). *Listeria monocytogenes* accounts for only 1% of all cases of bacterial meningitis, and is seen in infants, the elderly, and immunosuppressed patients.

Choice E: *Staphylococcus aureus* is seen in postsurgical and post-traumatic meningitis. *Staphylococcus epidermidis* accounts for 75% of shunt-related meningitis.

5. **The correct answer is D.** Patients with selective IgA deficiency may have circulating antibodies to IgA. Fatal anaphylaxis may ensue if they are transfused with blood products with serum containing IgA, although many patients with selective IgA deficiency are asymptomatic and never diagnosed. Symptomatic patients may have recurrent sinopulmonary infections and diarrhea, and also have an increased incidence of autoimmune and allergic diseases.

    AIDS (**choice A**) predisposes for infections and neoplasms, but not anaphylaxis.

    C1 esterase inhibitor deficiency (**choice B**) is an autosomal dominant disease characterized by recurrent attacks of colic and episodes of laryngeal edema, without pruritus or urticarial lesions. This disorder is also known as hereditary angioedema. It would not be expected to be associated with a blood transfusion but would occur throughout life.

    DiGeorge syndrome (**choice C**) is characterized by thymic aplasia and sometimes, hypoparathyroidism. The disorder is due to abnormal development of the third and fourth pharyngeal pouches.

    Wiskott-Aldrich syndrome (**choice E**) is a form of immunodeficiency associated with thrombocytopenia and eczema.

6. **The correct answer is E.** Urinary tract infections are the most common bacterial infections encountered during pregnancy, and *Escherichia coli* is the most commonly isolated organism. 70% of cases in the U.S. are caused

by P pili-positive strains. Pili are believed to be important mediators of attachment to the epithelium.

Bundle-forming pili (**choice A**) are found in enteroaggregative *E. coli* (EAEC).

GVVPQ fimbriae (**choice B**) are found in EAEC.

Heat labile toxins (**choice C**) are pathogenic factors in enterotoxic strains (ETEC).

Heat stable toxins (**choice D**) are pathogenic factors in ETEC or EAEC.

7. **The correct answer is E.** For many years, Whipple disease was suspected of having a bacterial etiology because bacterial forms could be seen on electron microscopy. However, the identity of the causative agent remained elusive. It has recently been found to be a bacterium, which is now named *Tropheryma whippelii*.

    Clostridium difficile (**choice A**) causes pseudomembranous colitis, generally after antibiotic administration.

    Enterotoxigenic *Escherichia coli* (**choice B**) is associated with tropical sprue.

    Isospora belli (**choice C**) is a cause of diarrhea in AIDS patients.

    Salmonella sp. (**choice D**) can cause diarrheal illness after ingestion of contaminated poultry or beef.

8. **The correct answer is B.** *Proteus* species produce urease, which raises the urinary pH and promotes the production of struvite stones.

    Escherichia coli (**choice A**) is by far the most common cause of urinary tract infections but is not responsible for the development of struvite stones.

    Pseudomonas aeruginosa (**choice C**) can also cause urinary tract infections, most commonly in hospitalized or immunocompromised patients (especially burn patients, patients on immunosuppressives/antimicrobials, and cystic fibrosis patients). It does not predispose to struvite stones.

    Staphylococcus saprophyticus (**choice D**) is a common cause of urinary tract infections in sexually active young women.

    Ureaplasma urealyticum (**choice E**) can produce urease (like *Proteus*), but it is responsible for urethritis, not stones.

9. **The correct answer is B.** This patient has a COMLEX-favorite disease: Goodpasture syndrome, which affects both the renal and pulmonary systems. In the kidney, it causes a rapidly progressive glomerulonephritis associated with antibodies directed against a collagen component of the glomerular basement membrane (anti-GBM antibody—a classic clue to this diagnosis). These antibodies

create a linear pattern on immunofluorescence. Note that they are also active against the basement membrane of respiratory alveoli, accounting for the pulmonary component of the disease.

Autoimmune reactions such as those found in Goodpasture syndrome, certain drug allergies, blood transfusion reactions, and hemolytic disease of the newborn, are classified as Type II hypersensitivities (antibody-mediated cytotoxicity). IgG or IgM antibody reacts with membrane-associated antigen on the surface of cells, causing activation of the complement cascade and, ultimately, cell destruction.

Type I (choice A) reactions (immediate, atopic, or anaphylactic) require an initial (sensitizing) exposure to an antigen. On re-exposure to the antigen, cross-linking of IgE receptors occurs on the surface of basophils and mast cells. The mast cells then release a variety of mediators, including histamine. Clinical syndromes include asthma, atopic dermatitis, eczema, and allergic rhinitis. Hives are characteristic of Type I hypersensitivity.

Type III (choice C) hypersensitivity (immune complex-mediated hypersensitivity) is caused by formation of antibody antigen complexes, which are filtered from the blood and activate complement. This results in the generation of C3b, which promotes neutrophil adherence to blood vessel walls. The complexes also generate C3a and C5a (anaphylatoxins), which lead to inflammation and tissue destruction. The hallmark signs of Type III sickness, which occur 7-14 days after exposure to the offending antigen, include urticaria, angioedema, fever, chills, malaise, and glomerulonephritis. Clinical syndromes include serum sickness (e.g., penicillin, streptomycin, sulfonamide, phenylbutazone hypersensitivity) and the Arthus response. Immune complexes are also observed in systemic lupus erythematosus (SLE). Type III glomerulonephritis (e.g., poststreptococcal glomerulonephritis) is characterized by a "lumpy bumpy" appearance on immunofluorescence using labeled antibody specific for immunoglobulin or complement.

Type IV (choice D) is also known as delayed-type hypersensitivity (DTH). Unlike the other types, which are mediated by antibody, DTH depends on TDTH cells that have been sensitized to a particular antigen. T cells react with antigen in association with MHC class I gene products and release lymphokines. Examples include tuberculin skin testing and contact dermatitis (e.g., poison ivy rash).

10. **The correct answer is C.** The patient has developed bacteremia; the description of the causative agent is consistent with a staphylococcal organism (catalase positive, gram-positive cocci that grow on mannitol

salt agar). The organism is most likely *Staphylococcus epidermidis* as it was not able to ferment mannitol and was not hemolytic. Both of those characteristics tend to rule out *Staphylococcus aureus*. **(choice B).** Two other tests that are commonly used are coagulase production and excretion of DNAse from colonies. *S. aureus* is positive in both tests, *S. epidermidis* is negative. *S. aureus* produces golden yellow colonies.

Enterococcus faecalis (choice A) might grow on the mannitol salt agar as it is relatively haloduric, but these organisms are catalase negative. The enterococci are extremely variable in hemolytic ability so this characteristic is not useful in species identification.

Both streptococcal organisms (choices D and E) are catalase negative and beta-hemolytic on sheep blood agar plates. Also, neither would grow on the mannitol salt agar. *Staphylococcus pyogenes* is sensitive to growth inhibition by bacitracin whereas *Staphylococcus agalactiae* (group B streptococci) is not.

11. **The correct answer is B.** Any time you see the development of diarrhea in the same question stem with "treated with antibiotics," you should immediately think of pseudomembranous colitis. This condition is caused by *Clostridium difficile* and typically occurs as a result of treatment with clindamycin or ampicillin. You would confirm your suspicion by sending a stool culture to be tested for the presence of the *C. difficile* toxin.

The most test-worthy side effect of chloramphenicol (choice A) is aplastic anemia, not diarrhea. In addition, you might have been able to eliminate this choice simply because of the extremely low probability that this patient would receive this antibiotic in the U.S.

The key side effects of gentamicin (choice C) include ototoxicity and nephrotoxicity.

Metronidazole (choice D) and vancomycin (choice E) do not cause pseudomembranous colitis; they are used to *treat* it.

12. **The correct answer is A.** Transplant rejection can be hyperacute (within minutes to hours), acute (usually within days, although it may appear later), or chronic (appearing 4-6 months after transplantation). Most acute rejection reactions are controlled, to some extent, by immunosuppressive therapy, so chronic rejection is more commonly seen. The patient described in this question is experiencing gradual renal failure over months, suggesting chronic rejection of the renal allograft. A renal biopsy from a patient experiencing chronic rejection typically shows intimal fibrosis in the vessels with fibrosis and tubular atrophy in the renal interstitium. Glomeruli may show ischemic changes, or may appear normal.

Linear deposition of immunoglobulin and complement in glomeruli (**choice B**) is a feature of Goodpasture syndrome (not a transplant rejection syndrome).

Neutrophils, immunoglobulin, and complement in blood vessels walls (**choice C**) are typical of hyperacute rejection, due to previous sensitization to an antigen found in the transplant.

A T-cell infiltrate (both CD4- and CD8-positive T cells) with interstitial edema (**choice D**) and hemorrhage characterizes acute cell-mediated rejection of an allograft. It would occur in a shorter time than that mentioned in this vignette.

Intimal thickening of vessels (**choice E**) due to proliferation of fibroblasts, myocytes, and foamy macrophages is a feature of subacute vasculitis, a common form of acute rejection generally seen in the first few months after transplantation.

13. **The correct answer is D.** This is one of the "higher order" questions the COMLEX favors. In this case, you need to figure out which disease the child has, which organism causes the disease, and which of the listed features is true of the microorganism. The disease in question is poststreptococcal glomerulonephritis, as evidenced by the smoky urine, hypertension, edema, and red blood cell casts in the urine sediment. The history of the prior sore throat is a tip-off that this is a nonsuppurative sequela of an infection due to *Streptococcus pyogenes* (group A β-hemolytic streptococci). *S. pyogenes* can be differentiated from *Streptococcus pneumoniae* and viridans streptococci by its hemolytic pattern; it is beta-hemolytic, whereas the others are alpha-hemolytic (**choice A**). It can be distinguished from the other beta-hemolytic streptococci by its sensitivity to the antibiotic bacitracin. Other important things to remember about *S. pyogenes* are its many virulence factors, including M protein, antiphagocytic capsule, hyaluronidase, streptolysins O and S, and erythrogenic toxins.

Choice B is incorrect because streptococci are catalase negative, whereas staphylococci are catalase positive.

Choice C is incorrect because *S. pyogenes* is coagulase negative. (In fact, there is no reason to perform a coagulase test on a catalase-negative organism.) The coagulase test is an important means of differentiating *Staphylococcus aureus*, which are coagulase positive, from all other species of *Staphylococcus*, which are coagulase negative. The only other medically important coagulase-positive organism is *Yersinia pestis*.

Choice E is incorrect because optochin is used to differentiate the viridans streptococci (resistant) from *S. pneumoniae* (sensitive).

14. **The correct answer is B.** The three major causes of neonatal meningitis are group B streptococci (*Streptococcus agalactiae*; **choice D**), *Escherichia coli* (**choice A**), and *Listeria monocytogenes*. All can be found in the vaginal tract of normal women and may contaminate the infant during passage through the birth canal. They colonize the upper respiratory tract and can cause pneumonia, septicemia, and/or meningitis in the neonate. They are readily distinguished on morphologic grounds; the streptococci are gram-positive cocci in chains, *E. coli* is a gram-negative rod, and *L. monocytogenes* is a gram-positive pleomorphic rod. There are other gram-positive rods that resemble *Listeria* (e.g., the diphtheroid bacilli found in the upper respiratory tract and on the skin); hence, a motility test is done to confirm the identification. *L. monocytogenes* is motile at room temperature but not when grown at 37 C. *L. monocytogenes* is also associated with drinking unpasteurized milk.

Neisseria meningitidis (**choice C**) is the most common cause of meningitis in school-aged children and young adults. It is a fastidious, nonmotile, gram-negative diplococcus that would be a very rare cause of meningeal disease in very young patients, such as this one.

Streptococcus pneumoniae (**choice E**) is a gram-positive coccus that grows in pairs and short chains. It is the number one cause of pneumonia, septicemia, and meningitis in the elderly. It would not be a common cause of neonatal meningitis.

15. **The correct answer is A.** This question relates to a COMLEX favorite side effect—the teeth mottling that occurs when a child is exposed to tetracycline *in utero*. You should remember that tetracycline is contraindicated in pregnancy and early childhood. Tetracycline is a bacteriostatic drug that binds to the 30s subunit of ribosomes, preventing aminoacyl-tRNA from binding with complementary mRNA. This inhibits peptide bond synthesis. Resistance is plasmid-mediated.

Inhibition of peptidyl transferase (**choice B**) occurs with chloramphenicol, a broad-spectrum bacteriostatic agent that binds to the 50s subunit of ribosomes. Resistance is plasmid mediated. It has high toxicity (gastrointestinal disturbances, aplastic anemia, and gray baby syndrome), so it is used mainly in severe infections or as a topical agent.

Interference with cell wall synthesis (**choices C and E**) occurs with penicillins and cephalosporins, the beta-lactam antibiotics. Resistance to these drugs appears in organisms that have developed beta-lactamases (penicillinases), enzymes that destroy the beta-lactam ring of these medications. The wider spectrum ampicillin, amoxicillin, ticarcillin, and carbenicillin are particularly penicillinase susceptible.

Large, cyclic, lactone-ring structures (**choice D**) describe the macrolides: erythromycin, azithromycin, and clarithromycin. They inhibit bacterial protein synthesis by reacting with the 50s ribosomal subunit and preventing the release of the uncharged tRNA. Resistance is plasmid mediated. Common side effects include gastrointestinal irritation, skin rashes, and eosinophilia. Erythromycin is a popular choice for patients with penicillin hypersensitivity. It is a cytochrome P450 inhibitor and therefore must be used with caution in patients taking other drugs.

16. **The correct answer is E.** The patient has hyperacute rejection due to the preformed anti-B ABO blood group antibody found in all type A positive individuals. Hyperacute rejection occurs within minutes to a few hours of the time of transplantation, and is due to the destruction of the transplanted tissue by preformed antibodies reacting with antigens found on the transplanted tissue that activate complement and destroy the target tissue. Preformed antibodies can also be due to presensitization to a previous graft, blood transfusion, or pregnancy.

Acute rejection due to antibody-mediated immunity (**choice A**) is incorrect because this patient had hyperacute rejection (immediate) occurring within minutes to hours, rather than days.

Acute rejection due to cell-mediated immunity (**choice B**) will not occur until several days or a week following transplantation. Acute rejection is due to type II and type IV reactions.

Chronic rejection, due to the presence of cell-mediated immunity to minor HLA antigens (**choice C**), occurs in allograft transplantation months to even years after the transplant. Chronic rejection is generally caused by both humoral and cell-mediated immunity.

An accelerated acute rejection, occurring in 3-5 days, can be caused by tissue infiltration and destruction by presensitized T lymphocytes and macrophages (**choice D**) and/or antibody-dependent, cell-mediated cytotoxicity (ADCC). Note that this is not a hyperacute reaction.

17. **The correct answer is E.** The disease described is measles (rubeola), which has the typical presentation described in the question stem. Measles is caused by a *Morbillivirus*, an RNA virus belonging to the Paramyxovirus family. Koplik's spots, which are pathognomonic for measles, are small, bluish-white spots on the buccal mucosa in the early stages of measles. These lesions appear just before the onset of the characteristic rash (which can also involve the extremities) and fade as the rash develops.

Leukoplakia is a premalignant condition characterized by adherent whitish patches on the gingiva (**choice A**) and other sites in the oral cavity.

Cold sores of the lips (**choice B**) are due to infection with Herpes viruses.

Candida infection (thrush) produces curdy white material loosely attached to an erythematous base (**choice C**).

Aphthous ulcers are large shallow ulcers of the oral mucosa (**choice D**), commonly known as canker sores.

18. **The correct answer is D.** Abscesses are often caused by *Staphylococcus aureus*. This organism may produce a penicillinase, an enzyme that cleaves the amide bond of beta-lactam antibiotics (the molecule shown is penicillin). The enzyme thus confers resistance to the beta-lactam antibiotics (penicillins and cephalosporins). Nafcillin (a semisynthetic penicillin) is very effective against penicillinase-producing *S. aureus*.

You should be familiar with other important enzymes and toxins produced by this organism, including heat-resistant enterotoxin, toxic shock syndrome toxin, exfoliatin (causes scalded-skin syndrome in children), alpha toxin (kills leukocytes), and coagulase.

19. **The correct answer is A.** *Bacillus cereus* contaminates grains, such as rice, and produces spores resistant to quick frying and steaming. If you see the words "fried rice" on the COMLEX, the odds are that the correct answer is *B. cereus*. The other most important clue for this etiology would be an onset of symptoms 1-2 hours after eating.

Campylobacter jejuni (**choice B**) causes enterocolitis with bloody diarrhea, crampy abdominal pain, malaise, and fever.

Clostridium botulinum (**choice C**) produces a constellation of signs and symptoms, including bulbar palsy, descending weakness or paralysis, progressive respiratory weakness, absence of fever, dry mucous membranes, and autonomic dysfunction.

Clostridium difficile (**choice D**) causes pseudomembranous colitis, classically resulting from clindamycin use.

Escherichia coli (**choice E**) comes in a variety of forms. The enterotoxigenic type is the most common cause of traveler's diarrhea.

20. **The correct answer is C.** The presence of sickle cell disease in a question stem is usually a significant clue. This question tests whether you know that patients with sickle cell anemia are more susceptible to osteomyelitis caused by *Salmonella*. (The patient's fever, bone pain, and x-ray results indicate osteomyelitis). *Staphylococcus aureus* (gram-positive coccus) is the most common cause of osteomyelitis overall, but 80% of osteomyelitis

cases in sickle cell patients are caused by *Salmonella*. If *Staphylococcus aureus* had not been ruled out on bone culture, you should have looked for it in the answer choices. Notice that you were required to know more than just the organism's name; you needed to know its distinguishing features. **Choice C** describes *Salmonella* (a gram-negative rod) accurately. *Salmonella* exists in more than 1800 serotypes and is known to contaminate poultry.

A comma-shaped organism that is sensitive to acidic pH (**choice A**) is *Vibrio cholerae*, a gram-negative rod that causes severe enterotoxin-induced diarrhea, with "rice-water" stools and dehydration. The toxin acts by stimulating adenylyl cyclase to overproduce cAMP in the brush border of the small intestine.

A facultative intracellular parasite (**choice B**) could be any one of a number of organisms. Facultative intracellular organisms survive inside cells when endocytosed but are capable of being grown on cell-free media. Examples include *Legionella* and *Listeria*.

A motile and oxidase positive organism (**choice D**) is *Pseudomonas*, a gram-negative rod that produces a polysaccharide slime layer. *P. aeruginosa* is the prototype and commonly colonizes the lungs of patients with cystic fibrosis. It is associated with production of blue-green pus because of its production of blue-green pigments.

A nonmotile, facultative anaerobe (**choice E**) could also be any of a number of organisms. The great majority of bacteria are facultative anaerobes, and of the gram-negative bacilli, *Shigella* and *Yersinia* would be examples of nonmotile genera.

21. **The correct answer is D.** This patient has cryptococcal meningitis, as evidenced by the "encapsulated organisms observable with India ink" in the CSF (a classic clue). *Cryptococcus* is a nondimorphic yeast, i.e., it exists only in the yeast form. Its capsule can be highlighted with India ink, and it reproduces by budding. It is found worldwide in bird droppings. It can also cause transient pulmonary illness in otherwise healthy individuals exposed to massive environmental doses.

The methenamine silver stain (**choice A**) is used primarily to demonstrate *Pneumocystis carinii* in tissues.

Branching septate hyphae (**choice B**) are characteristic of *Aspergillus fumigatus*, among other fungi.

Mycoses that exist in mycelial and yeast forms (dimorphism, diphasic; **choice C**) are *Histoplasma capsulatum, Coccidioides immitis, Blastomyces dermatitidis*, and *Sporothrix schenckii*.

Cryptococcus neoformans is not dimorphic and has a capsule (**choice E**).

22. **The correct answer is E.** *Histoplasma capsulatum* is a fungus common in soil contaminated with bird or bat droppings, especially in the Mississippi and Ohio River Valleys. Infection is usually asymptomatic or is associated with only mild symptoms; however, both the quantity inhaled and the immune status of the host determine the degree of symptoms.

Actinomyces israelii (**choice A**) is a branching, gram-positive rod that is part of the normal flora of the oral cavity. It can invade across fascial planes to produce abscesses with draining sinus tracts.

Aspergillus fumigatus (**choice B**) is a monomorphic fungus that is an opportunistic pathogen, especially in neutropenics.

Candida albicans (**choice C**) is part of the normal flora in humans and can be an opportunistic pathogen if there is a defect in cell-mediated immunity.

Coccidioides immitis (**choice D**) is a pathogenic fungus that can cause pneumonia if inhaled. Resolution occurs with the development of T-cell-mediated immunity. If this response is not raised, persistent or disseminated infection can occur. Pregnant women and individuals of African and Asian descent are at increased risk of disseminated infection. *C. immitis* is limited to the southwestern U.S. and northern Mexico.

23. **The correct answer is E.** The child most likely has chronic granulomatous disease (CGD), which results in recurrent staphylococcal infections (such as abscesses and furuncles) and an increased incidence of pneumonia due to *Serratia marcescens*. Organisms that cause recurrent infections in CGD patients are those that are catalase-positive. Neutrophils are unable to generate bacteria-killing superoxide radicals because of a lack of NADPH oxidase.

Aldolase B (**choice A**) cleaves fructose-1-phosphate to glyceraldehyde and dihydroxyacetone. Deficiency of aldolase B can produce hereditary fructose intolerance.

Galactokinase (**choice B**) phosphorylates galactose prior to the sugar's entry into the glycolytic pathway; deficiency of this enzyme can produce galactosemia.

Glucokinase (**choice C**) and hexokinase catalyze the first reaction in glycolysis. Their deficiency is not usually described, probably because these enzymes are so necessary that a significant deficiency would be incompatible with life.

Glucose-6-phosphate dehydrogenase (**choice D**) is the enzyme that starts the hexose monophosphate shunt; its deficiency causes a hemolytic anemia.

24. **The correct answer is B.** The patient likely has a candidal infection of the prosthetic aortic valve. That is why she did not respond favorably to antibacterial therapy, which

is known to promote fungal infection. Note that *Candida* tends to colonize foreign bodies, such as IV and Foley catheters, prosthetic valves, and ventricular shunts.

Actinomyces israelii (**choice A**) is known to cause cervicofacial infections in patients undergoing dental work. It is an anaerobe and would not favor an infection site in the bloodstream. It is the only bacterium on the list and is therefore least likely to be encouraged by a regimen of antibiotic therapy.

Histoplasma capsulatum (**choice C**) causes histoplasmosis, a pulmonary infection common in the midwestern river valleys. Multi-organ involvement is usually seen only in the immunocompromised. Transmission of the organism occurs through the inhalation of airborne microconidia (infectious spores). The organism is found in bird and bat droppings and in the soil.

Nocardia asteroides (**choice D**) is an aerobic filamentous bacterium that causes a chronic lobar pneumonia that may metastasize to the brain. It is more common in immunocompromised patients. It is found in soil and aquatic environments.

Trichophyton rubrum (**choice E**) is one of the organisms that commonly produce a variety of cutaneous mycoses, including tinea corporis (ringworm), tinea cruris (jock itch), and tinea pedis (athlete's foot).

25. **The correct answer is C.** Graft-versus-host disease is a feared complication of transplants of immunocompetent tissues from nonidentical (allogeneic) donors. It is thought to be caused by the transplantation of immune-competent T cells, which attack the host tissues. Elevation of alkaline phosphatase and bilirubin commonly occurs in this disorder. The fever and rash are also characteristic, as is the diarrhea observed in this patient.

Bacterial infection (**choice A**) might produce fever and diarrhea but would be unlikely to produce isolated elevations of alkaline phosphatase and bilirubin.

A blast crisis (**choice B**) would be unlikely, since high-dose whole body irradiation generally destroys the viable stem cells in the bone marrow.

Hyperacute graft rejection (**choice D**) is generally due to the presence of preformed antibody or prior exposure to an antigen (e.g., a prior transfusion or transplant from the donor), which is not suggested by the history in this case.

The symptoms described are not consistent with whole-body radiation toxicity (**choice E**), although diarrhea and skin changes would likely occur.

26. **The correct answer is E.** The combination of optochin sensitivity and positive Quellung reaction is characteristic of a single organism, *Streptococcus pneumoniae*. The other encapsulated organisms that have Quellung-positive reactions are *Haemophilus influenzae* (**choice B**), *Neisseria meningitidis*, and *Klebsiella pneumoniae* (**choice C**). However, none of these organisms are optochin-sensitive.

The other choices, *Escherichia coli* (**choice A**) and *Neisseria gonorrhoeae* (**choice D**), are not encapsulated.

27. **The correct answer is A.** Bacillary angiomatosis is a disease that occurs primarily in AIDS patients and is indicative of a defect in cell-mediated immunity. It is caused by either *Bartonella henselae* or *Bartonella quintana*. The domestic cat is the reservoir for these organisms, which are usually transmitted to humans via a cat scratch or bite. Patients with this illness usually have multiple skin lesions and extracutaneous manifestations involving liver and bone. Diagnosis is usually based on characteristic histopathologic findings, including plump "epithelioid" endothelial cells and mitotic figures. A macrolide, such as erythromycin or azithromycin, is the drug of choice for the infection.

Human papillomavirus (**choice B**) causes warts. It can present as sessile warts or as condylomata acuminata, which are fleshy soft growths that coalesce into large masses. When cellular immunity is depressed, as in AIDS, the condylomata acuminata proliferate.

Molluscum contagiosum (**choice C**) is caused by a poxvirus that is spread by close person-to-person contact. Infection produces a firm nodule that often becomes umbilicated and may resolve by discharging its contents. In AIDS, the lesions do not resolve, but enlarge and spread.

Rickettsia prowazekii (**choice D**) is the cause of epidemic typhus. It is spread by the human body louse *Pediculus humanis*. Its reservoirs are humans and flying squirrels.

Treponema pallidum (**choice E**) is the spirochete that causes syphilis. The primary lesion of syphilis is a chancre (a painless, indurated ulcer).

28. **The correct answer is C.** *Salmonella* spp., including *S. enteritidis* and *S. typhimurium*, produce a gastroenteritis or enterocolitis. Patients with decreased gastric acidity, sickle cell disease, or defects in immunity, and children younger than 4 years have a more severe course of disease. *Salmonella* spp. are carried in nature by animal reservoirs such as poultry, turtles, cattle, pigs, and sheep. The incubation period is 8-48 hours after ingestion of contaminated food or water.

Chlamydia psittaci (**choice A**) produces an interstitial pneumonitis accompanied by headache, backache, and a dry, hacking cough. A pale, macular rash is also found on the trunk (Horder's spots). Patients at risk include pet shop workers, pigeon handlers, and poultry workers.

Entamoeba histolytica (**choice B**) produces a diarrhea (frequently bloody or heme-positive), right lower quadrant crampy abdominal pain, and fever. Patients frequently have weight loss and anorexia. There is usually a history of travel outside the U.S. Most cases are chronic. Complications include liver abscesses.

Staphylococcus aureus (**choice D**) produces a self-limited gastroenteritis due to the production of preformed, heat-stable enterotoxins. The incubation period is 2-16 hours. The toxins enhance intestinal peristalsis and induce vomiting by a direct effect on the CNS.

Yersinia enterocolitica (**choice E**) usually produces a chronic enteritis in children. These patients have diarrhea, failure to thrive, hypoalbuminemia, and hypokalemia. Other findings include acute right lower quadrant abdominal pain, tenderness, nausea, and vomiting. The infection mimics appendicitis or Crohn disease.

29. **The correct answer is B.** Infection with hepatitis B virus (HBV) at birth or a very young age is associated with chronic HBV infection and the development of hepatocellular carcinoma later in life. In fact, infants born to hepatitis B surface antigen (HBsAg)-positive mothers are commonly infected, and approximately 90% become chronic carriers of the virus. In chronic carriers, hepatocellular carcinoma develops at an incidence more than 200 times higher than in noncarriers. The current recommendation for infants born of HBsAg-positive mothers is administration of hepatitis B immunoglobulin (HBIg) in the delivery room, with the first dose of the hepatitis B vaccine given at the same time or within 1 week. The second and third doses of the vaccine are then given at 1 and 6 months. With this protocol, 94% protection is achieved.

The Epstein-Barr virus (EBV; **choice A**) is the agent of heterophile-positive infectious mononucleosis. In children, primary EBV infection is often asymptomatic.

The measles virus (**choice C**) often causes a more severe disease in adults. The incidence of complications, including pneumonia, bacterial superinfection of the respiratory tract, bronchospasm, and hepatitis, is much higher in adults older than 20 than in children.

Poliovirus (**choice D**) causes asymptomatic or inapparent infections 95% of the time. Frank paralysis occurs in approximately 0.1% of all poliovirus infections. However, the probability of paralysis increases with increasing age.

Varicella zoster virus (**choice E**) is the agent of chickenpox and shingles. In immunocompetent children, it is a benign illness with a mortality of less than 2 per 100,000 cases. This risk is increased more than 15-fold in adults. Much of the increase is due to varicella pneumonitis, a complication that occurs more frequently in adults.

30. **The correct answer is A.** This patient has hereditary angioneurotic edema, which is caused by deficiency of C1 esterase inhibitor. Patients experience acute episodes of localized edema and colic. Stridor may occur because of airway obstruction due to laryngeal edema, the most dreaded complication of this condition. The disease is inherited as an autosomal dominant trait, explaining this patient's positive family history. Administration of epsilon-aminocaproate, an inhibitor of plasmin activation of C1, reduces the frequency of the episodes.

C3b inactivator (**choice B**) inhibits enzymes of the complement system.

Factor H (**choice C**) binds to C3b and C3b-containing convertases, precluding the binding of C3b to B. This interrupts the alternative pathway. Factor H also results in the dissociation of C3b from the Bb in the C3 and C5 convertases.

Carboxypeptidase (**choice D**) is a hydrolase that removes amino acids from the free carboxyl group at the end of a polypeptide chain.

Properdin (**choice E**) functions in the alternative pathway and recognizes a large range of microorganisms. Properdin places C3b on the microbial membrane, even in the absence of a specific antibody.

31. **The correct answer is D.** The patient died of rabies, caused by a rhabdovirus. Rabies infects the nervous system, causing extraordinary excitability, extreme thirst, pharyngeal spasms, and eventually death due to respiratory failure. Negri bodies (intracytoplasmic eosinophilic inclusions) are considered pathognomonic. It's a challenge to remember all the different viruses, but the tables on the following page should help.

RNA viruses	Examples
Picornaviruses	Polioviruses, echoviruses, coxsackie viruses, rhinoviruses, hepatitis A
Orthomyxoviruses	Influenza viruses
Paramyxoviruses	Rubeola virus, mumps virus, respiratory syncytial virus, parainfluenza viruses
Togaviruses	Equine encephalitis, rubella
Flaviviruses	Yellow fever, Dengue fever, hepatitis C, St. Louis encephalitis, Japanese encephalitis
Bunyaviruses	California encephalitis, hantavirus
Rhabdoviruses	Rabies
Coronaviruses	Common cold
Caliciviruses	Norwalk agent, hepatitis E
Arenaviruses	Lymphocytic choriomeningitis, Lassa fever
Filoviruses	Marburg, Ebola

DNA viruses	Examples
Reoviruses	Rotaviruses, orbiviruses
Retroviruses	HIV, HTLV
Hepadnavirus	Hepatitis B
Adenoviruses	Colds, diarrhea, conjunctivitis, pneumonia, flu-like syndromes
Papovaviruses	Human papillomavirus, BK, JC, SV40
Herpesviruses	Herpes simplex I and II, Epstein-Barr, varicella-zoster, cytomegalovirus
Poxviruses	Smallpox, molluscum contagiosum
Parvoviruses	Erythema infectiosum, marrow aplasia

32. **The correct answer is A.** Mucormycosis, to which diabetics are particularly vulnerable (perhaps because of the high glucose content of the diabetic nasal secretions), typically involves the nasal sinuses. It is especially dangerous because the organism can erode into the bones of the cranium, causing a life-threatening meningitis and/or encephalitis that is very difficult to treat.

Mucor can cause pneumonia (**choice B**), but this is not the most immediate threat.

Mucor can cause septicemia (**choice C**), but this usually occurs in more seriously ill patients and is not an immediate risk in this patient.

Mucor can cause a skin infection (**choice D**), but this generally occurs in conjunction with severe burns.

Mucor does not usually cause urinary tract infections (**choice E**).

33. **The correct answer is D.** *Mycoplasma pneumoniae* is a wall-less bacterium that causes interstitial pneumonia in young adults. Elevated cold agglutinins (a classic clue) are found in about half the patients. The cold agglutinins

are IgM antibodies. *M. pneumoniae* may be diagnosed by sputum or complement fixation.

Haemophilus (**choice A**) causes bronchopneumonia in infants and children and may occur in debilitated adults.

Klebsiella (**choice B**) causes a bronchopneumonia with patchy infiltrates involving one or more lobes. The cough is productive, and the sputum is bright red and gelatinous. It frequently occurs in debilitated patients, diabetics, and alcoholics. Note that these organisms are highly encapsulated and produce mucoid colonies on laboratory media.

Legionella (**choice C**) lives in contaminated water sources such as air conditioning systems. It causes an atypical pneumonia, most serious in elderly male smokers with high alcohol intake. It is not associated with cold agglutinin production.

Streptococcus pneumoniae (**choice E**) is the most common cause of pneumonia in the elderly population and in those with poor nutrition. It causes abscesses, productive cough, and rusty-colored sputum.

34. **The correct answer is D.** Rubella, also called German measles or 3-day measles, is a disease caused by a Togavirus, which is a small, enveloped, single-stranded, (+) linear RNA virus. Approximately 40% of patients are asymptomatic or have mild symptoms. In symptomatic patients, the clinical presentation typically consists of an erythematous rash that begins on the head and spreads downward to involve the trunk, and lasts for approximately 3 days. In addition to a transient rash, symptoms include fever, posterior cervical lymphadenopathy, and arthralgias. The greatest danger from rubella is to the fetus. If clinical rubella develops or seroconversion is demonstrated, there is a high risk of congenital abnormalities or spontaneous abortion. The risk varies from 40% to 60% if infection occurs during the first 2 months of gestation to 10% by the 4th month. Women of childbearing age should be warned not to become pregnant within 2-3 months from the time of immunization. Mild arthralgias and other symptoms may develop in 25% of immunized women. Enteroviral rashes may mimic rubella and rubeola.

Infectious mononucleosis (**choice A**) is caused by the Epstein-Barr virus, a herpesvirus. Classic findings include fever, exudative pharyngitis, generalized lymphadenopathy, severe malaise (most common complaint), and hepatosplenomegaly. A rash is not a characteristic feature unless the patient has been treated with ampicillin.

Lyme disease (**choice B**) is caused by the spirochete *Borrelia burgdorferi*. The disease is transmitted by the bite of the tick *Ixodes dammini*. Reservoirs in nature include the white-tailed deer and the white-footed mouse. The initial lesion is an annular rash with central clearing and a raised red border (erythema chronicum migrans) at the bite site. The rash is warm, but not painful or itchy. Patients also have fever, malaise, myalgias, arthralgias, headache, generalized lymphadenopathy, and, occasionally, neurologic findings.

Roseola (**choice C**) is caused by human herpesvirus 6. Other names include exanthem subitum or sixth disease. Children have a febrile period of 3-5 days with rapid defervescence followed by an erythematous maculopapular rash lasting 1-3 days.

Rubeola (**choice E**), or regular measles, is a disease caused by a paramyxovirus. Patients present with an upper respiratory prodrome and characteristic oral lesions (Koplik's spots) that precede the rash. The nonpruritic maculopapular rash begins on the face and spreads to the trunk and extremities, including palms and soles. The incubation period is 10-14 days. Patients also have a posterior cervical lymphadenopathy. The virus is not associated with risk to a fetus.

35. **The correct answer is B.** This is a multistep microbiology question that requires you to diagnose the illness, identify the microorganism, and remember its key feature. The first part should be easy: everything about this vignette suggests toxic shock syndrome. The organism in question is therefore *Staphylococcus aureus*, which is coagulase positive. All the other choices are classic features of other important pathogenic microorganisms:

Acid-fast organisms (**choice A**) are associated with mycobacteria. (In addition, *Nocardia* species are partially acid fast.)

EMB agar (**choice C**) refers to a selective and differential medium used to isolate and identify enteric gram-negative bacteria. Gram-positive bacteria will not grow on EMB agar because the addition of eosin inhibits their growth. Nonlactose fermenters will have colorless colonies; fermentation of this sugar will cause the colonies to appear pink or purple.

Thayer-Martin media (**choice D**) can be used for pathogenic *Neisseria* species. This growth medium contains the antibiotic vancomycin, which kills gram-positive organisms such as *Staphylococcus aureus*.

The Quellung reaction (**choice E**) can be used to identify the capsule type of a microorganism. Encapsulated microorganisms, like the pneumococci and *Haemophilus*, are mixed with specific antisera. If the antibodies recognize the microorganism's capsule type, the capsule will swell.

36. **The correct answer is A.** The children at this elementary school exhibit the classic signs of rubella (rash beginning on face and neck then spreading, posterior auricular and posterior cervical lymphadenopathy, pharyngeal injection). The rubella vaccine is composed of a live, attenuated virus. Measles, mumps, polio, smallpox, yellow fever, and adenovirus vaccines are other live, attenuated viral preparations.

The live, attenuated vaccine should confer enough immunity so that the addition of a specific immunoglobulin (**choice B**) would be unnecessary. Note that tetanus toxoid (an inactivated toxin) is often administered with anti-tetanus immunoglobulin in patients with tetanus-prone wounds who have not been previously vaccinated for tetanus.

Note that the Salk vaccine for polio is an example of a killed vaccine (**choices C and D**), whereas the Sabin vaccine (oral administration) is a live, attenuated vaccine (Sal**k** is **k**illed). The rabies vaccine used in humans is also a killed virus; however, veterinary vaccines against this virus are live, attenuated strains of the agent.

Specific immunoglobulin only (**choice E**) would confer passive immunity to the children, which might not effectively prevent disease in exposed children.

37. **The correct answer is C.** Ribavirin is an antiviral drug approved for the treatment of severe respiratory syncytial virus infection, the most common cause of pneumonia and bronchiolitis in children younger than 1 year. It should be given by aerosol.

Acyclovir (**choice A**) is a guanosine analog that is useful for the treatment of primary and recurrent herpes infections and herpes simplex virus encephalitis.

Ganciclovir (**choice B**) is a guanosine analog used in the treatment of cytomegalovirus retinitis and cytomegalovirus infections in AIDS patients.

Trifluorothymidine (**choice D**) is a thymidine analog used topically for the treatment of recurrent epithelial keratitis and primary keratoconjunctivitis due to herpes simplex viruses.

Zidovudine (**choice E**) is a thymidine analog that inhibits reverse transcriptase. It is active against human retroviruses, including HIV-1, HIV-2, and HTLV-I.

38. **The correct answer is D.** This infant is exhibiting passive immunity acquired from his mother *in utero*. IgG is the only class of immunoglobulins that can cross the placenta. As such, IgG molecules diffuse into the fetal circulation, providing immunity. This circulating maternal IgG protects the newborn during the first 4-6 months of life. Note that IgG is also capable of complement activation (a feature shared with IgM) and opsonization (unique to IgG).

IgA (**choice A**) functions in the secretory immune response. The secretory form of this immunoglobulin (sIgA) is found in tears, colostrum, saliva, breast milk, and other secretions. It is produced by the plasma cells in the lamina propria of the gastrointestinal, respiratory, and reproductive tracts.

IgD (**choice B**) functions as a cell surface antigen receptor, along with IgM monomers, on undifferentiated B cells. It does not reach appreciable plasma concentrations.

IgE (**choice C**) is involved in the allergic response and immediate hypersensitivity reactions. The Fc region of IgE binds to the surface of basophils and mast cells. Antigen cross-linking of two IgE molecules leads to mast cell degranulation and the release of leukotrienes, histamine, eosinophil chemotactic factors, and heparin.

IgM (**choice E**) is the first antibody detected in serum after exposure to antigen. IgM circulates as a pentamer and thus has five complement binding regions and ten antigen combining sites.

39. **The correct choice is B.** The presence of elevated ALT, HBsAg, anti-HBc, HBeAg, and bilirubin all point to active hepatitis B.

An asymptomatic carrier (**choice A**) would not have elevated ALT and bilirubin.

The absence of findings on physical examination rules out fulminant hepatitis B (**choice C**).

Recovery from acute self-limited HBV (**choice D**) is associated with the presence of anti-HBs and absence of HBsAg and HBeAg.

Someone who is vaccinated against HBV (**choice E**) has only anti-HBs in serum.

40. **The correct answer is B.** Tissue grafts in which the same individual acts as both the donor and recipient are termed autografts.

Allografts (**choice A**) refer to tissue transplants from one person to another genetically different individual.

Homograft (**choice C**) is not commonly used but is sometimes a synonym for allograft.

Isografts (**choice D**) refer to tissue transplants between genetically identical individuals (e.g., an identical twin donates her kidney to her twin sister).

Xenografts (**choice E**) refer to tissue transplants between species (e.g., baboon heart transplanted into a human).

41. **The correct answer is E.** While the commonly remembered association is that of inadequately cooked pork and trichinosis, the quality of purchased pork and the degree of cooking in this country are sufficiently high that pork-related trichinosis is quite uncommon. The more common scenario is actually the one described in the question stem, for two reasons. First, bear meat is not inspected, and it may often be served "rare," or relatively uncooked. The infected meat contains larvae that are released in the gastrointestinal tract after ingestion. The *Trichinella spiralis* larvae penetrate the intestinal mucosa and develop into adult worms in 30–40 hours. After reaching adulthood, they mate, and the females produce larvae that grow to maturity and seek out muscle in which to encyst (often in the orbital muscles) within approximately 5–8 days. The intestinal production of larvae may last up to 2 months, but may be shorter. Treatment is with mebendazole. (If you didn't know the answer to this question, you still might have noticed the presence of eosinophilia, which should have clued you in to the presence of a parasitic infestation, making trichinosis the only plausible answer.)

Anthrax (**choice A**) after eating bear meat is very unlikely. In addition, anthrax would not produce the described symptoms; instead, cutaneous lesions (95% of cases) or respiratory disease culminating in death (5% of cases; wool sorter's disease) would occur.

Bacillus cereus food poisoning (**choice B**) and *Escherichia coli* gastroenteritis (**choice D**) might lead to similar gastrointestinal symptoms but would not cause the eye findings nor eosinophilia.

Botulism (**choice C**) causes flaccid paralysis, not the symptoms described.

42. **The correct answer is E.** Many patients with *Yersinia enterocolitica* infection present with symptoms suggesting appendicitis (although constipation, rather than diarrhea, is common in appendicitis). Surgical exploration of the abdomen reveals mesenteric adenitis (involvement of the lymph nodes located in the mesentery), along with a normal appendix. Mesenteric adenitis is the tip-off that the patient has a *Y. enterocolitica* infection, and culture of the involved lymph nodes or of the stool is generally diagnostic.

Enteroinvasive *E. coli* (EIEC; **choice A**) causes fever, pain, diarrhea, and dysentery, usually following ingestion of contaminated cheese or water.

Salmonella (**choice B**) causes fever, pain, diarrhea, dysentery, bacteremia, and extraintestinal infections. It is commonly found in outbreaks due to a common contaminated food source (e.g., milk, beef, eggs, poultry).

Shigella (**choice C**) causes fever, pain, diarrhea, and dysentery in epidemics usually due to person-to-person spread.

Vibrio cholerae (**choice D**) causes cholera, characterized by watery, life-threatening diarrhea. It tends to spread in epidemics through third-world countries via contaminated water or shellfish.

43. **The correct answer is C.** This patient has primary subacute bacterial peritonitis, which commonly occurs in patients with alcoholic cirrhosis and ascites. Gram-negative bacilli in the normal flora, such as *Escherichia coli*, are the most likely causative agents.

Bacillus cereus (**choice A**) is a spore-forming, gram-positive rod. Its spores may germinate in rewarmed rice, causing food poisoning. It is not a normal flora organism.

Clostridium difficile (**choice B**) is a gram-positive rod that causes antibiotic-associated colitis (pseudomembranous colitis). It exists as normal flora in 2-10% of humans and is not likely to be a *common* cause of this presentation.

Entamoeba histolytica (**choice D**) is an intestinal protozoan that is frequent in the tropics and is prevalent in homosexual men. The liver is the most common site of systemic infection. It is not a normal flora organism.

Giardia lamblia (**choice E**) causes giardiasis, which presents with diarrhea, cramps, bloating, flatulence, malaise, weight loss, and occasional steatorrhea. It is not a normal flora organism.

44. **The correct answer is B.** The combination of repeated staphylococcal and streptococcal infections, normal phagocytic function, and normal delayed hypersensitivity responses is suggestive of Bruton hypogammaglobulinemia. The disease is characterized by an IgG level less than 100 mg/dL, other immunoglobulins deficient or absent, B cells deficient or absent, intact cellular (T-cell) immunity, and onset of infections after the 6th month of life, when maternal antibodies are no longer present. Therefore, B-cell-dependent areas, such as germinal centers, would be absent or greatly diminished in size and number.

Postcapillary venules (**choice A**) are not depleted in this disease.

The chemotactic response of neutrophils (**choice C**) is part of the phagocytic function assay, which was normal in the case presented.

Because T-cell functions are intact, the architecture of the portions of lymphoid tissues where T cells reside (e.g., paracortical areas, **choice D**; thymus-dependent areas, **choice E**) should be normal.

45. **The correct answer is D.** When you see *Chlamydia psittaci*, one word should come to mind—birds! Infection with this organism is an occupational hazard for anyone who works with birds (e.g., veterinarians, pet store employees), including poultry farmers.

Individuals who work with cats (**choice A**) would be at an increased risk for infection with *Pasteurella multocida* (which is acquired primarily through cat bites), *Bartonella henselae* (cat-scratch fever), and the protozoa *Toxoplasma gondii* (which can be acquired from ingestion of food contaminated with cat feces).

Florists (**choice B**) are at increased risk for infection with the fungus *Sporothrix schenckii*, a primary pathogenic fungus acquired by inoculation (e.g., a rose thorn puncturing the skin).

A person who works at a homeless shelter (**choice C**) would be at increased risk for infection with *Mycobacterium tuberculosis*, since this organism is spread through the air and is prevalent in the homeless community.

Slaughterhouse workers (**choice E**) are at an increased risk for infection with *Brucella*, a bacterium that is acquired by handling infected animals.

46. **The correct answer is C.** This patient has infectious mononucleosis due to cytomegalovirus (CMV). Patients present with symptoms similar to Epstein-Barr virus (EBV) infection (sore throat, fever, fatigue, cervical lymphadenopathy, and hepatomegaly), but their diagnostic workup (heterophile antibody, Epstein-Barr

titer) is negative for EBV. Though diagnosis of CMV depends on virus isolation in secretions, microscopic exam of epithelial cells reveals giant nuclei surrounded by clear zones (owl's eye nuclei), which are pathognomonic. Cytoplasmic inclusions also appear.

An enlarged nucleus with peripherally displaced chromatin (**choice A**) is seen in cells infected with human parvovirus B19, which causes Fifth disease (erythema infectiosum) in children. A classic clue to the diagnosis is the presence of a "slapped cheek" rash.

Conidia and septate hyphae (**choice B**) appear in aspergillosis, a lung disease that occurs mostly in the immunocompromised. A classic clue is the appearance of a "fungus ball" (aspergilloma) on chest x-ray, which appears as a large, round mass surrounded by air.

Multinucleated giant cells (**choice D**) appear in several viral infections, including measles (rubeola) and chickenpox (varicella).

Staining with India ink (**choice E**) is used on the CSF of patients with *Cryptococcus neoformans* CNS infection to highlight the yeast capsule.

47. **The correct answer is B.** Chancroid is a sexually transmitted disease (STD) that usually presents as a tender papule on the penis, which after 24 hours turns into a painful ulcer. It is associated with buboes.

    Choice A is also an STD that is a relapsing granulomatous anogenital infection. The lesions occur on the skin or mucous membranes, the genitalia, or perianal area. They are relatively painless, infiltrated nodules that do form ulcers.

    Choice C presents with a painless chancre on the genitalia.

    Choice D presents with superficial lesions, such as papules, vesicles, or ulcers that appear on the external genitalia. They are painless and disappear within a few days, leaving no scar. Inguinal buboes appear 1-4 weeks after exposure.

    Choice E presents with a painful cluster of vesicles around the genitalia that ulcerate and often have an erythematous base. It can be associated with a local adenopathy but is not associated with buboes.

48. **The correct answer is E.** This is the causative agent of chancroid.

    Choice A is the causative agent of herpes simplex.

    Choice B is the causative agent of granuloma inguinale.

    Choice C is the causative agent of lymphogranuloma venereum.

    Choice D is the causative agent of syphilis.

49. **The correct answer is E.** Ceftriaxone (250 mg IM) is the most appropriate drug used to treat chancroid. Because the patient has difficulty remembering to take his medication properly, you need to use a drug that can be given in a single dose, one time only. Ceftriaxone offers this advantage, as does azithromycin (1 g PO).

    Choice A is administered 500 mg PO QID for 21 days and is one of the drugs used to treat lymphogranuloma venereum or granuloma inguinale.

    Choice B is an antiviral drug used to treat herpes simplex viruses.

    Choice C is the drug of choice for treating lymphogranuloma venereum. An alternative would be tetracycline.

    Choice D is used to treat syphilis.

50. **The correct answer is C.** Syphilis has a 10% coinfection rate with chancroid.

    Choices A, B, D, and E have no known association with chancroid.

Microbiology/Immunology

1. Patients with the HLA-B27 antigen are known to have an increased risk of developing certain pathologic conditions. Which of the following infectious agents may cause a syndrome characterized by arthritis, conjunctivitis, and urethritis in an HLA-B27 positive patient?

   (A) *Borrelia burgdorferi*

   (B) *Chlamydia trachomatis*

   (C) Enterotoxigenic *Escherichia coli*

   (D) Group A β-hemolytic streptococci

   (E) *Trichomonas vaginalis*

2. A patient has chronic tissue changes at T11-L2. Which of the following is specifically associated with infection with *Schistosoma haematobium*?

   (A) Adenocarcinoma of the bladder

   (B) Adenocarcinoma of the renal pelvis

   (C) Squamous cell carcinoma of the bladder

   (D) Transitional cell carcinoma of the bladder

   (E) Transitional cell carcinoma of the renal pelvis

3. A 29-year-old woman diagnosed with AIDS has had a progressive blurring of vision in her right eye. On funduscopic examination, a small white opaque lesion is noted on the retina of her right eye. Structural examination reveals somatic dysfunction at T1-T4. Which of the following is the most appropriate therapy for this patient?

   (A) Acyclovir

   (B) Amantadine

   (C) Flucytosine

   (D) Ganciclovir

   (E) Zidovudine

4. A 45-year-old homeless man has a chronic cough and a cavitary lesion of the lung with T2-T7 somatic dysfunction. His sputum is positive for acid-fast bacilli. Which of the following is the principal form of defense by which the patient's body fights this infection?

   (A) Antibody-mediated phagocytosis

   (B) Cell-mediated immunity

   (C) IgA-mediated hypersensitivity

   (D) IgE-mediated hypersensitivity

   (E) Neutrophil ingestion of bacteria

5. A 10-year-old girl presents with sore throat and fever. She denies any cough or rhinorrhea. Physical examination reveals acute tissue changes at T1-T4. A throat culture grows bacitracin-sensitive bacterial colonies. The infecting organism would be protected from the lytic action of detergents by its

   (A) keratin-like proteins in the spore coat

   (B) lipopolysaccharide in the outer membrane

   (C) peptidoglycan layer

   (D) periplasmic space

   (E) Ca^{2+} chelators

6. A hospitalized patient with somatic dysfunction at T11-L2 complains of dysuria and suprapubic pain and is treated with ciprofloxacin. What is the mechanism of action of this antibiotic?

   (A) It inhibits dihydrofolate reductase

   (B) It inhibits DNA-dependent RNA polymerase

   (C) It inhibits protein synthesis by binding to the 30s ribosomal subunit

   (D) It inhibits protein synthesis by binding to the 50s ribosomal subunit

   (E) It inhibits topoisomerase II (DNA gyrase)

7. Two weeks after returning from a trip to New Delhi, India, a 35-year-old man presents to the emergency department complaining of daily fevers, headache, chills, and malaise. He recalls getting a number of flea bites on his ankles and calves during his trip. Physical examination reveals a maculopapular rash on his trunk, arms, and thighs. Which of the following is the most likely cause of this patient's condition?

   (A) *Bartonella henselae*

   (B) *Borrelia recurrentis*

   (C) *Coxiella burnetii*

   (D) *Ehrlichia chaffeensis*

   (E) *Rickettsia typhi*

8. A child in a developing country develops repeated eye infections with an organism that causes chronic conjunctivitis, scarring, eyelid deformities, pannus formation, and eventual blindness. Which of the following is a distinctive feature of the causative organism?

   (A) Also causes cat scratch fever

   (B) Antigen cross-reactivity with antibodies to *Proteus vulgaris*

   (C) Arthropod transmission

   (D) Bird reservoir

   (E) Reticulate body

9. A 34-year-old woman presents with fatigue, malaise, and swollen, tender joints. Physical examination is significant for a maculopapular eruption over sun-exposed areas, including the face. Examination of a peripheral blood smear reveals mild thrombocytopenia. Which of the following autoantibodies, if present, would be most specific for the diagnosis of the patient's disorder?

   (A) Anti-centromere antibody

   (B) Anti-IgG antibody

   (C) Antinuclear antibody

   (D) Anti-Sm (Smith antigen) antibody

   (E) Anti-SS-A (Ro) antibody

10. A 4-year-old girl presents with a maculopapular rash on her hands and feet and painful ulcers distributed anteriorly on her lips, palate, tongue, and buccal mucosa. Systemic features and lymphadenopathy are absent. Which of the following viruses is most likely to have caused this disorder?

    (A) Coronavirus

    (B) Coxsackievirus type A16

    (C) Herpes simplex virus type 1

    (D) Parainfluenza type 3

    (E) Rhinovirus

11. A patient with nuchal rigidity and headache undergoes lumbar puncture. The CSF contains markedly increased numbers of lymphocytes, leading to a presumptive diagnosis of viral meningitis. Which of the following groups of viruses is most likely to be involved?

    (A) Adenoviruses

    (B) Enteroviruses

    (C) Human papillomaviruses

    (D) Poxviruses

    (E) Reoviruses

12. While playing outside, an 8-year-old girl is bitten in the leg by a neighbor's cat. She presents the next day with fever and bone pain localized to her right calf. An x-ray film reveals a lytic lesion of the right tibia. Results of the bone culture are pending. Which of the following is the most likely pathogen?

    (A) *Brucella melitensis*

    (B) *Eikenella corrodens*

    (C) *Francisella tularensis*

    (D) *Pasteurella multocida*

    (E) *Yersinia pestis*

13. A 6-year-old boy presents to the pediatric clinic with fever and earache. He has just finished an unsuccessful course of amoxicillin. On physical examination, his right tympanic membrane appears injected. Structural examination reveals acute tissue changes at T1-T4. Which of the following is the most appropriate pharmacotherapy?

    (A) Amphotericin B

    (B) Bacitracin

    (C) Cefaclor

    (D) Erythromycin

    (E) Sulfamethoxazole

14. A 4-year-old boy presents to the emergency department with muscle spasms. Structural findings reveal spasmodic, warm, and boggy tissues throughout the whole body. His past medical history is significant for recurrent infections and neonatal seizures. Evaluation of his serum electrolytes reveals hypocalcemia. This patient would be most susceptible to which of the following diseases?

    (A) Chickenpox

    (B) Diphtheria

    (C) Gas gangrene

    (D) Gonorrhea

    (E) Tetanus

15. A patient develops fever and shortness of breath, and appears to be quite ill. Structural examination reveals somatic dysfunction of T2-T7 bilaterally. An x-ray film demonstrates bilateral interstitial lung infiltrates, and bronchial washings demonstrate small "hat-shaped" organisms visible on silver stain within the foamy alveolar exudate. Which predisposing condition is most likely present in this patient?

    (A) AIDS

    (B) Congestive heart failure

    (C) Pulmonary embolus

    (D) Rheumatoid arthritis

    (E) Systemic lupus erythematosus

16. A 30-year-old veterinarian visits her obstetrician for a first-trimester prenatal check-up. She has no complaints. Routine physical examination is significant only for mild cervical lymphadenopathy. She is prescribed spiramycin but is noncompliant. Her child is born with hydrocephalus and cerebral calcifications. Which of the following organisms is most likely responsible?

    (A) *Isospora belli*

    (B) *Leishmania donovani*

    (C) *Plasmodium vivax*

    (D) *Toxoplasma gondii*

    (E) *Trypanosoma cruzi*

17. A 38-year-old woman complains of cold and painful fingertips, as well as difficulty swallowing and indigestion. Physical examination is remarkable for a thickened, shiny epidermis over the entire body, with restricted movement of the extremities, particularly the fingers, which appear claw-like. Which of the following autoantibodies will likely be found in this patient's serum?

    (A) Anti-DNA topoisomerase I (anti-Scl-70)

    (B) Anti-double-stranded DNA (ds DNA)

    (C) Anti-IgG

    (D) Anti-Sm

    (E) Anti-SS-A

18. A 24-year-old AIDS patient develops chronic abdominal pain, low-grade fever, diarrhea, and malabsorption. Oocysts are demonstrated in the stool. Which of the following organisms is most likely the cause of the patient's diarrhea?

    (A) *Diphyllobothrium latum*

    (B) *Entamoeba histolytica*

    (C) *Giardia lamblia*

    (D) *Isospora belli*

    (E) Microsporidia

19. An African child develops massive unilateral enlargement of his lower face in the vicinity of the mandible. Biopsy demonstrates sheets of medium-sized blast cells with admixed larger macrophages. This type of tumor has been associated with which of the following?

    (A) Epstein-Barr virus and t(8;14)

    (B) Hepatitis B and t(9;22)

    (C) Herpesvirus and CD5

    (D) HIV and CD4

    (E) Human papillomavirus and t(2;5)

20. A 1-week-old girl with symptoms of vomiting and anorexia has a temperature of 102 F. A bulging fontanelle that has a cranial rythmn of 11 cycles per minute is noted on physical examination. Which of the following is the most likely causative agent?

    (A) *Haemophilus influenzae* type b

    (B) *Listeria monocytogenes*

    (C) *Neisseria meningitidis*

    (D) *Staphylococcus aureus*

    (E) *Streptococcus agalactiae*

21. A mailman gets a severe bite wound from a pit bull guarding a junkyard. The wound is cleansed and he receives a booster injection of tetanus toxoid and an injection of penicillin G. Several days later, the wound is inflamed and purulent. The exudate is cultured on blood agar and yields gram-negative rods. Antibiotic sensitivity tests are pending. Which of the following is the most likely pathogen?

    (A) *Bartonella henselae*

    (B) *Brucella canis*

    (C) *Clostridium tetani*

    (D) *Pasteurella multocida*

    (E) *Toxocara canis*

22. A 1-year-old girl presents with a 2-day history of fever, vomiting, and watery, nonbloody diarrhea. On physical examination, she appears dehydrated. Structural examination reveals acute tissue changes at T5-L2. Which of the following best describes the most likely infecting organism?

    (A) It has a complex double-stranded DNA genome

    (B) It has a partially double-stranded circular DNA genome

    (C) It has a segmented, double-stranded RNA genome

    (D) It has a single-stranded circular RNA genome

    (E) It has a single-stranded RNA genome

23. A 27-year-old, HIV-positive patient presents complaining of visual disturbances. The patient is referred to an ophthalmologist, who notes perivascular hemorrhage and bilateral retinal exudates. The virus responsible for this patient's retinitis belongs to which of the following viral families?

    (A) Adenovirus

    (B) Herpesvirus

    (C) Orthomyxovirus

    (D) Paramyxovirus

    (E) Retrovirus

24. A 78-year-old woman with a history of renal calculi and recurrent urinary tract infections presents with fever, chills, leukocytosis, and cloudy urine that has a pH of 8.2. A urine culture grows a lactose-negative, urease-positive, gram-negative rod. Which of the following microorganisms is most likely responsible for her infection?

    (A) *Enterococcus faecalis*

    (B) *Escherichia coli*

    (C) *Klebsiella pneumoniae*

    (D) *Proteus mirabilis*

    (E) *Pseudomonas aeruginosa*

25. A 25-year-old woman presents with pain and tenosynovitis of the wrists and ankles, and arthralgias of other joints. She notes two prior episodes similar to the present one. She just had her menstrual period during the previous week. Physical examination reveals ulcerated lesions overlying the wrists and ankles. These symptoms are likely due to deficiency of which of the following?

    (A) C1 esterase inhibitor

    (B) Ciliary function

    (C) Complement (C6-C8) components

    (D) Endothelial adhesion molecules

    (E) Eosinophils

26. An 8-month-old infant presents to the emergency department with a 1-day history of poor feeding and generalized weakness. The mother states that she often feeds the infant honey to pacify her. The toxin responsible for this presentation works by which of the following mechanisms?

    (A) It blocks the release of acetylcholine from the nerve terminal

    (B) It blocks the release of inhibitory neurotransmitters such as glycine and GABA

    (C) It has a subunit that inactivates an elongation factor by ADP-ribosylation

    (D) It is a lecithinase

    (E) It stimulates guanylate cyclase

27. A 36-year-old, HIV-positive, white man presents with a fever and progressive headache. He complains of recent forgetfulness and "spells," during which he smells a "harsh, bitter smell." An MRI of the brain shows multiple, spherical, ring-enhancing lesions in the left temporal lobe. Laboratory analysis of CSF is normal. Which of the following microorganisms is most likely responsible for his illness?

    (A) *Cryptococcus neoformans*

    (B) *Mycobacterium leprae*

    (C) *Pasteurella multocida*

    (D) *Pneumocystis carinii*

    (E) *Toxoplasma gondii*

28. A 57-year-old woman with a history of hypertension and arthritis is referred to a rheumatologist for evaluation. A complete blood count (CBC) is normal, and a mini-chem panel shows no electrolyte abnormalities. Her erythrocyte sedimentation rate (ESR) is elevated, and an antinuclear antibody test (ANA) is positive. Further antibody studies are performed, and the results are shown below.

Anti-histones	high titer
Anti-double-stranded DNA	not detected
Anti-single-stranded DNA	not detected
Anti-SSA	not detected
Anti-SSB	not detected
Anti-SCI-70	not detected
Anti-Smith	not detected
Anti-centromere	not detected
Anti-RNP	not detected

    Which of the following diseases is suggested by these results?

    (A) CREST syndrome

    (B) Diffuse form of scleroderma

    (C) Drug-induced lupus

    (D) Sjögren syndrome

    (E) Systemic lupus erythematosus (SLE)

29. An otherwise healthy patient who wears contact lenses develops a small ulceration of the eye. Which of the following organisms is most likely involved?

    (A) *Acanthamoeba*

    (B) Cytomegalovirus

    (C) Herpes simplex

    (D) *Toxocara*

    (E) *Toxoplasma*

30. A 32-year-old woman with increased frequency of urination, suprapubic pain, and dysuria for the past 3 days comes to the emergency department. She has no fever, nausea, or vomiting. She has acute somatic dysfunction at T11-L2. A Gram stain reveals gram-negative rods. Which of the following is the most likely pathogen?

    (A) *Escherichia coli*

    (B) *Neisseria gonorrhoeae*

    (C) *Shigella dysenteriae*

    (D) *Streptococcus pneumoniae*

    (E) *Treponema pallidum*

31. Gram stain of the sputum from a patient with lobar pneumonia involving the left lower lobe demonstrates gram-positive, encapsulated, lancet-shaped diplococci. Which of the following is the most probable causative organism?

    (A) *Haemophilus influenzae*

    (B) *Neisseria gonorrhoeae*

    (C) *Pneumocystis carinii*

    (D) *Staphylococcus aureus*

    (E) *Streptococcus pneumoniae*

32. A 12-year-old girl has a temperature of 102.5 F and a sore throat. Two days later, she develops a diffuse erythematous rash and is taken to her pediatrician. On physical examination, there is circumoral pallor, and an erythematous rash with areas of desquamation is noted. The myocardial damage that can follow this infection is produced in a manner similar to the damage associated with which of the following disorders?

    (A) Atopic allergy

    (B) Contact dermatitis

    (C) Graft-versus-host disease

    (D) Graves disease

    (E) Idiopathic thrombocytopenic purpura

33. A 27-year-old IV drug user presents with difficulty swallowing. Examination of the oropharynx reveals white plaques along the tongue and the oral mucosa. Which of the following best describes the microscopic appearance of the microorganism responsible for this patient's illness?

    (A) Budding yeast and pseudohyphae

    (B) Encapsulated yeast

    (C) Mold with nonseptate hyphae

    (D) Mold with septate hyphae

    (E) Nonencapsulated yeast

34. A 40-year-old, otherwise healthy gardener presents with several subcutaneous nodules on his right hand, where he had cut himself on rose thorns. Physical examination reveals several erythematous fluctuant lesions. Which of the following organisms is most likely responsible for his condition?

    (A) *Aspergillus*

    (B) *Malassezia*

    (C) *Onchocerca*

    (D) *Rhizopus*

    (E) *Sporothrix*

35. An alcoholic is brought to the emergency department in respiratory distress. A chest x-ray film demonstrates lobar consolidation of the right lower lung. There is somatic dysfunction at T2-T7 on the right side. Which of the following organisms should be highest on the differential diagnosis?

    (A) *Klebsiella pneumoniae*

    (B) *Legionella* spp.

    (C) *Mycoplasma pneumoniae*

    (D) *Pneumocystic carinii*

    (E) *Staphylococcus aureus*

36. A diabetic patient has chronic sinusitis that has not responded to a 6-week course of antibiotics. Structural examination reveals chronic somatic dysfunction at T1-T4. The physician should suspect infection with which of the following organisms?

    (A) *Actinomyces*

    (B) *Aspergillus*

    (C) *Cryptococcus*

    (D) *Mucor*

    (E) *Pneumocystis*

37. A mother brings her 3-year-old boy into the emergency department because he has developed a harsh, "barking" cough with hoarseness. The virus responsible for this child's illness belongs to which of the following families?

    (A) Papovavirus

    (B) Paramyxovirus

    (C) Parvovirus

    (D) Picornavirus

    (E) Poxvirus

38. A 12-year-old boy with sickle cell disease develops sudden onset of fever and chills accompanied by intense pain and tenderness over the distal tibia. X-ray films and CT scan of the distal leg reveal swelling of the subcutaneous tissue and bone demineralization. A clinical diagnosis of acute osteomyelitis is made. Blood cultures and bone biopsy are arranged to confirm the diagnosis and isolate the offending agent. Which of the following infectious agents will most likely be identified?

    (A) Group B streptococci

    (B) *Hemophilus influenzae*

    (C) *Mycobacterium tuberculosis*

    (D) *Pseudomonas aeruginosa*

    (E) *Staphylococcus aureus*

39. A 53-year-old woman with diarrhea and lower abdominal pain of 3 days' duration comes to her physician after various home remedies fail to relieve her symptoms. She denies any recent travel. There is blood and pus in her stool. Fecal cultures yield several flagellated, curved, oxidase-positive, gram-negative rods. Which of the following is the most likely pathogen?

    (A) *Campylobacter jejuni*

    (B) *Escherichia coli*

    (C) *Salmonella*

    (D) *Shigella*

    (E) *Vibrio cholerae*

40. A 15-year-old high school student and several of her friends ate lunch at a local Chinese restaurant. They all were served the daily luncheon special, which consisted of sweet and sour pork with vegetables and fried rice. All of the girls developed nausea, vomiting, abdominal pain, and diarrhea within 4 hours of eating lunch. Which of the following is the most likely cause of these symptoms?

    (A) *Bacillus cereus*

    (B) *Clostridium botulinum*

    (C) *Clostridium perfringens*

    (D) EHEC (enterohemorrhagic *Escherichia coli*)

    (E) *Staphylococcus aureus*

41. Three months after a needle-stick exposure to blood from a patient with hepatitis B, a nurse is evaluated for infection with the virus. Laboratory results reveal:

HBsAg	absent
anti-HBs antibody	absent
IgM anti-HBc	present
IgG anti-HBc	absent
HBeAg	absent

    On the basis of these results, which of the following most accurately describes the nurse's hepatitis B status?

    (A) She had been effectively vaccinated against hepatitis B before the needle-stick exposure occurred

    (B) She has mounted an inappropriate antibody response to hepatitis B as a result of an immunocompromised state

    (C) She is a carrier of hepatitis B

    (D) She is actively infected with hepatitis B

    (E) She was not infected with hepatitis B

42. A 32-year-old physician who has spent the past several years in New Guinea presents with ulcerating granulomata of his genital skin. Physical examination reveals somatic dysfunction at T10-T11. Microscopic evaluation of the papules with Wright-Giemsa stain reveals 1- to 2-μm, rounded structures contained within cystic areas of the cytoplasm of macrophages. Which of the following is the most likely pathogen?

   (A) *Calymmatobacterium donovani*

   (B) *Chlamydia trachomatis*

   (C) *Haemophilus ducreyi*

   (D) *Neisseria gonorrhoeae*

   (E) *Treponema pallidum*

43. A previously healthy 11-year-old girl develops a gastrointestinal infection with cramping and watery stools. After several days, she begins to pass blood per rectum and is hospitalized for dehydration. In the hospital, she has decreasing urine output with rising blood urea nitrogen (BUN). Total blood count reveals anemia and thrombocytopenia, and the peripheral smear is remarkable for fragmented red cells (schistocytes). Infection with which of the following bacterial genera is most likely responsible for this syndrome?

   (A) *Campylobacter*

   (B) *Clostridium*

   (C) *Salmonella*

   (D) *Shigella*

   (E) *Vibrio*

44. An 18-year-old college student presents to the student health center complaining of a sore throat and fever. He describes feeling tired for the past few days and reports a loss of appetite. On examination, he has pharyngitis with cervical lymphadenopathy. Osteopathic structural examination reveals acute tissue changes at T1-T4. Blood tests reveal lymphocytosis and the presence of heterophil antibodies. Which of the following best describes the virus responsible for his illness?

   (A) Double-stranded, enveloped DNA virus

   (B) Double-stranded, nonenveloped DNA virus

   (C) Single-stranded, enveloped RNA virus

   (D) Single-stranded, nonenveloped DNA virus

   (E) Single-stranded, nonenveloped RNA virus

Questions 45-50

SET A

Directions: For each numbered item (**patient presentation**), select the one lettered heading (**vector**) most closely associated with it. Each lettered heading may be selected once, more than once, or not at all.

   (A) *Ixodes scapularis*

   (B) *Anopheles*

   (C) tsetse fly

   (D) reduviid bug

   (E) sand fly

   (F) *Dermacentor andersoni*

45. Your patient recently traveled to Africa and has been bitten by a bug. He complains of high fevers, headaches, joint pain, diarrhea, cough, pruritus, and a papular skin rash.

46. Your patient was in New Jersey recently and was bitten by a tick. The bite mark became a raised erythematous lesion that expanded with central clearing. He complains of headaches and arthralgias.

47. Your patient recently returned from South America. He complains of difficulty swallowing. A radiologic consultation reported he has a megaesophagus. He remembers several bug bites.

48. While traveling in Montana a week ago, your patient was bitten by a tick during a hike. He complains of fever, chills, headache, nausea, vomiting, and a maculopapular rash that started on the wrist and ankles and has spread centrally.

49. While vacationing in Florida, your patient was bitten by a bug while canoeing at dusk in the Everglades. He complains of high fever, headache, nausea, vomiting, and neck stiffness.

50. While vacationing in Haiti, your patient was repeatedly bitten by bugs while walking on the beach in the evening. He complains of high fever, chills, diaphoresis, fatigue, headache, nausea, and vomiting.

Microbiology/Immunology

ANSWERS AND EXPLANATIONS

1.	B	26.	A
2.	C	27.	E
3.	D	28.	C
4.	B	29.	A
5.	C	30.	A
6.	E	31.	E
7.	E	32.	E
8.	E	33.	A
9.	D	34.	E
10.	B	35.	A
11.	B	36.	D
12.	D	37.	B
13.	C	38.	D
14.	A	39.	A
15.	A	40.	A
16.	D	41.	D
17.	A	42.	A
18.	D	43.	D
19.	A	44.	A
20.	E	45.	C
21.	D	46.	A
22.	C	47.	D
23.	B	48.	F
24.	D	49.	B
25.	C	50.	B

1. **The correct answer is B.** Reiter syndrome is a serious sequela that may follow enteric infections due to *Shigella*, *Salmonella*, *Yersinia*, or *Campylobacter* or sexually transmitted diseases caused by *Chlamydia* or *Ureaplasma*. Up to 80% of cases occur in HLA-B27 positive individuals. Male predominance is characteristic in cases following sexually transmitted infections. The role of infection is not clear, and infectious organisms have not been cultured from affected joints.

   Borrelia burgdorferi (**choice A**) is the causative agent of Lyme disease, a tick borne infection that manifests in three stages and involves the skin (erythema chronicum migrans), joints, heart, and meninges.

   Enterotoxigenic *Escherichia coli* (**choice C**) causes a self-limited enteric infection that manifests with watery diarrhea.

   Infection by group A β-hemolytic streptococci (**choice D**), usually a pharyngitis, may result in rheumatic heart disease characterized by carditis, migratory polyarthritis, erythema marginatum, subcutaneous nodules, and Sydenham chorea.

   Trichomonas vaginalis (**choice E**) causes a vaginitis associated with malodorous yellow-green discharge. The infection remains localized, and there are no systemic manifestations.

2. **The correct answer is C.** Carcinomas of the bladder and renal pelvis are usually transitional cell (**choices D and E**) carcinomas. However, *Schistosoma haematobium* infection (in which schistosomes lay eggs in the veins near the bladder, thereby inducing a marked inflammatory response) is associated with squamous metaplasia and squamous cell carcinoma of the bladder. Some authors have suggested that medications used to kill the worms may contribute to the etiology.

   Adenocarcinomas of the renal pelvis and bladder (**choices A and B**) are rare.

3. **The correct answer is D.** This patient most likely has cytomegalovirus (CMV) retinitis. The best drug treatment for this infection is ganciclovir.

   Acyclovir (**choice A**) is not effective in CMV infections. It is used more for HSV type 1 and 2 infections.

   Amantadine (**choice B**) is used either therapeutically or prophylactically for the influenza A virus.

   Flucytosine (**choice C**) is an antifungal agent.

   Zidovudine (**choice E**) is a first-line drug for the treatment of AIDS. The drug by itself is ineffective against CMV retinitis.

4. **The correct answer is B.** This patient has tuberculosis. The principal host defense in mycobacterial infections is cell-mediated immunity, which causes formation of granulomas. Unfortunately, in tuberculosis and many other infectious diseases characterized by granuloma formation, the organisms may persist intracellularly in the granulomas for years, and are a source of reactivation disease.

   Although antibody-mediated phagocytosis (**choice A**) is a major host defense against many bacteria, it is not the principal defense against mycobacteria.

   IgA-mediated hypersensitivity (**choice C**) does not exist. The only role of IgA is to prevent adherence of pathogens to mucosal surfaces.

   IgE-mediated hypersensitivity (**choice D**) is not involved in the body's defense against mycobacteria. It is important in allergic reactions.

   Neutrophil ingestion of bacteria (**choice E**) is a major host defense against bacteria but is not the principle defense against mycobacteria.

5. **The correct answer is C.** This girl has streptococcal pharyngitis. The infecting organism is group A beta-hemolytic streptococcus (*Streptococcus pyogenes*); its growth is inhibited by the placement of a bacitracin disk on the throat culture plate. (Beta-hemolysis occurs as the result of the bacterial hemolysin streptolysin S.) This is a gram-positive bacterium and therefore possesses a very thick peptidoglycan layer that would protect it from lysis by detergents. (Note that gram-positives also contain teichoic acid.) In contrast, gram-negatives have a thin peptidoglycan layer.

   Keratin-like proteins in the spore coat (**choice A**) and calcium ion chelators (dipicolinic acid; **choice E**) are found in spores formed by species of *Bacillus* and *Clostridium*. These protect the spores from the elements: dehydration, heat, chemicals, radiation, etc.

   Lipopolysaccharide in the outer membrane (**choice B**) and a periplasmic space (**choice D**) are found in gram-negative organisms. The lipopolysaccharide is an endotoxin, and the periplasmic space contains beta-lactamases in some species.

6. **The correct answer is E.** This is a straightforward question in which the introductory clinical details are really irrelevant. Ciprofloxacin and norfloxacin belong to a category of antibiotics called the fluoroquinolones. They are bactericidal and work by inhibiting topoisomerase II (DNA gyrase). They are effective against gram-negative rods and are the only oral agents effective against *Pseudomonas*. Ciprofloxacin is effective for treating urinary tract infections, gonorrhea, diarrheal diseases, and soft tissue infections. It is also used to treat *Pseudomonas* infections in cystic fibrosis.

Inhibition of dihydrofolate reductase (**choice A**) is the mechanism of action of trimethoprim, which is typically used in combination with sulfonamides (trimethoprim-sulfamethoxazole). Sulfonamides inhibit an earlier step in folate synthesis (dihydropteroate synthase), so the combination with trimethoprim is an effective "one-two" punch. Trimethoprim-sulfa is used in the treatment of *Shigella*, *Salmonella*, recurrent urinary tract infections, and *Pneumocystis carinii* pneumonia.

Inhibition of DNA-dependent RNA polymerase (**choice B**) is the mechanism of action of rifampin. Rifampin is used (along with other drugs) in the treatment of tuberculosis. You should also remember that rifampin can be used to treat individuals exposed to meningococcus or *Haemophilus influenzae* type B.

Inhibition of the 30s ribosomal subunit (**choice C**) is the mechanism of action of two important classes of antibiotics—the tetracyclines (tetracycline, doxycycline, demeclocycline) and the aminoglycosides (gentamicin, tobramycin, streptomycin, etc.). The tetracyclines inhibit the attachment of the aminoacyl-tRNA to the ribosome, whereas the aminoglycosides inhibit the formation of the initiation complex.

Inhibition of the 50s ribosomal subunit (**choice D**) is the mechanism of action of the macrolides (e.g., erythromycin), the lincosamides (e.g., lincomycin, clindamycin), and chloramphenicol. Chloramphenicol inhibits the 50s peptidyl transferase, whereas erythromycin blocks translocation.

7. **The correct answer is E.** The symptoms described are characteristic of endemic or murine typhus, caused by *Rickettsia typhi*. The vector is the rat flea, and the reservoirs are the rat and the rat flea. Unlike other rickettsial infections, *R. typhi* is frequently acquired in cities in the developing world with inadequate rodent control.

    Bartonella henselae (**choice A**) causes cat scratch disease and bacillary angiomatosis. Its reservoir is the domestic cat. The vector for the cat population is the cat flea, but most human infection is acquired through cat scratches or cat bites.

    Borrelia recurrentis (**choice B**) is a spirochete that causes louse-borne, relapsing fever. Humans are the only reservoir.

    Coxiella burnetii (**choice C**) is the cause of Q fever. It is acquired by inhalation, and its reservoirs are ticks, sheep, goats, and cattle.

    Ehrlichia chaffeensis (**choice D**) is a cause of human ehrlichiosis, which is characterized by leukopenia, thrombocytopenia, and anemia. It is transmitted by ticks, and deer are the reservoir.

8. **The correct answer is E.** The disease described is trachoma, which is caused by serovars A, B, and C of *Chlamydia trachomatis*. *C. trachomatis* causes a conjunctival and corneal infection that is spread in developing countries by eye-seeking flies. The lesions begin with formation of lymphoid follicles in the conjunctiva. With disease progression, there is tissue necrosis, granulation tissue deposition, and scar formation, leading to lacrimal duct obstruction and distortion of the eyelids. With the loss of an adequate tear system, the cornea becomes vulnerable to dehydration and opacification. Also, the vigorous inflammatory response can directly involve the cornea, with resulting opacity. In developed countries, chlamydial eye infections are often transmitted venereally, rather than by flies, and may cause conjunctivitis in neonates and in sexually active young adults. Humans are the only reservoir for *C. trachomatis*. *Chlamydia* are obligate intracellular parasites that have morphologically distinct infectious and reproductive forms. The infectious form is called the elementary body; the intracellular form is the reticulate body. *Chlamydia* are also distinctive in that they require host ATP and have a cell wall that lacks muramic acid. *C. trachomatis* also causes lymphogranuloma venereum (serovars L1, L2, and L3), inclusion conjunctivitis in infants (serovars D–K), and a variety of relatively nonspecific inflammations of the male and female genital tract (serovars D–K).

    Bartonella henselae causes cat scratch disease (**choice A**) and bacillary angiomatosis.

    The test described in **choice B** is the Weil-Felix test, which is used to identify rickettsia, not chlamydia.

    Choices C and D are incorrect because humans are the only known reservoir for *C. trachomatis*.

9. **The correct answer is D.** The patient described probably has systemic lupus erythematosus (SLE), which often presents with fatigue, malaise, fever, gastrointestinal symptoms, arthralgias, and myalgias. Hematologic abnormalities include anemia, leukopenia, lymphocytopenia, and thrombocytopenia. A circulating anticoagulant may prolong the activated partial thromboplastin time (APTT). Cutaneous manifestations include a malar rash and a generalized maculopapular eruption, both of which are photosensitive. Antibodies to the Smith antigen (core proteins of small ribonucleoproteins found in the nucleus) are present in only 20% to 30% of patients with SLE, but are quite specific for the disease, occurring only rarely in other autoimmune diseases.

    Anti-centromere antibody (**choice A**) is specific for the CREST (Calcinosis, Raynaud syndrome, Esophageal dysfunction, Sclerodactyly, and Telangiectasia) variant of progressive systemic sclerosis (scleroderma).

Rheumatoid factor is actually an autoantibody directed against the Fc portion of the IgG molecule (**choice B**). It is found in more than two-thirds of patients with rheumatoid arthritis.

Around 95% of patients with SLE develop antinuclear antibodies (ANA; **choice C**), so this test is quite sensitive but not very specific for SLE. ANA occur in patients with other inflammatory disorders, autoimmune diseases, and viral diseases, as well as in a number of normal individuals. Antibodies to double-stranded DNA are more specific for SLE but are not included as an answer choice.

Anti-SS-A antigen (**choice E**) refers to antibodies to certain ribonucleoproteins, which are fairly specific for Sjögren syndrome.

10. **The correct answer is B.** Hand-foot-and-mouth disease is characterized by the appearance of ulcers in the mouth and a maculopapular or vesicular rash on the hands and feet. It is most frequently caused by coxsackievirus type A16, although other coxsackieviruses have occasionally been implicated. The disease usually affects young children. Systemic features and lymphadenopathy are absent, and recovery is uneventful.

Coronavirus (**choice A**) is a cause of the common cold.

Herpes simplex virus type 1 (**choice C**) causes a variety of diseases, including gingivostomatitis, pharyngotonsillitis, herpes labialis, genital herpes, keratoconjunctivitis, and encephalitis. It may cause painful ulcers of the oral region, but it is unlikely to have caused the maculopapular rash described here.

Parainfluenza virus (**choice D**) is responsible for croup. Croup, or acute laryngotracheobronchitis, is an acute febrile illness with stridor, hoarseness, and cough.

Rhinovirus (**choice E**) is a member of Picornaviridae. It is the most common cause of the common cold.

11. **The correct answer is B.** Viral meningitis is relatively common, accounting for 10,000 cases of meningitis per year in the U.S. The vast majority of cases occur in individuals younger than 30 years. Usually, the symptoms are relatively mild, and death is uncommon. Enteroviruses, arboviruses, and type 2 herpes simplex virus are the most common causes of viral meningitis. Also, up to 10% of HIV patients develop an acute meningitis, typically at the time of seroconversion.

Adenovirus (**choice A**) infection is associated with upper respiratory tract infections (URIs), sinusitis, ocular disease, enteric infections, and bladder infections. It does not typically cause aseptic meningitis.

Human papillomaviruses (**choice C**) are associated with warts on the skin and genital areas.

Poxviruses (**choice D**) include the causative agents of smallpox, cowpox, and molluscum contagiosum. These agents do not typically cause meningitis.

Reoviruses (**choice E**) cause URIs, hepatitis, gastroenteritis, and encephalitis, but not meningitis.

12. **The correct answer is D.** This patient has osteomyelitis due to a cat bite that penetrated the periosteum. Whenever you see dog or cat bites in a question stem, consider *Pasteurella multocida* as a primary cause of wound infection. This organism is a short, encapsulated, gram-negative rod demonstrating bipolar staining. Rapidly arising cellulitis is particularly indicative of this organism.

Brucella melitensis (**choice A**) is a small, acapsular, gram-negative rod that causes brucellosis (undulant fever) and is associated with contact with goats or sheep. *Brucella abortus* and *Brucella suis* are variants associated with contact with cows and pigs, respectively. The organisms enter the body through the skin or through contaminated dairy products, such as unpasteurized imported goat's milk or cheeses.

Eikenella corrodens (**choice B**) is commonly found in human bites. It is a gram-negative rod that is part of the normal flora of the human mouth.

Francisella tularensis (**choice C**) is a small, pleomorphic, gram-negative rod that causes tularemia (rabbit fever). It occurs most commonly in rural areas. In the U.S., rabbits are the main reservoir for this organism, which is transmitted to humans by the *Dermacentor* tick or by contact with infectious animal tissues.

Yersinia pestis (**choice E**) is responsible for bubonic plague, which has been known to occur in the western U.S. Its main reservoir is the prairie dog, and its vector is the rat flea.

13. **The correct answer is C.** The drug of choice for otitis media in children is amoxicillin. In refractory cases, often due to bacterial resistance, switching to a different drug class is often effective. You must look for another medication that is effective against common organisms responsible for pediatric otitis media, such as *Streptococcus pneumoniae* (a gram-positive diplococcus) and *Haemophilus influenzae* (a gram-negative rod). A second-generation cephalosporin, such as cefaclor, should cover both and is the best choice. Consequently, it is commonly used in cases of amoxicillin-resistant otitis media. None of the other choices cover the proper spectrum of organisms.

Amphotericin B (**choice A**) is an antifungal polyene. It works by binding to ergosterol in the fungal cell membrane, creating an artificial pore. It is used to treat systemic mycoses such as those caused by *Aspergillus, Blastomyces, Candida, Coccidioides, Cryptococcus,* and *Histoplasma.*

Bacitracin (**choice B**) is a topical agent used to fight infection with gram-positive organisms. It interferes with cell wall synthesis.

Erythromycin (**choice D**) is a macrolide antibiotic that binds to the 23S rRNA portion of the 50S subunit of ribosomes, inhibiting release of uncharged tRNA and stopping protein synthesis. Though effective against *S. pneumoniae,* it is not particularly active against *H. influenzae.* Note that erythromycin may be used in amoxicillin-resistant otitis media, but only when administered with a sulfonamide such as sulfisoxazole.

Sulfamethoxazole (**choice E**) is a sulfonamide. It is bacteriostatic and works by inhibiting folic acid synthesis. It resembles p-aminobenzoic acid (PABA) structurally. When combined with trimethoprim (a dihydrofolate reductase inhibitor) it exerts a bactericidal effect and serves as the drug combination of choice for complicated urinary tract infections.

14. **The correct answer is A.** This boy probably has DiGeorge syndrome, as evidenced by his tetany (muscle spasms) due to hypocalcemia and his history of recurrent infections and neonatal seizures. The syndrome occurs because of an embryonic failure in the development of the third and fourth pharyngeal pouches. Patients have both hypoplastic parathyroids (producing hypocalcemia) and thymuses (producing T-cell deficiency and recurrent infections). Since cell-mediated immunity (which depends on T cells) is important in defense against infections caused by intracellular pathogens (such as viruses), patients with this condition are particularly susceptible to viral infections, such as chickenpox (varicella). They also have trouble with fungal pathogens (e.g., *Candida*) and mycobacteria.

Other clues to the diagnosis of DiGeorge syndrome include congenital cardiac defects, esophageal atresia, bifid uvula, short philtrum, hypertelorism, antimongoloid palpebral slant, mandibular hypoplasia, and low-set ears.

Diphtheria (**choice B**) is caused by *Corynebacterium diphtheriae,* which produces disease by the elaboration of a very potent exotoxin. Therefore, humoral immunity (antitoxin), which is not usually compromised in DiGeorge patients, is essential for defense against the organism. (Note that the *C. diphtheriae* exotoxin acts by causing the ADP-ribosylation of elongation factor-2

of eukaryotic cells, thereby inhibiting protein synthesis). The disease can be avoided by immunization with diphtheria toxoid.

Gas gangrene (**choice C**) is caused by *Clostridium perfringens,* which produces a potent alpha toxin that injures cell membranes. Therefore, humoral immunity would again play a predominant role in defense against this organism. Note that the disease occurs in wounds and would not be expected in an uninjured 4-year-old boy.

Gonorrhea (**choice D**) is caused by *Neisseria gonorrhoeae* and would not be expected in a 4-year-old boy unless there was evidence of sexual abuse. Virulence factors of this organism include pili, cell wall endotoxin and outer membrane, and IgA protease. Antibody responses, neutrophils, and complement are of prime importance in defense against gonococcal infections.

Tetanus (**choice E**) is caused by *Clostridium tetani* and serves as a tricky distracter, as you might have quickly associated the patient's muscle spasms with this answer choice. (This is why it is important to read the question stem carefully before prematurely jumping to the responses.) *C. tetani,* which gains entry through deep wounds, produces tetanus toxin (exotoxin) and can be prevented by immunization with tetanus toxoid.

15. **The correct answer is A.** This patient has *Pneumocystis carinii* pneumonia (PCP), which is caused by an agent now believed to be a fungus rather than a true bacterium. PCP is seen in immunocompromised patients, particularly those with AIDS, cancer, and, in children, prematurity or malnourishment. It can be the AIDS-defining illness.

Congestive heart failure (**choice B**) predisposes the patient to pulmonary edema.

Pulmonary embolus (**choice C**) can cause pulmonary infarction or sudden death.

Rheumatoid arthritis (**choice D**), particularly in miners, can cause formation of lung nodules similar to subcutaneous rheumatoid nodules.

Systemic lupus erythematosus (**choice E**) can cause pleuritis but is not associated with a significantly increased incidence of pneumonia.

16. **The correct answer is D.** Humans become infected with *Toxoplasma gondii* by ingesting cysts in contaminated food or through contact with cat feces. The veterinarian in question was therefore particularly at risk of infection. *T. gondii* is especially hazardous in pregnant women because the organism can be transmitted to the fetus through the placenta. (It is part of the ToRCHeS group of congenital infections—Toxoplasma, Rubella, CMV, Herpes/HIV, Syphilis). Since infected mothers

are usually asymptomatic, cases often go unnoticed. Occasionally, patients present with cervical lymphadenopathy, as did the veterinarian, and require treatment to prevent complications in the fetus. Though newborns are also often asymptomatic, they are at risk for developing the classic triad of chorioretinitis (at birth or later in life), hydrocephalus, and cerebral calcifications. Note that *T. gondii* is also a common cause of CNS infections (e.g., encephalitis) in HIV-positive patients.

Isospora belli (**choice A**) is an intestinal protozoan that causes watery diarrhea, particularly in immunocompromised patients. Fecal-oral transmission of oocysts allows invasion of small intestinal mucosa, destroying the brush border.

Leishmania donovani (**choice B**) causes kala-azar (visceral leishmaniasis), which is characterized by fever, weakness, weight loss, splenomegaly, and skin hyperpigmentation. It is prevalent in regions of the Mediterranean, Middle East, Russia, and China. The vector is the sandfly.

Plasmodium vivax (**choice C**) causes malaria and is transmitted by the female *Anopheles* mosquito, which introduces sporozoites into the blood. These differentiate into merozoites that destroy erythrocytes. Splenomegaly ensues. Other species of this organism that cause malaria are *P. malariae*, *P. ovale* and *P. falciparum* (which causes a more severe form of the disease). Note that sickle cell trait confers resistance to *P. falciparum*.

Trypanosoma cruzi (**choice E**) causes Chagas disease, characterized by unilateral facial edema and nodules, fever, lymphadenopathy, and hepatosplenomegaly. It affects cardiac muscle most severely and is a major cause of cardiac disease worldwide. The reduviid ("kissing") bug is the vector that infects humans by defecating in the bite wound. It is most prevalent in Central and South America, with rare cases in the southern U.S.

17. **The correct answer is A.** This patient has systemic sclerosis, also called scleroderma. Antibodies to topoisomerase I (anti-Scl-70) occur in up to 70% of patients with diffuse systemic sclerosis, but only rarely in other disorders. Systemic sclerosis is characterized initially by excessive fibrosis and edema of the skin, especially the hands and fingers, producing sclerodactyly (characteristic changes in the fingers, which resemble claws). Raynaud phenomenon is common. The diffuse type of systemic sclerosis generally spreads to include visceral organs, such as the esophagus (producing dysphagia), the lungs (producing pulmonary fibrosis), the heart (leading to heart failure or arrhythmia), and the kidneys (renal failure causes 50% of scleroderma deaths). Females are affected more than

males (3:1 ratio). A more restricted variant of systemic sclerosis, with a somewhat more benign course, is CREST syndrome (Calcinosis, Raynaud syndrome, Esophageal dysmotility, Sclerodactyly, and Telangiectasia), characterized by the presence of anti-centromere antibodies (although 10% of CREST patients will have anti-topoisomerase antibody as well).

Anti-ds DNA (**choice B**) and anti-Sm (Smith antigen; **choice D**) are characteristic of systemic lupus erythematosus (SLE) but are not common in patients with systemic sclerosis.

Rheumatoid factor is an autoantibody directed against IgG (**choice C**). It is found in patients with rheumatoid arthritis.

Anti-SS-A (**choice E**) is typically seen in Sjögren syndrome (although it may also be seen in SLE).

18. **The correct answer is D.** All of the organisms listed are protozoa. There are two intestinal protozoa specifically associated with AIDS that can cause transient diarrhea in immunocompetent individuals but can cause debilitating, and potentially life-threatening, chronic diarrhea in AIDS patients. These organisms are *Isospora belli* (treated with trimethoprim-sulfamethoxazole or other folate antagonists) and *Cryptosporidium parvum* (no treatment presently available).

Diphyllobothrium latum (**choice A**) is the fish tapeworm and occasionally causes diarrhea, which is not specifically associated with AIDS.

Entamoeba histolytica (**choice B**) and *Giardia lamblia* (**choice C**) are both causes of diarrhea, but they are not specifically associated with AIDS.

Microsporidia (**choice E**) are protozoa that cause diarrhea, but produce spores rather than oocysts.

19. **The correct answer is A.** The patient has Burkitt lymphoma. This high-grade B-cell lymphoma occurs endemically in Africa (it is the most common neoplasm in children in an equatorial belt that includes Africa and New Guinea) and sporadically in the U.S. and Europe. The sporadic form is often in an abdominal site and occurs in young adults. The African form of Burkitt lymphoma has been strongly associated with antibodies directed against Epstein-Barr virus; the association is weaker in sporadic cases. A characteristic translocation, t(8;14) (q24.l3;q32.33) has been described. Malaria infection is a cofactor.

Hepatitis B (**choice B**) is associated with hepatocellular carcinoma. t(9;22) is the Philadelphia chromosome, which is seen in some cases of chronic myelogenous leukemia (CML) and acute myelogenous leukemia (AML).

Herpesvirus (**choice C**) type 8 is associated with Kaposi sarcoma. CD5 is a marker seen in small lymphocytic and mantle cell lymphomas.

HIV (**choice D**) is linked to AIDS. Some patients also develop primary lymphomas (not usually Burkitt). CD4 is a marker for helper T cells and some T cell lymphomas.

Human papillomavirus (**choice E**) is linked with common warts, genital condylomata, and genital cancers. t(2;5) is linked to anaplastic large cell lymphoma.

20. **The correct answer is E.** The combination of vomiting, anorexia, high fever (above 100.4 F), and a bulging fontanel equals neonatal meningitis until proven otherwise. *Streptococcus agalactiae* (group B strep) and *Escherichia coli* (not an answer choice) are the most common causes in neonates up to 1 month of age. The next most reasonable response would have been *Listeria monocytogenes* (**choice B**), another, though less common, cause of neonatal meningitis.

Most cases of meningitis caused by *Haemophilus influenzae* (**choice A**) occur in children aged 6 months to 6 years; 90% of these cases result from the capsular type b strain. It has become much less prevalent now that the *H. influenzae* type b conjugate vaccine is routinely administered to infants.

Neisseria meningitidis (**choice C**) is the most common cause of <u>epidemic</u> meningitis. The two organisms most often associated with sporadic cases are *Haemophilus influenzae* and *Streptococcus pneumoniae* (the most common cause in adults older than 30).

Staphylococcus aureus (**choice D**) is not a common cause of meningitis, except in patients with CSF shunts. It is often responsible for abscesses, osteomyelitis, endocarditis, toxic shock syndrome, and food poisoning.

21. **The correct answer is D.** *Pasteurella multocida* is a gram-negative rod that is normal flora of the oral cavity of dogs and cats. It often causes a local abscess following introduction under the skin by an animal bite. Most cases occur in children who are injured while playing with a pet.

Bartonella henselae (**choice A**) is a very small, gram-negative bacterium that is closely related to the rickettsia, although it is able to grow on inert media. It is the cause of cat-scratch disease (a local, chronic lymphadenitis most commonly seen in children) and bacillary angiomatosis (seen particularly in AIDS patients). In this latter patient population, the organism causes proliferation of blood and lymphatic vessels causing a characteristic "mulberry" lesion in the skin and subcutaneous tissues of the afflicted individual.

Brucella canis (**choice B**) is a gram-negative rod that is a zoonotic agent. Its normal host is the dog, but when it gains access to humans, it causes an undulating febrile disease with malaise, lymphadenopathy and hepatosplenomegaly. The normal route of exposure is via ingestion of the organism.

Clostridium tetani (**choice C**) is a gram-positive spore-forming anaerobic rod. It causes tetanus [a spastic paralysis caused by tetanospasmin, which blocks the release of the inhibitory neurotransmitters glycine and gamma-aminobutyric acid (GABA)]. There may be no lesion at the site of inoculation, and exudation would be extremely rare.

Toxocara canis (**choice E**), a common intestinal parasite of dogs, is a metazoan parasite that causes visceral larva migrans. Young children are most likely to be affected, as they are most likely to ingest soil contaminated with eggs of the parasite.

22. **The correct answer is C.** Rotavirus is the most common cause of gastroenteritis in children aged 3 months to 2 years. It is most prevalent in the winter. Rotavirus, one of the reoviruses, looks like a wheel (which ROTAtes) and possesses a double-shelled icosahedral capsid with no envelope. Its genome consists of 11 segments of double-stranded RNA.

A complex double-stranded DNA genome (**choice A**) is found in enteric adenoviruses, the third most common cause of gastroenteritis in infants and children. This organism possesses an icosahedral nucleocapsid.

A partially double-stranded circular DNA genome (**choice B**) is characteristic of hepatitis B. Its envelope contains surface antigen (HBsAg). Its capsid is icosahedral and contains the genome along with DNA-dependent DNA polymerase, which also has reverse transcriptase activity.

A single-stranded circular RNA genome (**choice D**) is characteristic of hepatitis D virus. Its envelope consists of HBsAg. The virus is defective and can replicate only in cells infected with hepatitis B.

A single-stranded RNA genome (**choice E**) is characteristic of several viruses that cause gastroenteritis in children, including astrovirus and Norwalk virus. Astrovirus is the second most common cause of viral gastroenteritis in young children. Three structural proteins form its capsid. Norwalk virus is the most common cause of gastroenteritis outbreaks in older children and adults. Its capsid consists of one structural protein.

23. **The correct answer is B.** Retinitis in the setting of HIV is most likely caused by cytomegalovirus (CMV), which is a herpesvirus. Other herpesviruses include herpes simplex, varicella-zoster (chickenpox, shingles), and Epstein-Barr virus (mononucleosis).

The adenoviruses (**choice A**) can cause respiratory infections, pharyngitis, gastroenteritis, and conjunctivitis. They do not cause retinitis.

The orthomyxoviruses (**choice C**) include the influenza viruses.

The paramyxoviruses (**choice D**) include the viruses responsible for croup (parainfluenza), measles (rubeola), mumps, and respiratory syncytial virus.

The retroviruses (**choice E**) include HIV; however, retinitis in AIDS patients is usually due to an opportunistic infection with CMV.

24. **The correct answer is D.** *Proteus mirabilis* is a gram-negative rod that is a member of the family Enterobacteriaceae. It is lactose-negative and contains urease, which splits urea, raising the pH of the urine to create a more hospitable environment for the bacterium. Patients with stones are at increased risk for *Proteus* because the organism is able to hide in the stones, and patients with *Proteus* are more likely to get stones because the increased urinary pH contributes to their formation.

Enterococcus faecalis (**choice A**) is a gram-positive coccus that commonly causes urinary tract infections in elderly men with prostate problems.

Escherichia coli (**choice B**) is a lactose-positive, oxidase-negative, gram-negative rod that is the most common cause of community-acquired urinary tract infections.

Klebsiella pneumoniae (**choice C**) is a lactose-positive, oxidase-negative, gram-negative rod. It can cause urinary tract infections in patients with poorly controlled diabetes because glucose in the urine enhances growth of this microorganism.

Pseudomonas aeruginosa (**choice E**) is a gram-negative rod. It can easily be distinguished from the family Enterobacteriaceae because it is oxidase negative. It is an opportunistic pathogen that has an increased chance of causing urinary tract infections in patients who have catheters or are on antibiotics.

25. **The correct answer is C.** This patient has disseminated gonococcemia. Gonococcal arthritis and tenosynovitis typically involve both the upper and lower extremities equally. Vesicular skin lesions are characteristic of disseminated gonococcal disease. Females are at particular risk of gonococcemia during menstruation, since sloughing of the endometrium allows access to the blood supply, necrotic tissue enhances the growth

of *Neisseria gonorrhoeae*, and there is an alteration of the pH. Patients who have a C6-8 deficiency have both an increase risk of disseminated gonococcemia and a tendency to have multiple episodes. These patients are also at risk for bacteremia from *Neisseria meningitidis*.

C1 esterase inhibitor deficiency (**choice A**) can occur as an autosomal dominant disorder or is acquired. Patients have angioedema without urticaria. The syndrome is also associated with recurrent attacks of colic and episodes of laryngeal edema.

Ciliary dysfunction (**choice B**) is a marker of Kartagener syndrome (immotile cilia syndrome). The syndrome includes infertility, bronchiectasis, sinusitis, and situs inversus. It is an autosomal recessive disorder caused by abnormalities in the dynein arm of the cilia.

Endothelial adhesion molecule deficiency (**choice D**), or beta-2 integrin deficiency, is characterized by failure of neutrophils to express CD18 integrins on their surface. Patients have impaired phagocyte adherence, aggregation, chemotaxis, and phagocytosis of C3b-coated particles. Clinically, there is delayed separation of the umbilical cord, sustained agranulocytosis, recurrent infections of skin and mucosa, gingivitis, and periodontal disease.

Eosinophil deficiency (**choice E**) or eosinopenia occurs with stressors such as acute bacterial infection and following administration of glucocorticoids. There is no known adverse effect of eosinopenia.

26. **The correct answer is A.** The clinical history suggests infant botulism. The clue here is that the mother feeds the infant honey. *Clostridium botulinum* (a common honey contaminant) was ingested and produced toxin in the infant. The toxin, which blocks the release of acetylcholine from nerve terminals, is responsible for the floppiness. Acetylcholine is the neurotransmitter at the neuromuscular junction, and inhibition of release can lead to muscle weakness, failure to thrive, and, in more serious cases, respiratory impairment.

Glycine and GABA (**choice B**) release is inhibited by a toxin produced by *Clostridium tetani*. This leads to the muscular spasms of tetanus.

ADP-ribosylation of an elongation factor (**choice C**) is a mechanism of action of diphtheria and *Pseudomonas* exotoxins.

Alpha toxin from *Clostridium perfringens* is a lecithinase (**choice D**) responsible for the development of gas gangrene.

Guanylate cyclase (**choice E**) is stimulated by a heat-stable toxin produced by *Escherichia coli*.

27. **The correct answer is E.** The patient has cerebral toxoplasmosis. Toxoplasmosis is a major cause of neurologic symptoms in HIV-infected and other immunosuppressed patients. Domestic cats are the primary host for *Toxoplasma gondii* (a sporozoan) and shed cysts in their feces. Uncooked meats are another source of *Toxoplasma* infection. Symptoms in humans arise from the ingestion of these cysts, leading to invasion of the gut wall and subsequent systemic dissemination. Parasites that migrate to the brain cause multiple abscesses, particularly in the cortex and deep gray nuclei. Patients present with fever, headache, and focal neurologic symptoms. Ring-enhancing lesions are characteristic.

Cryptococcus neoformans (**choice A**) is an oval, budding yeast with a wide polysaccharide capsule. Infection results from the inhalation of the organism, which can then disseminate to the CNS (particularly in immunocompromised patients). CNS infection leads to a chronic meningitis characterized by high protein levels in the CSF. *C. neoformans* can be visualized in the CSF with an India ink preparation.

Mycobacterium leprae (**choice B**) causes leprosy and preferentially infects the skin and superficial nerves (because it prefers cooler temperatures).

Pasteurella multocida (**choice C**) is a gram-negative rod that is part of the normal oral flora of domestic dogs and cats. It causes a rapid onset cellulitis at the site of an animal bite.

Pneumocystis carinii (**choice D**) is a fungus that causes pneumonia, particularly in immunocompromised patients.

28. **The correct answer is C.** The single finding of high autoantibody titers to histones, without any other autoantibodies, is characteristic of drug-induced lupus. The most commonly implicated drugs are procainamide, hydralazine (given for hypertension), and isoniazid. Patients typically have milder disease than in systemic lupus erythematosus (SLE), and tend to have arthritis, pleuro-pericardial involvement, and, less commonly, rash. CNS and renal disease are not usually observed.

CREST syndrome (**choice A**) is a milder variant of scleroderma characterized by calcinosis, Raynaud phenomenon, esophageal dysmotility, sclerodactyly and telangiectasia. Anti-centromere antibodies are diagnostic.

The diffuse form of scleroderma (**choice B**), also known as systemic sclerosis, causes fibrosis of the skin and internal viscera. This disorder is characterized by anti-SCI-70 and often low titers of many other autoantibodies.

Sjögren syndrome (**choice D**) is characterized by dry eyes and dry mouth. Sjögren syndrome in isolation is characteristically positive for anti-SS-A and anti-SS-B. If it accompanies rheumatoid arthritis, anti-RNP will be positive as well.

SLE (**choice E**) is a multisystem disorder that is distinguished from drug-induced lupus by the presence of a wide variety of autoantibodies, including anti-double-stranded DNA (anti-dsDNA).

29. **The correct answer is A.** All the agents listed can infect the eyeball. The agent specifically associated with contact lens use is *Acanthamoeba*, which can infect lens solution. This amoeba is dangerous because it causes an intractable ulcerative keratitis that may progress to uveitis. If the lesion is suspected, the clinical laboratory should be notified, and specific directions for collecting samples for culture obtained. The parasites may be difficult to see in histologic sections or corneal scrapings.

Cytomegalovirus (**choice B**) and herpes (**choice C**) infections are most often seen in immunocompromised patients, particularly AIDS patients.

Circulating larvae of the helminth *Toxocara* (**choice D**) can lodge in the eye (particularly in the vitreous or retina); *Toxocara* infections are seen more commonly in children.

Toxoplasmosis (**choice E**) of the eye is most often congenital, but it can be acquired. It produces retinal scarring, not corneal ulceration.

30. **The correct choice is A.** This patient has the symptoms of a urinary tract infection (UTI). *Escherichia coli* is the leading cause of community-acquired UTIs. The proximity of the urinary tract to the anus facilitates colonization of the tract by fecal flora.

Other gram-negative rods causing UTIs include *Enterobacter cloacae*, *Klebsiella pneumoniae*, *Serratia marcescens*, *Proteus mirabilis*, and *Pseudomonas aeruginosa*.

None of the other choices listed cause UTIs.

31. **The correct answer is E.** This is the classic microscopic description of the pneumococcus *Streptococcus pneumoniae*, which is a common cause of lobar pneumonia. Most strains are still very sensitive to penicillins, although some drug-resistant strains have been isolated.

Haemophilus influenzae (**choice A**) is a gram-negative bacillus. Nontypeable strains may cause pneumonia in elderly patients with chronic respiratory disease.

Neisseria gonorrhoeae (**choice B**) is a gram-negative diplococcus that is not typically associated with pneumonia.

Pneumocystis carinii (**choice C**) is a small, hat-shaped fungus that is a common cause of pneumonia in HIV-positive patients.

Staphylococcus aureus (**choice D**) occurs as grapelike clusters of large, gram-positive cocci. It may cause pneumonia after surgery or after a viral respiratory infection, such as influenza, and is associated with empyema formation.

32. **The correct answer is E.** This is a case of rheumatic fever, which is an immunologically mediated sequela to *Streptococcus pyogenes* pharyngitis. It is a type II cytotoxic hypersensitivity, involving antibodies that bind to cardiac tissue, activate complement, and thereby cause cell destruction. It is therefore most similar to idiopathic thrombocytopenic purpura, which is also a form of type II cytotoxic hypersensitivity, in this case mediated by antibodies against platelets producing complement fixation and causing the clotting dyscrasia.

Atopic allergy (**choice A**) is a form of type I hypersensitivity, mediated by IgE antibodies, basophils, and mast cells.

Contact dermatitis (**choice B**) is a form of type IV hypersensitivity mediated by T cells and macrophages.

Graft-versus-host disease (**choice C**) is a form of type IV hypersensitivity mediated by T cells and macrophages.

Graves disease (**choice D**) is a form of type II hypersensitivity, but it is *not* cytotoxic in its action. Instead, antibodies to the TSH receptors on thyroid cells cause overstimulation of the gland and its eventual exhaustion.

33. **The correct answer is A.** This patient has *Candida* esophagitis. Any time a patient presents with dysphagia or odontophagia, along with white plaques in the oropharynx (thrush), you can assume that the *Candida* is affecting the esophagus as well. The fact that the patient is an IV drug user makes an opportunistic infection such as *Candida* more likely. *Candida* appears as budding yeast with pseudohyphae *in vivo*.

The other answer choices represent the morphology of other important opportunistic fungi:

Cryptococcus are encapsulated yeast (**choice B**). You should think about *Cryptococcus neoformans* when you're presented with an immunocompromised patient with neurologic symptoms. The classic clue is the presence of encapsulated organisms observable in an India ink preparation.

Mucor and *Rhizopus* are molds with nonseptate hyphae (**choice C**). You should think about *Mucor* when you are presented with a diabetic (especially ketoacidosis) or a leukemic patient with a severe sinus infection.

Aspergillus is a mold with septate hyphae (**choice D**). In immunocompromised patients, aspergillosis can present with acute pneumonia, often with cavitation (aspergillomas = fungus balls in the lungs).

Nonencapsulated yeast (**choice E**) is not the best answer because the history suggests *Candida*, which is a budding yeast with pseudohyphae. Nonencapsulating yeast is not known to infect the throat.

34. **The correct answer is E.** Whenever you see a question about a gardener who works with roses, think "*Sporothrix schenckii*." This organism is responsible for sporotrichosis, "rose gardener's disease." The organism enters through skin breaks in the fingers or hands, causing a chancre, papule, or subcutaneous nodule with erythema and fluctuance. Ulcerating lesions appear along lymphatic channels, but the lymph nodes are not commonly infected. Potassium iodide is the treatment of choice for the subcutaneous manifestations.

Aspergillus (**choice A**) causes pulmonary aspergillosis—a systemic mycotic infection. There is an allergic type that is caused by a hypersensitivity reaction to the organism and an infectious type that occurs more commonly in the immunocompromised. Hemoptysis is a common symptom.

Malassezia (**choice B**), specifically *M. furfur*, causes tinea versicolor, a superficial mycotic infection.

Onchocerca (**choice C**), specifically *O. volvulus*, causes river blindness. This organism is a helminth that is transmitted by black flies in Africa, Central America, and South America.

Rhizopus (**choice D**) causes rhinocerebral infections in diabetics with ketoacidosis.

35. **The correct answer is A.** Lobar pneumonia, in which an entire lobe of the lung becomes rapidly affected with pneumonia, is actually a relatively uncommon pattern for pneumonia. Common causative organisms include *Streptococcus pneumoniae* (pneumococcus), *Haemophilus influenzae*, and *Klebsiella pneumoniae*. *K. pneumoniae* is specifically associated with alcohol abuse, diabetes mellitus, and nosocomial infections.

Legionella spp. (**choice B**) most commonly causes a patchy atypical pneumonia not specifically associated with alcoholism. Instead, *Legionella* infection is associated with inspiration of aerosolized contaminated water.

Mycoplasma pneumoniae (**choice C**) causes extensive patchy infiltrates rather than lobar pneumonia. It is the most common cause of pneumonia in young adults.

Pneumocystis carinii (**choice D**) causes diffuse interstitial and alveolar infiltrates, typically in patients immunosuppressed by AIDS, cytotoxic drug therapy, or cancer.

Staphylococcus aureus (**choice E**) produces patchy infiltrates. Staphylococcal pneumonia may complicate influenza during epidemics, or it may be a nosocomial infection. It is associated with empyema formation.

36. **The correct answer is D.** There is a specific association between diabetes (particularly in brittle diabetics who may have episodes of ketoacidosis) and chronic sinusitis due to saprophytic Zygomycetes, including *Mucor* and *Rhizopus*. These fungi can spread rapidly from the sinuses to the nearby skull bones and brain, potentially causing massive tissue destruction and death. The term "rhinocerebral mucormycosis" is used in these cases. Less commonly, other sites may be involved (lung, gastrointestinal tract), depending on the port of entry. The physician should suspect mucormycosis in any patient with chronic sinusitis who appears unusually ill and does not respond to antibiotic therapy. Unfortunately, most cases are diagnosed at autopsy.

    Actinomyces (**choice A**) are part of the normal flora of the mouth. Actinomycosis also occurs in humans and may affect the cervicofacial region (typically following dental procedures or maxillofacial injuries), lungs, abdomen (typically following surgery, trauma, or intestinal penetration), or pelvis (related to IUD use). There is no specific association with diabetes mellitus.

    Aspergillus (**choice B**) can be present in the sinuses, and does have a somewhat increased incidence in diabetics, but is not the organism about which the physician should be most concerned.

    Cryptococcus (**choice C**) is found in pigeon feces and is usually introduced into the body via the respiratory tract. It can disseminate to the meninges and other sites in immunocompromised patients (often AIDS patients). It would not be of particular concern in this patient with sinusitis.

    Pneumocystis carinii (**choice E**) causes pneumonia in severely immunosuppressed patients, e.g., AIDS patients.

37. **The correct answer is B.** This question is difficult for two reasons. First, it asks for the viral family instead of the virus itself. Second, it includes distracters that all look alike. You probably realized that the child in question has croup (laryngotracheobronchitis); the classic clue here is the "barking cough." You might have remembered that the virus responsible for croup is the parainfluenza virus. The toughest part was remembering that parainfluenza virus (along with measles virus, mumps virus, and respiratory syncytial virus) belongs to the paramyxovirus family. These viruses all have negative-strand RNA and an enveloped helical nucleocapsid.

    The papovaviruses (**choice A**) are DNA viruses with a naked icosahedral nucleocapsid. This family includes the human papilloma viruses, which cause warts and are associated with penile, laryngeal, and especially, cervical cancer; the BK virus, which can affect immunosuppressed patients; the JC virus, which is associated

with progressive multifocal leukoencephalopathy; and the simian SV40 virus.

The parvoviruses (**choice C**) are small, single-stranded DNA viruses. Only one serotype (B19) causes diseases in humans: erythema infectiosum in children (characteristic "slapped cheek" rash), aplastic crises in patients with hemolytic diseases, and hydrops fetalis or stillbirth in anemic fetuses.

The picornaviruses (**choice D**) are positive single-stranded RNA viruses with a naked icosahedral nucleocapsid. This family includes the polioviruses, echoviruses, coxsackieviruses, enterovirus 72 (HepA virus), and rhinoviruses (common cold).

The poxviruses (**choice E**) are double-stranded DNA viruses. This family includes the viruses responsible for smallpox and molluscum contagiosum.

38. **The correct answer is D.** Pyogenic osteomyelitis may result from hematogenous dissemination or local spread from a contiguous infectious focus. Patients with sickle cell disease are prone to osteomyelitis, and *Pseudomonas aeruginosa* is the most common etiologic agent in this condition. Bone pain, fever, and x-ray evidence of early bone demineralization and soft tissue swelling are the presenting clinical picture.

    Hemophilus influenzae (**choice B**) and group B streptococci (**choice A**) are the most common causes of osteomyelitis occurring in infants.

    Osteomyelitis caused by *Mycobacterium tuberculosis* (**choice C**) most commonly affects vertebral bones and develops in 3% of cases of disseminated tuberculosis. A chronic destructive infection of the lumbar vertebrae that tracks down along the iliopsoas muscle into the soft tissue of the inguinal fossa is referred to as *Pott disease*.

    Staphylococcus aureus (**choice E**) accounts for approximately 90% of all cases arising in patients without specific predisposing conditions.

39. **The correct choice is A.** *Campylobacter* is a motile, curved, oxidase-positive, gram-negative rod with polar flagella. The illness typically begins 1-7 days following ingestion of the organism. The presentation is usually lower abdominal pain and diarrhea with blood and pus. The illness is self-limited after 3-5 days and can last up to 2 weeks. The organisms grow optimally at 42 C under microaerophilic conditions.

    Escherichia coli (**choice B**) is a flagellated gram-negative, oxidative-negative organism. It is not a common cause of bloody diarrhea in this age group.

    Salmonella (**choice C**) and *Shigella* (**choice D**) are incorrect because they are oxidase negative.

Vibrio cholerae (**choice E**) has many physical features in common with *C. jejuni*. However, *V. cholerae* is not enteroinvasive and does not produce bloody diarrhea, but "rice water" stools.

40. **The correct answer is A.** *Bacillus cereus* produces a self-limited diarrhea due to ingestion of the preformed enterotoxin in contaminated fried rice and seafood. The incubation period is typically around 4 hours. The degree of vomiting is greater than the diarrhea. *B. cereus* is also associated with keratitis, producing a corneal ring abscess.

Clostridium botulinum (**choice B**) produces a neurotoxin that blocks the release of acetylcholine, resulting in a symmetric descending paralysis that may lead to respiratory complications causing death. Symptoms include blurred vision, photophobia, dysphagia, nausea, vomiting, and dysphonia. Most cases are associated with the ingestion of contaminated home-canned food.

Clostridium perfringens (**choice C**) produces a severe diarrhea with abdominal pain and cramping (sometimes called "church picnic" diarrhea). The incubation period is 8-24 hours after ingesting contaminated meat, meat products, or poultry. The meats have usually been cooked, allowed to cool, and then warmed, which causes germination of the clostridial spores.

EHEC—Enterohemorrhagic *Escherichia coli* (**choice D**), produces a bloody, noninvasive diarrhea due to the ingestion of verotoxin found in undercooked hamburger at fast food restaurants. The 0157:H7 serotype typically produces this syndrome. Some patients develop a life-threatening complication called hemolytic-uremic syndrome.

Staphylococcus aureus (**choice E**) produces a self-limited food poisoning syndrome with nausea, vomiting, and abdominal pain followed by diarrhea beginning 1-6 hours after ingestion of the enterotoxin. The organism is found in foods such as potato salad, custard, milk shakes, and mayonnaise.

41. **The correct answer is D.** The nurse's elevated IgM anti-HBc indicates that she was infected with hepatitis B. Formerly, HBsAg (surface antigen) and anti-HBsAg (antibody to surface antigen) were used exclusively to determine this. Typically, HBsAg is positive for up to 6 months, and anti-HBsAg is positive for years after that. Unfortunately, this simple scheme has the disadvantage that many patients have a 2-week to 4-month "window" period, when the surface antigen (HBsAg) and the antibody (anti-HBs) are not detectable. Presumably, for a relatively brief period, HBsAg production exactly matches antibody production, and the two coprecipitate such that neither free species is present in adequate concentration to be detectable. This problem can be circumvented either by serial measurements of HBsAg

and anti-HBs, or by concurrent measurement of other antigens and antibodies, including HBeAg, anti-HBe, and anti-HBc (HBcAg is not reliable). During the window period, IgM anti-HBc may be the only marker of recent HBV infection, as it is in this nurse.

If the nurse had been effectively vaccinated for hepatitis B (**choice A**), she would have had an elevated anti-HBs antibody level and no HBsAg present in the serum. Anti-HBc antibody would have been absent as well.

The antibody response to hepatitis B infection was appropriate in this person, which argues against immunocompromise (**choice B**).

Carriers (**choice C**) have elevated HBsAg and may have persistently elevated HBeAg (in approximately 10% of cases). IgG anti-HBc (not IgM) predominates in these chronic patients.

Had she not been infected with hepatitis B at all (**choice E**), IgM anti-HBc would be absent.

42. **The correct answer is A.** This patient presents with the classic findings of granuloma inguinale (Donovanosis). The clue that he had traveled to New Guinea clinches the diagnosis (granuloma inguinale is common in India and New Guinea and rare in the U.S.). This is a chronic, sexually transmitted disease (STD) that presents with ulcerating granulomata of the genital skin and mucous membranes. On biopsy, there is granulation tissue and microabscesses with macrophages containing diagnostic Donovan bodies (small, rounded coccobacilli within cystic areas of the cytoplasm seen with Wright-Giemsa stain). This disease is caused by the bacterium *Calymmatobacterium donovani*.

Chlamydia trachomatis (**choice B**) causes lymphogranuloma venereum, an STD that is rare in the U.S. but common in the tropics. It can present with genital or anorectal lesions or regional lymphadenopathy. Cytoplasmic inclusion bodies would be seen in epithelial cells.

Haemophilus ducreyi (**choice C**) causes chancroid, an STD that presents with a painful chancre and regional lymphadenopathy. Remember that "ducreyi" makes you "cry" (because it's painful).

Neisseria gonorrhoeae (**choice D**) causes gonorrhea. There may be purulent inflammation or abscesses.

Treponema pallidum (**choice E**) causes syphilis. Patients usually present with cutaneous manifestations followed by widespread dissemination. It occurs in three stages: primary syphilis is associated with a painless chancre; secondary syphilis is associated with condyloma lata; and tertiary syphilis involves the brain (neurosyphilis) and the aorta (aneurysm) with the development of gummas.

43. **The correct answer is D.** This patient has hemolytic-uremic syndrome (HUS), a complication of the Shiga toxin or Shiga-like toxin (exotoxins released by *Shigella* species and the enterohemorrhagic *Escherichia coli*). In children, HUS usually develops after a gastrointestinal or flu-like illness and is characterized by bleeding, oliguria, hematuria, and microangiopathic hemolytic anemia. Presumably the Shiga toxin is toxic to the microvasculature, producing microthrombi that consume platelets and RBCs, and may fragment the red cell membrane.

The incorrect choices are all bacteria that may produce an enterocolitis but do not elicit HUS.

A long-term consequence of *Campylobacter* (**choice A**) infection is a reactive arthritis or full-blown Reiter syndrome.

Clostridial enterocolitis is produced by *Clostridium difficile* (**choice B**), a normal inhabitant of the gut that produces pseudomembranous colitis when other gut flora are suppressed by treatment with antibiotics.

In the U.S., *Salmonella* infections (**choice C**) are almost all nontyphoid inflammatory diarrhea, producing a simple enterocolitis that may proceed to sepsis in some cases. Typhoid fever (produced by *Salmonella typhi* and *Salmonella paratyphi*) causes a protracted illness that progresses over several weeks and includes rash and very high fevers, but not HUS.

Vibrio (**choice E**) infections produce copious amounts of watery diarrhea. The major risk of cholera and other *Vibrio* enteritides is shock due to hypovolemia or electrolyte loss.

44. **The correct answer is A.** In this case, the patient has all the hallmarks of mononucleosis (the heterophil antibodies should have confirmed your suspicion from the history and physical). Mononucleosis is caused by the Epstein-Barr virus, which, in turn, belongs to the herpesvirus family. The herpesviruses are enveloped viruses with double-stranded DNA. Remember that, in addition to Epstein-Barr virus, the herpesvirus family also includes herpes simplex (1 and 2), varicella-zoster (chickenpox, shingles), and cytomegalovirus (infection in immunocompromised patients). Cytomegalovirus also causes infectious mononucleosis, but the heterophil test is negative in these patients.

There are two families of viruses that are nonenveloped with double-stranded DNA (**choice B**): papovaviruses and adenoviruses.

There are many families of viruses that are enveloped with single-stranded RNA (**choice C**): arenaviruses, bunyaviruses, coronaviruses, filoviruses, flaviviruses, paramyxoviruses, orthomyxoviruses, retroviruses, rhabdoviruses, and togaviruses.

Parvoviruses are the only family of DNA virus with single-stranded DNA. They do not have an envelope (**choice D**).

There are two families of RNA virus that are single-stranded without an envelope (**choice E**): caliciviruses and picornaviruses.

45. **The correct answer is C.** West African sleeping sickness is caused by *Brucei gambiense*, a flagellated protozoan parasite transmitted to humans by the tsetse fly. The symptoms are as described in the scenario

46. **The correct answer is A.** Lyme disease is commonly found in the northeastern United States and is transmitted most commonly in that area by *Ixodes scapularis* (tick). The rash is known as erythema migrans, which is caused by the spirochete *Borrelia burgdorferi*.

47. **The correct answer is D.** Chagas disease is a zoonosis caused by the protozoan parasite *Trypanosoma cruzi* and is transmitted by the reduviid bug found only in the Americas from southeastern United States to southern Argentina. Romano sign is the classic finding in an acute case of Chagas disease (a painless edema of the palpebrae and periocular tissues).

48. **The correct answer is F.** Rocky Mountain spotted fever was originally found in Montana and Idaho; hence its name. It is now found throughout the western United States. In that area, the most common vector for transmission is *Dermacentor andersoni* (tick). The causative microorganism is *Rickettsia rickettsii*, an obligate intracellular parasite.

49. **The correct answer is B.** West Nile virus is transmitted by several types of mosquitoes in Florida, one of which is the *Anopheles*. The disease has no effective treatment or vaccine. It may develop into an encephalitis and possible death.

50. **The correct answer is B.** Malaria is a protozoan disease transmitted by the *Anopheles* mosquito. In Haiti, *Plasmodium falciparum* is the most common infectious agent.

Pathology and Pathophysiology

1. A 75-year-old man with a 5-year history of stable angina pectoris is brought to the emergency department with severe chest pain. EKG reveals profound ST segment elevations, and the CK-MB level is elevated. On stabilization, the patient is admitted to the coronary care unit for further management. Several days later, the patient again complains of chest pain. Physical examination is significant for fever, loud pericardial friction rub, mild pulmonary rales, 1+ pitting edema of the lower extremities, and acute tissue-texture changes paraspinally at levels T2-T7. Which of the following is the most likely diagnosis?

    (A) Caseous pericarditis

    (B) Fibrinous pericarditis

    (C) Hemorrhagic pericarditis

    (D) Serous pericarditis

    (E) Suppurative pericarditis

2. A 46-year-old woman presents to her physician complaining of weakness and fatigue. On physical examination, her physician notices a 10-lb weight gain since her last visit 6 months ago. Her blood pressure is 160/100 mm Hg. Blood tests reveal serum Na^+ 155 mEq/L, K^+ 2.8 mEq/L, and decreased serum renin. There is somatic dysfunction at T10 bilaterally. Which of the following is the most likely diagnosis?

    (A) Cushing syndrome

    (B) Diabetes mellitus

    (C) Pheochromocytoma

    (D) Primary aldosteronism

    (E) Secondary aldosteronism

3. A patient has a linear pruritic vesicular rash on his forearm. Which of the following disorders is mediated by a type IV hypersensitivity reaction and is the most likely diagnosis?

    (A) Bullous pemphigoid

    (B) Contact dermatitis

    (C) Dermatitis herpetiformis

    (D) Discoid lupus erythematosus

    (E) Urticaria

Questions 4-7

CASE A

A 41-year-old obese woman with a history of biliary colic presents with right upper quadrant discomfort and pain in her right shoulder after eating a fatty meal. Physical examination is significant for marked right upper quadrant tenderness during inspiration. The structural examination reveals T5-T9 are $NS_L R_R$.

4. Which of the following structures is most likely involved in producing her shoulder pain?

    (A) Expiratory motor neuron

    (B) Inspiratory motor neuron

    (C) Intercostal nerve

    (D) Phrenic nerve

    (E) Vagus nerve

5. The most appropriate diagnostic test to order for this patient would be

    (A) abdominal plain film

    (B) CT scan of gallbladder

    (C) ultrasound of gallbladder

    (D) endoscopic retrograde cholangiopancreatography

    (E) hepatic iminodiacetic acid scan

6. The diagnostic test you ordered confirmed your diagnosis. Your patient's pain is worsening and her WBC count is 13,000/mm^3. The most appropriate treatment would be

    (A) open hemicolectomy
    (B) open appendectomy
    (C) laparoscopic appendectomy
    (D) laparoscopic cholecystectomy
    (E) open cholecystectomy

7. After the patient has had the above surgery and is fully recovered, you still find the same somatic dysfunction. You wish to use a direct muscle energy treatment to correct it. To what level of the spine would you localize your treatment?

    (A) T5
    (B) T6
    (C) T7
    (D) T8
    (E) T9

8. On a routine physical examination for medical insurance, a midsystolic ejection murmur is detected in the pulmonic area of a 35-year-old female executive. The cardiac examination also reveals a prominent right ventricular cardiac impulse and wide and fixed splitting of the second heart sound. An EKG shows right axis deviation, and a chest x-ray film shows enlargement of the right ventricle and atrium. Which of the following is the most likely diagnosis?

    (A) Aortic stenosis
    (B) Atrial septal defect
    (C) Mitral regurgitation
    (D) Mitral stenosis
    (E) Pulmonary valve stenosis

9. A 5-year-old boy, hospitalized for cellulitis, exhibits global denudation of the skin resulting from splitting of the epidermis at the stratum granulosum. Which of the following is the most likely diagnosis?

    (A) Impetigo
    (B) Melasma
    (C) Scalded skin syndrome
    (D) Tinea corporis
    (E) Vitiligo

10. A 6-month-old child has an eye surgically enucleated because it contains a retinoblastoma. To which of the following structures should the pathologist pay particular attention when evaluating the specimen?

    (A) Anterior chamber
    (B) Cornea
    (C) Lens
    (D) Optic nerve
    (E) Vitreous

11. Conjoined twins are born attached at the chest. Examination of the placenta would likely reveal which of the following arrangements of the fetal membranes?

    (A) Diamnionic, dichorionic
    (B) Diamnionic, fused dichorionic
    (C) Diamnionic, monochorionic
    (D) Monoamnionic, dichorionic
    (E) Monoamnionic, monochorionic

12. A 36-year-old man with ulcerative colitis develops pruritus and fatigue. Alkaline phosphatase is elevated. The biliary tree appears beaded on barium radiograph, and there is somatic dysfunction at the T5-T8 spinal levels. Which of the following is the most likely diagnosis?

    (A) Acute cholecystitis
    (B) Cholesterolosis
    (C) Chronic cholelithiasis
    (D) Gallstone ileus
    (E) Sclerosing cholangitis

13. A 14-year-old boy presents with a 1-month history of knee pain and a 6-pound weight loss. He is pale and afebrile. Physical examination reveals somatic dysfunction of T10-L2. An x-ray film reveals a densely sclerotic lesion in the distal femur extending from the growth plate into the diaphysis. The periosteum is lifted, forming an angle with the cortex. The surrounding soft tissue resembles a "sunburst" on the radiograph. Which of the following is the most likely diagnosis?

    (A) Nonossifying fibroma
    (B) Osteochondroma
    (C) Osteomyelitis
    (D) Osteosarcoma
    (E) Paget disease

14. A gastroenterologist performs a colonoscopy on a patient with a family history of gastric and colon cancer and discovers multiple polyps. Biopsy of one lesion reveals a benign hamartoma. On physical examination the patient is noted to have dark pigmentation of the buccal mucosa and lips. The structural examination reveals ropy, fibrotic tissue in the lumbar spine. What is the most likely diagnosis?

    (A) Adenomatous polyposis coli
    (B) Gardner syndrome
    (C) Peutz-Jeghers (PJ) syndrome
    (D) Turcot syndrome
    (E) Somatic dysfunction of T1-T4.

15. A 36-year-old gravid woman notes vaginal bleeding. Ultrasound reveals small grape-like cystic structures without evidence of a developing embryo. A diagnosis of complete hydatidiform mole is made at the hospital. Further analysis is most likely to reveal that

    (A) the genotype of the mole is 46, XX and is completely paternal in origin
    (B) the genotype of the mole is triploid
    (C) human chorionic gonadotropin (hCG) levels are markedly decreased
    (D) serum levels of alpha fetoprotein are elevated
    (E) two or more sperm fertilized the ovum

16. A 22-year-old man with fatigue, recurrent fever, and enlarged cervical lymph nodes has numerous atypical lymphocytes in his peripheral blood smear. A biopsy from the patient's enlarged node shows expansion of lymphoid follicles with preservation of the underlying architecture. Numerous atypical lymphocytes are present in the paracortical areas. Which of the following is the most likely diagnosis?

    (A) AIDS
    (B) Burkitt lymphoma
    (C) Hodgkin disease
    (D) Mononucleosis
    (E) Non-Hodgkin lymphoma

17. A 70-year-old man experiences continuous lower abdominal discomfort with alternating constipation and diarrhea. The physical examination reveals chronic tissue-texture changes at T12-L2. His symptoms seem to improve on a high-fiber diet. If exploratory surgery were performed, which of the following would the surgeon most likely see?

    (A) An inflamed and fibrosed appendix
    (B) Multiple diverticula of the rectosigmoid colon
    (C) Normal small and large intestine
    (D) Thick, rubbery small and large intestinal walls
    (E) A trabeculated, dilated bladder

18. A 45-year-old man is diagnosed with primary hypoaldosteronism. Which of the following laboratory results is most consistent with this diagnosis?

	Serum sodium	Serum potassium	Serum bicarbonate	Urine sodium	Urine potassium
(A)	↓	↑	↓	↑	↓
(B)	↓	↑	↑	↑	↓
(C)	↓	↓	↓	↑	↑
(D)	↑	↓	↑	↓	↑
(E)	↑	↑	↑	↓	↓

19. A 29-year-old woman with a history of pelvic inflammatory disease presents to the emergency department with severe left lower quadrant crampy pain and spotting, and amenorrhea for the past two cycles. Physical examination reveals a left adnexal mass with tenderness to palpation. Structural examination is notable for somatic dysfunction at T12-L2. The beta-human chorionic gonadotropin (hCG) level is elevated. Further studies would most likely reveal an implantation at which of the following locations in the fallopian tube?

(A) Ampulla

(B) Fimbriae

(C) Infundibulum

(D) Isthmus

(E) Uterine segment

20. A 13-year-old boy presents to the emergency department with a deep skin abrasion on his knee. He states that it has not stopped bleeding since it happened during recess approximately 20-30 minutes ago. Physical examination reveals a well-developed, well-nourished adolescent. There are multiple purpura over his legs and arms, and a few scattered petechiae on his chest and gums. His bleeding time = 22 minutes, platelets = 300,000/mm³, and hemoglobin = 11g/dL. A trial of cryoprecipitate transfusion does not improve his bleeding time, but a normal platelet transfusion does. Which of the following is the correct diagnosis?

(A) Bernard-Soulier syndrome

(B) Henoch-Schönlein purpura

(C) Idiopathic thrombocytopenic purpura

(D) Thrombotic thrombocytopenic purpura

(E) Von Willebrand disease

21. A patient with respiratory failure secondary to poliomyelitis is placed on a respirator accidentally set at too high a rate. Which of the following changes in arterial blood gas studies would you expect to see?

	P_{O_2}	P_{CO_2}	pH
(A)	Markedly decreased	Slightly decreased	Increased
(B)	Markedly increased	Markedly increased	Decreased
(C)	Markedly increased	Slightly decreased	Decreased
(D)	Normal or slightly increased	Markedly decreased	Increased
(E)	Normal or slightly increased	Slightly decreased	Decreased

22. A 27-year-old man presents with recurrent episodes of intensely pruritic vesicles symmetrically distributed on his trunk. On electron microscopy, granular deposition of IgA and complement is noted at the dermoepidermal junction. Which of the following underlying conditions predisposes patients to the described skin disorder?

(A) Celiac sprue

(B) Lactase deficiency

(C) Tropical sprue

(D) Ulcerative colitis

(E) Whipple disease

23. A 54-year-old diabetic patient comes in for osteopathic treatment and microproteinuria. There is somatic dysfunction at T11-L1. Which of the following histologic changes in the kidney would be caused by proteinuria?

    (A) Antibody deposition in the glomeruli

    (B) Complement deposition in the glomeruli

    (C) Hyaline droplets in the renal tubular epithelium

    (D) Increased mesangial cells in the glomeruli

    (E) Neutrophils in the glomeruli

24. Biopsy of a skin lesion shows marked intercellular edema that splays apart adjacent cells, leaving only thin dark lines between the cells. What is this process called?

    (A) Acantholysis

    (B) Acanthosis

    (C) Hyperkeratosis

    (D) Parakeratosis

    (E) Spongiosis

25. A 25-year-old, previously healthy man notices that he now develops painful muscle cramps after strenuous exercise. After shoveling 2 feet of snow off his driveway, his urine turns red, and he consults a physician. Which of the following genetic conditions does the patient most likely have?

    (A) Gaucher disease

    (B) McArdle syndrome

    (C) Niemann-Pick disease

    (D) Tay-Sachs disease

    (E) von Gierke disease

26. A 40-year-old alcoholic woman presents with intense pruritus and fatigue. Her medical history is significant for hypothyroidism. Physical examination reveals a slightly enlarged liver, xanthomas, and chronic somatic dysfunction of T1-T4. Laboratory studies show a cholesterol of 538 mg/dL and an alkaline phosphatase of 571 IU/L. Which of the following serum values would most likely be elevated?

    (A) Alpha-fetoprotein

    (B) Antimitochondrial antibody

    (C) HBs antigen

    (D) Prothrombin time

    (E) Serum transaminases

27. A 56-year-old man presents with higher-than-normal language output and frequent paraphasic errors. Neurologic testing reveals that his comprehension of auditory and visual language is severely disturbed. He also exhibits an inability to repeat language. This patient has which of the following types of aphasia?

    (A) Broca (expressive)

    (B) Conduction

    (C) Global

    (D) Transcortical sensory

    (E) Wernicke (receptive)

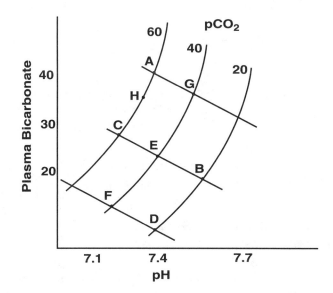

28. A 31-year-old stockbroker drives to a high-altitude mountain resort to do some rock-climbing. Later that day, he experiences headache, fatigue, dizziness, and nausea. Which point on the graph above best corresponds to the relationship between plasma bicarbonate, pH, and P_{CO_2} in this patient?

    (A) A

    (B) B

    (C) C

    (D) D

    (E) E

29. A 45-year-old woman presents with recent onset of blood-tinged discharge from the right nipple. The nipple appears slightly retracted, and a ill-defined subareolar nodule can be appreciated on palpation. Mammographic examination reveals linear shadows attributable to calcification. An excisional biopsy is performed. Microscopically, the lesion consists of markedly dilated ducts that contain inspissated secretion and are surrounded by fibrosis and chronic inflammation. Focal calcium deposition is present. Which of the following is the most likely diagnosis?

   (A) Abscess

   (B) Adenocarcinoma

   (C) Fat necrosis

   (D) Fibrocystic changes

   (E) Mammary duct ectasia

30. A 54-year-old male nonsmoker comes to the office for his annual physical. The physical examination is significant for somatic dysfunction at T2-T7. If these changes were due to cancer, then which of the following is most probable?

   (A) Bronchioloalveolar carcinoma

   (B) Bronchogenic adenocarcinoma

   (C) Large cell anaplastic carcinoma

   (D) Small cell (oat cell) carcinoma

   (E) Squamous cell carcinoma

31. The 10-year-old daughter of a United Nations ambassador in Turkey develops a severe sore throat, which resolves after a few days. Ten days later, the mother notices dark stains on the child's underwear and takes her to the pediatrician. A urine sample appears smoky, and red cell casts are noted in the urinary sediment. Physical examination reveals acute tissue-texture changes at T11-L1. If a renal biopsy were obtained from this child it would probably show

   (A) dense deposits

   (B) fusion of podocyte foot processes

   (C) linear deposition of IgG

   (D) mesangial IgA deposits

   (E) subepithelial humps

32. A 37-year-old woman presents to her physician complaining of difficulty reading and fatigue. She reports having had a "pins and needles" feeling in her left arm several months ago that resolved without treatment. On examination, visual field deficits and mild hyperreflexia are noted. The structural examination reveals no acute somatic dysfunction. MRI confirms the suspected diagnosis. Which of the following is the underlying mechanism of this patient's disease?

   (A) Antibodies to acetylcholine receptors

   (B) Axonal degeneration

   (C) Demyelination of the peripheral nerves

   (D) Loss of oligodendrocytes

   (E) Loss of Schwann cells

33. A blood sample from a patient with polycythemia vera is sent for complete blood count. Which of the following blood components is most likely to be reported within normal limits?

   (A) Lymphocytes

   (B) Neutrophils

   (C) Platelets

   (D) Red blood cells

   (E) White blood cells

34. A 60-year-old man suddenly becomes completely blind in one eye, and angiography demonstrates occlusion of the central retinal artery. Which of the following is the most likely cause of the occlusion?

   (A) Atheroma or embolism

   (B) Cranial (temporal) arteritis

   (C) Hypertension

   (D) Polycythemia vera

   (E) Tumor

35. A 55-year-old man with a history of recurrent calcium-containing renal stones presents to the emergency department with excruciating flank pain and blood in the urine. Physical examination reveals acute and chronic somatic dysfunction at T11-L1 bilaterally. This patient is likely to have which of the following underlying disorders?

   (A) Anemia of chronic disease

   (B) Chronic *Proteus* infection

   (C) Factor VIII deficiency

   (D) Hyperaldosteronism

   (E) Hyperparathyroidism

36. A 26-year-old woman accidentally inhales a peanut while laughing hysterically at a comedy club. Her friends bring her to a nearby emergency department, where it is revealed that the peanut lodged in her right mainstem bronchus. Which of the following is true about the blood flowing through the area of lung distal to the peanut?

    (A) The amount of dissolved oxygen is greater than normal

    (B) The oxygen dissociation curve is left-shifted

    (C) The P_{CO_2} is lower than normal

    (D) The pH is lower than normal

    (E) The P_{O_2} approaches that of arterial blood

37. A 40-year-old man who recently immigrated from Japan presents to his physician with abdominal discomfort characterized by sensations of fullness and mild pain after eating. He was previously diagnosed with a gastric ulcer, which has been refractory to traditional treatment. Physical examination reveals chronic left-sided tissue-texture changes at T5-T9. Biopsy of the lesion reveals gastric carcinoma. The cancer is most likely located in which of the following regions of the stomach?

    (A) Antropyloric region

    (B) Apex of the cardia

    (C) Greater curvature of the body

    (D) Lesser curvature of the body

    (E) Within 6 cm of the gastroesophageal junction

38. A viscerosomatic reflex at T1-T4 could be caused by myocardial ischemia and is an early manifestation of a heart attack. Pathologically, the earliest evidence that a myocardial infarction has occurred consists of

    (A) infiltration of the myocardium with leukocytes

    (B) intercellular edema with "wavy change" of affected myocytes

    (C) necrosis with preservation of cell outlines

    (D) proliferation of fibroblasts

    (E) a softened, yellow plaque on the endocardial surface

39. A 65-year-old woman with an 8-year history of type 2 diabetes dies in the hospital. She had no other significant medical history. Which of the following was the most likely cause of death?

    (A) Diabetic ketoacidosis

    (B) Infection

    (C) Myocardial infarction

    (D) Renal failure

    (E) Stroke

40. A 21-year-old woman attempts suicide by taking an overdose of barbiturates. On arrival in the emergency department, her blood pressure is 95/65 mm Hg, and her pulse is 105/min. The physician in the intensive care unit orders arterial blood gases. Which of the following values would you expect in this patient?

    (A) $P_{O_2} = 45$, $P_{CO_2} = 45$, pH = 7.45

    (B) $P_{O_2} = 55$, $P_{CO_2} = 70$, pH = 7.50

    (C) $P_{O_2} = 65$, $P_{CO_2} = 35$, pH = 7.45

    (D) $P_{O_2} = 75$, $P_{CO_2} = 60$, pH = 7.30

    (E) $P_{O_2} = 98$, $P_{CO_2} = 60$, pH = 7.20

41. An accident in a dry cleaning facility exposed an employee to massive amounts of carbon tetrachloride, both on the skin and by inhalation. Physical examination reveals somatic dysfunction at T5-T9. Severe damage to which of the following organs is most likely to occur?

    (A) Heart

    (B) Intestine

    (C) Kidney

    (D) Liver

    (E) Stomach

42. A 65-year-old man complains of weakness, weight loss, and bone pain. He reports having progressive difficulty seeing. Physical examination is significant for hepatosplenomegaly and lymphadenopathy. Serum protein electrophoresis reveals an M-protein spike, with an elevated serum IgM level. Bone marrow aspiration shows intensely eosinophilic plasma cells. Urine contains Bence-Jones proteins. Which of the following is the most likely diagnosis?

    (A) Heavy chain disease
    (B) Monoclonal gammopathy of undetermined significance
    (C) Multiple myeloma
    (D) Plasmacytoma
    (E) Waldenström macroglobulinemia

43. A patient has a lymphoproliferative disorder containing mature B cells that mark weakly with kappa light chain on the plasma membrane, strongly with CD5, strongly with CD23, and weakly with CD22. Which of the following is the most likely diagnosis?

    (A) Chronic lymphocytic leukemia
    (B) Hairy cell leukemia
    (C) Non-Hodgkin lymphoma
    (D) Prolymphocytic leukemia
    (E) Sézary syndrome

44. The EKG of a 60-year-old man reveals QRS intervals of 0.14 seconds with distinctly abnormal configurations. Physical exam is significant for paradoxical splitting of the second heart sound. Which of the following conduction defects is likely in this patient?

    (A) Complete AV block
    (B) First-degree AV block
    (C) Mobitz Type I AV block
    (D) Mobitz Type II AV block
    (E) Wolff-Parkinson-White syndrome

45. A 56-year-old man presents with complaints of gnawing pain in the mid-epigastrium, with occasional radiation to the back. He also notes a 15-pound weight loss over the past 3 months. Structural examination reveals cool, ropy tissues at T5-T8. The clinician suspects pancreatic carcinoma. Which of the following tumor markers would aid in confirming this diagnosis?

    (A) Alpha-fetoprotein (AFP)
    (B) CA-125
    (C) Carcinoembryonic antigen (CEA)
    (D) Human chorionic gonadotropin (hCG)
    (E) Prostate-specific antigen (PSA)

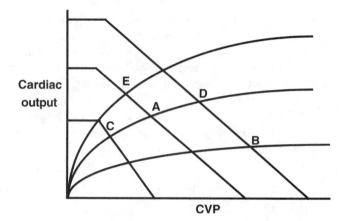

46. A 19-year-old man is brought into the emergency department with a gunshot wound to his leg. He is pale and tachypneic, his blood pressure is 90/65 mm Hg, and his pulse is weak and rapid at 130/min. This man's condition corresponds to which point (A–E) on the above graph?

    (A) A
    (B) B
    (C) C
    (D) D
    (E) E

47. A 25-year-old drug abuser with history of gonorrhea presents with fever and shortness of breath. Pulse oximetry reveals hypoxia. Physical examination reveals chronic somatic dysfunction at T2-T7. A chest x-ray film is significant for bilateral interstitial infiltrates. Which of the following findings is consistent with the most likely diagnosis?

    (A) Acid-fast organisms in sputum

    (B) Appearance of Curschmann spirals in mucus plugs

    (C) Elevated serum cold agglutinins

    (D) Positive methenamine-silver stain of lung tissue

    (E) Presence of Charcot-Leyden crystals in sputum

48. A 46-year-old woman who is clearly jaundiced is seen in clinic. Physical examination reveals cool, ropy, fibrotic tissue at T6-T8 on the right side. Laboratory tests reveal conjugated hyperbilirubinemia. Urine bilirubin levels are significantly above normal, while urine urobilinogen levels are significantly below normal. Which of the following mechanisms is the most likely cause of her jaundice?

    (A) Blockage of the common bile duct

    (B) Deficiency of glucuronyl transferase

    (C) Hemolytic anemia

    (D) Hepatocellular damage

    (E) A somatovisceral reflex

49. A 35-year-old woman complains of vomiting dark, greenish material approximately 1 hour after eating. An osteopathic structural examination reveals chronic tissue changes at T5-T9. She is scheduled for a barium meal to evaluate the upper portion of the gastrointestinal tract. She denies pain and is anicteric. Which of the following is the most likely cause of this woman's condition?

    (A) Annular pancreas

    (B) Esophageal atresia

    (C) Gallstones

    (D) Meckel's diverticulum

    (E) Pyloric stenosis

50. A 57-year-old man presents with painless swelling in his neck. Physical examination is remarkable for splenomegaly. Biopsy of the neck mass reveals a neoplasm containing small, cleaved cells that recapitulate the normal follicular architecture of lymph nodes. Which of the following mechanisms is most likely involved in the development of this patient's neoplasm?

    (A) Amplification of L-*myc*

    (B) Homozygous loss of *p53*

    (C) Over-expression of *bcl-2*

    (D) Point mutation in *ras* decreasing its GTPase activity

    (E) Reciprocal translocation between chromosome 9 and 22

Pathology and Pathophysiology

ANSWERS AND EXPLANATIONS

1.	B		26.	B
2.	D		27.	E
3.	B		28.	B
4.	D		29.	E
5.	E		30.	B
6.	D		31.	E
7.	C		32.	D
8.	B		33.	A
9.	C		34.	A
10.	D		35.	E
11.	E		36.	D
12.	E		37.	A
13.	D		38.	B
14.	C		39.	C
15.	A		40.	D
16.	D		41.	D
17.	B		42.	E
18.	A		43.	A
19.	A		44.	D
20.	A		45.	C
21.	D		46.	C
22.	A		47.	D
23.	C		48.	A
24.	E		49.	A
25.	B		50.	C

1. **The correct answer is B.** Pericarditis is inflammation of the pericardium. Fibrinous pericarditis is the most frequent form of pericarditis associated with myocardial infarction. Clinically, it may present as a loud pericardial friction rub with chest pain, fever, and, occasionally, symptoms of congestive heart failure (CHF).

   Caseous pericarditis (**choice A**) is usually caused by tuberculosis.

   Hemorrhagic pericarditis (**choice C**) is usually associated with tuberculosis or a malignant neoplasm.

   Serous pericarditis (**choice D**) is usually caused by an immunologic reaction, tumor, uremia, or viral infection; it can also be idiopathic.

   Suppurative pericarditis (**choice E**) may be caused by bacterial, fungal, or parasitic infections, and can clinically present with systemic signs of infection (fever, malaise) and a soft friction rub.

2. **The correct answer is D.** Primary aldosteronism (Conn syndrome) is a condition of hyperaldosteronism originating in the adrenal gland. The causes include an aldosterone-secreting adrenocortical adenoma, hyperplasia of the zona glomerulosa, and, very rarely, an adrenal carcinoma. It is characterized by hypertension secondary to sodium retention, hypokalemia, and a decreased serum renin due to a negative feedback of increased blood pressure on renin secretion.

   Cushing syndrome (**choice A**) is the result of increased glucocorticoid production, particularly cortisol. Physical signs typically include "moon facies," truncal obesity, "buffalo hump," and purple abdominal striae.

   Diabetes mellitus (**choice B**) is a condition of inadequate insulin production that presents with hyperglycemia and ketoacidosis.

   Pheochromocytoma (**choice C**) is a rare tumor of chromaffin cells occurring most commonly in the adrenal medulla. The tumor secretes epinephrine and norepinephrine, resulting in secondary hypertension.

   Secondary aldosteronism (**choice E**) results from activation of the renin-angiotensin system caused by renal ischemia, edema, and renal tumors. In contrast to primary aldosteronism, secondary aldosteronism is associated with increased serum renin.

3. **The correct answer is B.** Contact dermatitis is a form of *eczematous dermatitis*, characterized clinically by itchy vesicular eruption and histologically by epidermal spongiosis and chronic dermal inflammation. Contact dermatitis is initiated by hypersensitivity to an antigen that is taken up by Langerhans cells. These antigen-presenting cells process antigens and present them to naïve CD4 positive (helper) T lymphocytes. Antigen re-exposure

leads to recruitment of helper T cells and release of cytokines that mediate the inflammatory response.

   Bullous pemphigoid (**choice A**) is mediated by different types of autoantibodies that react with components of desmosomes or hemidesmosomes, disrupting intercellular junctions and resulting in bulla formation. Thus, the immune mechanism of these conditions can be regarded as type II hypersensitivity reactions.

   Dermatitis herpetiformis (**choice C**) is a blistering disease that develops in individuals allergic to gliadin, a gluten component. IgA and IgG antibodies react with gliadin and deposit in the tips of dermal papillae, leading to inflammation and bulla formation. Type III hypersensitivity therefore appears to be the prevalent immunologic mechanism.

   Discoid lupus erythematosus (**choice D**) is the localized cutaneous form of systemic lupus erythematosus. Skin lesions are associated with immune complex deposition along the dermal-epidermal junction. This is a form of type III hypersensitivity reaction.

   Urticaria (**choice E**) is mediated by IgE-triggered degranulation of mast cells, which may follow exposure to a number of antigens, e.g., food, drugs, and pollen. This is a classic example of a type I hypersensitivity reaction.

4. **The correct answer is D.** This patient likely has cholelithiasis, with possible acute cholecystitis. The typical patient is "fat, female, fertile, and older than 40." The right upper quadrant tenderness on inspiration is called Murphy's sign and is characteristic of biliary inflammation. In this patient, inflammation of the gallbladder might produce irritation of the central diaphragmatic pleura, which is innervated by the phrenic nerve. The dermatome of the nerve root of the phrenic nerve (C3-C5) includes the right shoulder.

   The expiratory motor neurons (**choice A**) are located in the lower medulla. They operate only during forced expiration to initiate contraction in expiratory muscles via alpha motor fibers.

   The inspiratory motor neurons (**choice B**) are located in the upper part of the medulla and send impulses via alpha motor fibers to the muscles of inspiration. They play no role in Murphy's sign.

   The intercostal nerves (**choice C**) innervate the costal and peripheral portions of the diaphragmatic pleura.

   The vagus nerve (**choice E**) mediates the Hering-Breuer (stretch-inflation) reflex of breathing.

5. **The correct answer is E.** The hepatic iminodiacetic acid (HIDA) scan is useful in demonstrating the obstructed cystic duct that is the cause of this patient's suspected acute cholecystitis. This study is reliable as long as the

bilirubin is less than 5 mg/dL (98% sensitivity and 81% specificity for acute cholecystitis). Because no laboratory studies are given, you may assume that the bilirubin is less than 5 mg/dL.

Plain films of the abdomen (**choice A**) may show radiopaque gallstones in 15% of cases. This would be good for demonstrating cholelithiasis, but because of the patient's symptoms, we suspect an acute cholecystitis, x-ray would not demonstrate the cystic duct.

CT scan of the gallbladder (**choice B**) or x-ray is used for the diagnosis of porcelain gallbladder. This test is not specific or sensitive enough to confirm the diagnosis.

Ultrasound of the gallbladder (**choice C**) may show the presence of gallstones but is not specific for acute cholecystitis, having 67% sensitivity and 82% specificity.

Endoscopic retrograde cholangiopancreatography (ERCP) (**choice D**) is the most direct and accurate means of determining the cause, location, and extent of obstruction in choledocholithiasis. Our patient has acute cholecystitis, however.

6. **The correct answer is D.** The patient has acute cholecystitis and the surgery of choice is laparoscopic cholecystectomy. This procedure is preferred over open cholecystectomy (**choice E**) because of reduced postsurgical complications; it is the least invasive and results in less scarring.

All other choices are incorrect because they are indicated for different diagnoses. Open hemicolectomy (**choice A**) is indicated for cancer of the colon. An open (**choice B**) and laparoscopic (**choice C**) appendectomy are for appendicitis.

7. **The correct answer is C.** When treating a neutral curve dysfunction, the key vertebra for treatment is located in the middle of the curve; as T7 is the middle of the curve, all other answer choices are incorrect.

8. **The correct choice is B.** The classic findings in atrial septal defect are a prominent right ventricular cardiac impulse, a systolic ejection murmur heard in the pulmonic area and along the left sternal border, and fixed splitting of the second heart sound. These findings are due to an abnormal left to right shunt through the defect, creating a volume overload on the right side. The increase in volume on the right side creates the flow murmur, the dilatation of the right-sided chambers, and the delayed closure of the pulmonic valve, all of which are present in this case.

Aortic stenosis (**choice A**) is also associated with a systolic ejection murmur. The murmur is usually loudest at the right sternal border and radiates upward to the jugular notch. This condition is associated with left ventricular hypertrophy.

Mitral regurgitation (**choice C**) would present with a systolic murmur as well. However, left atrial enlargement would be seen before right ventricular enlargement.

Mitral stenosis (**choice D**) would present with an "opening snap" and a diastolic murmur.

Pulmonary valve stenosis (**choice E**) causes an increase in right ventricular pressure resulting in right ventricular hypertrophy and pulmonary artery dilatation. A crescendo-decrescendo murmur may be heard if the stenosis is severe. Right atrial enlargement would not be present.

9. **The correct answer is C.** Scalded skin syndrome is a pediatric condition caused by an exfoliative toxin produced by *Staphylococcus aureus* (which is a common cause of cellulitis). The toxin splits the epidermis at the level of the stratum granulosum, causing global denudation of the skin. Scalded skin syndrome is not associated with suntanning or sunburn.

Impetigo (**choice A**) is a superficial skin infection, usually caused by group A beta-hemolytic streptococci or staphylococci. Classic clues are eroded pustules covered by honey-colored crusts. Impetigo may lead to post-streptococcal glomerulonephritis, a sign of which is red cell casts in the urine.

Melasma (**choice B**) consists of irregular patches of hyperpigmentation on the face. It most commonly appears during pregnancy and may not completely regress.

Tinea corporis (**choice D**) is a fungal infection. It is also known as "ringworm" because it presents as an expanding round lesion with an erythematous circinate border.

Vitiligo (**choice E**) is characterized by irregular patchy depigmentation of the skin that exhibits melanocyte deficiency microscopically. It is possibly autoimmune in origin and may be related to stress. It is not associated with sun exposure and is a chronic condition.

10. **The correct answer is D.** Retinoblastomas are aggressive, malignant neoplasms derived from embryonic neuronal cells. Fortunately, they are rare. These tumors present in early childhood, often within the first 3 months of life. Retinoblastomas are very dangerous both because they can metastasize widely via a hematogenous route and because they show a marked propensity to invade the optic nerve and tract into the brain, where they quickly become inoperable. The pathologist should pay particular attention to the cut end of the optic nerve to make sure that the entire retinoblastoma was removed.

11. **The correct answer is E.** This question may seem a bit challenging, but you have all the information you need to answer it. The type of fetal membranes produced in identical twin pregnancies depends on the timing of the twinning process. The chorion forms before the amnion, so the possible combinations for all twin pregnancies are monoamnionic and monochorionic, diamnionic and monochorionic, and diamnionic and dichorionic (with the chorions either separate or fused). The first two possibilities are seen only in identical twins, the last one can be seen in both identical and fraternal twins. Exactly what happens depends on the precise point at which twinning occurs.

Very early separation (at the two-cell stage) produces completely separate membranes with duplication of both the amnion and chorion (**choice A**).

Slightly later separation results in two amnions and fused chorions (**choice B**).

Separation at a later stage, when the inner cell mass is present, produces twins with one chorion and two amnions (**choice C**). Very late separation results in one chorion and one amnion. Conjoined (Siamese) twins result from a very late twinning event, so the placenta will be monoamnionic and monochorionic.

Monoamnionic and dichorionic placentas (**choice D**) are not usually seen, as the chorion forms before the amnion.

12. **The correct answer is E.** Young men with ulcerative colitis are at increased risk for developing primary sclerosing cholangitis (PSC), a chronic cholestatic condition that leads to fibrosis of the bile ducts. A classic clue to the diagnosis is a beaded appearance of the biliary tree on barium radiograph.

Patients with acute cholecystitis (**choice A**) present with acute onset of right upper quadrant pain, fever, tenderness, and leukocytosis.

Cholesterolosis (strawberry gallbladder; **choice B**) refers to lipid foci deposited in the gallbladder wall. It is asymptomatic and unrelated to cholelithiasis.

Cholelithiasis (gallstones; **choice C**) is commonly asymptomatic but can cause biliary colic and may progress to acute cholecystitis.

Gallstone ileus (**choice D**), due to obstruction of the small bowel by gallstones, is associated with air in the biliary tree on abdominal radiograph.

13. **The correct answer is D.** This patient has osteosarcoma, a malignant bone tumor that produces osteoid and bone. Prognosis is poor. X-ray reveals bone destruction, soft tissue with "sunburst" appearance, and Codman's triangle (periosteal elevation that forms an angle with the cortex of the bone)—all classic clues to the diagnosis. Other hints were the patient's weight loss and pallor, which should have raised your suspicion that a malignancy existed. Choice D is the only malignant process among the answer choices. This tumor usually occurs in the 2nd or 3rd decades of life. At the same time, it is the most common bone tumor in the elderly and is often associated with Paget disease (**choice E**). A classic histologic finding for osteosarcoma is the presence of anaplastic cells with osteoid (a pink amorphous material that is variably mineralized).

Nonossifying fibroma (**choice A**), also known as fibrous cortical defect, is a common developmental abnormality seen in the bones of the lower extremities of children. This is a non-neoplastic lesion of bone cortex that is composed of fibrous connective tissue and usually resolves spontaneously. X-ray reveals irregular, well-demarcated radiolucent defects in the bony cortex with an intact subperiosteal shell of bone. In the metaphysis, there are whorls of connective tissue. These fibromas do not cross the epiphyses of bone, which distinguishes them from giant cell tumors of bone.

Osteochondromas (**choice B**) are hereditary multiple exostoses (bony metaphyseal projections capped with cartilage) that may be asymptomatic or may produce deformity and compromise the blood supply of bone. Five percent of them progress to sarcomas. If a patient presents with exostoses, sebaceous cysts, dermoid tumors, and colonic polyps, the likely diagnosis is Gardner syndrome.

Osteomyelitis (**choice C**) usually produces fever, localized pain, erythema, and swelling. The patient in question is afebrile, which decreases the likelihood of this diagnosis. Though x-ray films may show periosteal elevation, more specific findings would be expected in a patient with this condition, such as sequestrum (necrotic bone fragment), involucrum (new bone that surrounds the area of inflammation), and Brodie's abscess (localized abscess formation in the bone).

Paget disease (**choice E**), also known as osteitis deformans, is due to excessive bone resorption with replacement by soft, poorly mineralized matrix (osteoid) in a disorganized array. It generally affects the skull, pelvis, femur, and vertebrae. Skull involvement might produce deafness by impinging on the cranial nerves. Malignant transformation to osteosarcoma is seen in 1% of cases. X-ray reveals enlarged, radiolucent bones. Lab tests reveal extremely elevated alkaline phosphatase. If you see a patient who is older than 40 and has bone fracture, hearing loss, and increased alkaline phosphatase, suspect Paget disease. Note that this disease rarely occurs in the young and could have been ruled out as a possible answer by virtue of the patient's age.

14. **The correct answer is C.** All the choices are familial polyposes. The classic clue for Peutz-Jeghers (PJ) syndrome is the melanin pigmentation of the buccal mucosa and lips (the palms and soles may also be darkened). PJ presents with polyps of the entire gastrointestinal tract (thus the appearance of colonic lesions), but the small intestine is usually most severely affected. The polyps of PJ are hamartomas and are not premalignant, although there is an increased incidence of stomach, breast, and ovarian cancer associated with this disease.

Adenomatous polyposis coli (**choice A**) is also called familial multiple polyposis. Like PJ, it is inherited in an autosomal dominant fashion. Polyps typically begin in the rectosigmoid area and spread to the entire colon. Because almost all patients go on to develop cancer, colectomy is recommended once the diagnosis is made.

Gardner syndrome (**choice B**) refers to colonic polyps in the setting of other neoplasms (e.g., bone, skin) and desmoid tumors. Risk of colon cancer is close to 100%.

Turcot syndrome (**choice D**) is characterized by colonic polyps associated with brain tumors such as gliomas and medulloblastomas.

Somatic dysfunction of T1–T4 (**choice E**) is incorrect because this is the viscerosomatic reflex level for the heart and lungs. The correct level is at T12–L2.

15. **The correct answer is A.** A complete hydatidiform mole is characterized by elevated human chorionic gonadotropin (hCG) and grape-like cystic structures filling the uterus with no detectable embryo on ultrasound. The genotype of a complete hydatidiform mole is purely paternal, caused by fertilization of an egg that has lost its chromosomes. Hydatidiform mole is associated with increasing maternal age and may be a precursor to choriocarcinoma.

Triploidy and even tetraploidy are characteristics of partial moles (**choice B**). Partial moles are thought to be due to fertilization of an egg with two different sperm, one with an X and one with a Y chromosome, typically leading to triploidy.

hCG levels are increased relative to normal values for dates, rather than decreased (**choice C**), in a molar pregnancy.

Alpha fetoprotein (AFP; **choice D**) is a marker for endodermal yolk sac tumors, embryonal tumors in men, and hepatocellular carcinoma. It is made by the fetus. In a complete hydatidiform mole, AFP is not detectable since there is no fetus.

Two or more sperm may fertilize an ovum, leading to a triploid fetus and partial mole (**choice E**).

16. **The correct answer is D.** Infectious mononucleosis is a benign infection caused by the Epstein-Barr virus (EBV), a herpesvirus. Although B lymphocytes are infected by the virus, the characteristic atypical cells are activated cytotoxic and suppressor T cells—thus the paracortical location (T cell zone) in the lymph node. Lymph nodes in viral infections show expansion of germinal centers without loss of normal architecture. All lymphomas, including Burkitt, Hodgkin, and non-Hodgkin lymphomas, destroy the normal architecture of the lymph node.

AIDS (**choice A**) is associated with a number of neoplastic and infectious processes that may alter the lymph node structure. The characteristic lymph node changes in AIDS are progressive transformation of the germinal centers, not paracortical hyperplasia.

Burkitt lymphoma (**choice B**) produces a sea of monotonous, mitotically active cells in a "starry sky" appearance.

Hodgkin lymphoma (**choice C**) also can show nodular or diffuse patterns but is characterized by the presence of Reed-Sternberg cells.

Other non-Hodgkin lymphomas (**choice E**) show either a nodular appearance or diffuse sheets of cells that replace the germinal centers.

17. **The correct answer is B.** This is a presentation of colonic diverticulosis, although only about 20% of affected individuals develop clinical symptoms. Patients are typically older than 40. The diverticula are small, flask-like outpouchings of the colonic mucosa and submucosa. They are often found at sites of focal weakness of the colonic wall, particularly adjacent to the taeniae coli, where the nerves and arterial vasa recta penetrate the inner circular muscle coat. High-fiber diets appear to improve the symptoms, but it is unclear whether such diets can impede disease progression. Note that irritable bowel syndrome may also present with alternating constipation and diarrhea, but is more common in younger females. No organic changes are evident in this disease.

An inflamed appendix (**choice A**) is more likely to be seen in a younger individual.

Crohn disease, which produces rubbery small and large intestinal walls (**choice D**), usually presents at a much younger age, with intermittent attacks of abdominal pain and relatively mild diarrhea.

A dilated bladder (**choice E**) would produce urinary rather than colonic symptoms.

18. **The correct answer is A.** Aldosterone is an adrenal hormone that maintains intravascular volume by promoting sodium and water reabsorption at the distal

convoluted tubule. Hypoaldosteronism results in salt-wasting, thereby decreasing serum sodium and increasing urine sodium. Since water follows sodium, the patient may develop orthostatic hypotension or become frankly hypotensive. In response to the electrical gradient established by sodium reabsorption, aldosterone induces the passive secretion of potassium at the distal convoluted tubule, promoting potassium excretion. Hypoaldosteronism would, in contrast, increase serum potassium and decrease urine potassium. Aldosterone causes hydrogen ions to be actively secreted into the distal tubule. Therefore, in hypoaldosteronism, H⁺ ions are retained, creating a metabolic acidosis (decreased serum bicarbonate).

A comment on strategy: A good way to approach this question is to break it down into parts. Begin by looking for answer choices in which the serum sodium values are decreased. This allows you to eliminate **choices D and E**. Next, look for increased urine sodium. This does not allow you to eliminate any more choices, so you must move on and look for increased serum potassium. **Choice C** can now be eliminated. As both of the remaining choices show decreased urinary potassium, decreased serum bicarbonate is the deciding factor, and the correct answer is **choice A**.

19. **The correct answer is A.** This patient has an ectopic (tubal) pregnancy. Patients with a history of pelvic inflammatory disease are more susceptible to this disorder. The ampulla is the most common site of fertilization within the fallopian tube, as well as the most common site for tubal pregnancy. It is the longest region of the tube and has thin walls.

The fimbriae (**choice B**) of the fallopian tubes are highly unlikely locations for tubal pregnancy. They are mucosal ridges located at the funnel-shaped end of the oviduct that are covered with ciliated cells. They beat toward the mouth of the tube, "brushing" the ovum released from the ovary into the fallopian tube.

The infundibulum (**choice C**) is the technical term for the "funnel-shaped end of the fallopian tube." It opens to the peritoneal cavity.

The isthmus (**choice D**) is the narrow, thick-walled segment of the fallopian tube nearest to the uterine wall.

The uterine (interstitial) segment (**choice E**) is the portion of the tube that traverses the uterine wall. Ectopic pregnancies occurring here are at particularly high risk for catastrophic rupture.

20. **The correct answer is A.** Bernard-Soulier syndrome is an autosomal recessive disease of platelet adhesion that causes prolonged bleeding times in the presence of normal platelet counts. These patients' platelets cannot bind to subendothelial collagen properly because of a deficiency or dysfunction of the glycoprotein Ib-IX complex. Clinically the patients have impaired hemostasis and recurrent severe mucosal hemorrhage. The only treatment for an acute episode is a transfusion of normal platelets. This patient has a slightly decreased hemoglobin because of blood loss.

Henoch-Schönlein purpura (**choice B**) is a self-limited autoimmune vasculitis that affects children and young adults, usually following an upper respiratory infection. Affected individuals develop purpuric rashes on the extensor surfaces of their arms, legs, and buttocks. They also have abdominal pain and hematuria from glomerulonephritis. Despite the tendency toward hemorrhage, the bleeding times and platelet count would be normal.

Idiopathic thrombocytopenic purpura (**choice C**) causes an increase in the bleeding time, but, as the name implies, platelet counts are decreased. There is bleeding from small vessels, especially of the skin, gastrointestinal tract, and genitourinary tract. Purpura and petechiae frequently develop. It is considered a self-limited autoimmune disorder, typically affecting children after a recent viral infection.

Thrombotic thrombocytopenic purpura (**choice D**), which is characterized by an increased bleeding time but a decreased platelet count, is a rare disorder of unknown etiology. It is thought to be initiated by endothelial injury, which releases certain procoagulant materials into the circulation, causing platelet aggregation. It causes purpura, fever, renal failure, microangiopathic hemolytic anemia, and microthrombi, generally in young women. In this disorder, platelet transfusion is actually contraindicated, as it can precipitate thrombosis.

Von Willebrand disease (**choice E**) causes increased bleeding times with normal platelet counts. It is the most common inherited bleeding disorder, caused by a defect in von Willebrand factor, which aids the binding of platelets to collagen. Even though the platelets themselves are normal, binding is impaired, thus a platelet transfusion would not correct the problem. Cryoprecipitate, a plasma fraction rich in von Willebrand factor, would help in the case of von Willebrand disease but would not help with Bernard-Soulier syndrome.

21. **The correct answer is D.** This situation is analogous to the voluntary hyperventilation that can occur during anxiety. CO_2 is "blown off," potentially leading to a markedly decreased P_{CO_2} with resulting increase in pH (dissolved CO_2 combines with water to form carbonic acid, which lowers pH). In an individual with normal lungs, the hemoglobin becomes nearly fully saturated

(97.5%) during the normal passage of blood through the alveolar capillaries. So, hyperventilation does not usually change P_{O_2} significantly.

22.   **The correct answer is A.** Patients with celiac sprue (nontropical sprue or gluten-sensitive enteropathy) are prone to the development of dermatitis herpetiformis, the dermatologic diagnosis in this patient. This gastrointestinal malabsorption syndrome is caused by an allergic, immunologic, or toxic reaction to the gliadin component of gluten and has a genetic predisposition. There is reversal of symptoms of celiac sprue with a gluten-free diet.

Hint: Even if you were unaware of the association between celiac sprue and dermatitis herpetiformis, the mention of IgA and complement as an element in the skin pathology should have increased your suspicion that the associated condition was immunologically related.

Lactase deficiency (**choice B**) is the most common disaccharidase deficiency (lactase is absent from the brush border of the small intestine). It results in milk intolerance, with symptoms of bloating, diarrhea, and cramping following ingestion of dairy products.

Tropical sprue (**choice C**) is a disorder of malabsorption of unknown etiology that may be caused by enterotoxigenic *Escherichia coli*. There is a high incidence in the tropics, where it occasionally occurs in epidemics. Treatment is with tetracycline and folic acid.

Ulcerative colitis (**choice D**) is associated with a dermatologic condition called pyoderma gangrenosum. This disorder is characterized by blue-red ulcerations that surround purulent necrotic bases.

Whipple disease (**choice E**) is a systemic disorder characterized by clumps of periodic acid-Schiff (PAS)-positive macrophages (full of and surrounded by small bacilli) in the lamina propria of intestines and in mesenteric lymph nodes. It also leads to malabsorption and responds to tetracycline.

23.   **The correct answer is C.** In cases of proteinuria, hyaline (dark-staining) droplets can be found in the epithelium of the proximal convoluted tubule. These droplets are protein-containing, pinocytotic vesicles that have fused with lysosomes (to produce phagolysosomes). This change is a sensitive histologic indicator of proteinuria.

Glomerular changes (**choices A, B, D, and E**) can cause proteinuria, but are not usually produced by it.

24.   **The correct answer is E.** Spongiosis is the name used for intercellular edema of the epidermis. Fluid accumulates between the cells, pulling them apart. However, the intercellular connections (desmosomes) remain largely

intact. This produces a distinctive microscopic appearance in which each cell is surrounded by a broad white band with tiny dark cross-stripes, somewhat reminiscent of a closed zipper.

Acantholysis (**choice A**) is the process of cell separation seen in some blistering diseases. The intercellular connections are broken in acantholysis, producing "rounded-up" cells that are dissociated from each other.

Acanthosis (**choice B**) is a marked thickening of the epidermis due to an increase in the number and size of the epithelial cells.

Hyperkeratosis (**choice C**) is an increase in the thickness of the superficial keratin layer of the epidermis.

The term parakeratosis (**choice D**) is used when nuclei are present in the normally anuclear superficial keratin layer.

25.   **The correct answer is B.** This is a typical clinical history for patients with the glycogen storage disease (glycogenosis) known as McArdle syndrome (type V glycogenosis). These patients are deficient in muscle phosphorylase and accumulate glycogen in skeletal muscle tissue without accumulating glycogen in the liver. Their muscles are typically weak, owing to impaired energy production, although they may never have specifically noticed this (on careful questioning, they may instead say they never liked exercise). Obvious clinical onset is typically in the 20s, and measurement of very low serum lactate in these patients during exercise is helpful in establishing the diagnosis. Myoglobinuria (with reddish urine) may occur. The heart is typically not particularly affected, and longevity is normal. A similar presentation can be seen in muscle phosphofructokinase deficiency (type VII glycogen storage disease) and in mild forms of the generalized glycogenosis known as Pompe disease (type II glycogenosis).

Gaucher disease (**choice A**) is a lysosomal disorder of cerebroside metabolism that typically involves the reticuloendothelial system; the brain is not affected.

Niemann-Pick disease (**choice C**) is a lysosomal disorder of sphingomyelin metabolism that typically involves the CNS and the reticuloendothelial system.

Tay-Sachs disease (**choice D**) is another lysosomal storage disease with defective ganglioside degradation. It principally affects the brain.

von Gierke disease (**choice E**) is a hepatorenal form of glycogen storage disease that is not compatible with normal longevity.

26.   **The correct answer is B.** Primary biliary cirrhosis is an autoimmune disease associated with elevated antimitochondrial antibodies. Note that Hashimoto thyroiditis,

an autoimmune disease that is the most common cause of hypothyroidism, is also associated with increased levels of this antibody.

Elevated alpha-fetoprotein (**choice A**) is associated with hepatocellular carcinoma.

HBs antigen (**choice C**) is usually elevated in active hepatitis B (unless the patient is tested during the window period).

Elevated prothrombin time (**choice D**) and increased serum transaminases (**choice E**) are indicative of liver failure. These values are usually normal in primary biliary cirrhosis.

27. **The correct answer is E.** The question stem describes Wernicke, or receptive, aphasia. It is caused by a lesion in Wernicke's area, which is located in the posterior part of the superior temporal gyrus of the language-dominant hemisphere.

Broca (expressive) aphasia (**choice A**) is a disorder primarily of language output. Speech is slow and effortful, phrase length is short, and the patient tends to use only common nouns, verbs, and, occasionally, adjectives. Comprehension is relatively intact. Repetition is generally disturbed comparable to the amount of spontaneous output. It is produced by a lesion of Broca's area, which is in the posterior part of the inferior frontal gyrus of the language-dominant hemisphere.

Conduction aphasia (**choice B**) is produced by a lesion in the arcuate fasciculus, which is in the posterior inferior part of the parietal lobe of the language-dominant hemisphere. This effectively disconnects Broca's area from Wernicke's area, resulting in the inability to repeat.

Global aphasia (**choice C**) occurs with the destruction of Broca's area, Wernicke's area, and the arcuate fasciculus, resulting in a combination of both Broca and Wernicke aphasias.

Transcortical sensory aphasia (**choice D**) is similar to Wernicke aphasia (**choice E**), but the ability to repeat is preserved. The lesion is generally posterior or superior to Wernicke's area.

28. **The correct answer is B.** Acute mountain sickness is caused by hypoxemia and alkalosis due to exposure to high altitude. Hyperventilation occurs in response to the hypoxemia, which helps bring the oxygen saturation back toward normal, but "blows off" excessive amounts of CO_2, producing acute respiratory alkalosis.

Choice A represents respiratory acidosis with renal compensation or metabolic alkalosis with respiratory compensation.

Choice C represents uncompensated respiratory acidosis.

Choice D represents either metabolic acidosis with respiratory compensation or respiratory alkalosis with renal compensation.

Choice E represents metabolic acidosis.

29. **The correct answer is E.** Mammary duct ectasia may simulate cancer clinically. It is a disorder of premenopausal age that manifests often with nipple retraction or inversion and sometimes with nipple discharge. Characteristic histologic features include marked dilatation (ectasia) of large ducts with fibrosis and chronic inflammation. The pathogenesis is obscure but may be a reaction to stagnant colostrum.

Abscesses (**choice A**) develop most often in the lactating breast and are associated with an exquisitely painful mass with systemic signs of infection. *Staphylococcus aureus* is the most common etiologic agent.

The histologic features of the lesion exclude a diagnosis of adenocarcinoma (**choice B**), which is composed of atypical cells arranged in duct-like or glandular structures.

Fat necrosis (**choice C**) refers to a focus of necrotic adipose tissue with secondary histiocytic infiltration. Physical findings may mimic cancer. It is often related to localized trauma.

Fibrocystic changes (**choice D**) are among the most common breast changes and include varying combinations of cysts, fibrosis, apocrine metaplasia, calcification, chronic inflammation, and epithelial hyperplasia. The latter, if florid or associated with atypia, is associated with an increased risk of cancer transformation.

30. **The correct answer is B.** Bronchogenic adenocarcinoma is only weakly associated with smoking. This disorder is the most common lung cancer seen in nonsmokers and in women.

Bronchioloalveolar carcinoma (**choice A**) is a relatively uncommon form of carcinoma of the lung. It arises in the lung periphery and does not appear to be clearly related to smoking.

Large cell (anaplastic) carcinomas (**choice C**) are unusual and probably represent undifferentiated variants of squamous cell and bronchogenic adenocarcinomas.

Small cell (oat cell) carcinoma (**choice D**) is very strongly associated with smoking.

Squamous cell carcinoma (**choice E**) is very strongly associated with smoking.

31. **The correct answer is E.** The history suggests streptococcal pharyngitis, followed by poststreptococcal glomerulonephritis. Subepithelial humps composed of

proteinaceous material can be seen projecting outward from the outer capillary wall to the urinary space by light or electron microscopy. Granular deposits of IgG and C3 can be seen by immunofluorescence microscopy.

Dense deposits (**choice A**) are characteristic of type II membranoproliferative glomerulonephritis.

Fusion of podocyte processes (**choice B**) is seen in minimal change disease.

Linear deposition of IgG (**choice C**) is seen in Goodpasture syndrome.

Mesangial IgA deposits (**choice D**) are characteristic of Berger disease.

32. **The correct answer is D.** This woman presents with the classic signs and symptoms of multiple sclerosis (MS). A key to the diagnosis is different neurologic signs that are separated by space and time. (Another classic clue might have been oligoclonal bands on electrophoresis of the CSF.) MS is a demyelinating disease of the CNS, characterized by loss of oligodendroglial cells, which are responsible for producing myelin in the CNS. Diagnosis can be confirmed by an MRI revealing sharply delineated regions of demyelination (plaques) throughout the CNS white matter (especially in periventricular areas).

Antibodies to acetylcholine receptors (**choice A**) have been implicated in the etiology of myasthenia gravis, not MS.

MS is generally characterized by axonal preservation, rather than degeneration (**choice B**).

Demyelination of peripheral nerves (**choice C**) occurs in a number of diseases (e.g., Guillain-Barré), but not in MS. Guillain-Barré is characterized by ascending muscle weakness, areflexia, and paralysis.

Oligodendrocytes are responsible for producing myelin in the CNS; Schwann cells (**choice E**) are responsible for myelination in the peripheral nervous system and are not affected in MS.

33. **The correct answer is A.** Polycythemia vera is an example of a myeloproliferative disorder, a neoplastic disease of multipotential myeloid stem cells with the capacity to differentiate into erythrocytes, megakaryocytes, or granulocytes. The only hematologic cell line that is not increased in polycythemia vera is the lymphocytic line, and the lymphocyte count is generally normal. The complications of polycythemia vera are generally due to increased blood viscosity and a tendency toward thrombosis. Without regular phlebotomy, death usually occurs within months of diagnosis.

Clonal expansion of granulocyte precursors leads to markedly increased neutrophil counts (**choice B**) and white blood cell counts (**choice E**).

Increased megakaryocyte production often produces platelet counts (**choice C**) above 500,000 cells/mL.

Dramatic increases in erythroid cell production (**choice D**) dominate the hematologic picture in polycythemia vera, and patients may have hematocrits as high as 60%.

34. **The correct answer is A.** The point of this question is that sometimes the obvious explanation is the correct one. Occlusion of the central retinal artery rapidly causes irreversible blindness with loss of the inner retinal layers. (The photoreceptor rod and cone cells are maintained by the pigment epithelium.) The site of occlusion is typically just posterior to the cribriform plate. A garden-variety atheroma or embolism is overwhelmingly the most common cause of central retinal artery occlusion.

Despite all of the teaching about the risk of blindness in temporal arteritis (**choice B**), this disorder causes only 10% of central retinal artery occlusions.

Hypertension (**choice C**) is more likely to cause bleeding than thrombosis.

Polycythemia vera (**choice D**) could (rarely) cause occlusion because of increased blood viscosity and a tendency for thrombosis.

Tumor (**choice E**) might also cause retinal artery thrombosis, but this would be far rarer than atheroma.

35. **The correct answer is E.** This patient is experiencing the very painful passage of a renal stone, which is often accompanied by hematuria. His history of recurrent urolithiasis with calcium-containing stones implies a disorder in the regulation of calcium concentration. Hyperparathyroidism is associated with increased parathormone (PTH) levels, which can produce hypercalcemia, hypercalciuria, and, ultimately, renal stones.

Anemia of chronic disease (**choice A**) does not produce calcium stones. It is an attractive distracter because the patient presents with a chronic condition and hematuria. Note that urinary blood loss is not usually significant enough to produce an anemic state.

Chronic *Proteus* infection (**choice B**) would produce struvite (magnesium-ammonium phosphate), not calcium stones. Staghorn calculi are also seen.

Factor VIII deficiency (**choice C**) occurs in hemophilia, a hereditary clotting disorder. It is not associated with calcium stones.

Hyperaldosteronism (**choice D**) results in potassium depletion, sodium retention, and hypertension. Primary hyperaldosteronism (Conn syndrome) is associated with adrenocortical adenomas in 90% of patients and is characterized by decreased renin. Secondary hyperaldosteronism results from excessive stimulation by angiotensin II, which is caused by excess renin production (plasma renin-angiotensin levels are high). Neither condition is associated with renal stones.

36. **The correct answer is D.** This woman sustained an obstruction of a major airway such that the area of the lung distal to the obstruction was perfused, but not ventilated. In this area of lung, there will be no gas exchange, and the V/Q ratio will approach zero. As a result, the P_{O_2} and P_{CO_2} of the pulmonary blood (and alveolar gas) approaches that of venous blood (P_{O_2} = 40 mm Hg, P_{CO_2} = 45 mm Hg). Therefore, the P_{O_2} will be lower, and the P_{CO_2} will be higher than normal. Because the P_{CO_2} is high, pH will be low.

The amount of dissolved oxygen will be lower than normal, not greater (**choice A**). Dissolved oxygen is equal to 0.003 mL O_2/100 mL blood times P_{O_2}. Because the P_{O_2} is low in this situation, so must be the dissolved oxygen.

P_{CO_2} will be elevated and pH will be diminished in this lung area. Both of these factors cause the curve to shift to the right, not to the left (**choice B**).

P_{CO_2} will be higher than normal, not lower (**choice C**).

P_{O_2} is decreased and approaches that of venous blood, not arterial blood (**choice E**).

37. **The correct answer is A.** Gastric carcinomas involve the antropyloric region in 50% to 60% of cases. Note that gastric carcinoma is the most common malignancy in Japan and typically presents with early satiety and pain after eating large meals.

Gastric carcinoma occurs at the apex of the cardia (**choice B**) in 25% of cases. These patients generally present with dysphagia due to esophageal outlet obstruction.

The greater curvature of the body (**choice C**) is involved in only about 12% of cases of gastric carcinoma. However, when an ulcerating lesion does occur in this region, it is quite likely to be malignant.

The antropyloric region is involved more often than the lesser curvature of the body (**choice D**), where lesions typically present with symptoms of peptic ulcer, not early satiety.

Gastric carcinoma occurs much more commonly in the antropyloric region than near the gastroesophageal junction (**choice E**).

Although the lesser curvature of the antropyloric region is a favored site, any nonhealing ulcer at any site in the stomach should be biopsied, as it may be cancer.

38. **The correct answer is B.** The earliest microscopic signs of a myocardial infarct are intercellular edema and "wavy change" at the periphery of the affected area. The wavy change in the myocytes is thought to be due to the effects of nearby, intact myocyte contraction on the ischemic myocytes situated at the periphery of the lesion. Such changes can be observed as early as 1 hour after infarction.

Neutrophilic infiltration (**choice A**) is observed within about 12 hours of infarction.

Necrosis with preservation of cell outlines (**choice C**) is a definition of coagulative necrosis, the type that characterizes the myocardium. Coagulative necrosis appears within the first days after an infarct but is not evident during the first hour or so, when wavy change is apparent.

Proliferation of fibroblasts (**choice D**) is a component of scar formation, which occurs weeks after an infarct (if the patient survives).

A softened, yellow plaque (**choice E**) is generally visible about 1 week after infarction.

39. **The correct answer is C.** Myocardial infarction is the leading cause of death in diabetics. The advanced glycosylated products associated with long-standing diabetes mellitus accelerate the atherosclerotic process. Other risk factors for coronary artery disease (CAD) include hypertension, smoking, hypercholesterolemia, family history of CAD at a young age, male sex, or being a postmenopausal female.

Diabetic ketoacidosis (DKA; **choice A**) carries a high mortality rate for type 1 diabetics. However, this patient had type 2 diabetes, which is associated with hyperosmolar coma, not with DKA.

Although the remaining choices (**choices B, D, and E**) are all common causes of morbidity and mortality in diabetics, myocardial infarction is the most frequent cause.

40. **The correct answer is D.** Barbiturate overdose causes respiratory depression, resulting in carbon dioxide retention (producing increased P_{CO_2} and decreased pH) and hypoxemia (decreased P_{O_2}). In other words, the patient has respiratory acidosis. You should look for low P_{O_2}, high P_{CO_2}, and acidotic pH. **Choices A, B, C, and E** do not fulfill these requirements. Note that **choice C** might be expected in a patient who is hyperventilating to the point of respiratory alkalosis: diminished O_2 (the usual drive for hyperventilation in nonpsychiatric hyperventilation), diminished CO_2, and mildly alkalotic pH.

41. **The correct answer is D.** The most important risk to this patient is liver damage by free radical species derived from carbon tetrachloride (CCl_4), notably

CCl_3. These species are produced when the hepatic P-450 microsomal system attempts to degrade the CCl_4. They can cause severe, sometimes fatal, fatty liver damage by reacting with the polyenoic (multiple double bonds) acids present in the membrane phospholipids. The reaction is particularly harmful because peroxides are often formed as a byproduct. Peroxides can be autocatalytic, in that the peroxide radicals themselves form new free radicals capable of more damage to membranes and other cellular structures. Clinically, patients may have an extremely rapid (30 min to 2 hours) decline in hepatic function after the carbon tetrachloride exposure. Other organs are not affected to the same degree, because of the relatively lower concentration of the toxic metabolites there.

42. **The correct answer is E.** The challenge in answering this question arises from the difficulty in differentiating the very similar diseases that cause monoclonal gammopathy. The key to answering correctly is making sure not to use only one piece of information as the sole distinguishing factor. You must look at the whole picture—clinical presentation, physical exam, and laboratory findings—just as will be expected when you practice medicine in the future. This 65-year-old patient has Waldenström macroglobulinemia (WM), a disease resulting from neoplasms of lymphocytoid plasma cells that produce monoclonal IgM. Peak incidence is between ages 60 and 70. This patient's symptoms and signs are due to hypergammaglobulinemia and tumorous infiltration (weakness, weight loss, bone pain, hepatosplenomegaly, and lymphadenopathy). His visual disturbance is a symptom of blood hyperviscosity (this creates a resistance to blood flow that may create dysfunction in organs supplied by small arteries such as the retinal artery). The M-protein spike found on serum protein electrophoresis is consistent with WM but not specific for it since this result is also associated with the other answer choices. The intensely eosinophilic plasma cells discovered on bone marrow aspiration are known as "flame cells" and are classic for WM. Although Bence-Jones proteins in the urine are classically associated with multiple myeloma (MM; **choice C**), they are also found in about 10% of patients with WM. This highlights the importance of not jumping to the answers prematurely.

Heavy chain disease (**choice A**) occurs rarely, when a neoplastic clone of plasma cells or lymphocytes produces a monoclonal alpha, gamma, or M chain.

Patients with monoclonal gammopathy of undetermined significance (**choice B**) are generally asymptomatic. Incidence increases with age. Patients with this disorder have a predisposition for developing myeloma, lymphoma, amyloidosis, or WM. They should be followed with periodic evaluations for serum and urine immunoglobulins.

Patients with multiple myeloma (**choice C**) present with susceptibility to infection, proteinuria, bone pain, and hypercalcemia. Renal insufficiency commonly develops. Peak incidence is from age 50 to 60. Tumor-secreted osteoclast-activating factor (OAF) results in osteolytic lesions and "punched out" defects on x-ray films. Bone marrow aspiration would reveal plasma cells in various stages of maturation that may resemble lymphoid precursors with cytoplasmic inclusions (Russell bodies).

Plasmacytoma (**choice D**), or solitary myeloma, is a rare, isolated plasma cell neoplasm in bone or soft tissues. If the primary cancer is in bone, it is likely to disseminate; extraosseous tumors tend to remain localized.

43. **The correct answer is A.** The immunophenotype of chronic lymphocytic leukemia is distinctive among clonal B-cell disorders. There is usually strong expression of both CD5 and CD23, and weak expression of surface immunoglobulin (either kappa or lambda chain) and CD22.

In contrast, other disorders that contain mature B cells, such as hairy cell leukemia (**choice B**), non-Hodgkin lymphoma (**choice C**), including follicular and mantle cell lymphomas, and prolymphocytic leukemia (**choice D**), typically have strong expression of surface immunoglobulin and CD22. There is usually absent expression of CD5 (may be seen in prolymphocytic leukemia and some non-Hodgkin lymphomas) and CD23 (may be seen in some non-Hodgkin lymphomas).

Sézary syndrome (**choice E**) is a form of T-cell lymphoma/leukemia.

44. **The correct answer is D.** This patient has bundle branch block, as implied by the QRS interval greater than 0.12 seconds and by paradoxical splitting of the second heart sound. Mobitz II block is frequently associated with bundle branch block. Mobitz II block is characterized on EKG by a constant PR interval before failure of AV conduction occurs. The anatomic site of this type of block is usually below the AV node.

Complete AV block (**choice A**) represents the failure of any impulses to be conducted from the atria to the ventricles. The ventricles are depolarized by an AV nodal or ventricular escape rhythm. It is manifested by a slow ventricular rate, wide pulse pressure, a variable first heart sound, and prominent jugular venous pulsations.

First-degree AV block (**choice B**) represents a delay in conduction of the impulse from the atria to the ventricles, due most commonly to abnormalities in the AV node. It is reflected by a prolonged PR interval, usually exceeding 0.20 seconds.

Mobitz Type I AV block (Wenckebach; **choice C**) is usually due to a problem in the AV node and can result from a variety of cardiac or systemic disorders, including myocardial infarction.

Wolff-Parkinson-White syndrome (**choice E**) is also known as pre-excitation syndrome because conduction occurs by way of an auxiliary pathway between the atria and ventricles. Findings on EKG include a short PR interval and a delta wave (slurred QRS upstroke).

45. **The correct answer is C.** Tumor markers can be very helpful in narrowing the possible primary sources for metastatic lesions. Carcinoembryonic antigen (CEA) can be seen in any tumor derived from gut epithelium, notably colon cancer and pancreatic cancer. Tumor markers should not be used as the primary tool for cancer diagnosis, but they have considerable utility in the confirmation of the diagnosis, as well as for monitoring recurrence or response to therapy.

Alpha-fetoprotein (AFP; **choice A**) is seen in hepatocellular carcinoma, embryonal cell tumor of the testis, and malignant teratoma.

CA-125 (**choice B**) is produced by ovarian cancer.

The beta subunit of human chorionic gonadotropin (hCG; **choice D**) is seen in choriocarcinoma, hydatidiform mole, and germinoma.

Prostate-specific antigen (PSA; **choice E**) is seen in prostatic carcinoma.

You should also remember that serum elevations of many of these markers can also be seen in some benign conditions of similar tissues. hCG, for example, is elevated normally in pregnancy.

46. **The correct answer is C.** This is essentially a Frank-Starling curve that plots cardiac output against central venous pressure (CVP). This patient is in hemorrhagic shock due to trauma. Both cardiac output and CVP should be reduced.

Point A represents normality.

Point B represents diminished cardiac output despite elevated preload and implies intrinsic cardiac pathology (cardiogenic shock).

Point D represents a state in which cardiac output increases normally in response to increased preload.

Point E represents elevated cardiac output despite diminished preload and corresponds to septic shock.

47. **The correct answer is D.** This patient has two major risk factors for HIV: drug abuse and a prior sexually transmitted disease (STD), implying high-risk behav-

ior. *Pneumocystis carinii* is the most common cause of pneumonia in HIV-positive patients and is diagnosed by demonstration of organisms via methenamine-silver stain or fluorescent antibody in lung tissue. Bilateral interstitial infiltrates are characteristic of this disease.

Acid-fast bacteria found in the sputum (**choice A**) is associated with tuberculosis (TB), which is also commonly found in HIV-positive patients. Primary TB is usually asymptomatic, whereas reactivation of the infection (secondary TB) is associated with chronic cough, hemoptysis, fever, weight loss, and night sweats. The presence of both a calcified peripheral lung nodule (Ghon complex) and a calcified perihilar lymph node is characteristic of this disease.

Curschmann spirals in mucus plugs (**choice B**), which are shed epithelia that have assumed a spiral configuration, and the presence of Charcot-Leyden crystals (**choice E**), which are eosinophils and membrane proteins forming a crystalloid collection, are characteristic of asthma.

Elevated serum cold agglutinins (IgMs; **choice C**) are found in 50% of patients with *Mycoplasma pneumoniae* infection, the most common cause of pneumonia in young adults. Clinical features include fever, malaise, and a dry hacking cough. Twenty percent of patients with adenovirus exhibit this finding as well.

48. **The correct answer is A.** Cholestasis due to obstruction of the common bile duct results in an increase in serum conjugated bilirubin, an increase in urine bilirubin, and a decrease in urine urobilinogen. This form of jaundice is caused by a deficit in bilirubin excretion, since the process of bilirubin conjugation is normal. Because the conjugated bilirubin cannot be excreted through the biliary tree, it refluxes back into the serum, resulting in increased serum and urine bilirubin levels. In addition, because very little (if any) of the bilirubin is excreted into the gastrointestinal tract, there is very little urobilinogen produced by the enteric flora, resulting in decreased urobilinogen levels.

A deficiency in glucuronyl transferase (**choice B**) would result in impaired bilirubin conjugation, leading to an unconjugated hyperbilirubinemia.

Increased erythrocyte destruction caused by hemolytic anemia (**choice C**) would release more free bilirubin into the bloodstream than the liver could immediately process, resulting in a predominantly unconjugated hyperbilirubinemia.

Hepatocellular damage (**choice D**) results in a mixed conjugated/unconjugated bilirubinemia, since the hepatic mechanisms for both bilirubin conjugation and excretion are disrupted.

This is a viscerosomatic reflex of the gallbladder, not a somatovisceral reflex (**choice B**).

49. **The correct answer is A.** An annular pancreas may exert pressure on the duodenum, causing the patient to vomit bile-stained material. This condition is the result of the ventral pancreatic bud's failure to migrate normally.

Esophageal atresia (**choice B**) is diagnosed shortly after birth. Milk cannot reach the stomach and is therefore quickly regurgitated in an undigested state.

The lodging of one or more gallstones (**choice C**) in the extrahepatic biliary apparatus may cause indigestion, severe pain, and jaundice.

Meckel's (ileal) diverticulum (**choice D**) is persistence of a portion of the embryonic vitelline duct (yolk stalk). It is usually asymptomatic but may cause bleeding or ulceration because of the presence of ectopic gastric tissue.

Pyloric stenosis (**choice E**) is a congenital thickening of the smooth muscle in the wall of the pyloric portion of the stomach. It is usually diagnosed in infants following episodes of projectile vomiting.

50. **The correct answer is C.** This patient has a non-Hodgkin lymphoma of the follicular type. *Bcl-2* is a very important gene that normally acts to prevent apoptosis, or programmed cell death. In approximately 85% of B-cell lymphomas (especially follicular and undifferentiated), this gene is over-expressed as a result of a translocation [t(14;18)(q32;q21)] that links *bcl-2* (at 18q21) to the Ig heavy chain gene (14q32). It is thought that the resultant over-expression of *bcl-2* causes other mutations, which then produce the frank lymphoma.

Amplification of L-*myc* (**choice A**) is associated with the development of small cell (oat cell) carcinoma of the lung.

Homozygous loss of *p53* (**choice B**) is associated with a number of different kinds of human neoplasms, including colon, breast, and lung cancer.

Point mutation in *ras* (**choice D**) may alter its ability to bind GTPase activating proteins (GAPS), thereby preventing termination of the signal transduced by the *ras* protein. The net result is excessive activation of a mitogenic cellular pathway, as well as tumor formation. Approximately 30% of human tumors are associated with *ras* mutations.

Reciprocal translocation between chromosome 9 and chromosome 22 (**choice E**) forms the Philadelphia chromosome, which is associated with chronic myelocytic leukemia.

Pathology and Pathophysiology

1. A teenage boy with a history of peripheral neuropathy and ocular abnormalities has multiple purplish nodules diffusely over his skin. Other family members have been similarly affected, as shown in the pedigree above. Laboratory tests reveal the young man has a deficiency of α-galactosidase A. Biopsy of the skin lesions would most likely reveal that they were

   (A) basal cell carcinomas

   (B) cavernous hemangiomas

   (C) cystic hygromas

   (D) neurofibromas

   (E) squamous cell carcinomas

2. A neonate develops marked unconjugated hyperbilirubinemia. No hemolysis can be demonstrated, and other liver function tests are normal. No bilirubin is found in the urine. This infant's condition continues to deteriorate, and he dies at 2 weeks of age. To which of the following conditions did the infant most likely succumb?

   (A) Crigler-Najjar syndrome, Type I

   (B) Crigler-Najjar syndrome, Type II

   (C) Dubin-Johnson syndrome

   (D) Gilbert syndrome

   (E) Rotor syndrome

3. A 59-year-old man complains of headache and decreasing visual ability. History reveals that the patient has also "outgrown" his pants and shirts within the past year. The man exhibits a marked overbite and somatic dysfunction at T1-T3. Which of the following is the best method to diagnose this patient?

   (A) Measuring growth hormone (GH) and insulin growth factor-1 (IGF-1) levels before and after administrating glucose

   (B) Measuring resting corticotropin (ACTH) levels

   (C) Measuring resting prolactin levels

   (D) Measuring the patient's height and comparing it with last year's value

   (E) Measuring the patient's shoe size and comparing it with last year's value

4. A 36-year-old alcoholic man is brought to the emergency department because he is jaundiced and exhibits inappropriate somnolence. Past medical history is significant for depression and seizures, both of which are well controlled with medications. Physical exam is significant for icterus, asterixis, tachypnea, and chronic somatic dysfunction at T5-T9 on the right side. Slit lamp examination reveals greenish-golden crescents on the cornea. AST is 2489 IU/L, ALT is 4873 IU/L, bilirubin is 29 mg/dL, alkaline phosphatase is 112 IU/L, hematocrit is 29%, prothrombin time (PT) is 19.1 seconds, and serum ceruloplasmin is decreased. Which of the following is the most likely diagnosis?

   (A) Alcoholic hepatitis

   (B) Budd-Chiari syndrome

   (C) Drug-induced hepatitis

   (D) Hepatitis B

   (E) Wilson disease

5. A 9-year-old Mexican girl develops rapid, purposeless movements, an expanding erythematous rash, and subcutaneous nodules 3 weeks after recovery from a severe sore throat. A biopsy of the subcutaneous nodules would most likely reveal

(A) caseous necrosis with epithelioid cells and Langhans giant cells

(B) fibrinoid necrosis with lymphocytes, macrophages, and Anitschkow cells

(C) focal collections of hemosiderin-laden macrophages

(D) lymphoid nodules with a "starry-sky" appearance

(E) Reed-Sternberg cells in a background of lymphocytes with occasional eosinophils

Questions 6-8

CASE A

A 55-year-old man presents with a 5-year history of type 2 diabetes mellitus.

6. The patient has tissue texture changes at T1-T4. What is the most likely complication of diabetes mellitus that could contribute to his somatic dysfunction?

(A) Fatty liver
(B) Intermittent claudication
(C) Motor neuropathy
(D) Retinopathy
(E) 3+ proteinuria

7. Which of the following measures is most effective in preventing or delaying the complications abovementioned?

(A) Funduscopic examination
(B) Maintaining the Hb_{A1c} at less than 7%
(C) Maintaining the Hb_{A1c} at greater than 11%
(D) Performing a glucose tolerance test
(E) Morning spot albumin/creatinine ratio test

8. Your patient returns in 2 weeks complaining of edema in the lower extremities. Which of the following medications is the most likely cause of his edema?

(A) Glipizide
(B) Tramadol
(C) Captopril
(D) Rosiglitazone
(E) Simvastatin

9. A 20-year-old man presents with an enlarged right testicle that was undescended at birth but had self-corrected by age 1. Physical examination reveals T10FRS$_R$. Serum AFP is elevated. A testicular tumor is biopsied and reveals multiple mitoses, along with hemorrhage and necrosis. The surgeon decides to perform an orchiectomy because the tumor type is not particularly radiosensitive. Which of the following is the most likely diagnosis?

(A) Embryonal carcinoma
(B) Interstitial cell tumor
(C) Seminoma
(D) Sertoli cell tumor
(E) Leydig cell tumor

Questions 10-11

CASE B

A 28-year-old woman complains of fatigue, irritability, and headaches. On physical examination stools are guaiac-negative. On further testing, microcytic hypochromic anemia is found.

10. The most common etiology is

(A) gastrointestinal bleed
(B) menorrhagia
(C) alcohol abuse
(D) cancer
(E) systemic lupus erythematosus

11. What will the peripheral blood smear look like 1 month after iron therapy is begun for a patient with iron deficiency anemia?

(A) Almost all larger than normal erythrocytes
(B) Almost all normal erythrocytes
(C) Almost all small, but no longer hypochromic, erythrocytes
(D) Almost all small hypochromic erythrocytes
(E) A mix of small hypochromic and normal erythrocytes

12. A 35-year-old man presents to the physician with intensely pruritic skin lesions on his axillary folds, nipples, waistband, wrists, interdigital spaces of the hand, and genitalia. Linear burrows are apparent in affected areas. Which of the following is the most likely diagnosis?

    (A) Dermatitis herpetiformis
    (B) Lichen planus
    (C) Photosensitivity
    (D) Scabies
    (E) Seborrhea

13. A patient complains to her physician that she feels lightheaded and has even fainted during defecation. This is most probably an example of syncope due to which of the following mechanisms?

    (A) Anoxia
    (B) Hyperventilation
    (C) Hypovolemia
    (D) Sinus node disease
    (E) Valsalva mechanism

14. Radiographic studies of a 2-year-old child brought to an emergency department reveal a new fracture of the humerus and evidence of multiple old fractures in ribs and long bones of the extremities. A social worker wants to initiate prosecution of the parents for child abuse, but an alert emergency department physician notices that, despite the broken arm, the toddler shows minimal bruising. A very careful, directed, physical examination reveals that the toddler has "peculiar teeth," a blue tinge to the sclera, and unusually mobile joints. The physician suspects a disease that is characterized by an abnormality of which of the following biochemical functions?

    (A) Collagen type I synthesis
    (B) Collagen type II synthesis
    (C) Collagen type III synthesis
    (D) Collagen type IV synthesis
    (E) Collagen type V synthesis

Questions 15-16

CASE C

A 35-year-old roofer presents to his primary care physician complaining of dyspnea and chronic dry cough. Structural examination reveals stiff, fibrotic, cool, ropy tissues at T2-T7. A chest x-ray film reveals pulmonary hyperinflation with honeycombing and calcified parietal pleural plaques.

15. Which of the following is the most likely diagnosis?

    (A) Anthracosis
    (B) Asbestosis
    (C) Berylliosis
    (D) Byssinosis
    (E) Silicosis

16. The bronchial lavage of this patient most likely would reveal

    (A) macrophages containing black cytoplasm
    (B) corkscrew-shaped casts
    (C) rhomboid-shaped crystals within eosinophils
    (D) concentrically arranged layer of squamous cells
    (E) beaded, dumbbell-shaped protein iron complexes

17. A concerned mother brings her 6-year-old son to the pediatrician because he has developed a "puffy face." On examination, the child has a blood pressure of 90/60 mm Hg, marked periorbital edema, and pitting edema of both the hands and feet. Cardiac examination is unremarkable, and he has no splenomegaly or signs of liver disease. On structural examination, there is somatic dysfunction at T11-L1. Laboratory values are notable for decreased serum albumin and increased total cholesterol. A urinalysis reveals 4+ proteinuria but no red blood cells, white blood cells, or casts. Which of the following is the most likely diagnosis?

    (A) Goodpasture syndrome
    (B) minimal change nephropathy
    (C) poststreptococcal glomerulonephritis
    (D) systemic lupus erythematosus
    (E) Wegener granulomatosis

18. A 50-year-old industrial chemist presents with painless hematuria. On further questioning he also describes urinary frequency and urgency. Physical examination reveals a chronic paraspinal tissue change at T11-L2. After additional testing, a diagnosis of bladder cancer is made. The patient's cancer is most likely which of the following types?

    (A) Adenocarcinoma

    (B) Papilloma

    (C) Sarcoma

    (D) Squamous cell carcinoma

    (E) Transitional cell carcinoma

19. A 42-year-old man previously diagnosed with kidney stones complains of gnawing, burning epigastric pain. On questioning, he also notes moderate to severe diarrhea. Physical examination reveals chronic somatic dysfunction at T5-T9. Measurement of the patient's basal gastric acid output reveals that it is markedly elevated. These symptoms are likely the result of which of the following neoplastic syndromes?

    (A) Familial polyposis coli

    (B) Multiple endocrine neoplasia type I (MEN I)

    (C) MEN IIA

    (D) MEN IIB

    (E) MEN III

20. A patient took DES in 1960. Her daughter has an increased risk for developing which of the following cancers?

    (A) Bladder cancer

    (B) Endometrial carcinoma

    (C) Ovarian carcinoma

    (D) Renal cell carcinoma

    (E) Vaginal clear cell adenocarcinoma

Questions 21-22

CASE D

A 65-year-old man with a history of smoking and alcohol abuse complains of poor appetite and difficulty swallowing both solid and liquid foods over the course of the past 4 months. He has lost 20 lb and occasionally vomits blood. Structural examination reveals T2-T7 NR_RL. A mass is detected in his esophagus and is subsequently biopsied.

21. What is the most likely histologic appearance of the biopsy?

    (A) Glandular epithelium associated with desmoplasia

    (B) Malignant tumor of mesenchymal origin

    (C) Squamous cell morphology

    (D) Tumor derived from all three germ layers

    (E) Tumor of epithelial origin demonstrating transitional cell morphology

22. Preventive measures to reduce the risk for the above-mentioned condition would be to

    (A) lose weight

    (B) drink red wine

    (C) quit tobacco and alcohol use

    (D) smoke cigars instead of cigarettes

    (E) eat soft foods and liquids

23. A 7-year-old boy with chickenpox is given aspirin to reduce his fever. He develops severe vomiting, mental status changes, and seizures, and eventually falls into a coma. A quick, osteopathic structural examination reveals acute tissue changes at T5-T9. Which of the following would you expect to see on a biopsy specimen of his liver?

    (A) Diffuse fibrosis with areas of regeneration

    (B) Fatty change

    (C) Hemosiderin deposits

    (D) Hepatocyte necrosis

    (E) Mallory bodies

Questions 24-25

<u>CASE E</u>

An 18-year-old Japanese woman presents to her physician with fever and conjunctivitis. Physical exam is significant for oral erythema and fissuring along with a generalized maculopapular rash and cervical lymphadenopathy. The patient's 3-year-old sister experienced the same symptoms 1 week ago.

24. Which of the following is the most likely diagnosis?

   (A) Henoch-Schönlein purpura

   (B) Kawasaki disease

   (C) Polyarteritis nodosa

   (D) Rheumatic fever

   (E) Takayasu arteritis

25. The above patient should be monitored for what associated complication?

   (A) Glomerulonephritis

   (B) Coronary artery aneurysm

   (C) Renal failure

   (D) Mitral stenosis

   (E) Blindness

26. This woman and her sister should have what diagnostic study performed to prevent this possible complication?

   (A) Renal biopsy

   (B) Echocardiogram

   (C) Renal scan

   (D) Cardiac catheterization

   (E) Eye examination

27. The pharmacologic treatment of the 3-year-old child would be to administer

   (A) acetaminophen

   (B) ibuprofen

   (C) aspirin

   (D) propranolol

   (E) retinol

28. A 24-year-old man presents to his physician with gynecomastia and testicular enlargement. Physical examination reveals somatic dysfunction at T10-T11. Serum urine and human chorionic gonadotropin (hCG) levels are elevated. Biopsy of the testicular mass reveals a cytotrophoblastic and syncytiotrophoblastic structure. Which of the following is the most likely diagnosis?

   (A) Choriocarcinoma

   (B) Sertoli cell tumor

   (C) Teratoma

   (D) Yolk sac tumor

   (E) Leydig cell tumor

Questions 29-30

<u>CASE F</u>

A 68-year-old, well-developed, well-nourished black man presents to the emergency department complaining of shortness of breath. He denies chest pain. He has no significant past medical history and takes no medications. Structural examination reveals chronic somatic dysfunction at T1-T4. A chest x-ray film shows clear lung fields, mild cardiomegaly, and a widened thoracic aorta with linear calcifications. An MRI of the chest shows aortic dilatation in the thorax, extending proximally, with atrophy of the muscularis and wrinkling of the intimal surface.

29. What is the most likely etiology of this condition?

   (A) Atherosclerosis

   (B) Hypertension

   (C) Marfan syndrome

   (D) Syphilis infection

   (E) Takayasu arteritis

30. This patient should have been treated previously with which of the following medications?

   (A) Simvastatin

   (B) Propranolol

   (C) Aortic bypass graft

   (D) Benzathine penicillin G

   (E) Corticosteroids

31. Bronchoalveolar lavage is performed in a patient with long-standing congestive heart failure exacerbated by periodic acute pulmonary edema. Which of the following findings would be consistent with this patient's history of cardiac failure?

    (A) Charcot-Leyden crystals

    (B) Curschmann spirals

    (C) Fat-laden macrophages

    (D) Ferruginous bodies

    (E) Iron-laden macrophages

32. A young man presents to his physician's office for a physical examination. He is concerned because his father died of a heart attack in his late 40s. The physician finds that the patient has elevated serum cholesterol and LDL levels, but his VLDL and triglyceride levels are normal. Osteopathic structural exam reveals T3 NR$_L$S. Further investigation reveals an LDL receptor deficiency. This patient has which of the following types of hyperlipidemia?

    (A) I

    (B) IIa

    (C) IIb

    (D) III

    (E) IV

33. A 28-year-old woman presents to the physician complaining of syncopal episodes that last a few minutes. She is not taking any medications and has no previous medical history. EEG and EKG studies are performed and are unremarkable. An echocardiogram shows a single ball-shaped mass dangling in the left atrium near the mitral valve. Which of the following is the most likely diagnosis?

    (A) Angiosarcoma

    (B) Mesothelioma

    (C) Myxoma

    (D) Rhabdomyoma

    (E) Rhabdomyosarcoma

34. An infant born at 33 weeks' gestation exhibits signs of respiratory distress at birth. Her mother had gestational diabetes. Which of the following would have indicated lung immaturity in the fetus prior to birth?

    (A) <0.5 L of amniotic fluid

    (B) Alpha-1 antitrypsin deficiency in amniotic fluid

    (C) Amniotic lecithin:sphingomyelin ratio less than 2:1

    (D) Elevated maternal HbA$_{1c}$

    (E) Elevated maternal serum alpha-fetoprotein (AFP)

35. A patient is observed to have an abnormal breathing pattern characterized by cyclical changes in tidal volume. The tidal volume first increases and then decreases to the point of apnea. What term best describes this breathing pattern?

    (A) Apneustic

    (B) Biot's

    (C) Cheyne-Stokes

    (D) Hysterical

    (E) Kussmaul

36. A cyanotic infant is discovered to have a ventricular septal defect, an overriding aorta, right ventricular hypertrophy, and complete pulmonic stenosis. Which of the following accompanying congenital anomalies permits survival in this patient?

    (A) Bicuspid aortic valve

    (B) Ostium secundum defect

    (C) Patent ductus arteriosus

    (D) Patent foramen ovale

    (E) Preductal coarctation of aorta

37. A 45-year-old man presents to the physician with muscle cramps, perioral numbness, and irritability over the past 3-4 months. Physical examination reveals chronic somatic dysfunction at T1-T4. Laboratory results reveal hypocalcemia, normal albumin level, mild hypomagnesemia, and hyperphosphatemia. Parathyroid hormone (PTH) level is decreased. Alkaline phosphatase level is normal. Which of the following is most likely causing this clinical scenario?

    (A) Bone metastases

    (B) Hashimoto thyroiditis

    (C) Hypervitaminosis D

    (D) Hypomagnesemia

    (E) Previous subtotal thyroidectomy

38. A 32-year-old woman with one child has tried unsuccessfully to conceive for the past 2 years. She tells her physician that she has had problems putting on weight and is often anxious and irritable. On physical examination, her thyroid is enlarged with no palpable nodules. Structural examination reveals chronic tissue-texture change paraspinally at T1-T4. Which of the following laboratory findings would be most suggestive of a diagnosis of secondary hyperthyroidism?

    (A) Decreased thyroxine-binding globulin (TBG)
    (B) Elevated triiodothyronine (T3)
    (C) Elevated thyroxine (T4)
    (D) Elevated thyroid-stimulating hormone (TSH)
    (E) Presence of serum thyroid-stimulating autoantibodies

39. A hospitalized man with hemoglobinuria and symptoms of anemia undergoes a complete hematologic evaluation. The reticulocyte count is elevated. The remaining laboratory results are pending. Which of the following diagnoses is most consistent with the information available thus far?

    (A) Chronic renal disease
    (B) Folate deficiency
    (C) G6PD deficiency
    (D) Iron deficiency
    (E) Pernicious anemia

40. A 62-year-old man presents with progressive, pruritic erythroderma, exfoliation, and lymphadenopathy. Peripheral smear reveals T cells with cerebriform nuclei. Which of the following is the most likely diagnosis?

    (A) Burkitt lymphoma
    (B) Histiocytic lymphoma
    (C) Lymphoblastic lymphoma
    (D) Lymphocytic lymphoma
    (E) Sézary syndrome

41. A 32-year-old man with a history of chronic drug abuse presents to his primary care physician complaining of uncontrollable shaking in his hands. He moves very slowly and walks with a stooped posture and shuffling gait. Physical examination reveals cogwheel rigidity, a pill-rolling tremor, and masked facies. His condition deteriorates, and he eventually dies. Structures similar to which of the following would be expected on autopsy?

    (A) Hirano bodies
    (B) Lewy bodies
    (C) Lipofuscin granules
    (D) Negri bodies
    (E) Neurofibrillary tangles

42. A 45-year-old woman complains of difficulty speaking, chewing, and swallowing. She experiences generalized weakness that increases with effort and as the day goes on. Symptoms are significantly improved after taking neostigmine. Autoantibodies responsible for causing the patient's condition are directed against which of the following?

    (A) Acetylcholine receptors
    (B) Double-stranded DNA
    (C) Dystrophin
    (D) Erythrocyte surface antigens
    (E) Myelin

43. A patient has severe arthritis involving the lower back. Physical examination reveals decreased flexion and extension, as well as stiff, ropy, fibrotic soft tissues of the lumbar spine. The sacroiliac joints are tender to palpation. Before making a diagnosis of ankylosing spondylitis, the patient should be questioned about which of the following diseases?

    (A) Carcinoid syndrome
    (B) Celiac disease
    (C) Crohn disease
    (D) Peptic ulcer
    (E) Whipple disease

44. A 3-year-old child develops severe generalized edema following a viral infection. On the basis of clinical chemistry tests, a renal biopsy is performed, with normal light microscopic findings. Which of the following abnormal laboratory values might be expected in this individual?

(A) Decreased alpha$_2$ globulin levels

(B) Decreased fibrinogen

(C) Increased serum calcium levels

(D) Low serum albumin levels

(E) Red blood cell casts in the urine

45. A patient with long-standing hypertension dies in a car accident. At autopsy, multiple, small, cavitary lesions are observed in the basal ganglia and chronic tissue changes at T2-T8. This finding is most consistent with pathology of which of the following arteries?

(A) Anterior cerebral

(B) Lateral striate

(C) Posterior cerebral

(D) Superior cerebellar

(E) Vertebral

46. A 75-year-old man with angina pectoris has recurrent episodes of atrial tachycardia (240/min). A rapid sequence of normal QRS waves is seen on EKG. The episodes are controllable by the patient's performance of vagal maneuvers. Which of the following is the most likely etiology of this arrhythmia?

(A) Atrial reentry

(B) Automatic atrial conduction

(C) AV dissociation

(D) AV nodal reentry

(E) Wandering atrial pacemaker

Questions 47-49

CASE G

47. A 2-year-old girl has an infection. A complete blood count reveals increased numbers of the white blood cell type shown above. Which of the following diseases is most consistent with this laboratory result?

(A) Bronchiolitis

(B) Cellulitis

(C) Diphtheria

(D) Epiglottitis

(E) Pertussis

48. What is the most likely pathogen?

(A) *Corynebacterium diphtheriae*

(B) *Haemophilus influenzae*

(C) *Bordetella pertussis*

(D) Respiratory syncytial virus

(E) *Streptococcus* Group C

49. The most appropriate treatment would be

(A) direct laryngoscopy, antitoxin, and erythromycin

(B) penicillin G, increased fluids, and acetaminophen

(C) erythromycin, increased fluids, rest, and acetaminophen

(D) hospitalization, ceftizoxime, and dexamethasone

(E) hydration, humidification of evaporated air, and ventilatory support

50. A 25-year-old woman is discovered on physical exam to have a midsystolic click and a high-pitched heart murmur. Somatic dysfunction is noticed at T2 $F_R S_L$ and T4 $F_R S_L$. Which of the following additional cardiovascular findings is she most likely to exhibit?

   (A) Atrial fibrillation
   (B) Decreased peripheral pulse pressure
   (C) Premature ventricular contractions
   (D) Slowed carotid upstroke
   (E) Wide pulse pressure

Pathology and Pathophysiology

ANSWERS AND EXPLANATIONS

1.	B	26.	B
2.	A	27.	C
3.	A	28.	A
4.	E	29.	D
5.	B	30.	D
6.	D	31.	E
7.	B	32.	B
8.	D	33.	C
9.	A	34.	C
10.	B	35.	C
11.	E	36.	C
12.	D	37.	E
13.	E	38.	D
14.	A	39.	C
15.	B	40.	E
16.	E	41.	B
17.	B	42.	A
18.	E	43.	C
19.	B	44.	D
20.	E	45.	B
21.	C	46.	D
22.	C	47.	A
23.	B	48.	D
24.	B	49.	E
25.	B	50.	C

1. **The correct answer is B.** Fabry disease is a lysosomal storage disease with sex-linked genetics caused by deficiency of a-galactosidase, which leads to the accumulation of ceramide trihexoside in many tissues (reticuloendothelial, myocardial, ganglion, renal glomeruli and tubules, and connective tissue). Fabry disease is characterized by angiokeratoma corporis diffusum (cavernous hemangioma with epidermal keratosis), thickened blood vessels (with risk of myocardial infarction and stroke), and progressive renal failure and hypertension in adult life.

Multiple basal cell carcinomas (**choice A**) are seen in familial basal cell nevus syndrome, which is not a lysosomal storage disease.

Cystic hygromas (**choice C**) are seen in Turner syndrome and are associated with a "webbed" neck.

Neurofibromas (**choice D**) are seen in neurofibromatosis.

Multiple squamous cell carcinomas (**choice E**) are seen in skin badly damaged by the sun or radiation, in xeroderma pigmentosa, and in albinism.

2. **The correct answer is A.** All the diseases listed are inherited disorders of bilirubin metabolism, and they are usually discussed together. Crigler-Najjar syndrome (**choices A and B**) and Gilbert syndrome (**choice D**) are both unconjugated hyperbilirubinemias, whereas Dubin-Johnson syndrome (**choice C**) and Rotor syndrome (**choice E**) are conjugated hyperbilirubinemias. Crigler-Najjar syndrome (particularly the type I variant) is rare and extremely serious (with the presentation given in the question stem), whereas Gilbert syndrome is completely benign. The type II variant of Crigler-Najjar is intermediate in severity between Gilbert and the Type I. Dubin-Johnson and Rotor syndromes are also relatively benign; Dubin-Johnson is distinguished from Rotor syndrome by the presence of a black pigment of unknown composition in the liver.

3. **The correct answer is A.** Acromegaly is most commonly caused by a pituitary adenoma. Acromegalic persons secrete excessively high levels of growth hormone (GH) and insulin growth factor-1 (IGF-1) from pituitary gland tissue. These hormones are not suppressed by glucose, as they would be in a normal person.

Measuring resting corticotropin (ACTH) levels (**choice B**) may be indicated in a person with Cushing syndrome.

Measuring resting prolactin levels (**choice C**) would be indicated in a person with a suspected prolactinoma.

Measuring the height (**choice D**) of a 59-year-old patient would not be indicated. Acromegaly, or excess GH, in individuals who have already experienced closure of bone growth centers results in a broadening of the skeletal bones, not a lengthening. Lengthening of skeletal bones occurs in gigantism, before the closure of bone growth centers.

Measuring a patient's shoe size and comparing it with last year's size (**choice E**), although indicative of a broadening of skeletal bones, is not a clinically used standard for the diagnosis of acromegaly.

4. **The correct answer is E.** Acute liver failure (implied by the abnormal liver function tests) in this young patient with depression strongly suggests Wilson disease (WD). In conjunction with a low serum ceruloplasmin level, the presence of Kayser-Fleischer rings (greenish-golden crescents on the cornea) on slit lamp examination is diagnostic of WD.

Alcoholic hepatitis (**choice A**) very rarely causes elevation of transaminases in the range of 3000-4000, but it is classically associated with an AST twice the value of the ALT.

Budd-Chiari syndrome (**choice B**), or hepatic vein thrombosis, is a rare condition that presents with abdominal pain, large, tender liver, and ascites. Micropathology is similar to chronic passive congestion of the liver, with central hemorrhagic necrosis and rupture at Disse's spaces. The liver develops a "nutmeg" appearance, which is also seen in patients with severe heart failure.

Drug-induced hepatitis (**choice C**) may be caused by phenytoin, which the patient may have been taking for seizures. However, drug-induced hepatitis usually presents with fever, rash, joint pain, and eosinophilia, which are not evident in this patient. Other medications causing drug-induced hepatitis include isoniazid, methyldopa, and halothane.

Patients with hepatitis B (**choice D**) typically present with nausea, vomiting, malaise, diarrhea, and dark urine. Jaundice, tender hepatomegaly, and low-grade fever may be evident on physical exam. Serum transaminases are usually elevated, but serum ceruloplasmin would likely be normal. The detection of hepatitis antigens and antibodies in serum is diagnostic.

5. **The correct answer is B.** The history of a recent severe sore throat in a young person is a classic clue suggesting rheumatic fever. The histologic description given is that of an Aschoff body, which classically occurs in the heart in rheumatic heart disease. Erythema marginatum (the expanding erythematous rash) and Sydenham chorea (rapid, purposeless movements) also accompany this disorder. The subcutaneous nodules characteristic of rheumatic fever are basically "giant" Aschoff bodies.

Caseous necrosis with epithelioid cells and Langhans giant cells (**choice A**) are characteristic of the granulomas of tuberculosis.

Hemosiderin-laden macrophages (**choice C**) may be found in chronic passive congestion of the liver.

Burkitt lymphoma is characterized by dense collections of lymphoid cells with macrophages intermixed. The macrophages often have a clear space around them, giving the tissue a "starry sky" appearance (**choice D**).

Reed-Sternberg cells (**choice E**) are characteristic of Hodgkin lymphoma. Occasional eosinophils are often admixed with the proliferating lymphocytes in this disorder.

6. **The correct answer is D.** Diabetic retinopathy usually precedes the development of diabetic nephropathy and proteinuria (**choice E**).

    Fatty liver (**choice A**) occurs in alcohol abuse and toxic insults to the liver. It is not associated with diabetes.

    Intermittent claudication (**choice B**) and coronary artery disease, when solely associated with diabetes and no other risk factors (e.g., hypertension, smoking), usually occur later in the disease.

    Motor neuropathy (**choice C**) is rare in diabetes and usually occurs later in the disease (at about 10 years). It is usually manifested by foot or wrist drop (peroneal and radial nerve palsies, respectively).

7. **The correct answer is B.** Maintaining the Hb_{Alc} at 7% or less indicates tight sugar control, which reduces or prevents retinopathy.

    Although a funduscopic examination (**choice A**) would certainly discover the disease, it would not prevent or delay the onset of it.

    Choice C would accelerate and worsen the retinopathy.

    Performing a glucose tolerance test (**choice D**) would be helpful in the diagnosis of hypoglycemia.

    Choice E is indicated for microscopic proteinuria, indicating kidney damage secondary to diabetes mellitus.

8. **The correct answer is D.** Rosiglitazone has been demonstrated to cause edema in patients.

    Choices A, B, C, and E are not known to have edema as a side effect.

9. **The correct answer is A.** Embryonal carcinomas occur most commonly in the 20-30 age group and are more aggressive than seminomas. These tumors present with testicular enlargement, and 30% have metastasized at the time of diagnosis. Serum AFP is usually elevated. They are less radiosensitive than seminomas.

    Interstitial (Leydig) cell tumors (**choices B and E**) can produce androgens, estrogens, or corticosteroids. In children, they often present with masculinization or feminization. In adults, they often present with gynecomastia. Microscopically, tumor cells resemble normal Leydig cells with round nuclei, eosinophilic cytoplasm, and lipid granules. Approximately half the tumors contain cigar-shaped crystalloids of Reinke.

    Seminomas (**choice C**) occur most commonly in the fourth decade of life. Microscopic exam reveals sheets of uniform polyhedral cells divided by fibrous septa of connective tissue; lymphocytes and multinucleated giant cells may also be present. These tumors are highly radiosensitive.

    Sertoli cell tumors (**choice D**) can produce small amounts of androgens or estrogens, but usually not enough to cause endocrinologic changes. They may present with testicular enlargement. Microscopic exam reveals uniform, tall, polyhedral cells with clear cytoplasm, growing in cords resembling spermatic tubules.

10. **The correct answer is B.** This patient has iron deficiency anemia, and in a young female the most common cause is heavy menstruation.

    Although **choices A, C, D, and E** can cause anemia, they are not the most common etiology of iron deficiency anemia.

11. **The correct answer is E.** Erythrocytes have a life-span of about 110 days in the bloodstream. Since the circulating erythrocytes have no nucleus, produce no RNA, and make no protein, there is no way for the circulating erythrocytes to utilize the newly available iron. Thus the older cells, many of which will still remain in the bloodstream, will have an unchanged appearance after iron therapy. The erythrocytes newly released into the bloodstream had an adequate iron supply during their development and will consequently be normal. The result is that the peripheral blood smear shows a mixture of normal red cells and hypochromic, microcytic red cells.

12. **The correct answer is D.** This pattern of lesions is seen in scabies, a contagious skin disease characterized by intense itching. Scabies is caused by infestation with small, burrowing mites (*Sarcoptes scabiei*).

    Dermatitis herpetiformis (**choice A**) typically affects the scalp, shoulders, anterior surface of the knees, elbows, and the small of the back.

    Lichen planus (**choice B**) affects the mouth, anterior forearms, genitalia, the small of the back, and the posterior aspect of the leg below the knee.

    Photosensitivity (**choice C**) produces skin changes in the face and anterior neck except below the chin, the back of the neck, and the dorsum of the hands.

    Seborrheic rashes (**choice E**) affect the scalp, posterior surface of the head, neck, and shoulders, the perianal region, chin, groin, umbilicus, and sternum.

13. **The correct answer is E.** Syncope has a broad differential diagnosis, since fainting can be produced by a wide variety of mechanisms. All of the mechanisms listed in the answers can produce syncope, but only the Valsalva mechanism (in which high intra-abdominal pressures trigger a reflex fall in cardiac output) is specifically associated with defecation. This mechanism can also produce fainting during weight-lifting and with the use of wind instruments.

Anoxic "seizures" (nonepileptic; **choice A**) are fainting spells that occur because a patient holds his/her breath while experiencing severe pain or intense emotion.

Hyperventilation (**choice B**), typically related to anxiety, can also cause fainting.

Patients who are hypovolemic (**choice C**) because of medical reasons (e.g., hemorrhage, acute sodium or water loss, burns, Addison disease) tend to be hypotensive and may faint.

Patients with cardiac arrhythmias (**choice D**) are prone to fainting spells.

14. **The correct answer is A.** The child has the most common variant (type I) of osteogenesis imperfecta, which is an autosomal dominant genetic defect in the synthesis of type I collagen, due to decreased synthesis of the procollagen alpha$_1$(1) amino acid chain. This defect (unlike that of the perinatal, lethal, type II form of osteogenesis imperfecta) is compatible with survival but does cause skeletal fragility, dentinogenesis imperfecta (abnormal teeth), blue sclera, joint laxity, and hearing impairment. Unfortunately, a number of children with this defect have been removed from their parents because of "abuse," only to have the broken bones continue in the new environment. Type I collagen is found in skin, bone, tendons, and most other organs.

Type II collagen (**choice B**) is found in cartilage and vitreous humor.

Type III collagen (**choice C**) is found in blood vessels, uterus, and skin.

Type IV collagen (**choice D**) makes basement membranes.

Type V collagen (**choice E**) is a minor component of interstitial tissues and blood vessels. There are also type VI-XI collagens, which are minor constituents of various tissues.

15. **The correct answer is B.** This question concerns a COMLEX-favorite topic—pneumoconioses. Be sure to know the classic clues associated with each of the answer choices to this question. Asbestosis is a disease caused by a family of fibrous silicates commonly found in shipyards, insulation, and roofing industries. Many years after exposure, patients complain of dyspnea and chronic dry cough, along with recurrent respiratory infections (especially viral) and weight loss. A classic pathologic finding is lower lobe interstitial fibrosis with septal wall widening that is worse near the periphery of the lung. Chest x-ray film often reveals hyperinflation of the normal parenchyma leading to "honeycombing." Calcified parietal pleural plaques are also commonly present. Secondary bronchiectasis may complicate the picture.

Anthracosis (**choice A**) is due to the inhalation of carbonaceous particles by city dwellers, cigarette smokers, and miners. Deposition of carbon dust can be seen as black pigment in lung parenchyma, pleura, and lymph nodes. When isolated, it is not associated with systemic disease.

Berylliosis (**choice C**) is due to heavy exposure to airborne beryllium or its salts. Because of its high tensile strength and resistance to heat and fatigue, beryllium is used in the electronic, ceramic, aerospace, and nuclear energy industries. Disease due to beryllium probably represents a type IV hypersensitivity reaction, with noncaseating granuloma formation and eventual fibrosis. There is increased risk of bronchogenic carcinoma.

Byssinosis (**choice D**) is a type of hypersensitivity pneumonitis that can occur with exposure to cotton, linen, or hemp. It is associated with histamine-related bronchospasm.

Silicosis (**choice E**) occurs with prolonged exposure to silica dust (mining, glass production, sand blasting, farming, and road construction). This insidious disease can progress to respiratory failure and death and is associated with increased risk for tuberculosis. Classic x-ray findings include calcified lymph nodes that produce an "eggshell" pattern. The disease initially involves the upper lobes and perihilar region. Pleural involvement creates dense fibrous plaques and adhesions that may obliterate the pleural cavities. Uninvolved parenchyma tends to be hyperinflated and emphysematous.

16. **The correct answer is E.** These are known as asbestos bodies (ferruginous bodies).

Anthracotic macrophages (**choice A**), which contain black cytoplasmic carbon particles, are associated with smoking.

Curschmann spirals (**choice B**) are mucous plugs present in bronchial lavage and are associated with COPD.

Charcot-Leyden crystals (**choice C**) are derived from enzymes present within eosinophils and are associated with asthma.

Choice D is known as squamous pearls, which are layers of keratinized proteins. They are dislodged squamous cells from the bronchial epithelium and are considered normal in a specimen from a bronchial lavage.

17. **The correct answer is B.** This boy has nephrotic syndrome: edema, heavy proteinuria with a benign urinary sediment, hypoalbuminemia, and hypercholesterolemia. Of the choices listed, only minimal change nephropathy is a recognized cause of nephrotic syndrome. It is the most common cause of nephrotic syndrome in children.

None of the other choices are consistent with the clinical history; they are causes of nephritis, not nephrosis. Remember that nephritic patients present with hypertension, moderate proteinuria, hematuria, and an active urinary sediment with red blood cell casts.

18. **The correct answer is E.** In this item, the clinical information is really just "window dressing" for the actual question. All you are being asked is, "What is the most common type of cancer seen in the bladder?" The answer is that 90% of primary bladder cancers are transitional cell carcinomas, derived from bladder urothelium (a transitional cell epithelium). Let's take a moment to review the classic clues associated with bladder carcinoma: exposure to industrial chemicals, cigarette smoking, and infection with *Schistosoma haematobium* (predisposes to squamous cell type). Remember that a patient's occupation is usually stated for a reason.

All of the other answer choices are quite rare by comparison.

19. **The correct answer is B.** Pancreatic islet tumors, which may produce gastrin and secondarily Zollinger-Ellison syndrome, are a feature of multiple endocrine neoplasia type I (MEN I). Other features of MEN I are tumors of the parathyroid (the resulting hypercalcemia and hypercalciuria leads to kidney stones), adrenal <u>cortex</u>, and pituitary gland. In general, the tumors in the MEN syndromes may be expressed at different times in a patient's life, and not all patients exhibit the full syndromes.

Endocrine tumors are not a feature of familial polyposis coli (**choice A**), which is instead characterized by colonic polyps and colon cancer.

MEN type IIA (**choice C**) features tumors of the adrenal <u>medulla</u> (pheochromocytoma), medullary carcinoma of the thyroid, and parathyroid hyperplasia or adenoma.

MEN type IIB (**choice D**) closely resembles type IIA but also includes mucosal neuromas, and less often includes parathyroid diseases.

MEN type III (**choice E**) is now considered to be the same as MEN type IIB.

20. **The correct answer is E.** Diethylstilbestrol, or DES, is an estrogen analog that was prescribed in the 1950s-1970s for prevention of spontaneous abortion. The progeny of woman taking DES were often diagnosed with clear cell vaginal or cervical adenocarcinoma, which is rarely seen in unexposed women.

Bladder cancer (**choice A**) is often seen in individuals exposed to beta-naphthalene dyes or phenacetin.

Endometrial carcinoma (**choice B**) is seen in individuals on long-term estrogen therapy, but was not seen in the progeny of DES-treated women.

Ovarian carcinoma (**choice C**) is increased in nulliparous women and in those with a family history of the disorder.

Renal cell carcinoma (**choice D**) has been linked to such epidemiologic factors as smoking. The incidence is increased in patients with von Hippel-Lindau syndrome.

21. **The correct answer is C.** The most common esophageal cancer is squamous cell in origin (although the incidence of adenocarcinoma is rising). Recall that the esophageal mucosa consists of stratified, nonkeratinized, squamous epithelium. Smoking and alcohol increase the risk for the development of esophageal squamous cell carcinoma. Suspect cancer when there are signs like rapid weight loss in a short period of time and symptoms such as dysphagia, hematemesis, and anorexia.

Glandular epithelium (**choice A**) is associated with adenocarcinoma, which is often associated with Barrett's esophagus. This is not as common as squamous cell carcinoma, especially in smokers.

A mesenchymal tumor (**choice B**) is a sarcoma.

A teratoma can be derived from all three germ layers (**choice D**), e.g., a dermoid cyst in the ovary.

Transitional cell morphology (**choice E**) is found in the urinary system and not in the esophagus, unless a urinary tract tumor was metastatic to that location.

22. **The correct answer is C.** This patient has esophageal cancer and should have been advised to quit alcohol use and smoking, which are known to increase the risk for developing esophageal squamous cell carcinoma.

The patient has lost weight already because of his condition; this is a symptom and would not be a preventative measure (**choice A**).

Drinking red wine (**choice B**) may be helpful for the heart, but as mentioned, alcohol increases the risk for developing esophageal cancer.

Although some believe that smoking cigars (**choice D**) is safer than smoking cigarettes, the fact is that it is even worse than cigarette smoking.

Eating soft foods and liquids (**choice E**) would not be preventative.

23. **The correct answer is B.** This is a two-step question. First, you need to make a diagnosis. In this case, the combination of viral illness plus aspirin followed by neurologic symptoms should have led you straight to the diagnosis of Reye syndrome. Next, what are the liver changes associated with this condition? The answer is that the liver will characteristically show microvesicular fatty changes. Note that the neurologic symptoms result from encephalopathy and that the brain will develop cerebral edema that may lead to herniation.

Diffuse fibrosis, with areas of regeneration (**choice A**), is characteristic of cirrhosis.

Hemosiderin deposits (**choice C**) would be seen in patients with hemochromatosis.

There is no hepatocyte necrosis (**choice D**) in Reye syndrome, although mitochondrial effects can be seen on electron microscopy.

Mallory bodies (**choice E**) can be seen in alcoholic hepatitis, Wilson disease, hepatocellular carcinoma, and primary biliary cirrhosis. They are not seen in Reye syndrome.

24. **The correct answer is B.** This patient presents with five of the six clinical criteria associated with Kawasaki disease: fever, conjunctivitis, oral involvement, rash, and cervical lymphadenopathy. Edema, erythema, or desquamation of the hands and feet is the sixth sign. (Fulfillment of at least five criteria is necessary to make the diagnosis.) The disease usually occurs in children younger than 4 years, but has been reported in patients up to 34 years of age. Multiple members of the same household might be affected. The syndrome was first described in Japan and is still more common there. The etiology is still unknown, but a viral or immunologic basis for the disease is suggested suspected. The disease involves inflammation and necrosis of the blood vessel wall and possible aneurysm formation. The most hazardous potential complication is the development of coronary aneurysm, thrombosis, or rupture.

Henoch-Schönlein purpura (**choice A**) is a hypersensitivity angiitis that occurs in children. It is characterized by nonthrombocytopenic purpura, skin lesions, joint involvement, colicky abdominal pain, and renal lesions. A classic clue to the diagnosis is the appearance of lesions on the extensor surfaces of the limbs and across the buttocks.

Polyarteritis nodosa (**choice C**) is a systemic necrotizing vasculitis. Though the disease is most common in young adults (which may have led you to choose this answer), patients present with low-grade fever, weakness, and weight loss. They may also have abdominal pain, hematuria, renal failure, hypertension, and leukocytosis.

Rheumatic fever (**choice D**) is a recurrent inflammatory disease that typically follows streptococcal pharyngitis. Onset is typically 1-3 weeks after infection. The major Jones criteria are migratory polyarthritis, erythema marginatum, Sydenham chorea, subcutaneous nodules, and carditis. The minor criteria are previous rheumatic fever, elevated temperature, arthralgias, prolonged PR interval, elevated erythrocyte sedimentation rate (ESR), leukocytosis, and elevated C-reactive protein. These are very testable concepts (not only on the COMLEX but also during your pediatrics rotation), so memorize them.

Takayasu arteritis (**choice E**) is a granulomatous inflammation of medium-to-large arteries, often branches of the aortic arch. Although it commonly affects Asian women between the ages of 15 and 45 (which might have led you to choose this answer), its clinical presentation includes ocular disturbances, neurologic abnormalities, and weak pulses in the upper extremities. Weakness, fever, malaise, and arthralgias may also occur.

25. **The correct answer is B.** This patient has Kawasaki syndrome; the most serious complication is a ruptured coronary artery aneurysm.

All other choices are associated with other diseases.

26. **The correct answer is B.** Both patients should receive serial echocardiograms monitoring specifically for coronary artery aneurysm.

All other choices are appropriate for other diseases.

27. **The correct answer is C.** Even though the patient is 3 years old and normally should not be given aspirin, this is one disease in which aspirin therapy has been shown to reduce the risk for the severe complications of Kawasaki disease, especially coronary artery aneurysm. The benefits of aspirin therapy far outweigh the risk for Reye syndrome, but the patient also should be monitored for the symptoms of this condition.

Although **choices A and B** help reduce the fever, they do not prevent the complications.

Choices D and E are not helpful in preventing the complications of Kawasaki syndrome.

28. **The correct answer is A.** Choriocarcinomas are most common in men aged 15-25 years. These tumors are highly malignant and are associated with gynecomastia or testicular enlargement. Laboratory studies typically show elevated serum and urine human chorionic gonadotropin (hCG) levels.

Sertoli (**choice B**) and Leydig (**choice E**) cell tumors can produce small amounts of androgens or estrogens, but usually not enough to cause endocrinologic changes. They may present with testicular enlargement. Microscopic exam reveals uniform, tall, polyhedral cells with clear cytoplasm, growing in cords resembling spermatic tubules.

Teratomas (**choice C**) can occur at any age but are most common in infants and children. This type of tumor appears as a testicular mass. Microscopically, it may show differentiation into any of the three germ layers: endoderm, mesoderm, or ectoderm.

Yolk sac tumors (**choice D**) are most common in infants and children; they are rare in adults. They can also coincide with embryonal carcinomas. Serum AFP is elevated.

29. **The correct answer is D.** Although rare now because of advances in treatment, syphilitic aortitis and aneurysm are still seen, especially in underserved populations. This complication generally occurs 10-40 years after initial infection. The vasa vasorum of the aorta undergoes obliterative endarteritis, leading to atrophy of the muscularis and elastic tissues of the aorta and dilatation. Linear calcifications are often seen in the ascending aorta by x-ray. The intimal wrinkling or "tree barking" is also a common feature. Syphilitic aneurysm can be associated with respiratory distress, cough, congestive heart failure, and, rarely, rupture.

Atherosclerosis (**choice A**) is the most common cause of aortic aneurysms. These are most often located in the abdominal aorta, distal to the renal arteries. Intimal wrinkling and linear calcifications are not seen.

Hypertension (**choice B**) is usually responsible for dissecting aneurysms located within 10 cm of the aortic valve. Patients present with sudden chest pain that is usually severe and tearing in nature. The chronic hypertension causes a cystic medial necrosis, allowing the separation of vessel layers.

Marfan syndrome, an autosomal dominant connective tissue disorder (**choice C**), is also associated with dissecting aneurysms, usually of the ascending aorta. The patients are often very tall with arachnodactyly and ligamentous laxity. Their life-span is generally shortened. This patient's description and age are not consistent with this diagnosis.

Takayasu arteritis (**choice E**) is a syndrome characterized by ocular disturbances and weak pulses in the arms. It occurs most frequently in young females. It is considered a giant cell arteritis and does not cause aneurysms.

30. **The correct answer is D.** This patient has been diagnosed with tertiary syphilis and would have benefited greatly from early administration of benzathine penicillin G to prevent this late-stage complication of syphilitic aortic dissection.

Choices A, B, C, and E would have done nothing to prevent the formation of the aortic dissection because they are not effective against the causative agent of syphilis, *Treponema pallidum*.

31. **The correct answer is E.** Many different types of structures and cells, normal and pathologic, can be found in bronchial and alveolar cavities. These can be observed in bronchial washings obtained by bronchoalveolar lavage—a procedure in which buffered saline is injected into a peripheral bronchus and then reaspirated. Hemosiderin-laden macrophages, or *heart failure cells*, indicate prior episodes of pulmonary edema or intra-alveolar hemorrhage of any cause (e.g., Goodpasture syndrome).

Charcot-Leyden crystals (**choice A**) are rhomboid structures derived from enzymes present within eosinophils. They are commonly found in patients with allergic conditions (asthma).

Curschmann spirals (**choice B**) are corkscrew-shaped casts resulting from mucus plugs present in smaller bronchi and commonly found in association with chronic obstructive disease.

Fat-laden macrophages (**choice C**) have been observed in cases of lipid pneumonia.

Ferruginous bodies (**choice D**) are needle-shaped structures surrounded by an iron-protein coat. Ferruginous bodies are also known as *asbestos bodies*, since asbestos is the most common (although not the sole) source of these structures.

32. **The correct answer is B.** There are many clues in the question that should have guided you to this choice. The laboratory findings are classic for type IIa hyperlipidemia. These patients have LDL receptor deficiencies and are at a great risk of advanced coronary atherosclerosis. Since it is autosomal dominant, the patient's father could have been affected as well.

Type I hyperlipidemia (**choice A**), or familial hyperchylomicronemia, is caused by a lipoprotein lipase deficiency. These patients have high serum triglycerides and normal cholesterol. They do not have a substantially higher risk of atherosclerosis.

Type IIb hyperlipidemia (**choice C**), or familial combined hyperlipidemia, presents as elevated serum LDL, VLDL, cholesterol, and triglycerides. These patients have an increased incidence of atherosclerosis.

Type III hyperlipidemia (**choice D**), or familial dysbetalipoproteinemia, presents as increased serum cholesterol and triglycerides. The mode of inheritance is not understood, but apoprotein E is affected and the risk of atherosclerosis is great.

Type IV hyperlipidemia (**choice E**), or familial hyper-triglyceridemia, presents as increased triglycerides with normal cholesterol and LDL. The disease may be sporadic and is possibly associated with an increased risk for atherosclerosis.

33. **The correct answer is C.** The vignette illustrates a typical presentation for a tumor of the heart. Primary cardiac tumors are rare and usually require a intensive work-up to pinpoint the diagnosis. Seventy-five percent of primary cardiac tumors are benign; among these, myxoma is the most common. The tumors are usually single, and the most common location is the left atrium. They may cause syncopal episodes or even shock and death due to obstruction by a "ball valve" mechanism.

Angiosarcoma (**choice A**) is a malignant tumor of vascular origin that can occur as a primary cardiac tumor. It is the most common malignant primary cardiac tumor, but it is still very rare. Angiosarcoma usually affects the right side of the heart.

Mesothelioma (**choice B**) is a benign tumor of mesothelial origin that can rarely present as a primary cardiac tumor. It is usually a small intramyocardial tumor that presents with disturbances of the conduction system of the heart.

Rhabdomyoma (**choice D**) is a benign tumor of muscle origin. It can occur as a primary cardiac tumor, typically in infants and children, in whom it may be associated with tuberous sclerosis. It usually occurs in the ventricles.

Rhabdomyosarcoma (**choice E**) is a malignant neoplasm that can also occur as a rare primary cardiac tumor. It is of muscle origin and usually affects the right heart.

34. **The correct answer is C.** Neonatal respiratory distress syndrome (hyaline membrane disease) occurs in premature infants as the result of a deficiency in pulmonary surfactant (composed primarily of dipalmitoyl lecithin). This is due to inadequate lecithin synthesis by immature type II pneumocytes. It can be diagnosed before birth by analyzing the amniotic fluid: a lecithin:sphingomyelin ratio greater than 2:1 and the presence of phosphatidylglycerol implies lung maturity. The syndrome is the most common cause of death in premature neonates. Risk factors include birth before the 37th week of gestation, birth by cesarean section, and maternal diabetes.

Less than 0.5 L of amniotic fluid (**choice A**) is the definition of oligohydramnios, which can be associated with renal agenesis. (Failure of the fetal kidneys to produce urine will result in a low amniotic fluid volume.)

Alpha-1 antitrypsin deficiency in amniotic fluid (**choice B**) is not associated with lung immaturity. However, deficiency of this enzyme is associated with both emphysema and liver failure in adults.

Elevated maternal HbA$_{1c}$ (**choice D**) would indicate poor glycemic control in the mother and a potentially increased risk for fetal abnormalities, but it does not serve as direct evidence of lung immaturity.

Elevated maternal serum alpha-fetoprotein (AFP; **choice E**) would be expected in fetal neural tube defects. A low maternal AFP is associated with fetal Down syndrome.

35. **The correct answer is C.** Cheyne-Stokes breathing is characterized by the pattern described in the question stem, and is considered an ominous prognostic sign when observed in a seriously ill patient. This form of respiratory dysfunction suggests that central respiratory mechanisms are no longer functioning adequately.

Apneustic breathing (**choice A**) is seen after head trauma and is characterized by inspiratory breath-holding that lasts many seconds, followed by brief exhalations.

Biot's breathing (**choice B**) is seen in some patients with CNS disease (e.g., meningitis). It consists of periods of normal breathing interrupted suddenly by periods of apnea.

Hysterical breathing (**choice D**) may produce hyperventilation, i.e., rapid, intense breathing that causes the PaCO$_2$ to decrease.

Kussmaul breathing (**choice E**) occurs in diabetic coma and consists of continuous, rapid, deep breathing.

36. **The correct answer is C.** The ductus arteriosus connects the aorta with the pulmonary artery. If it remains patent after birth, it allows oxygenated blood to flow from the aorta to the pulmonary artery. In this patient, who has tetralogy of Fallot with complete right ventricular outflow obstruction, this anastomosis is a crucial source of blood to the pulmonary vasculature.

A bicuspid aortic valve (**choice A**) may be asymptomatic but can lead to infective endocarditis, left ventricular overload, and sudden death. It is a common cause of aortic stenosis. It would not benefit a patient with tetralogy of Fallot in any way.

Ostium secundum defect (**choice B**) is the most common form of atrial septal defect (ASD). ASD is an acyanotic congenital heart disease that would not improve cardiovascular function in a patient with tetralogy of Fallot.

A patent foramen ovale (**choice D**) is a slit-like remnant of communication between the left and right atria in the fetus. It is usually not of clinical significance.

A preductal coarctation of the aorta (**choice E**) involves narrowing of the aorta proximal to the opening of the ductus arteriosus. This would prevent adequate blood flow through a possible life-preserving patent ductus arteriosus and would result in the patient's death.

37. **The correct answer is E.** This patient is experiencing symptoms of hypocalcemia secondary to diminished parathyroid hormone (PTH) secretion. This must always be considered in a patient who undergoes total or subtotal thyroidectomy, because the parathyroids are nestled in the tissue surrounding the thyroid gland. Surgical attempts to leave portions of the parathyroids intact are sometimes unsuccessful. Other causes of decreased PTH include neck irradiation, autoimmune phenomena (polyglandular autoimmune syndromes), dysembryogenesis (as in DiGeorge syndrome), and heavy metal damage (Wilson disease, hemosiderosis, hemochromatosis).

Bone metastases (**choice A**) would cause hypercalcemia, as a result of osteolysis.

Hashimoto thyroiditis (**choice B**) is the most common cause of hypothyroidism and results in decreased thyroid hormone and elevated thyroid-stimulating hormone (TSH) levels. Serum calcium and PTH should be normal.

Hypervitaminosis D (**choice C**) would cause hypercalcemia.

Hypomagnesemia (**choice D**) may cause a functional hypoparathyroidism, because magnesium is needed for PTH activity in tissue. In such a case, however, actual PTH levels would not be decreased. Severe hypomagnesemia (levels below 0.4 mmol/L [1 mg/dl] blocks release of PTH, but mild hypomagnesemia can actually enhance PTH release.

38. **The correct answer is D.** Secondary hyperthyroidism presents in a similar clinical fashion to primary hyperthyroidism. However, secondary hyperthyroidism is the result of a pituitary hyperfunction resulting in an excess production of thyroid-stimulating hormone (TSH) and a secondary elevation of thyroid hormones T4 and T3. Some of the symptoms of hyperthyroidism include nervousness, anxiety, heat intolerance, increased sweating, tachycardia, amenorrhea, and infertility.

Decreased thyroxine-binding globulin (TBG; **choice A**) is not by itself diagnostic.

Elevated T3 (**choice B**) and T4 (**choice C**) are found in both secondary and primary hyperthyroidism.

The presence of serum thyroid-stimulating autoantibodies (**choice E**) is diagnostic of Graves disease, a cause of primary hyperthyroidism.

39. **The correct answer is C.** Hemoglobinuria means that there is hemoglobin in the urine and suggests hemolysis in a patient with symptoms of anemia. The patient's reticulocytosis further supports this suspicion. Reticulocytosis refers to an increase in the number of circulating reticulocytes. Reticulocytes are immature red blood cells that typically constitute approximately 1% of circulating red blood cells. The reticulocyte count is used to differentiate between anemias due to decreased erythropoiesis (low reticulocyte count since marrow can't produce reticulocytes) and anemias secondary to blood loss or peripheral red blood cell destruction (hemolysis; reticulocyte count elevates as marrow tries to compensate).

Of the choices listed, only G6PD deficiency leads to hemolysis. (In the absence of G6PD, there is a deficiency of NADPH and, therefore, a deficiency of reduced glutathione. This causes oxidative stress on the erythrocyte that leads to hemolysis.) Other causes of hemolytic anemia include hereditary spherocytosis, sickle cell disease, thalassemias, autoimmune hemolytic anemia, red blood cell trauma, and paroxysmal nocturnal hemoglobinuria.

All the distracters would lead to anemia secondary to decreased erythropoiesis and would therefore be associated with low reticulocyte counts.

Chronic renal disease (**choice A**) results in decreased production of the hormone erythropoietin, leading to decreased reticulocyte (and therefore erythrocyte) production.

Folate deficiency (**choice B**) results in decreased red blood cell production and a megaloblastic anemia characterized by macrocytic red blood cells and hypersegmented neutrophils.

Iron deficiency (**choice D**) results in a microcytic, hypochromic anemia. An elevated reticulocyte count after administration of ferrous sulfate would indicate improvement of the anemia with therapy.

Pernicious anemia (**choice E**) refers to vitamin B_{12} malabsorption secondary to antibodies against intrinsic factor or intrinsic factor receptors. B_{12} deficiency leads to megaloblastic anemia.

40. **The correct answer is E.** Sézary syndrome is a rare chronic disease associated with progressive, pruritic erythroderma, exfoliation, and lymphadenopathy. It is related to the cutaneous T-cell lymphoma mycosis fungoides, and may be a leukemic variant of this condition.

Burkitt lymphoma (**choice A**) is endemic in Africa and sporadic in the U.S. It usually affects children or young adults. In Africa, it often arises in the mandible or max-illa. In the U.S., it often arises in the abdomen. It is related to EBV infection, which may act as a mitogen, initiating a sustained polyclonal activation of B cells. This eventually leads to a neoplastic proliferation of a single B-cell clone after a chromosomal translocation occurs. Microscopic examination reveals a uniform sea of moderately large cells with round nuclei, multiple nucleoli, moderately basophilic cytoplasm with lipid-containing vacuoles, frequent mitoses, and many macrophages with ingested debris ("starry sky pattern").

Histiocytic lymphoma (choice B) is one of the most common non-Hodgkin lymphomas. It is usually diffuse but may be nodular. The diffuse form typically presents with nodal involvement (usually on one side of the diaphragm), extranodal involvement (gastrointestinal tract, skin, brain, bone), or, rarely, liver and spleen involvement. Microscopic examination shows large tumor cells with vesicular nuclei and prominent nucleoli. The cells may be pleomorphic.

Lymphoblastic lymphoma (choice C) is a diffuse lymphoma that is most common in adolescents and young adults, but there is a bimodal age distribution with a second peak in the 70s. The male:female ratio is 2.5:1. The disease is often associated with a mediastinal mass (thymoma), suggesting thymic origin for the neoplastic cells. These cells often express T-cell markers and resemble the lymphoblasts of ALL. They have uniform size, scant cytoplasm, delicate chromatin, and absent nucleoli. The nuclear membrane may be loculated or convoluted. There are frequent mitoses.

Lymphocytic lymphoma (choice D) occurs in two forms: well-differentiated (WDLL) and poorly differentiated (PDLL). WDLL usually affects older patients, who present with generalized lymphadenopathy and mild hepatosplenomegaly. Microscopic examination reveals small round lymphocytes with scant cytoplasm, dark nuclei, and rare mitoses. PDLL patients are usually middle-aged or older. Most present with lymphadenopathy and with infiltration of bone marrow, liver, and spleen at the time of diagnosis. Microscopic examination reveals atypical lymphocytes, often larger than in WDLL. Nuclei are irregular, angular, and indented, and have coarse chromatin. Mitoses are rare.

41. **The correct answer is B.** This patient has irreversible parkinsonism induced by a contaminant of illicit drugs—methylphenyltetrahydropyridine (MPTP), a meperidine analog. The parkinsonism is caused by the drug's destruction of dopaminergic neurons in the substantia nigra. The clinical signs and symptoms described in the question are classically associated with parkinsonism. Lewy bodies are neuronal inclusions that are characteristic of Parkinson disease. The latest research suggests that structures resembling immature

Lewy bodies appear in MPTP-induced parkinsonism.

Hirano bodies (choice A) are intraneuronal, eosinophilic rod-like inclusions in the hippocampus that are associated with Alzheimer disease. They may occur in normal elderly brains as well.

Lipofuscin granules (choice C) are pigmented cytoplasmic inclusions that commonly accumulate with aging. They are believed to be residual bodies derived from lysosomes.

Negri bodies (choice D) are intracytoplasmic inclusions that are pathognomonic for rabies. They are found in the pyramidal cells of the hippocampus, the brainstem, and the Purkinje cells of the cerebellum.

Neurofibrillary tangles (choice E) consist of intracytoplasmic degenerated neurofilaments and are seen in patients with Alzheimer disease. Amyloid plaques are also commonly seen in these patients.

42. **The correct answer is A.** The patient has myasthenia gravis (MG), which typically produces weakness worsening over the course of the day. It often affects the eye muscles and can produce diplopia. Neostigmine, an acetylcholinesterase inhibitor, would temporarily improve the patient's condition, which is associated with antibodies against nicotinic acetylcholine receptors present on skeletal muscle.

Antibodies to double-stranded DNA (choice B), as well as anti-Smith antibodies, are found specifically in systemic lupus erythematosus. Peripheral nuclear staining is observed on immunofluorescence.

Antibodies to dystrophin (choice C) do not produce recognized pathology. Abnormal or absent dystrophin, resulting from mutations in the X chromosome, is associated with Becker and Duchenne muscular dystrophy, respectively. Pelvic girdle weakness and ataxia are classic symptoms.

Antibodies to erythrocyte surface antigens (choice D) can be found in warm antibody autoimmune hemolytic anemia. Patients with this condition would have a positive direct Coomb's test.

Antibodies to myelin (choice E) may play a role in multiple sclerosis, which is presumed to be of autoimmune etiology. This demyelinating disease is characterized by the spontaneous appearance and remission of symptoms such as hyperreflexia, weakness, spasticity, dysarthria, tremor, ataxia, and visual disturbances. Neostigmine would not produce any improvement.

43. **The correct answer is C.** Ten to twenty percent of patients with Crohn disease and ulcerative colitis develop an arthritis that resembles ankylosing spondylitis. Similar arthropathies are seen in psoriasis or Reiter

syndrome (arthritis, urethritis, conjunctivitis, and rash following chlamydial infection), as well as related syndromes seen following *Shigella, Salmonella,* or *Yersinia* enterocolitis. The other answers are distracters.

44. **The correct answer is D.** This child has minimal change disease, which is the major cause (more than 90% of cases) of nephrotic syndrome in children aged 2-6 years. The most prominent clinical chemistry finding in these patients is massive proteinuria. The urinary protein in minimal change disease, in contrast to other causes of nephrotic syndrome, is often composed predominantly of albumin. Many other clinical chemistry changes may also be seen, including decreased serum albumin levels, hyperlipidemia, increased serum levels of alpha$_2$- and beta-globulins, decreased IgG, and increased fibrinogen. Minimal change disease characteristically shows normal or near normal appearance of the glomeruli by light microscopy and extensive fusion of foot processes of the glomerular podocytes by electron microscopy. A point not always recognized by beginners is that the podocyte alterations may represent a reaction to, rather than a cause of, the proteinuria (e.g., an attempt to "seal the holes" in the glomerulus), since varying degrees of foot process fusion (together with more specific features) may sometimes be seen in other glomerular diseases associated with the nephrotic syndrome.

Alpha$_2$-globulin levels (**choice A**) are increased, rather than decreased, in minimal change disease.

Fibrinogen levels are increased, rather than decreased (**choice B**).

Serum calcium levels (**choice C**) are typically decreased in the nephrotic syndrome, possibly because of renal loss of vitamin D binding protein.

Red blood cell casts in the urine (**choice E**) are indicative of glomerulonephritis, rather than the nephrotic syndrome.

45. **The correct answer is B.** The lateral striate arteries are penetrating branches of the middle cerebral artery that supply the caudate, putamen, globus pallidus, and internal capsule. Lacunar infarcts, small cavitary lesions that commonly occur in the distribution of the lateral striate and lenticulostriate arteries, are relatively common in the context of long-standing hypertension. The basal ganglia and thalamus are favorite sites for lacunar infarcts.

The anterior cerebral artery (**choice A**) supplies the medial surface of the cerebral hemispheres extending from the frontal pole to the parieto-occipital sulcus. It therefore supplies the leg and foot area of the motor and sensory cortices.

The posterior cerebral artery (**choice C**) supplies the occipital lobe, which contains the visual cortex. Occlusion of this vessel results in contralateral hemianopia with macular sparing. This vessel also supplies the inferior surface of the temporal lobe (which contains the hippocampal formation) and the thalamus, and provides the major blood supply to the midbrain.

The superior cerebellar artery (**choice D**) supplies the superior cerebellar peduncle, the superior surface of the cerebellum, and the deep cerebellar nuclei. It also supplies the dorsolateral tegmentum of the rostral pons.

The vertebral artery (**choice E**), a branch of the subclavian artery, gives rise to the posterior inferior cerebellar artery (PICA) and the anterior spinal artery. PICA supplies the dorsolateral quadrant of the medulla and the inferior surface of the cerebellum. The anterior spinal artery supplies the anterior two thirds of the spinal cord.

46. **The correct answer is D.** This patient has paroxysmal supraventricular tachycardia (PSVT), which is a regular, rapid (150-250/min) arrhythmia originating in the atria or AV node. AV nodal reentry is the most common cause of this arrhythmia (about 70% of patients). In this condition, the AV node is pathologically divided into two functional pathways. The electrical impulse usually proceeds anterograde down the slow pathway and retrograde up the fast pathway. The P waves are recorded nearly simultaneously with the QRS complexes (which occur in rapid sequence) and are therefore obscured on EKG. This arrhythmia is commonly seen in older patients, about half of whom have underlying heart disease. Reentry PSVTs can be reverted to normal sinus rhythm by interrupting the reentry pathway. For example, the performance of vagal maneuvers often improves the condition by increasing AV nodal refractoriness.

Atrial reentry (**choice A**) causes about 10% of all PSVTs. The reentrant pathway is in the atria. The P wave is recorded before the QRS complex. This arrhythmia is frequently associated with organic heart disease.

Automatic atrial conduction (**choice B**) results in about 5% of PSVTs. Often, these are not paroxysmal, last days to years, and are resistant to treatment. The P wave has an abnormal configuration.

AV dissociation (**choice C**) is caused by accelerated junctional rhythms, in which a normally latent pacemaker in the AV nodal area depolarizes at a regular, accelerated rate of 60-150/min. When the rate of the accelerated pacemaker approaches the rate of the SA node, the ectopic impulses are often conducted to the ventricles only, while the atria remain under the control of the SA node, producing AV dissociation.

Wandering atrial pacemaker (**choice E**) is a usually benign arrhythmia. The dominant pacemaker "wanders" from one atrial focus to another and in and out of the SA node.

Test-taking strategy: If you are unsure of an answer to a question, have tried to reason through the problem to no avail, and believe you must randomly guess, choose the "most common" item from among the given answer choices. Remember, the COMLEX tends to test common concepts, so the odds should be in your favor.

47. **The correct answer is A.** The figure shown depicts a lymphocyte. Lymphocytosis is commonly associated with viral infections; therefore, you should have looked for a viral disease in the answer choices. Bronchiolitis in a 2-year-old is most likely caused by respiratory syncytial virus (RSV). The rest of the diseases listed have bacterial etiologies.

Cellulitis (**choice B**) is a bacterial infection usually attributed to *Staphylococcus* or *Streptococcus*.

Diphtheria (**choice C**) is due to *Corynebacterium diphtheriae*.

Epiglottitis (**choice D**) in a 2-year-old is most likely due to Haemophilus influenzae.

Pertussis (**choice E**) is caused by *Bordetella pertussis*.

48. **The correct answer is D.** This is the classic presentation of infection with respiratory syncytial virus.

Choice A is associated with diphtheria.

Choice B is associated with epiglottitis.

Choice C is associated with pertussis.

Choice E is one of the causative agents of bacterial cellulitis infections.

49. **The correct answer is E.** The most appropriate treatment is predominantly supportive care for RSV infections. There are no known antiviral drugs available for this condition.

Choice A is the correct treatment for diphtheria.

Choice B is the treatment for cellulitis of *Streptococcus* origin.

Choice C is the treatment for pertussis.

Choice D is one of the accepted treatments for epiglottitis.

50. **The correct answer is C.** A midsystolic click and a high-pitched heart murmur in a young woman is the classic presentation of mitral valve prolapse. Patients are usually asymptomatic, but may have dyspnea, tachycardia, chest pain, syncope, eventual congestive heart failure, or, rarely, sudden death. Prolapse may coincide with tricuspid or pulmonary valve disease or with psychiatric conditions such as anxiety or depression. Complications include atrial thrombosis, calcification, infective endocarditis, emboli to the brain, rupture of chordae, mitral regurgitation, arrhythmias, and premature ventricular contractions (PVCs).

Atrial fibrillation (**choice A**) may result from chronic mitral stenosis. This valvular disease is associated with an early diastolic opening snap.

Decreased peripheral pulse pressure (**choice B**) and slowed carotid upstroke (**choice D**) are seen in aortic valve stenosis. A systolic ejection click is associated with this valvular disease.

Wide pulse pressure (**choice E**) is seen clinically as bounding pulses. It is associated with aortic valve insufficiency.

Pathology and Pathophysiology

1. A patient presents to his physician because of a chronic cough. He notes occasional streaks of blood in his sputum. Osteopathic structural examination reveals T2-T7 somatic dysfunction. A chest x-ray film reveals multinodular, cavitating lesions in the apical posterior segments of both lungs, with evident satellite lesions. The condition described is likely to occur in the apices of the lungs, rather than in the base, because the apices

   (A) are better perfused

   (B) are more acidic

   (C) contain more alveolar macrophages

   (D) have a higher P_{O_2}

   (E) ventilate better

2. A 50-year-old man presents to his physician with diarrhea, flushing, and wheezing. Physical examination is significant for a grade II/VI diastolic murmur located at the right sternal border at the 4th intercostal space. Which of the following substances is most likely to be elevated in this patient's urine?

   (A) 5-Hydroxyindoleacetic acid (5-HIAA)

   (B) Homovanillic acid (HVA)

   (C) Phenylalanine

   (D) Selegiline

   (E) Vanillylmandelic acid (VMA)

3. Many patients with cirrhosis, particularly alcoholic cirrhosis, develop gynecomastia, testicular atrophy, and impotence. Structural examination shows development of chronic somatic dysfunction at T5-T9 on the right. Which of the following is thought to be the underlying mechanism producing these changes?

   (A) Both decreased testosterone secretion and decreased extraction of androstenedione

   (B) Decreased hepatic extraction of androstenedione

   (C) Increased estrogen secretion by Leydig cells

   (D) Increased estrogen secretion by Sertoli cells

   (E) Testosterone deficiency alone

4. A 29-year-old woman comes to her physician's office complaining of headaches, fatigue, and weakness over the past several months. Physical examination is significant for pallor, tachycardia, dizziness on standing up, and koilonychia.

   Laboratory studies show:

Hemoglobin	10.2 g/dL
Hematocrit	30.8%
Serum iron	24 mg/dL
Serum ferritin	30 ng/mL
Total iron binding capacity	713 mg/dL

   A peripheral blood smear would likely show which of the following?

   (A) Macrocytosis with hypersegmented neutrophils

   (B) Microcytosis with basophilic stippling

   (C) Microcytosis with hypochromia

   (D) Numerous schistocytes

   (E) Normocytic normochromia

5. A 27-year-old African American man visits his primary care physician because of recent onset of "yellowness in the whites of his eyes." His recent history is significant for a "chest cold," for which he is taking trimethoprim-sulfamethoxazole; he is also taking fluoxetine for depression. On examination, the sclera are icteric and the mucosa beneath the tongue appears yellow. No hepatosplenomegaly is present.

Laboratory studies are as follows:

Hemoglobin	11.1 g/dL
Hematocrit	34%
Total bilirubin	6.2 mg/dL
Conjugated (direct) bilirubin	0.8 mg/dL
Alkaline phosphatase	77 U/L
AST (SGOT)	24 U/L
ALT (SGPT)	22 U/L

The most likely cause of this patient's jaundice is which of the following?

(A) Acute infectious hepatitis

(B) Cholestatic liver disease

(C) Drug reaction from fluoxetine

(D) Drug reaction from trimethoprim-sulfamethoxazole

(E) Somatic dysfunction at L2-L5

6. Autopsy investigations on a 70-year-old man with a history of peripheral vascular disease reveal an atherosclerotic plaque in the left anterior descending coronary artery, which results in 80% luminal stenosis. This atheroma is covered by a smooth endothelial lining without evidence of thrombosis, ulceration, or hemorrhage. The remaining coronary vessels are relatively spared. Which of the following clinical syndromes would most likely have resulted from this pathologic lesion?

(A) Chest pain awakening the patient in the early morning

(B) Chest pain occurring with progressive frequency and severity

(C) Chest pain precipitated by exercise and consistently relieved by rest

(D) Progressive development of congestive heart failure without chest pain

(E) Prolonged (more than 30 minutes) chest pain accompanied by shock

7. A newly pregnant patient is given folate supplements that have been shown to reduce the risk of which of the following fetal abnormalities?

(A) Arnold-Chiari malformations

(B) Germinal matrix hemorrhage

(C) Holoprosencephaly

(D) Neural tube defects

(E) Syringomyelia

8. A patient develops an acute febrile illness with shivers, nonproductive cough, and pleuritic chest pain. Five days later, he presents to the emergency department after abruptly having "coughed up" nearly a cup of blood-stained sputum. Osteopathic structural examination reveals chronic tissue-texture changes at T2-T7 bilaterally. Which of the following is most likely to be seen on a chest x-ray film?

    (A) Blunting of diaphragmatic costal angles

    (B) A cavity with a fluid level

    (C) Complete opacification of one lobe with no additional findings

    (D) Patchy consolidation centered on bronchi

    (E) Prominent bronchi that can be followed far out into the lung fields

Questions 9-10

<u>CASE A</u>

A 30-year-old woman has chronic, silver-white, scaly patches with an erythematous border on the skin of her knees and elbows.

9. Which of the following is the most likely etiology of this condition?

    (A) Autoimmune disease

    (B) Bacterial disease

    (C) Fungal disease

    (D) Granulomatous disease

    (E) Large vessel vasculitis

10. The above condition can be clinically identified by which of the following?

    (A) KOH preparation

    (B) Christmas tree distribution pattern bleeding

    (C) Removal of scale results in pinpoint bleeding

    (D) Avulsion of epidermis on gentle pressure

    (E) Tzanck smear

11. An infant born with a congenital infection has excessive growth of new bone on the anterior surface of the tibia with anterior bowing of the bone. This finding is due to which of the following processes?

    (A) Neoplastic cortical bone deposition

    (B) Neoplastic medullary bone deposition

    (C) Neoplastic periosteal bone deposition

    (D) Reactive medullary bone deposition

    (E) Reactive periosteal bone deposition

12. A 22-year-old man is evaluated for mitral regurgitation due to mitral valve prolapse. Examination reveals a tall, slender young man with long extremities and long tapering fingers. Pupillary dilation followed by slit-lamp examination reveals bilateral dislocation of the lenses of the eyes. Structural examination reveals viscerosomatic changes at T1-T4. This patient is potentially at increased risk for development of which of the following?

    (A) Aortic dissection

    (B) Lisch nodules

    (C) Noncaseating granulomata

    (D) Progressive dementia

    (E) Rapidly progressive renal failure

13. A 6-cm length of rectosigmoid colon containing a 2-cm diameter sessile polyp is surgically removed. On sectioning, the lesion shows finger-like papillae with cores of scant lamina propria. The surfaces of the papillae are covered by dysplastic columnar epithelium with considerable nuclear pleomorphism. No glandular structures are seen in the base of the lesion or in the adjacent muscle tissue. The margins of the specimen are free of dysplastic epithelium. What further therapy does this person most likely require?

    (A) Adjunct chemotherapy

    (B) Complete colectomy

    (C) Radiation therapy

    (D) Resection of regional lymph nodes

    (E) No further therapy is required

14. A 65-year-old man presents with a productive cough and difficulty breathing. Physical examination reveals multiple thoracic and rib dysfunction. His sputum culture is positive for encapsulated gram-positive cocci, which are often seen in pairs. The patient's dyspnea is primarily due to which of the following mechanisms?

    (A) Inadequate perfusion

    (B) Inadequate ventilation

    (C) Increased airway resistance

    (D) Increased lung compliance

    (E) Poor oxygen diffusion

15. A previously healthy 20-year-old woman presents to the emergency department with fever, jaundice, and confusion. Her examination is notable for a temperature of 102 F, scleral icterus, scattered petechiae on her palate and extremities, and disorientation on mental status examination. Laboratory studies reveal a platelet count of 20,000/mm³, a hemoglobin of 8 g/dL, an elevated indirect bilirubin level, and a creatinine of 5 mg/dL. Her prothrombin time (PT) and partial thromboplastin time (PTT) are both normal. Her peripheral blood smear reveals decreased platelets and numerous fragmented red blood cells. Which of the following is the most likely diagnosis in this patient?

    (A) Autoimmune hemolytic anemia
    (B) Disseminated intravascular coagulation (DIC)
    (C) Idiopathic thrombocytopenic purpura (ITP)
    (D) Thrombotic thrombocytopenic purpura (TTP)
    (E) Von Willebrand disease

16. A 52-year-old man is brought into the emergency department by his wife because he has been complaining of a severe headache. Physical examination reveals ptosis of the right eyelid with the right eye facing down and out. There is a fixed and dilated right pupil with an inability to accommodate. Structural examination reveals acute tissue-texture changes at T1-T4. Subarachnoid blood appears on non contrast CT scan. Magnetic resonance angiography (MRA) would be expected to reveal an aneurysm of which of the following arteries?

    (A) Anterior cerebral
    (B) Anterior communicating
    (C) Middle cerebral
    (D) Posterior communicating
    (E) Posterior inferior cerebellar

17. During a routine pediatric examination, a 12-year-old boy is noted to be in growth arrest. The child is obese and has multiple small bruises on his arms and legs. The patient has difficulty rising from a crouching position. Measurements of blood pressure demonstrate hypertension when compared with age-based standards. This patient most likely has which of the following disorders?

    (A) Diabetes mellitus
    (B) Graves disease
    (C) Hypothyroidism
    (D) Parathyroid adenoma
    (E) Pituitary microadenoma

18. A 15-year-old white boy presents with a hemarthrosis of the right knee joint and a recent history of protracted bleeding from cuts or scrapes. He has no family history of bleeding disorders. The patient also notes a long history of chronic abdominal discomfort and diarrhea, which has been worse for the past 6 months, occasionally accompanied by fever. Physical examination reveals a patient at the 5th percentile for both height and weight; an actively bleeding rectal fissure is also noted. Both prothrombin time (PT) and the partial thromboplastin time (PTT) are prolonged. Laboratory evaluation of the blood is likely to reveal low levels of which of the following?

    (A) Factor VIII
    (B) Factor IX
    (C) Factors II, VII, IX, and X
    (D) Factors II, V, VII, IX, and X
    (E) von Willebrand factor

19. A 63-year-old woman presents to her physician complaining of right facial numbness and weakness. Six months earlier she presented with moderate diplopia. Neurologic examination reveals a decrease of all sensation over the right face. There is decreased strength and bulk of the right masseter and temporalis muscles, decreased abduction of the right eye, and weakness of all facial muscles on the right. Structural examination reveals chronic somatic dysfunction at T1-T4. What would testing of the corneal reflex most likely reveal?

    (A) A consensual reflex but no direct reflex of the left eye

    (B) A consensual reflex but no direct reflex of the right eye

    (C) A direct reflex and a consensual reflex of the left eye

    (D) A direct reflex and a consensual reflex of the right eye

    (E) No direct reflex and no consensual reflex of the right eye

20. A 30-year-old patient presents to a physician because his morning urine had a dark red-brown color. He describes having had several months of increasing weakness and dyspnea on exertion, several episodes of cramping abdominal pain, and a recent cold. Physical examination reveals pallor and mild jaundice. Osteopathic structural examination reveals chronic tissue changes on the right side of T5-T9 spinal levels. A urine sample appears yellow and clear. Which of the following additional tests is most likely to yield an abnormal result?

    (A) Urine complete cell count

    (B) Urine free hemoglobin

    (C) Urine free myoglobin

    (D) Urine hemosiderin

    (E) Urine red cell count

21. Primary immunodeficiencies can be investigated by injecting tetanus toxoid into the medial aspect of the thigh, followed by ipsilateral inguinal node biopsy 7 days later. If this test is performed on an immunocompetent individual, which of the following would be the predominant change observed in the biopsied lymph node?

    (A) Follicular hyperplasia

    (B) Necrotizing lymphadenitis

    (C) Paracortical lymphoid hyperplasia

    (D) Sinus histiocytosis

    (E) Stellate abscesses

22. A 16-year-old boy sustains multiple fractures over the course of an intramural basketball season and is referred to a radiologist. X-ray examination of the boy's upper extremities reveals diffusely sclerotic bones with enlarged, flask-shaped radial and ulnar metaphyses. The boy's father had a similar condition as a child, but he lived in a rural area and was not further evaluated. The boy's condition is most likely due to which of the following?

    (A) Deficiency of vitamin D

    (B) Deficient osteoblastic activity

    (C) Deficient osteoclastic activity

    (D) Deficient synthesis of type I collagen

    (E) Primary hyperparathyroidism

23. A 32-year-old woman with insomnia undergoes an electroencephalogram (EEG) in a sleep disorder clinic. At 3:00 AM, the EEG technician notes that the woman is exhibiting vertex waves, sleep spindles, and K complexes. Which stage of sleep is she in at this time?

    (A) REM

    (B) Stage 1

    (C) Stage 2

    (D) Stage 3

    (E) Stage 4

24. A patient with a history of hypocholesteremia has acute tissue change at T1-T4. The presence of which of the following features in an atherosclerotic plaque indicates that it has become a complicated lesion?

    (A) Cholesterol crystals

    (B) Chronic inflammatory cells

    (C) Intimal smooth muscle

    (D) Lines of Zahn

    (E) Necrotic cell debris

25. A 40-year-old woman with polycythemia vera develops progressive severe ascites and tender hepatomegaly over a period of several months. Liver function tests are near normal. Which of the following tests would be most likely to establish the probable diagnosis?

    (A) Endoscopic retrograde cholangiopancreatography

    (B) Hepatic venography

    (C) Serum alpha-fetoprotein

    (D) Serum ceruloplasmin studies

    (E) Serum iron studies

26. A 4-year-old girl is brought to her pediatrician for a check up. The child's skin is slightly jaundiced, and she has mild splenomegaly. Physical examination reveals that there is tissue-texture change paraspinally at T5-T9. Her hemoglobin and hematocrit are reduced. Her mean corpuscular volume is 90 μm^3, and her reticulocyte count is 7%. A Coombs test is performed and is negative. A hemoglobin electrophoresis shows an abnormal component, constituting less than 25% of the total. A blood smear shows inclusion bodies within the RBCs. Which of the following is the most likely diagnosis?

    (A) Beta thalassemia

    (B) Heinz body anemia

    (C) Hereditary spherocytosis

    (D) Pernicious anemia

    (E) Sickle cell anemia

27. A high school basketball player passes out in the middle of a game. He is rushed to the emergency department, where he regains consciousness. He claims that just before he fainted, he had difficulty breathing and experienced palpitations. On physical examination, he has a bifid apical impulse and a coarse systolic murmur at the left sternal border. On structural examination, there is chronic somatic dysfunction at T1-T4. The echocardiogram reveals ventricular hypertrophy with asymmetric septal thickening. Which of the following would increase the intensity of his heart murmur?

    (A) Elevating his legs

    (B) Increasing sympathetic tone

    (C) Performing the Valsalva maneuver

    (D) Squatting

    (E) Rib-raising treatment for <3 lower rib levels

28. An MRI reveals a cerebellomedullary malformation in which the vermis of the cerebellum and the medulla are elongated and flattened and protrude through the foramen magnum into the vertebral canal. Which of the following is the most likely diagnosis?

    (A) Arnold Chiari malformation

    (B) Dandy-Walker syndrome

    (C) Holoprosencephaly

    (D) Lissencephaly

    (E) Polymicrogyria

    (F) Schizencephaly

29. Two weeks after starting a course of methicillin, a pneumonia patient develops fever, hematuria, proteinuria, skin rash, and eosinophilia. Physical examination reveals acute muscle spasms at T10-T11 paraspinally. Which of the following is the most likely diagnosis?

    (A) Acute interstitial nephritis

    (B) Acute renal tubular necrosis

    (C) Crescentic glomerulonephritis

    (D) Minimal change disease

    (E) Pyelonephritis

Questions 30-32

CASE B

A woman is brought into the emergency department following an automobile accident in which her chest was hit by the steering wheel. Physical examination reveals multiple ecchymosis on the chest wall, with exhalation dysfunction of several ribs. Her blood pressure is 120/90 mm Hg. When she inhales, her systolic blood pressure drops to 100 mm Hg.

30. This finding defines which of the following terms?

    (A) Pulsus alternans

    (B) Pulsus bisferiens

    (C) Pulsus paradoxus

    (D) Pulsus parvus

    (E) Pulsus tardus

31. After several hours in the emergency department you notice your patient has distended neck veins and a pulse of 140 beats/min. Blood pressure is 60/30 and heart sounds are decreased. The most likely diagnosis is

    (A) cor pulmonale

    (B) tension pneumothorax

    (C) acute pulmonary embolism

    (D) cardiac tamponade

    (E) traumatic pneumothorax

32. The most appropriate management of this condition would be

    (A) oxygen by way of nasal cannula

    (B) pericardiocentesis

    (C) Swan-Ganz catheter

    (D) placement of thoracotomy tube

    (E) simple aspiration

33. A 13-year-old girl complaining of visual deficits is diagnosed with a brain tumor. The mass is detectable on x-ray by the presence of opaque calcifications. MRI reveals destruction of more than 75% of the anterior pituitary gland. Which of the following clinical manifestations would be most likely in this patient?

    (A) Amenorrhea and galactorrhea

    (B) Bilateral exophthalmos and palpitations

    (C) Coarse facial features and enlarged hands and feet

    (D) Polydipsia, polyuria, and low urine osmolality

    (E) Weight gain, sluggishness, and depression

34. A 47-year-old alcoholic presents with fever and a tender, enlarged liver. Structural examination reveals T5-T9 NR$_R$S$_L$. His AST is 150 U/L, and his SGPT ALT is 70 U/L. His prothrombin time is 25 seconds, and his partial thromboplastin time is 30 seconds. This patient has a deficiency of which of the following clotting factors?

    (A) II

    (B) V

    (C) VII

    (D) VIII

    (E) IX

Questions 35-36

CASE C

A 23-year-old construction worker presents to the emergency department after falling down on his outstretched right hand. Structural examination reveals tenderness, erythema, and warmth and swelling of the right hand and wrist. There is a decreased range of all motion in the wrist. The patient is unable to perform muscle testing due to internal pain. An x-ray film reveals a fracture of one of the wrist bones.

35. The physician is concerned about the risk for avascular necrosis. Which of the following bones was fractured?

    (A) Capitate

    (B) Lunate

    (C) Pisiform

    (D) Scaphoid

    (E) Trapezoid

36. The most appropriate management of this above-mentioned fractured bone would be

    (A) rest, ice, and elevation

    (B) Ace bandage

    (C) immobilization with a Spica cast

    (D) counterstrain

    (E) indirect myofascial release

37. A 50-year-old woman presents with complaints of difficulty rising from a chair and combing her hair. Physical examination is remarkable for erythema and edema of cheeks, eyelids, and the backs of her hands. The lesions have a distinctive mauve color, and mauve papules are noted on the knuckles. Approximately 30% of patients with this disorder also may have

    (A) abnormal circulating lymphocytes with cerebriform nuclei

    (B) bacillary bodies in macrophages in the lamina propria of the intestine

    (C) flattening and blunting of villi in the jejunum

    (D) a mutation in a skeletal muscle protein

    (E) an underlying malignancy

38. A patient presents to a dermatologist because of skin changes. The skin is hyperpigmented and thickened and feels velvety. Multiple skin tags are present. The changes are worst in the axillae, groin, and anogenital area, but are very widespread. Somatic dysfunction is noted at T2-T8 bilaterally. This patient should be specifically evaluated for which of the following diseases?

    (A) Hepatic cirrhosis

    (B) Lung cancer

    (C) Polycystic renal disease

    (D) Systemic lupus erythematosus

    (E) Ulcerative colitis

39. A 48-year-old woman presents to the physician with lower back pain. She states that she has had the pain for about 2 weeks and that it has become steadily more severe. Osteopathic structural examination reveals acute and chronic somatic dysfunction at L3-L5. An x-ray film shows a lytic bone lesion in her lumbar spine. Review of systems reveals the recent onset of mild headaches, nausea, and weakness. Her CBC shows a normocytic anemia, and her erythrocyte sedimentation rate is elevated. Urinalysis shows heavy proteinuria, and a serum protein electrophoresis shows a monoclonal peak of IgG. Which of the following is responsible for this patient's spinal lesion?

    (A) Light chain immunoglobulin

    (B) Lymphoplasmacytoid proliferation

    (C) Osteoblast activating factor

    (D) Osteoclast activating factor

    (E) Primary amyloidosis (AL)

40. Biopsy of a 4-mm rough, tan, and slightly raised skin lesion on the face of a 65-year-old man demonstrates atypical basal cells with eosinophilic cytoplasm but persistent intercellular bridges. The stratum corneum is thickened, and parakeratosis is present; the remainder of the epidermis is thinned. Which of the following features would also probably be seen in the dermis?

    (A) Benign nevus cells

    (B) Blue-gray elastic fibers

    (C) Large numbers of spindle-shaped fibroblasts

    (D) Malignant nevus cells

    (E) Touton giant cells

41. During a bitterly cold winter, an elderly couple is found dead in their apartment. All their windows are closed, and their leaky old furnace is on full. Which of the following is the primary mechanism by which the toxin involved led to the death of this couple?

    (A) Decreasing intracellular calcium

    (B) Inhibition of cytochrome oxidase

    (C) Inhibition of Na^+/K^+ ATPase

    (D) Irreversible binding to hemoglobin

    (E) Stimulation of cellular apoptosis

42. A 25-year-old-man presents with weight loss, abdominal pain, and bloody diarrhea. There are Chapman reflex points bilaterally along the iliotibial bands. Sigmoidoscopy/colonoscopy reveals mucosal erythema and ulceration extending in a continuous fashion proximally from the rectum. Which of the following pathologic findings would also be characteristic of this patient's illness?

    (A) Bowel wall thickening

    (B) Cobblestone appearance of mucosa

    (C) Fistulas

    (D) Pseudopolyps

    (E) Transmural lesions

43. A 50-year-old woman complains of a lump in her breast. Biopsy of the breast mass reveals loss of cell differentiation and lack of tissue organization. Which of the following terms best corresponds to this finding?

    (A) Anaplasia

    (B) Desmoplasia

    (C) Dysplasia

    (D) Hyperplasia

    (E) Metaplasia

44. An infant who developed to term has major developmental malformations of his visceral organs. These are usually due to problems that occur at which of the following fetal ages?

    (A) 0-4 weeks
    (B) 4-8 weeks
    (C) 8-16 weeks
    (D) 16-24 weeks
    (E) 24-40 weeks

45. A 62-year-old indigent woman with a long history of uncontrolled hypertension presents to the emergency department with headache, vomiting, and patchy loss of vision. Physical examination reveals somatic dysfunction at T1-T4. Her blood pressure is 210/155 mm Hg, and her blood chemistry reveals marked azotemia. Which of the following would most likely be associated with her condition?

    (A) Berry aneurysm
    (B) Granulomatous arteritis
    (C) Hyperplastic arteriolitis
    (D) Phlebosclerosis
    (E) Thromboangiitis obliterans

46. A 40-year-old female diabetic has glycosuria. This finding may be attributed to inadequate glucose reabsorption at which of the following sites?

    (A) Collecting duct
    (B) Distal convoluted tubule
    (C) Glomerulus
    (D) Loop of Henle
    (E) Proximal convoluted tubule

47. A patient had a baby with the hydrops fatales form of thalassemia. Which of the following genotypes is associated with this condition?

	Beta-Chain Genes	Alpha-Chain Genes
(A)	Four abnormal	Two normal
(B)	Two abnormal	Four normal
(C)	Two normal	Four abnormal
(D)	Two normal	Two normal
(E)	Four abnormal	Two abnormal

48. A 3-year-old patient with short stature has hepatosplenomegaly, skeletal abnormalities, mental retardation, and corneal clouding. Electron microscopy of lysosomes reveals laminated structures. Which of the following substances would accumulate in this patient?

    (A) Galactocerebroside
    (B) Glucocerebroside
    (C) GM$_2$ ganglioside
    (D) Heparan sulfate
    (E) Sphingomyelin

49. A Japanese patient comes to the office for a consult on a viral disease. This oncogenic virus has been implicated in the pathogenesis of which of the following diseases?

    (A) Acute lymphocytic leukemia
    (B) Acute myelogenous leukemia
    (C) Adult T-cell leukemia
    (D) Chronic myelogenous leukemia
    (E) Hairy cell leukemia

50. A patient develops a pea-sized, translucent nodule on the wrist, which when excised shows cystic degeneration of connective tissue without a true cell lining. Which of the following is the most likely diagnosis?

    (A) Ganglion cyst
    (B) Gout
    (C) Pseudogout
    (D) Synovial cyst
    (E) Villonodular synovitis

Pathology and Pathophysiology

ANSWERS AND EXPLANATIONS

1.	D	26.	B
2.	A	27.	C
3.	A	28.	A
4.	C	29.	A
5.	D	30.	C
6.	C	31.	D
7.	D	32.	B
8.	B	33.	E
9.	A	34.	C
10.	C	35.	D
11.	E	36.	C
12.	A	37.	E
13.	E	38.	B
14.	E	39.	D
15.	D	40.	B
16.	D	41.	D
17.	E	42.	D
18.	C	43.	A
19.	E	44.	B
20.	D	45.	C
21.	A	46.	E
22.	C	47.	C
23.	C	48.	D
24.	D	49.	C
25.	B	50.	A

1. **The correct answer is D.** The presentation is typical for reactivation pulmonary tuberculosis. The patient may also note fever, malaise, and weight loss. The high P_{O_2} found in the upper portion of the lungs provides a favorable environment for growth of *Mycobacterium tuberculosis*, leading to reactivation tuberculosis. (In contrast, primary tuberculosis tends to occur in the lower and middle lobes, where small infectious particles are most likely to lodge after being inhaled.)

   Ventilation increases from the top to the bottom of the lung, so **choice E** is wrong. Perfusion increases even more rapidly than ventilation, so **choice A** is also wrong. As a result, the ventilation-perfusion ratio decreases from the top to the bottom of the lung. The higher ratio at the apex of the lung results in a relatively elevated P_{O_2} at that location.

   The apex of the lung has a higher pH than the base, so **choice B** is wrong. Because the ventilation-perfusion ratio is higher at the apex, P_{CO_2} would be lower, thus increasing the pH.

   Regional differences in the density of alveolar macrophages (**choice C**) are not known to cause the described predisposition.

2. **The correct answer is A.** 5-Hydroxyindoleacetic acid (5-HIAA) is a metabolite of serotonin, a major secretory product of carcinoid tumors. The signs and symptoms of carcinoid syndrome include diarrhea, flushing, and wheezing. The cardiac abnormalities are commonly concentrated in the right heart because carcinoid secretory products are degraded or detoxified in the lung.

   Homovanillic acid (HVA; **choice B**) is a breakdown product of dopamine through the monoamine oxidase (MAO) or catechol-*o*-methyltransferase (COMT) metabolism pathways.

   Phenylalanine (**choice C**) is an essential amino acid that is used to synthesize tyrosine, the precursor of the catecholamines (dopamine, norepinephrine, and epinephrine).

   Selegiline (**choice D**) is a MAO-B inhibitor that inhibits the degradation of dopamine. It is used in the treatment of Parkinson disease.

   Vanillylmandelic acid (VMA; **choice E**) is a metabolite of epinephrine that is elevated in the urine of individuals with pheochromocytoma.

3. **The correct answer is A.** The secondary sexual changes seen in alcoholic cirrhosis appear to be due to both decreased testicular secretion of testosterone and decreased hepatic extraction of the androgen androstenedione. Thus, androstenedione is available for extrasplanchnic aromatization (occurring mostly in peripheral adipose tissue) to form compounds with estrogenic activity.

   Choices B and E do not fully explain the secondary sexual changes.

   Although tumors of Leydig and/or Sertoli cells may excrete both androgens and estrogens, the normal Leydig (**choice C**) and Sertoli cells (**choice D**) do not usually secrete estrogens.

4. **The correct answer is C.** This is a classic description of iron deficiency anemia (up to 20% of adult women are iron deficient!). Iron deficiency anemia is very common in menstruating women and is associated with the signs and symptoms described (fatigue, weakness, pallor). It can also be associated with epithelial changes, such as brittle nails and atrophic tongue. The typical laboratory values are those presented, along with a decreased reticulocyte count. On peripheral blood smear, the RBCs are small (microcytic) and pale (hypochromic, due to low hemoglobin levels from inadequate iron stores).

   Vitamin B_{12}/folate deficiency would produce macrocytosis with hypersegmented neutrophils (**choice A**).

   Lead poisoning would produce microcytosis with basophilic stippling (**choice B**).

   Schistocytes (**choice D**) are RBC fragments seen when the cells are destroyed by shearing forces in the vascular system, such as those present in prosthetic heart valves and microangiopathic hemolytic anemias.

   Iron-deficiency anemia is a microcytic hypochromic anemia. Normocytic normochromia (**choice E**) can be for normal blood or an early stage of iron-deficiency anemia.

5. **The correct answer is D.** This man has glucose-6-phosphate dehydrogenase (G6PD) deficiency (as do 10% of African-American males). G6PD serves to protect the RBC from oxidative damage by maintaining high intracellular levels of NADPH. People of Mediterranean descent can also have G6PD deficiency, but to a much greater degree. Therefore, hemolytic episodes in this population are more severe (and can be fatal) as compared with those of the African-American type, which are usually mild and self-limited. Common oxidative stressors that initiate hemolysis are drug reactions (especially sulfa drugs), febrile illnesses, and fava bean ingestion.

   Acute infectious hepatitis (**choice A**) would more likely present with abdominal pain, hepatomegaly, and high elevations of AST and ALT (often into the 1,000s).

   Cholestatic liver disease (**choice B**) more often presents with elevation of alkaline phosphatase, along with mild AST and ALT elevations. This patient has elevated unconjugated bilirubin levels, as in hemolytic disorders. Both hepatocellular (hepatitis) and cholestatic liver disease cause more conjugated (as opposed to unconjugated) hyperbilirubinemia.

The most common side effects of fluoxetine (a selective serotonin reuptake inhibitor; **choice C**) are anxiety, agitation, and insomnia.

Somatic dysfunction at L2-L5 (**choice E**) has no bearing on this patient's diagnosis.

6. **The correct answer is C.** The atherosclerotic lesion described here is referred to as *fixed coronary obstruction*, which becomes clinically manifest with chest pain when increased myocardial demand cannot be compensated by vasodilatation. This usually occurs when the obstruction is more than 75% the cross-sectional area of the lumen, unless there are additional predisposing factors. Fixed coronary artery obstruction manifests with *stable angina*, i.e., chest pain triggered by exercise or emotional strain and promptly relieved by rest.

    Chest pain that awakens a patient in the early morning (**choice A**) is characteristic of *Prinzmetal angina*, which is due to coronary artery vasospasm and is not often associated with atherosclerotic lesions.

    Chest pain occurring with progressive frequency and severity (**choice B**) refers to *unstable angina*, in which chest pain manifests with relatively unpredictable patterns. Pain becomes increasingly frequent and less responsive to rest or medication. This form is related to plaque rupture, hemorrhage, ulceration, and superimposed thrombosis.

    Progressive development of congestive heart failure without chest pain (**choice D**) defines chronic ischemic heart disease, which is usually due to involvement of all three coronary branches and associated with diffuse loss of myofibers and fibrosis throughout the ventricles.

    Prolonged (more than 30 minutes) chest pain accompanied by shock (**choice E**) is most likely due to myocardial infarction. This is usually caused by occlusive thrombosis complicating acute plaque changes, such as ulceration or rupture.

7. **The correct answer is D.** Neural tube defects result from failure of the primitive neural tube to close, which may affect either end of the neuraxis and lead to anomalies involving both the neural tissue and overlying skin and bone. Anencephaly and encephalocele may develop at the cranial end, whereas various forms of spina bifida, myelomeningocele, and meningocele occur at the caudal end. Folate deficiency has been linked to neural tube defects. Elevated alpha-fetoprotein in the maternal blood allows antenatal diagnosis.

Arnold-Chiari malformations (**choice A**), which affect the craniospinal junction, have two forms. Type 1 is frequent but usually asymptomatic and consists of downward displacement of the cerebellar tonsils. Type 2 is much more complex and manifests with early signs and symptoms of hydrocephalus.

Germinal matrix hemorrhage (**choice B**) is one cause of perinatal brain injury and consists of hemorrhage within the germinal matrix, the periventricular layer of neuronal and glial precursors. This injury affects premature infants and may lead to significant neurologic impairment or death.

Holoprosencephaly (**choice C**) is a severe malformation in which lack of separation between hemispheres leads to a single central ventricle. It is usually associated with trisomy 13.

Syringomyelia (**choice E**) refers to the formation of an ependymal-lined cavity within the spinal cord, parallel to and connected with the central canal. It is associated with Arnold-Chiari type 1, traumas, or spinal tumors and leads to progressive neurologic deficits.

8. **The correct answer is B.** This is a classic presentation of a pulmonary abscess. Chronic courses with less severe symptoms (with intermittent improvement following short courses of antibiotics) are also sometimes seen, particularly if the diagnosis was not suspected. A chest x-ray film typically shows pneumonic opacification in which a cavity, often with a fluid level, is visible. Pulmonic abscesses can be caused by anaerobes (most common, particularly if aspiration initiated the abscess), gram-negative aerobic bacilli, and staphylococci. Therapy is based on the organisms isolated and should be continued for at least 4-6 weeks. In cases that fail to resolve, the possibility of coexisting carcinoma should be considered.

    Choice A is the x-ray appearance of pleural effusion.

    Choice C is the x-ray appearance of lobar pneumonia.

    Choice D is the x-ray appearance of bronchopneumonia.

    Choice E is the x-ray appearance of bronchiectasis.

9. **The correct answer is A.** The patient has psoriasis. This chronic disease, which affects 1 to 2% of people in the U.S., typically involves the elbows, knees, scalp, intergluteal cleft, penis, and lumbosacral area. Well-established lesions show extensive parakeratotic scales overlying a thinned or absent stratum granulosum. The mitotic rate in the underlying epidermis is increased, and mitotic figures can be seen well above the basal cell layer. Collections of neutrophils (Munro abscesses) can be seen within the parakeratotic stratum corneum. The pathogenesis of psoriasis is not well understood, but evidence has been accumulating that autoimmunity may play a role. The theory

is that exogenous or endogenous damage to the stratum corneum of the skin exposes antigens against which complement-fixing autoantibodies are directed. Activation of the complement cascade draws neutrophils to the site, further damaging the stratum corneum and perpetuating the process. The damage also triggers release of proliferative factors for epidermal cells, leading to increased epithelial turnover, hyperplasia, and scale formation (an alternative theory is that the underlying process begins with an enhanced ability of the endothelial cells of the superficial dermal microvessels to recruit neutrophils).

Bacterial (**choice B**) or fungal (**choice C**) diseases may trigger psoriasis but are not the primary etiologies.

Psoriasis is not associated with granuloma formation (**choice D**), but rather with the formation of microabscesses (Munro abscesses—see above) in the stratum corneum.

Large vessel vasculitis (**choice E**) does not seem to play a role in the pathogenesis of psoriasis.

10. **The correct answer is C.** The patient is diagnosed with psoriasis; Auspitz sign should clue you in to the diagnosis.

Choice A is for the identification of fungal infections.

Choice B is the distribution pattern for pityriasis rosea.

Choice D is the Nikolsky sign and is indicative of pemphigus vulgaris.

Choice E is used to diagnose herpesvirus infections.

11. **The correct answer is E.** The infant has congenital syphilis. The tibial deformity develops when spirochetes localize in the periosteum, where they produce an active inflammation with many plasma cells. This then causes a massive, reactive, periosteal deposition of bone on the medial and anterior surfaces of the tibia ("saber shin"). "Saddle nose" deformity, another feature of congenital syphilis, is due to inflammatory destruction of the nasal and palatal bones. Gummas, in which a central necrotic focus is surrounded by layers of granulomatous and nonspecific chronic inflammation, can also be found in and near the saber shin and saddle nose.

The bone changes are not neoplastic (**choices A, B, and C**), and involvement of the medulla (**choice B and D**) and cortical layer of the bone is less marked than are the periosteal changes.

12. **The correct answer is A.** This young man is displaying features of Marfan syndrome, a genetic (often autosomal dominant) disease of connective tissues that affects the skeleton (tall stature, long fingers and toes, hyperextensible joints), eyes (often subluxation of the lenses bilaterally), and the cardiovascular system (cystic medial necrosis predisposing to aortic dissection, or

aortic valve incompetence). Marfan syndrome is due to mutations in the fibrillin gene, leading to defects in the structure of elastic tissue.

Lisch nodules (**choice B**) are pigmented nodules found on the iris of the eye. They are associated with type I neurofibromatosis.

Noncaseating granulomata (**choice C**) can be seen in a variety of disorders, including sarcoidosis and berylliosis.

Progressive dementia (**choice D**) is a feature of a number of disorders, including Alzheimer disease, Huntington disease, and Pick disease.

Rapidly progressive renal failure (**choice E**) is not a feature of Marfan disease. It occurs in a number of other disorders, such as Goodpasture disease.

13. **The correct answer is E.** The patient has a villous adenoma, which has been adequately treated by complete resection. If dysplastic epithelium had been found at the surgical resection margins, re-excision to remove the dysplastic epithelium would be required, since villous adenomas are considered to be a premalignant condition.

Adjunct chemotherapy (**choice A**) or radiation therapy (**choice C**) are not indicated since villous adenoma is a premalignant condition rather than an actual malignancy.

Complete colectomy (**choice B**) is typically performed for inflammatory bowel disease rather than for carcinoma of the colon, and would certainly not be indicated for the treatment of villous adenoma.

The presence of clearly invasive glands would have indicated that the patient had a true adenocarcinoma, and examination of regional lymph nodes (**choice D**) would be required to evaluate the extent of the disease.

14. **The correct answer is E.** The patient has pneumococcal pneumonia. In many bacterial pneumonia's, alveoli in large areas of the lungs fill with viscous fluid containing proteinaceous debris and many neutrophils. This filling limits the rate at which oxygen can diffuse into the capillary bed and, in many filled alveoli, may even completely block oxygen diffusion into the bloodstream.

Inadequate ventilation (**choice B**) is not initially as important as poor diffusion.

Changes in perfusion (**choice A**), airway resistance (**choice C**), and lung compliance (**choice D**) usually play lesser roles, although a perfusion/ventilation mismatch may also develop as blood is shunted through poorly ventilated lung tissue.

15. **The correct answer is D.** This woman is exhibiting the classic pentad of thrombotic thrombocytopenic purpura (TTP)—fever, encephalopathy, renal dysfunction,

thrombocytopenia, and microangiopathic hemolytic anemia.

Autoimmune hemolytic anemia (**choice A**) can cause anemia and an elevated indirect bilirubin, but generally produces only mild symptoms, is not associated with thrombocytopenia, and does not cause fragmentation of red blood cells on the peripheral smear.

Disseminated intravascular coagulation (DIC; **choice B**) can cause thrombocytopenia and microangiopathic hemolytic anemia, but is also associated with prolongation of both the prothrombin time (PT) and activated partial thromboplastin time (PTT).

Idiopathic thrombocytopenic purpura (ITP; **choice C**) causes thrombocytopenia with minimal symptoms along with normal hemoglobin and PT/PTT. The peripheral smear in ITP reveals only a decreased number of platelets.

Von Willebrand disease (**choice E**) is an inherited coagulopathy that causes abnormal bleeding. The PTT is typically prolonged.

16. **The correct answer is D.** Aneurysm of the posterior communicating artery is the second most common aneurysm of the circle of Willis (anterior communicating artery is most common) and can result in third cranial nerve palsy (paralysis). The oculomotor nerve (CN III) innervates the levator palpebrae muscle. CN III paralysis would therefore result in ptosis (drooping of the upper eyelid). CN III also innervates all of the extraocular muscles, except for the superior oblique (CN IV) and the lateral rectus muscles (CNVI). Thus, CN III palsy would result in unopposed action of the superior oblique and lateral rectus muscles, causing the affected eye to look down and out. CN III also supplies parasympathetic innervation to the sphincter muscle of the iris (which constricts the pupil) and to the ciliary muscle. Interruption of this pathway leads to a dilated and fixed pupil and to paralysis of accommodation.

The symptoms described probably resulted from subarachnoid hemorrhage (SAH), in this case, due to rupture of a posterior communicating artery aneurysm. A classic clue to the diagnosis is a patient presenting with "the worst headache of his or her life." When you are presented with a case of sudden severe headache, SAH should rank highly on your differential diagnosis list.

The anterior cerebral artery (**choice A**) supplies the medial surface of the cerebral hemisphere, from the frontal pole to the parieto-occipital sulcus. Occlusion may produce hypesthesia and paresis of the contralateral lower extremity.

The anterior communicating artery (**choice B**) connects the two anterior cerebral arteries. It is the most common

site of aneurysm in the circle of Willis and may cause aphasia, abulia (impaired initiative), and hemiparesis.

The middle cerebral artery (**choice C**) supplies the lateral convexity of the cerebral hemisphere, including Broca's and Wernicke's speech areas and the face and arm areas of the motor and sensory cortices. It also gives rise to the lateral striate arteries, which supply the internal capsule, caudate, putamen, and globus pallidus. The middle cerebral artery is the most common site of stroke.

The posterior inferior cerebellar artery (**choice E**) supplies the dorsolateral medulla and the inferior surface of the cerebellar vermis. Occlusion may result in Wallenberg syndrome: cerebellar ataxia, hypotonia, loss of pain and temperature sensation of the ipsilateral face, absence of corneal reflex ipsilaterally, contralateral loss of pain and temperature sensation in the limbs and trunk, nystagmus, ipsilateral Horner syndrome, dysphagia, and dysphonia.

17. **The correct answer is E.** The child has features of Cushing syndrome, which can be caused by excess corticotropin (ACTH), due to pituitary adenoma or ectopic ACTH production, or can occur independently of ACTH production, due to adrenal adenoma, adrenal carcinoma, alcohol, or exogenous steroids. The presentation of Cushing syndrome, as classically stressed to medical students, includes truncal obesity, moon facies, and "buffalo hump." However, these features cannot always be clearly distinguished from ordinary obesity, particularly in unusual populations such as children. It is consequently of great help to be aware of other features that may suggest the diagnosis. Children with Cushing syndrome almost inevitably have growth arrest, which may, as in this patient, be the initial diagnostic clue that more than simple obesity is present. Some children also show precocious puberty, secondary to androgen excess. Features present in both children and adults that are particularly helpful in discriminating Cushing syndrome from obesity include easy bruising and a mild proximal myopathy that can be demonstrated by asking the patient to rise from a crouching position. Hypertension is another prominent feature, which tends to be more common in patients with Cushing syndrome than in those who are obese. A predisposition to infections can be another helpful clue. Other features that can be present (usually in adult cases) include psychiatric abnormalities, most commonly depression and lethargy; osteoporotic vertebral collapse leading to lost height, seen in longstanding Cushing syndrome; red-purple striae of the abdomen or thighs; plethorics appearance secondary to skin thinning; and, sometimes, skin pigmentation in ectopic ACTH syndrome and with some pituitary

tumors. Once Cushing syndrome is suspected, it can be investigated with a variety of endocrine techniques, including urinary free cortisol, dexamethasone suppression tests, and plasma ACTH, and can be treated surgically if an adrenal or pituitary tumor is found.

18. **The correct answer is C.** Low levels of factors II, VII, IX, and X are seen in vitamin K deficiency, leading to prolonged prothrombin time (PT) and partial thromboplastin time (PTT). Vitamin K deficiency is occasionally severe enough in obstructive jaundice, pancreatic disease, or small bowel disease to cause a bleeding diathesis. This patient has evidence of small bowel disease and a history suggestive of Crohn disease (chronic abdominal discomfort, diarrhea and fever). Crohn disease, which is also characterized by rectal fissures, growth retardation, and malabsorption, causes malabsorption of fat-soluble vitamins (A, D, E, K) by several mechanisms. It most often involves the terminal ileum, which is responsible for the recycling of bile acids necessary for the transport and proper absorption of lipids. Small intestinal Crohn disease itself can cause malabsorption by reducing the surface area available for absorption of nutrients. Finally, the disease can cause the development of fistulae, which can lead to exclusion of loops of bowel, also reducing available absorptive surface area.

Factor VIII deficiency (**choice A**) is the cause of hemophilia A. This answer is incorrect because hemophilia A is characterized by an elevated PTT but a normal PT, since only factor VIII is involved. Although hemophilia A can cause gastrointestinal hemorrhage and pain, a 6-month crisis with abdominal discomfort as the only symptom would be extremely rare. Also, hemophilia would likely be characterized by black tarry stools rather than diarrhea. Hemophilia A is inherited as an X-linked recessive; thus, affected individuals are usually male, whereas carriers are female.

Low levels of factor IX (**choice B**) is the cause of Christmas disease. Like hemophilia A, factor IX deficiency is characterized by prolonged APTT and normal PT. Specific coagulation factor assays distinguish these two diseases, as they are otherwise identical in both presentation and inheritance.

Low levels of factors II, V, VII, IX, and X (**choice D**) could be characteristic of liver disease, but in such a case both PT and APTT would be elevated. Note that in liver disease, all other factors (except for Factor VIII) would also be low.

Low levels of von Willebrand's factor (**choice E**) cause a prolonged or normal APTT, a normal PT, and a prolonged bleeding time. Von Willebrand disease is inherited in an autosomal dominant pattern with incomplete penetrance.

19. **The correct answer is E.** This woman has lesions of the right trigeminal (CN V; right facial numbness, decreased bulk of the right masseter and temporalis muscles), right abducens (CN VI; diplopia, decreased abduction of the right eye), and right facial (CN VII; weakness of all facial muscles on the right) nerves. A corneal reflex is elicited by touching a cotton wisp to the eye, resulting in bilateral blinking. The afferent limb of this reflex is carried by CN V (V1), and the efferent limb is mediated by CN VII. Touching the cotton to this patient's right eye would not produce blinking in either eye. The right eye would not blink because of CN V and CN VII lesions, and the left eye would not blink because of a lesion of CN V. Touching cotton to the left eye would result in blinking of the left eye, but not the right (lesion of right CN VII).

20. **The correct answer is D.** The patient has paroxysmal nocturnal hemoglobinuria (PNH), which can cause a striking hemoglobinuria with red-brown to black urine and an elevated urine hemosiderin level. The condition usually presents between 20 and 40 years of age. The hemoglobinuria is intermittent, but a regular, rhythmic nocturnal pattern is actually observed in only a minority of patients. PNH is an acquired disease, and, surprisingly, may be related to erythroleukemia. (The erythrocytes that lyse in PNH appear to be derived from a clone arising from somatic mutation.) Factors that may trigger lysis include infection (even with the common cold), menstruation, surgical procedures, exposure to cold, vaccines, and possibly "stress." These patients are prone to venous thrombosis (thought to result from inappropriate platelet activation), which may be the cause of the abdominal pain that is frequently experienced. Thrombosis and thromboembolism are the most frequent immediate cause of death in PNH patients, with the intrahepatic veins being a favorite site for thrombosis (producing Budd-Chiari syndrome). Other complications include pigment gallstones (secondary to chronic hemolysis) and granulocytopenia, leading to frequent infections.

Urine complete cell counts (**choice A**) are generally uninformative.

In practice, urine hemosiderin levels are a more reliable indicator of the condition than urine free hemoglobin (**choice B**), which is typically present only during episodes of frank hemolysis. Because the patient's urine sample was yellow, it is unlikely that he is experiencing hemolysis at the present time; however, in all likelihood, the urine would still contain hemosiderin.

Myoglobin (**choice C**) would not be expected to be present in the urine in PNH.

Urine red cell counts (**choice E**) are generally uninformative.

21. **The correct answer is A.** The antigenic challenge in this case would result in activation of B-lymphocytes and production of antigen-specific immunoglobulins. The B-dependent areas of lymph nodes would consequently become hyperplastic. These are the germinal centers of lymphoid follicles, where maturation of B-cells takes place. Thus, a picture characterized by enlargement of germinal centers develops. This is called follicular hyperplasia.

Necrotizing lymphadenitis (**choice B**) is seen in a few specific infections (namely tularemia, bubonic plague, anthrax, and typhoid fever) and in Kikuchi lymphadenitis, a rare noninfectious form.

Paracortical lymphoid hyperplasia (**choice C**) refers to hyperplasia of the interfollicular zones, which are predominantly populated by T-cells. This change is seen in response to phenytoin, viral infections, and antiviral vaccinations.

Sinus histiocytosis (**choice D**) is characterized by enlarged lymphatic sinuses filled with reactive histiocytes. This nonspecific change is seen frequently in nodes draining sites with chronic infections or a neoplasia.

Stellate abscesses (**choice E**) occur in nodes involved by cat-scratch disease, tularemia, and lymphogranuloma venereum.

22. **The correct answer is C.** The patient described is exhibiting signs of osteopetrosis, characterized by abnormally brittle bones with increased density throughout the body. In this condition, the ends of long bones also show a characteristic widening (Erlenmeyer flask deformity) on x-ray films. Deficient osteoclast activity underlies this rare hereditary disorder. In the autosomal dominant form, which this boy (and his father) presumably has, the defect is fairly mild, characterized by multiple fractures and anemia (due to filling of the medullary cavities of bone with immature bone). The autosomal recessive form is much more severe, with only a few afflicted children surviving into infancy.

Deficiency of vitamin D (**choice A**) causes rickets in children and osteomalacia in adults. Both are characterized by inadequate mineralization of an exuberant cartilage matrix.

Deficient osteoblastic activity (**choice B**) would produce decreased bone density, not increased density, as in this patient.

Deficient synthesis of type I collagen (**choice D**) underlies some forms of osteogenesis imperfecta. This disorder is characterized by multiple fractures; however, these fractures are related to the production of smaller amounts of abnormal bone, rather than too much bone, as in osteopetrosis.

Hyperparathyroidism (**choice E**) produces characteristic bone demineralization, in contrast to the diffuse, symmetric, skeletal sclerosis seen in osteopetrosis.

23. **The correct answer is C.** Stage 2 sleep is characterized by low-amplitude, mixed-frequency EEG activity with more theta waves than Stage 1. In addition, vertex waves (sharply contoured potentials at the vertex), sleep spindles (short bursts of 12-16 Hz activity), and K complexes (high-amplitude waves with superimposed sleep spindles) occur intermittently. Muscle tone is slightly reduced, and eye movements are absent.

REM sleep (**choice A**) is characterized by low-amplitude, mixed-frequency activity. Ponto-geniculo-occipital (PGO) spikes, which are transient, larger amplitude potentials, occur over the occipital areas. There are also episodic bursts of rapid eye movements (REMs), and skeletal muscle tone is decreased.

Stage 1 sleep (**choice B**), or drowsiness, is characterized by a transition from alpha rhythms (relaxed wakefulness) to theta rhythms. Electromyographic (EMG) activity is decreased, compared with relaxed wakefulness, and there are slow, roving eye movements.

Stages 3 (**choice D**) and 4 (**choice E**) are also known as slow-wave sleep. They are characterized by high-amplitude slow waves, especially delta waves. Eye movements are absent, and EMG activity is decreased compared with relaxed wakefulness.

24. **The correct answer is D.** Complicated lesions indicate advanced atherosclerotic disease. They arise in atherosclerotic plaques and render them more susceptible to sudden occlusion and acute infarction of the supplied tissues. Commonly, the plaque ulcerates or ruptures, and the exposed surfaces, being highly thrombogenic, precipitate thrombus formation. Thrombi are typified by the lines of Zahn, alternating layers of platelets and fibrin (the pale lines), and layers of blood (the dark lines). Beyond thrombus formation, other features of a complicated plaque include hemorrhage into the lesion itself, and microembolism by cholesterol crystals or calcified debris. Furthermore, the weakened media underlying the plaque may develop an aneurysmal dilatation. In general, the clinical significance of atherosclerosis is related to the consequences of complicated lesions.

The incorrect options all include features of atheromatous plaques but do not indicate complicated lesions:

Beneath the endothelium of a plaque there is a fibrous cap composed of smooth muscle (**choice C**), chronic inflammatory cells (**choice B**), and lipid laden macrophages (foam cells), as well as extracellular material.

The core of the lesion, which lies between the intima and the media, is composed of necrotic cellular debris (**choice E**), with cholesterol crystals (**choice A**), calcium, and more foam cells.

25. **The correct answer is B.** The clinical presentation is most consistent with Budd-Chiari syndrome (hepatic vein obstruction), which may occur as a complication of thrombogenic and myeloproliferative disorders including polycythemia vera. The presentation illustrated is the most common; alternative presentations include fulminant liver failure and cases in which intractable abdominal pain is the most prominent initial finding. Hepatic venography is the best technique of those listed to demonstrate the occlusion of the hepatic venous system.

Endoscopic retrograde cholangiopancreatography (**choice A**) is most useful in demonstrating lesions of the biliary tree.

Serum alpha-fetoprotein (**choice C**) is a marker for hepatocellular carcinoma.

Ceruloplasmin (**choice D**) levels are decreased in Wilson disease.

Serum iron studies (**choice E**) are useful when considering hemochromatosis as a cause of cirrhosis.

26. **The correct answer is B.** Heinz body anemia is an autosomal dominant disease that causes an abnormal hemoglobin variant. The mutant hemoglobin precipitates within the RBC, forming an inclusion, or Heinz body. The RBC is then either phagocytosed or removed by the spleen. Patients present with hemolytic anemia, jaundice, splenomegaly, and dark colored urine. The MCV is normal, and electrophoresis usually reveals the abnormal component as a small percentage of the total. The reticulocyte count is increased as the body tries to make new blood to compensate. If the Coombs test were positive, this would indicate that the problem was extracorpuscular.

Beta thalassemia (**choice A**), an inherited defect in or absence of the beta chain of hemoglobin, causes a microcytic, rather than a normocytic, anemia. It results in red cells containing excess alpha globin chains that form insoluble aggregates, leading to hemolysis. The presenting symptoms are anemia, jaundice, splenomegaly, hepatomegaly, and certain developmental abnormalities, depending on the subtype of the disease.

Hereditary spherocytosis (**choice C**) can cause a normocytic anemia with an increased reticulocyte count, but the hemoglobin electrophoresis would be normal in these patients. Jaundice and splenomegaly are often

present. The disease is caused by an autosomal dominant defect in the erythrocyte membrane spectrin molecule that makes the cell less pliable and more easily destroyed.

Pernicious anemia (**choice D**) causes a megaloblastic anemia, ruled out in this patient by the normal MCV. It presents in children younger than 10 years (juvenile form) or in adults in the 6th decade. It is caused by lack of intrinsic factor from the gastric mucosa, causing a lack of vitamin B_{12} uptake in the terminal ileum. Patients present with pallor, slight jaundice, tachycardia, a smooth red tongue, diarrhea, and possibly CNS symptoms.

Sickle cell anemia (**choice E**) causes a microcytic, rather than normocytic, anemia. It is a hereditary disorder characterized by a substitution of valine for glutamic acid in the beta hemoglobin chain. With hypoxemia, the red cell changes to a sickle shape. Patients present with pain, jaundice, splenomegaly, and anemia.

27. **The correct answer is C.** This patient has hypertrophic cardiomyopathy (idiopathic hypertrophic subaortic stenosis)—the most common cause of sudden cardiac death in young patients. It usually causes problems during exertion. Clues to the diagnosis include dyspnea, palpitations, bifid apical impulse, coarse systolic murmur at the left sternal border, and ventricular hypertrophy with asymmetric septal thickening on echocardiogram. Left ventricular outflow obstruction typically plays an important role in the pathophysiology of this condition. Maneuvers that decrease preload, such as the Valsalva maneuver, will accentuate the heart murmur because they result in less ventricular filling, contributing to greater outflow obstruction.

Elevating his legs (**choice A**), increasing sympathetic tone (**choice B**), squatting (**choice D**), and rib-raising (**choice E**) would all increase venous return and therefore diminish the murmur.

28. **The correct answer is A.** The findings in this patient indicate the presence of an Arnold Chiari malformation. There are also variable defects of the hindbrain and skeletal structure. Hydrocephalus and myelomeningocele are often present.

In Dandy-Walker syndrome (**choice B**), the cerebellar vermis is hypoplastic or aplastic, and the posterior fossa is instead filled with a large cyst produced by expansion of the roofless (lacking the cerebellar vermis) fourth ventricle.

Holoprosencephaly (**choice C**) is a failure of the prosencephalon to cleave, also leading to a defect of midline facial development. The most severe form results in cyclopia. In the form that results from trisomy 13 (Patau syndrome) there are bilateral cleft lip and palate, low-set ears, microcephaly, ocular anomalies, hypotelorism, mental retardation, convulsions, deafness, and ventricular septal defects.

Lissencephaly (**choice D**) is agyria, which means "smooth brain." The cerebral hemispheres are devoid of gyri or sulci.

Polymicrogyria (**choice E**) describes a brain in which the gyri are too small and too numerous.

Schizencephaly (**choice F**) is characterized by symmetric clefts that extend from the cortical surface to the underlying ventricle. The cleft is generally hypoplastic.

29. **The correct answer is A.** This is a typical presentation for drug-induced acute interstitial nephritis, which usually resolves when the offending drug is removed. Half of the cases progress to acute renal failure. Additional offending drugs include other penicillin derivatives, sulfonamides, and some diuretics.

    Acute renal tubular necrosis (**choice B**) has been associated with exposure to aminoglycosides, amphotericin, and methoxyflurane.

    Crescentic glomerulonephritis (**choice C**) is not typically associated with methicillin exposure, but rather with immunologic mechanisms or unknown causes.

    Minimal change disease (**choice D**), or lipoid nephrosis, is an important cause of the nephrotic syndrome in children and is sometimes associated with a recent respiratory infection or a vaccination.

    Pyelonephritis (**choice E**) is a tubulointerstitial kidney disease caused by bacterial infection, with elements of obstruction or vesicoureteral reflux in many cases.

30. **The correct answer is C.** Pulsus paradoxus is defined as a fall in systolic blood pressure >10 mm Hg on inspiration. It can be associated with cardiac tamponade and chronic obstructive pulmonary disease (COPD).

    Pulsus alternans (**choice A**) is a repeated variation in the amplitude of the pulse pressure. It can be associated with profound left ventricular dysfunction.

    Pulsus bisferiens (**choice B**) is a double pulsation occurring during systole. It can be associated with aortic regurgitation and hypertrophic cardiomyopathy.

    Pulsus parvus (**choice D**) is a weak pulse upstroke caused by diminished stroke volume. It can be associated with hypovolemia, aortic stenosis, mitral stenosis, and left ventricular failure.

    Pulsus tardus (**choice E**) is a delayed pulse upstroke. It can be associated with aortic stenosis.

31. **The correct answer is D.** This is the classic presentation of cardiac tamponade: distended neck veins, tachycardia, hypotension, and diminished heart sounds.

    Choice A presents with severe dyspnea, diaphoresis, pallor, S3 gallop, and jugular venous distension on inspiration (Kussmaul sign).

    Tension pneumothorax (**choice B**) commonly occurs spontaneously in young adults. It presents with sharp chest pain, asymmetric chest movements, dyspnea, cyanosis, neck vein distension, and tracheal deviation.

    Choice C usually occurs when a venous thrombus in the deep veins of the legs dislodges and enters the pulmonary arterial circulation. It also can cause acute cor pulmonale. Signs and symptoms are identical to those presented, except there is no decrease in heart sounds.

    In traumatic pneumothorax (**choice E**), in addition to the symptoms mentioned, there are broken ribs and other damage.

32. **The correct answer is B.** Pericardiocentesis is the most appropriate management of this condition and is used to aspirate the blood that is tamponading the heart.

    Choice A would be helpful, but is certainly not the appropriate management because it would not remove the cause of the tamponade.

    Choice C is used for hemodynamic monitoring of the pulmonary capillary wedge.

    Choice D is used to repair a severe pneumothorax.

    The insertion of a 16-gauge cannula into the second anterior intercostal space at the midclavicular line (**choice E**) is used to withdraw air manually until a tension pneumothorax is resolved.

33. **The correct answer is E.** This patient has panhypopituitarism induced by her brain mass This condition is associated with decreased serum levels of thyroid-stimulating hormone (TSH), adrenocorticotropic hormone (ACTH), follicle-stimulating hormone (FSH), luteinizing hormone (LH), prolactin, and growth hormone. The x-ray findings (opaque calcifications) and patient description suggest a craniopharyngioma, the most common pituitary tumor in children. Note that nonsecreting-chromophobe adenomas may also present with hypopituitarism. Weight gain, sluggishness, and depression are all signs of hypothyroidism, resulting from the decreased TSH levels caused by anterior pituitary hypofunction.

    Amenorrhea and galactorrhea (**choice A**) are associated with hyperpituitarism, which is most often associated with a pituitary adenoma that secretes prolactin, growth hormone, or ACTH.

Bilateral exophthalmos and palpitations (**choice B**) are symptoms of Graves disease. This condition is associated with a decrease in TSH, which occurs in response to elevated thyroid hormone levels; it is not a result of anterior pituitary hypofunction.

Coarse facial features and enlarged hands and feet (**choice C**) are signs of acromegaly, which may result from increased growth hormone levels associated with hyperpituitarism.

Polydipsia, polyuria, and low urine osmolality (**choice D**) are symptoms of diabetes insipidus. Central diabetes insipidus is associated with disorders of the posterior pituitary or the hypothalamus (decreased antidiuretic hormone [ADH]). Remember that nephrogenic diabetes insipidus stems from renal unresponsiveness to ADH, not from diminished levels of the hormone.

34. **The correct answer is C.** This vignette had some clinical information that was irrelevant in terms of answering the question. This is a common COMLEX question format—providing a clinical context for a straightforward basic science question. It is important that you don't spend too much time analyzing data (for example the liver function tests in this case) before you've read the actual question. This is especially true on the even longer vignettes you may occasionally see on the test.

To answer this question, you need to know that the prothrombin time (PT) measures the extrinsic pathway, that the partial thromboplastin time (PTT) measures the intrinsic pathway, and which of the factors listed is unique to the extrinsic system (so that a deficiency would elevate the PT without affecting the PTT). The only factor listed that is unique to the extrinsic pathway is factor VII. The reason that the PT is elevated in patients with liver damage (alcoholic hepatitis in this patient) is that all the coagulation factors (with the exception of factor VIII) are synthesized solely by the liver. The reason the PT is elevated before the PTT is affected is that factor VII has the shortest circulating half-life of any of the coagulation factors. You should be aware that in severe liver damage, the PTT eventually will also rise as the patient develops a deficiency in all the coagulation factors (except VIII).

Factors II (**choice A**) and V (**choice B**) are part of the final common pathway and are not unique to either the intrinsic or extrinsic systems. Deficiencies in any of these factors would elevate both the PT and the PTT.

Factors VIII (**choice D**) and IX (**choice E**) are exclusive to the intrinsic pathway. Patients with deficiencies in any of these factors (e.g., hemophilia) will have elevated PTTs with normal PTs.

Here are some useful mnemonics:

To remember that PT measures the extrinsic pathway: PET.

To remember that PTT measures the intrinsic pathway: PITT.

To remember the factors in the final common pathway: $1 \times 2 \times 5 = 10$ (factors I, II, V, and X).

35. **The correct answer is D.** Suspect fracture of the scaphoid (navicular) bone in any young adult who has "fallen on an outstretched hand" (classic clue). The physician was concerned about the risk of avascular necrosis because, in some people, the blood supply of the bone is located distally, and a fracture will deprive the proximal region of the bone of its arterial nourishment. Osteoarthritis is a common complication of scaphoid fractures that do not heal properly.

The lunate bone (**choice B**) is commonly dislocated in patients who have fallen on an outstretched hand. Median nerve injury is a frequently associated occurrence.

The capitate (**choice A**), pisiform (**choice C**), and trapezoid (**choice E**) bones of the wrist are less commonly associated with falls on an outstretched hand.

36. **The correct answer is C.** This is the treatment of choice for a fracture of the scaphoid bone; it immobilizes the bone and promotes its healing.

Choices A, B, D, and E are certainly all acceptable treatments that can be added to the spica cast to promote faster healing, but they are not the treatments of choice.

37. **The correct answer is E.** This is a typical presentation of dermatomyositis. Approximately 30% of middle-aged patients who present with this condition have an underlying malignancy. A wide variety of cancers, particularly adenocarcinomas, can cause dermatomyositis. The mauve papules are known as Gottron's sign and, together with the eyelid involvement, are helpful in distinguishing the rash of dermatomyositis from that of systemic lupus erythematosus.

Abnormal lymphocytes with cerebriform nuclei (**choice A**) circulate in Sézary syndrome, which is a leukemic variant of mycosis fungoides, a cutaneous T-cell lymphoma.

Bacillary bodies in macrophages within the intestinal lamina propria (**choice B**) are characteristic of Whipple disease.

Flattening and blunting of villi in the jejunum (**choice C**) are characteristic of celiac sprue, or gluten-sensitive enteropathy.

Duchenne-type muscular dystrophy is caused by a mutation in a skeletal muscle protein (**choice D**), dystrophin.

38. **The correct answer is B.** The condition described is acanthosis nigricans. Mild forms are common and may be associated with obesity and endocrine abnormalities. More extensive forms, such as in this patient, may be associated with malignant disease: usually an adenocarcinoma (often lung), less commonly a lymphoma. The pattern is important to recognize because the eruption may precede other symptoms of the malignancy by several years.

39. **The correct answer is D.** The disease described above is multiple myeloma, a plasma cell neoplasm in which the neoplastic plasma cells elaborate a single, or monoclonal, type of immunoglobulin. In this case, and most commonly, IgG is produced. Patients with this disease are usually older than 40 and may have normocytic anemia. They often complain of skeletal pain from lytic bone lesions and may report headaches and nausea caused by hyperviscosity of the blood due to the excessive amounts of immunoglobulins. The lytic bone lesions are caused by the production of osteoclast activating factor by the neoplastic plasma cells. This can also lead to hypercalcemia.

    Immunoglobulin light chains (**choice A**) are Bence Jones proteins. They are often overproduced in multiple myeloma and are filtered in the urine. They are not usually detected in serum unless there is renal impairment, but they can be detected in the urine by electrophoresis and immunofixation. They do not cause bony lytic lesions.

    Lymphoplasmacytoid proliferation (**choice B**), describes a normal type of B lymphocyte that is morphologically between a lymphocyte and a plasma cell. Lymphoplasmacytoid lymphocytes produce IgM; in Waldenstrom macroglobulinemia, they undergo neoplastic proliferation and produce IgM peaks. Bone lesions are not seen in this disease.

    Osteoblast activating factor (**choice C**) would not produce osteolytic lesions and is not seen in multiple myeloma. There is a rare osteoblastic variant of multiple myeloma with dense bony osteosclerosis rather than lytic lesions, but osteoblast activating factor has not been shown to be involved.

    Primary amyloidosis (AL; **choice E**), is a primary light-chain type of amyloidosis associated with multiple myeloma. The insoluble proteinaceous deposits occur in the tongue, heart, kidney, and skin. This does not cause bony lytic lesions.

40. **The correct answer is B.** The lesion described is an actinic keratosis. This common premalignant lesion is caused by solar damage, which also characteristically damages the elastic fibers (changing their color in stained tissue to blue gray) of the superficial dermis.

Benign nevocellular nevus cells (**choice A**) are found in common moles (nevocellular nevi).

Large numbers of spindle-shaped fibroblasts (**choice C**) are found in dermatofibromas.

Malignant nevus cells (**choice D**) are found in melanoma.

Touton giant cells (**choice E**) are found in xanthomas.

41. **The correct answer is D.** This couple died of carbon monoxide poisoning. Carbon monoxide has approximately 240 times the affinity for hemoglobin than does oxygen. In a sense, the hemoglobin-CO dissociation curve is shifted very far to the left compared with the hemoglobin-O_2 dissociation curve. This means that the binding of hemoglobin to carbon monoxide is virtually irreversible. (The carbon monoxide that cigarette smokers inhale is cleared only when senescent red cells are phagocytized in the spleen and the hemoglobin is degraded.) In addition, the carbon monoxide shifts the hemoglobin-O_2 dissociation curve to the left, making the unloading of O_2 to the tissues very difficult. When too much hemoglobin is tied up with carbon monoxide, the person dies. The carbon monoxide-hemoglobin complex has a bright red color; a distinctive feature of carbon monoxide poisoning that can be helpful either at autopsy or in living patients is that this color makes the skin and organs also appear bright cherry red.

Generally, intracellular calcium levels increase, rather than decrease (**choice A**), with cellular injury or death.

Cytochrome oxidase is inhibited by cyanide (**choice B**).

Ouabain is an example of a poison that inhibits the Na+/K+ ATPase (**choice C**).

Apoptosis (programmed cell death) is stimulated (**choice E**) by certain genes (e.g., *p53, ced 3,4*), glucocorticoids, and aging.

42. **The correct answer is D.** This is a question that tests your ability to distinguish between ulcerative colitis (UC) and Crohn disease. First, you need to figure out which one this patient has. The key clues here are the bloody diarrhea (much more common in UC), the rectal involvement, and, especially, the continuous nature of the mucosal damage. Once you've figured out that the patient has UC, you need to identify the answer choice that is characteristic of UC. The correct answer is pseudopolyps, which are inflammatory polyps found in ulcerative colitis and not Crohn disease.

All the other choices are features of Crohn disease. Especially diagnostic is the transmural nature of the inflammation, which can lead to the development of fissures and fistulas. Remember also that although Crohn disease can involve any part of the gastrointestinal tract, it typically does not involve the rectum and is usually found in the terminal ileum and/or colon. In contrast to UC, the lesions are discontinuous (skip lesions).

43. **The correct answer is A.** Anaplasia is a loss of cell differentiation and tissue organization. It is associated with malignancy and is an ominous prognostic sign.

Desmoplasia (**choice B**) is excessive fibrous tissue formation in tumor stroma.

Dysplasia (**choice C**) is abnormal atypical cellular proliferation.

Hyperplasia (**choice D**) is an increase in the number of cells.

Metaplasia (**choice E**) is a reversible change of one cell type to another, usually in response to irritation.

44. **The correct answer is B.** During the 4th to 8th weeks, organogenesis is still occurring, but a defect during this time is usually not lethal. Unfortunately, a woman may be inadvertently exposed to teratogens during the early part of this period, when she may not even realize that she is pregnant.

Anomalies occurring during the first 4 weeks of life (**choice A**) typically cause intrauterine death.

Choices C, D, and E: Organogenesis has already occurred by these ages.

45. **The correct answer is C.** This patient has developed malignant hypertension, a syndrome of end-organ damage associated with long-standing hypertension, usually occurring with blood pressures greater than 200/140 mm Hg. Severe elevations of blood pressure are frequently associated with hyperplastic arteriolitis (truly an arteriolosclerosis), typified by concentric, laminated smooth muscle proliferation narrowing the arteriolar lumen (onion skinning). Necrotizing arteriolitis, characterized by fibrinoid degeneration and acute inflammation in the arteriolar wall, may also be seen.

Berry aneurysms (**choice A**) arise at points of weakness in the arterial media, especially branch points in the circle of Willis. Although hypertension may play a role in atherosclerosis and the development of dissecting aortic aneurysms, berry aneurysms are believed to be congenital.

Granulomatous arteritis (**choice B**) is typical of several large and medium vessel diseases, especially giant cell arteritis, Takayasu arteritis, and Wegener granulomatosis. It is identified histologically with mural inflammation with clusters of macrophages, often containing multinucleated giant cells. The arteriolar inflammation in malignant hypertension involves neutrophils, not granulomata.

Phlebosclerosis (**choice D**) is the characteristic change in varicose veins, in which dilated and tortuous veins show elastic degeneration and calcifications in the venous media.

Thromboangiitis obliterans (**choice E**), also known as Buerger disease, is a disease of cigarette smokers. It is characterized by segmental vascular occlusion with luminal thrombus formation and microabscesses within small to medium-sized arteries and veins in the extremities.

46. **The correct answer is E.** The proximal convoluted tubule is the site of reabsorption (via Na^+/glucose cotransporters) of nearly 100% of the glucose filtered at the glomerulus. In diabetes mellitus, sugar spills into the urine when the proximal convoluted tubule's capacity for reabsorption is exceeded.

The collecting duct (**choice A**) is the site of reabsorption of water (and urea) when antidiuretic hormone (ADH) is present.

The distal convoluted tubule (**choice B**) is one of the sites of sodium reabsorption.

The glomerulus (**choice C**) is the site of filtration of the plasma entering via the afferent arteriole.

In the initial part of the loop of Henle (**choice D**), water moves out into the hypertonic interstitium. In the ascending limb, sodium and chloride are reabsorbed, but water cannot follow, so the filtrate becomes more hypotonic.

47. **The correct answer is C.** Hydrops fetalis is a form of alpha-thalassemia, which results from deletion of the four genes responsible for alpha-chain synthesis. Deletion of one gene produces a silent carrier. Deletion of two genes causes alpha-thalassemia trait (with a mild hypochromic anemia; **choice D**). Deletion of three genes results in HbH disease (with hemolysis), and deletion of four genes leads to the condition known as hydrops fetalis and death *in utero*. Beta-thalassemia is due to a genetic abnormality at a single site that results in defects in mRNA processing. Since a person receives genetic material from both parents, the patient can have 0, 1, or 2 abnormal genes at this site, but not four (**choices A and E**). Homozygotes for beta-thalassemia (**choice B**) have beta-thalassemia major. Heterozygotes have beta-thalassemia minor.

48. **The correct answer is D.** This patient has a mucopolysaccharidosis, which exists in several different forms. In Hurler syndrome and Sanfilippo syndrome, lysosomes contain characteristic laminated structures on electron microscopy. In Hurler syndrome, a defect in α-L-iduronidase causes accumulation of heparin and dermatan

sulfate. In Sanfilippo syndrome, heparan sulfate accumulates.

Accumulation of galactocerebroside (**choice A**) occurs in Krabbe disease, which is due to galactocerebrosidase deficiency.

Accumulation of glucocerebroside (**choice B**) occurs in Gaucher disease, which is due to defects in β-glucocerebrosidase. The reticuloendothelial cells and CNS are affected.

Accumulation of GM_2 ganglioside (**choice C**) occurs in Tay-Sachs disease because of hexosaminidase A deficiency. The swollen ganglion cells of the retina contribute to a classic sign of Tay-Sachs—the macular cherry-red spot.

Accumulation of sphingomyelin (**choice E**) in a variety of organs occurs in Niemann-Pick disease, which is due to a defect in sphingomyelinase.

49. **The correct answer is C.** The only disease listed that has been established as related to an oncogenic virus is adult T-cell leukemia. This disease is endemic in Japan. It is caused by the human T-cell leukemia virus known as HTLV-1.

For the COMLEX, you should also be aware of the other neoplastic diseases thought to be caused by viruses: Burkitt lymphoma (Epstein-Barr virus), hepatocellular carcinoma (hepatitis B virus), cervical/penile/anal carcinoma (human papillomavirus), and Kaposi sarcoma. Note: Kaposi sarcoma is associated with HIV but is now thought to be caused by a specific Kaposi sarcoma-associated herpesvirus—HHV 8 (human herpesvirus type 8).

50. **The correct answer is A.** Ganglion cysts are common, benign degenerations of connective tissue that are almost always located near a joint capsule or tendon sheath, often in the wrist. Ganglion cysts characteristically lack a true lining, which distinguishes them morphologically from synovial cysts.

Gout (**choice B**) and pseudogout (**choice C**) produce crystal deposition rather than fluid-filled cavities.

A synovial cyst (**choice D**) is due to herniation of synovium through a joint capsule and is characteristically lined by synovium.

Villonodular synovitis (**choice E**) is a benign, synovial proliferation that produces a shaggy mass in the synovium.

Pathology and Pathophysiology

1. Following an upper respiratory infection, a 5-year-old develops large purpuric lesions on the buttocks and extensor surfaces of the arms and legs. The patient also has abdominal pain, vomiting, and arthralgias. There is somatic dysfunction at T10-L1. Dipstick analysis of the urine shows microscopic hematuria. Renal biopsy would probably show which of the following distinctive features?

   (A) IgA in the mesangial region

   (B) Marked interstitial nephritis

   (C) Subepithelial electron-dense deposits

   (D) Tumor

   (E) Vasculitis

2. A 29-year-old man presents with hemoptysis and hematuria. Structural examination reveals acute somatic dysfunction at T11-L1 bilaterally. Renal biopsy shows inflammation of the glomeruli. An x-ray film shows focal pulmonary infiltrates. Which of the following is likely to be found with an immunofluorescence study of the glomeruli and alveoli?

   (A) Electron-dense humps on the epithelial side of basement membrane

   (B) Linear IgG deposits on alveolar and glomerular basement membranes

   (C) Mesangial deposition of IgA

   (D) Spike and dome IgG deposits on the glomerular basement membrane

   (E) Capillary basement-membrane thickening

3. A farmer develops acute attacks of fever, dyspnea, cough, and leukocytosis whenever he works around wet, harvested hay. On physical examination, there is somatic dysfunction at T2-T8 bilaterally. Lung biopsy would be most likely to show which of the following?

   (A) Alveoli filled with dense, amorphous, proteinaceous material

   (B) Ferruginous bodies

   (C) Interstitial pneumonitis with eosinophils, and interstitial fibrosis

   (D) Interstitial pneumonitis with lymphocytes, plasma cells, and macrophages, and interstitial fibrosis

   (E) Linear immune deposition along the alveolar basement membrane

4. A 50-year-old man has hepatic steatosis. Which of the following is the most common cause of this condition in industrialized nations?

   (A) Alcohol abuse

   (B) Carbon tetrachloride exposure

   (C) Diabetes mellitus

   (D) Malnutrition

   (E) Obesity

5. A 25-year-old man presents to his physician after finding a lump in the left side of his neck. He also states that he has recently lost 10 pounds and sometimes awakens dripping in sweat. Biopsy of a cervical node reveals Reed-Sternberg cells. The remainder of his workup reveals nodal involvement limited to the neck and axilla. How should his disease be staged?

   (A) IIA

   (B) IIB

   (C) IIIA

   (D) IIIB

   (E) IVA

6. A patient with a history of easy bruising is diagnosed with Bernard-Soulier syndrome. Which of the following would you expect to find in this patient?

   (A) Decreased circulating von Willebrand factor (vWF)

   (B) Prolonged bleeding time

   (C) Prolonged partial thromboplastin time (PTT)

   (D) Prolonged prothrombin time (PT)

   (E) Thrombocytopenia

7. A normal ovum is fertilized by two separate sperm. All genetic material is retained. Which of the following terms best describes the product of this conception?

   (A) Complete hydatidiform mole

   (B) Normal infant

   (C) Partial hydatidiform mole

   (D) Placenta accreta

   (E) Placenta previa

8. A neurologic examination of a 47-year-old woman reveals a normal corneal reflex in her right eye, but no consensual corneal reflex in her left eye. Which of the following additional findings might be expected?

   (A) Absence of pupillary light reflex of the left eye

   (B) Hyperacusis of the left ear

   (C) Inability to abduct the right eye

   (D) Loss of pain and temperature of the left face

   (E) Loss of taste from the anterior two thirds of the right tongue

9. A 25-year-old woman presents with a 12-month history of palpitations, intermittent diarrhea, anxiety, and a 1-month history of "bulging of both eyes." The physical examination reveals chronic tissue changes at T1-T4. What is the most likely cause of her symptoms?

   (A) Graves disease

   (B) Hashimoto thyroiditis

   (C) Multinodular toxic goiter

   (D) Papillary carcinoma

   (E) Subacute thyroiditis

10. A 38-year-old woman has anemia. Which of the following is most likely the cause of her hypochromic microcytic anemia?

    (A) Folate deficiency

    (B) Hereditary spherocytosis

    (C) Iron deficiency anemia

    (D) Sickle cell anemia

    (E) Vitamin B_{12} deficiency

11. Which of the following is thought to be a major contributor to the cachexia often experienced by patients with advanced cancer?

    (A) Clathrin

    (B) Histamine

    (C) Interferon

    (D) Interleukin 2

    (E) Tumor necrosis factor (TNF)

12. A 47-year-old alcoholic presents with acute upper left abdominal pain with tenderness on palpation. The pain is referred to his back at the T5-T9 spinal level. Laboratory results reveal a low serum calcium level. His hypocalcemia probably reflects which of the following?

    (A) Caseous necrosis

    (B) Coagulative necrosis

    (C) Enzymatic fat necrosis

    (D) Gangrenous necrosis

    (E) Liquefactive necrosis

13. A 70-year-old woman presents to her physician prior to beginning chemotherapy for newly diagnosed small cell lung carcinoma. Her examination is notable for obesity, blood pressure of 180/110 mm Hg, facial hair, abdominal striae, and an acneiform rash on her chest and back. Structural examination reveals chronic somatic dysfunction at T10. Laboratory values are normal except for a serum glucose of 250 mg/dL. Her chest x-ray film shows a right perihilar mass and severe diffuse osteoporosis. Which of the following most likely accounts for her physical examination, laboratory, and x-ray findings?

    (A) Adrenal gland destruction by metastases

    (B) Anterior pituitary gland disruption by metastases

    (C) Ectopic production of corticotropin (ACTH)

    (D) Ectopic production of gastrin

    (E) Ectopic production of parathyroid hormone (PTH)

Questions 14-15

CASE A

A 35-year-old woman presents to her physician with paresthesias of the left shoulder and arm. She has also noticed a hard, bony structure on the left side of her neck above the clavicle. Osteopathic structural examination is significant for a positive Adson test.

14. Which of the following diagnoses best accounts for her symptoms?

    (A) Horner syndrome

    (B) Osteopetrosis

    (C) Pancoast tumor

    (D) Shoulder dislocation

    (E) Thoracic outlet obstruction

15. To confirm this diagnosis, you perform which of the following?

    (A) Tinel test

    (B) Speed test

    (C) Apley scratch test

    (D) Adson test

    (E) Drop arm test

16. A young girl develops dilation of the lateral ventricles as a consequence of a massive astrocytoma involving the cerebellum and compressing the fourth ventricle. Which of the following is the most likely diagnosis?

    (A) Arnold Chiari malformation

    (B) Communicating hydrocephalus

    (C) Dandy-Walker syndrome

    (D) Noncommunicating hydrocephalus

    (E) Syringomyelia

17. A 60-year-old alcoholic with a 50 pack-year history of smoking presents with hoarseness and dysphagia. Physical examination reveals cervical lymphadenopathy. Laryngoscopy reveals an ulcerated nodule on the laryngeal surface. Osteopathic structural examination reveals ropy, cool, fibrotic tissue at the T1-T4 spinal level. Which of the following is the most likely diagnosis?

    (A) Adenocarcinoma

    (B) Anaplastic carcinoma

    (C) Malignant papilloma

    (D) Squamous cell carcinoma

    (E) Transitional cell carcinoma

18. A patient presents to the emergency department in the middle of the night with acute abdominal pain. Which of the following descriptions of the patient's pain would be consistent with a diagnosis of diverticulitis?

    (A) Burning substernal pain after meals

    (B) Severe, diffuse ache in the periumbilical region

    (C) Steady ache in the left lower quadrant with referral to the back at the T12-L2 spinal level

    (D) Steady, boring epigastric pain with referral to the back at the T5-T9 spinal level

    (E) Sudden, severe pain in the lower quadrant with referral to the flank

Questions 19-20

<u>CASE B</u>

A 60-year-old alcoholic who appears malnourished presents to his physician complaining of shortness of breath and gasping for air on awakening. Cardiac exam reveals an S3 heart sound, a diastolic murmur, and jugular venous distention. Pulmonary rales and peripheral edema are evident. Structural examination reveals chronic somatic dysfunction at T1-T4.

19. An echocardiogram would be expected to reveal which of the following?

    (A) A carotid pulse tracing with spike and dome configuration

    (B) Bilateral atrial enlargement and ventricular thickening

    (C) Depressed left ventricular function with pericardial effusion

    (D) Left and right ventricular dilatation with poor contraction throughout

    (E) Left ventricular hypertrophy with asymmetric septal hypertrophy

20. This patient's lower extremity edema is being treated by the consulting cardiologist. He asks you what you could do osteopathically to help reduce the edema. Your first treatment would be to perform a

    (A) thoracic pump

    (B) pétrissage of the lower extremities

    (C) effleurage of the lower extremities

    (D) thoracic inlet fascia release

    (E) pedal pump

21. A 67-year-old man presents with decreased sensation and tingling in his fingers and toes. He appears fatigued and malnourished. Physical examination is remarkable for hyperactive deep tendon reflexes, spasticity, and the presence of Romberg sign. Blood tests reveal a hematocrit of 22% and a hemoglobin level of 6 mg/dL. What other hematologic values would be expected in this patient?

	MCV	Reticulocyte Count	WBC Count	Folate Level	Target Cells	Hypersegmented Neutrophils
(A)	65	Increased	Low	Normal	None	None
(B)	85	Normal/Low	Normal	Low	None	Present
(C)	110	Normal/Low	Low	Normal	None	Present
(D)	115	Increased	Normal	Normal	None	Present
(E)	120	Increased	Normal	Normal	Present	None

22. A 64-year-old man presents with increased language output, most of which is incomprehensible. Neurologic testing reveals that he cannot comprehend verbal or written language. What is the location of his lesion?

    (A) Basal ganglia

    (B) Frontal lobe

    (C) Occipital lobe

    (D) Parietal lobe

    (E) Temporal lobe

23. A 68-year-old woman who recently had a cholecystectomy develops a temperature of 103 F and has persistent drainage from her biliary catheter. Structural examination reveals acute tissue changes at T11-L1 bilaterally. She is given cephalothin and gentamicin for 10 days. Her serum creatinine level increases to 7.6 mg/dL. Her urine output is 1.3 L/day and has not diminished over the past few days. There is no history of hypotension, and her vital signs are normal. Renal ultrasonography shows no evidence of obstruction. The most likely etiology of the patient's condition is which of the following?

    (A) Acute glomerulonephritis

    (B) Acute renal failure secondary to cephalothin

    (C) Gentamicin nephrotoxicity

    (D) Renal artery occlusion

    (E) Sepsis

24. A 52-year-old woman complains of sudden visual abnormalities. She has a 30 pack-year history of smoking, as well as hypertension, and hypercholesterolemia. A head CT shows a lesion in the right occipital lobe, and an angiogram reveals an embolic stroke of the right posterior cerebral artery. Which of the following types of visual deficits is she most likely experiencing?

    (A) Bitemporal hemianopia

    (B) Left homonymous hemianopia

    (C) Left superior quadrantanopia

    (D) Right homonymous hemianopia

    (E) Right superior quadrantanopia

25. A 40-year-old woman complains of arthralgia, fatigue, and depression. During the workup, a bone mass was found. Pathology found that it was a bone mass resulting from accumulation of osteoclasts, reactive multinucleated giant cells, and hemosiderin deposits in areas of microfractures is characteristic of which of the following endocrine abnormalities?

    (A) Cushing syndrome

    (B) Graves disease

    (C) Hyperparathyroidism

    (D) Hypoparathyroidism

    (E) Hypothyroidism

Questions 26-27

CASE C

An abdominal x-ray performed on a 54-year-old man demonstrates a large, irregular, calcified mass with multiple broad projections filling one renal pelvis. The structural examination reveals chronic somatic dysfunction at the T11-L1 paraspinal area.

26. Which of the following laboratory findings might be expected in this patient?

    (A) Decreased urine pH

    (B) Hypercalcemia

    (C) Hyperuricemia

    (D) Increased ammonia concentration in the urine

    (E) Increased cystine concentration in the urine

27. At which spinal level would you expect a viscerosomatic reflex to occur if the left renal pelvis was involved?

    (A) Right paraspinal musculature at T5-T9

    (B) Left paraspinal musculature at T5-T9

    (C) Right paraspinal musculature at T11-L1

    (D) Left paraspinal musculature at T11-L1

    (E) Left paraspinal musculature at L3-L4

Questions 28-29

CASE D

In a patient with headache and nuchal rigidity, a lumbar puncture reveals grossly bloody CSF with elevated pressure, high protein, and low glucose.

28. Which of the following is the most likely diagnosis?

(A) Amyloid angiopathy

(B) Hypertensive vascular changes

(C) Rupture of a berry aneurysm

(D) Tear of bridging veins

(E) Tear of middle meningeal artery

29. Osteopathic manipulative treatment of this patient's headache would include

(A) OA decompression

(B) CV4

(C) frontal lift

(D) parietal lift

(E) no cranial treatment

30. A premature infant develops progressive difficulty breathing over the first few days of life. Deficient surfactant synthesis by which of the following cell types may have contributed to the infant's respiratory problems?

(A) Alveolar capillary endothelial cells

(B) Bronchial mucous cells

(C) Bronchial respiratory epithelium

(D) Type I pneumocytes

(E) Type II pneumocytes

31. A chronic alcoholic presents with confusion, impaired balance, and nystagmus. Administration of thiamine leads to rapid symptomatic improvement. Which of the following neuropathologic changes accounts for this presentation?

(A) Axonal degeneration of posterior and lateral columns of spinal cord

(B) Demyelination affecting the central region of basis pontis

(C) Demyelination involving corpus callosum and anterior commissure

(D) Hemorrhagic necrosis of mammillary bodies and periaqueductal gray matter

(E) Loss of neocortical neurons, Purkinje cells, and hippocampal pyramidal neurons

32. An HIV-positive, 38-year-old woman is suspected of having a B-cell lymphoma. Which of the following pathologic findings would be most likely in this patient?

(A) Greatly elevated levels of serum IgM

(B) Positive Epstein-Barr virus (EBV) titer

(C) Presence of Bence-Jones proteins in a urine sample

(D) Presence of Reed-Sternberg cells in a lymph node biopsy

(E) Translocation between chromosomes 9 and 22 in white blood cells

33. A 59-year-old construction worker has a history of asbestos exposure and chronic tissue-texture changes at T2-T7. Which of the following malignancies is most likely to occur in this man?

(A) Bladder carcinoma

(B) Bronchogenic carcinoma

(C) Lymphoma

(D) Malignant mesothelioma

(E) Scrotal carcinoma

34. A 76-year-old man presents to his physician complaining of an inability to empty his bladder for the past 3 days and a continual leakage of urine for the past 2 days. Structural examination reveals somatic dysfunction at T11-L1 bilaterally and a backward sacral torsion. A cystometrogram reveals that his bladder has an abnormally large capacity, and an MRI reveals a lesion limited to the sacral spinal cord. Which of the following is the most likely diagnosis?

(A) Automatic neurogenic bladder

(B) Autonomous neurogenic bladder

(C) Motor neurogenic bladder

(D) Sensory neurogenic bladder

(E) Uninhibited neurogenic bladder

Questions 35-37

<u>CASE E</u>

A 70-year-old woman undergoes a bilateral hip replacement for osteoarthritis.

35. Which of the following pathologic changes will the removed femoral heads most likely demonstrate?

(A) Marked synovial proliferation with pannus formation

(B) Multiple small fractures in the cartilage

(C) Multiple white flecks in the synovium

(D) No visible change

(E) Pus covering the articular surface

36. After a successful surgery the patient complains of a cough and a feeling of anxiousness. Physical examination reveals distended neck veins, dyspnea, tachypnea, and a pulse of 128 beats/min. Chest x-ray is normal. The most likely diagnosis is

(A) pneumonia

(B) cardiac tamponade

(C) atelectasis

(D) myocardial infarct

(E) pulmonary embolism

37. The above diagnosis could be confirmed by which of the following?

(A) Cardiac catheterization

(B) Pericardiocentesis

(C) Troponin I and T levels

(D) Sputum cultures

(E) V̇/Q̇ lung scan

38. A 60-year-old man who is being evaluated for abdominal pain and a 30-lb weight loss undergoes endoscopy, which demonstrates a broad region of the gastric wall in which the rugae are flattened. Biopsy of this area shows infiltration by numerous polygonal tumor cells with small, dark, round, or ovoid nuclei pushed to the margin of the cell by large, clear, cytoplasmic structures. These cells might be expected to have which of the following properties?

(A) Keratohyalin granules observed by electron microscopy

(B) Melanosomes and premelanosomes by electron microscopy

(C) Positive staining for gastrin by light microscopy

(D) Positive staining for leukocyte common antigen by light microscopy

(E) Positive staining for mucin by light microscopy

39. A 30-year-old woman is diagnosed with cervical intraepithelial neoplasia (CIN) associated with a previous viral infection. Which of the following viral products is (are) implicated in producing this type of dysplasia?

(A) EBNA proteins

(B) E1A and E1B proteins

(C) E6 and E7 proteins

(D) Large tumor antigen

(E) Not discernible from the information given

40. A tall man with gynecomastia and testicular atrophy has a testicular biopsy that shows sparse, completely hyalinized seminiferous tubules with a complete absence of germ cells and only rare Sertoli cells. Leydig cells are present in large clumps between the hyalinized tubules. Which of the following genetic disorders should be suspected?

(A) Testicular feminization syndrome

(B) Trisomy 18

(C) Trisomy 21

(D) 45,XO

(E) 47,XXY

Questions 41-43

<u>CASE F</u>

A male infant begins to have persistent, projectile, nonbilious vomiting at age 2-3 weeks.

41. Which of the following conditions is likely responsible for these symptoms?

   (A) Caroli disease
   (B) Cystic fibrosis
   (C) Diaphragmatic hernia
   (D) Gastric ulcer
   (E) Pyloric stenosis

42. On physical examination the above condition would reveal a

   (A) palpable mass in the left iliac fossa
   (B) palpable olive-sized abdominal mass
   (C) pulsatile abdominal mass
   (D) palpable, tender, sausage-shaped abdominal mass
   (E) large fecal mass palpable in the left lower abdomen

43. The appropriate study was performed and it demonstrated

   (A) a single fine line of barium in the pyloric canal
   (B) an apple core
   (C) a copious amount of mucous plugs
   (D) a loop of bowel above the diaphragm
   (E) a coiled spring appearance

44. A patient with severe iron-deficiency anemia refractory to oral ferrous sulfate therapy is given multiple blood transfusions in preparation for surgery. She develops hemosiderosis. Which of the following microscopic findings would be expected?

   (A) Hepatocytes damaged by intracellular iron accumulation
   (B) Intense lysosomal staining with methylene blue
   (C) Storage of excess copper in hepatocytes
   (D) Yellow-brown granules in cell cytoplasm
   (E) Hemosiderin-laden macrophages

Questions 45-46

<u>CASE G</u>

Over a span of years, an individual develops thickening of the fascia of one palm, which eventually causes a flexion contracture of the hand, most markedly involving the fourth and fifth fingers.

45. The patient most probably has which of the following conditions?

   (A) Desmoid
   (B) Dupuytren contracture
   (C) Neurofibroma
   (D) Peyronie disease
   (E) Plantar fibromatosis

46. The abovementioned condition is commonly associated with

   (A) cocaine abuse
   (B) marijuana abuse
   (C) opioid abuse
   (D) amphetamine abuse
   (E) alcohol abuse

47. A patient presents with hypertension, hypernatremia, hypokalemia, low renin levels, and metabolic alkalosis. Which of the following is the most likely diagnosis?

   (A) Bartter syndrome
   (B) Conn syndrome
   (C) Kimmelstiel-Wilson syndrome
   (D) Sheehan syndrome
   (E) Waterhouse-Friderichsen syndrome

48. A 64-year-old man with atherosclerosis suffers an embolic stroke that leaves him with a left leg paresis. Physical examination reveals a Babinski sign on the left and diminished sensation over his left leg. Blockade of which of the following vessels is responsible for his symptoms?

   (A) Left anterior cerebral artery
   (B) Left middle cerebral artery
   (C) Left posterior cerebral artery
   (D) Right anterior cerebral artery
   (E) Right middle cerebral artery

49. A 4-year-old child with chronic tonsillitis presents with a swollen cervical lymph node. Osteopathic structural examination reveals chronic tissue changes at T1-T4. Biopsy of the node would most likely reveal which of the following?

    (A) Acute nonspecific lymphadenitis

    (B) Follicular hyperplasia form of chronic nonspecific lymphadenitis

    (C) Hodgkin lymphoma

    (D) Paracortical lymphoid hyperplasia form of chronic nonspecific lymphadenitis

    (E) Sinus histiocytosis form of chronic nonspecific lymphadenitis

50. A 70-year-old woman dies 3 days after admission to the ICU. The clinical picture is characterized by fever, purulent sputum, and pulmonary infiltrates on chest radiograph. An autopsy shows patchy areas of consolidation in both lungs, with neutrophilic exudate filling bronchi and bronchioles on microscopic examination. Gram staining reveals colonies of small gram-negative bacilli. Which of the following is the most likely diagnosis?

    (A) Anaerobic pneumonia

    (B) Community-acquired pneumonia

    (C) Hospital-acquired pneumonia

    (D) Lipid pneumonia

    (E) Primary atypical pneumonia

Pathology and Pathophysiology

ANSWERS AND EXPLANATIONS

1.	A	26.	D
2.	B	27.	D
3.	D	28.	C
4.	A	29.	E
5.	B	30.	E
6.	B	31.	D
7.	C	32.	B
8.	B	33.	B
9.	A	34.	B
10.	C	35.	B
11.	E	36.	E
12.	C	37.	E
13.	C	38.	E
14.	E	39.	C
15.	D	40.	E
16.	D	41.	E
17.	D	42.	B
18.	C	43.	A
19.	D	44.	D
20.	D	45.	B
21.	C	46.	E
22.	E	47.	B
23.	C	48.	D
24.	B	49.	B
25.	C	50.	C

1. **The correct answer is A.** The presentation in the question stem is classic for Henoch-Schönlein purpura. The distinctive renal biopsy finding is deposition of IgA (together with IgG and complement) in the mesangium of the glomeruli. IgA can also be present in small dermal vessels within the characteristic skin lesions, which consist of subepidermal hemorrhages with necrotizing vasculitis. Vasculitis (**choice E**) can also be present in gastrointestinal organs (hence the abdominal symptoms) but is not present in the kidney. The condition typically occurs in young children, between the ages of 3 and 8 years, but it can occur in adults. Adults are more likely to develop severe renal disease with crescentic glomerulonephritis. The clinical course is variable; patients who have more extensive renal damage and proteinuria are more likely to progress to eventual renal failure. Some patients have recurrent hematuria for years.

   Subepithelial electron dense "humps" (**choice C**) are a feature of post-streptococcal glomerulonephritis, which can also follow an upper respiratory infection but differs from Henoch-Schönlein purpura by the absence of vasculitis and purpura.

   Interstitial nephritis (**choice B**) and tumor (**choice D**) are distracters that are unrelated to Henoch-Schönlein purpura.

2. **The correct answer is B.** This is a classic case of Goodpasture syndrome, which is autoimmune in origin and characterized by hemorrhagic pneumonitis leading to hemoptysis and glomerulonephritis progressing to renal failure. Most cases involve the presence of anti-basement membrane antibodies. It occurs mostly in young men. Under immunofluorescence, there are linear deposits of IgG on alveolar and glomerular basement membranes.

   Electron-dense humps (**choice A**) are found with electron microscopy, not immunofluorescence. These humps are found in poststreptococcal glomerulonephritis; immunofluorescence in this case would show C3, IgM, and IgG granular deposits.

   Mesangial deposition of IgA (**choice C**) occurs in Berger disease or IgA nephropathy.

   Spike and dome IgG deposits (**choice D**) are found in membranous nephropathy, a cause of the nephrotic syndrome.

   Capillary basement-membrane thickening (**choice E**) is found in diabetic glomerulosclerosis.

3. **The correct answer is D.** Hypersensitivity pneumonitis constitutes a spectrum of interstitial lung disorders that occur in response to a variety of environmental (often occupational) antigens. Farmer's lung, which this patient has, is one example of a hypersensitivity pneumonitis and is related to antigens found in the spores of thermophilic actinomycetes, which grow in warm, moist hay. Other examples of hypersensitivity pneumonitis include pigeon breeder's lung (bird excreta), humidifier lung (thermophilic bacteria), and mushroom picker's lung. Although one might expect to see eosinophils, the interstitial pneumonitis is instead composed of lymphocytes, plasma cells, and macrophages. Long-standing cases additionally show permanent disease features that may include interstitial fibrosis, obliterative bronchiolitis, and granuloma formation.

   Alveoli filled with dense, amorphous, proteinaceous material (**choice A**) are a feature of pulmonary alveolar proteinosis.

   Ferruginous bodies (**choice B**) are a feature of asbestosis.

   Interstitial pneumonitis with eosinophils and interstitial fibrosis (**choice C**) is a feature of Loeffler syndrome.

   Linear deposition of antibody and complement along the alveolar basement membrane (**choice E**) is a feature of Goodpasture syndrome.

4. **The correct answer is A.** All the conditions listed can cause steatosis (fatty change) of the liver. In industrialized nations, however, the most common cause is alcohol abuse. The steatosis may take the form of either microsteatosis (multiple, very small, lipid vacuoles) or macrosteatosis (a single, large, coalesced lipid vacuole in each cell); the two forms may also coexist. The triglyceride accumulation underlying the changes is related to alcohol-induced damage to mitochondrial and microsomal functions that normally degrade triglycerides.

5. **The correct answer is B.** This patient has Hodgkin disease (Reed-Sternberg cells were the classic clue), affecting more than one lymph node region but limited to one side of the diaphragm. This corresponds to Stage II (Stage I is only one node region; Stage III is both sides of diaphragm; Stage IV means disseminated disease to nonlymphoid organs). The A/B designation depends on the presence of constitutional symptoms such as weight loss, fever, chills, or night sweats. A = no constitutional symptoms, and B = presence of constitutional symptoms. Therefore, this patient has Stage IIB disease.

6. **The correct answer is B.** Bernard-Soulier syndrome is caused by a deficiency in the platelet membrane glycoprotein GPIb. GPIb serves as the platelet receptor for von Willebrand factor (vWF), which, in turn, is required for normal platelet adhesion to exposed col-

lagen. A defect in platelet adhesion will result in a prolonged bleeding time. Remember that the bleeding time is a measure of platelet plug formation; it is not related to the functioning of the coagulation cascade.

Although vWF will not be able to bind to platelets in patients with Bernard-Soulier, the amount of vWF will not be affected (**choice A**).

As noted above, platelet adhesion defects do not affect the functioning of the coagulation cascade; thus, patients with Bernard-Soulier will have a normal PTT (**choice C**) and PT (**choice D**).

Bernard-Soulier represents a qualitative, not a quantitative, platelet defect. These patients do not have thrombocytopenia (**choice E**).

7. **The correct answer is C.** Hydatidiform moles can be considered an aberrant form of pregnancy. The moles are found in the uterus and are characterized by dilated chorionic villi and production of human chorionic gonadotropin (hCG). Moles are subclassified into partial moles (which contain a triploid genome derived from the egg and two sperm) and complete moles (which contain a diploid genome derived completely from one duplicated or two separate sperm with loss of maternal genetic material; **choice A**). The two types can be distinguished grossly (partial moles have fewer enlarged villi) and microscopically (partial moles often have blood vessels containing fetal erythrocytes). Treatment is by removal of the mole with follow-up of serum hCG levels.

Fertilization of an egg by two sperm is not generally associated with placental abnormalities (**choices D and E**).

8. **The correct answer is B.** The first trick to this question is to determine where the lesion is. The corneal reflex is tested by touching a cotton wisp to the eye. A normal response would be blinking of the ipsilateral eye as well as the contralateral eye (consensual reflex). The afferent limb of the corneal reflex is contained within the ophthalmic division of the ipsilateral ophthalmic nerve (V1), the efferent limb is by both (right and left) facial nerves (VII). This woman had a normal corneal reflex in her right eye, indicating a normal right V1 and right VII. However, she lacked a consensual reflex, indicating an abnormal left VIIth nerve. The next trick to this question is to determine what other signs a lesion in the left VIIth nerve could produce. A lesion in the left VIIth would also produce hyperacusis (increased sensitivity to sound) in the left ear because of paralysis of the stapedius muscle, which ordinarily dampens sound transmission through the middle ear.

Absence of a pupillary light reflex of the left eye (**choice A**) could be caused either by a lesion of the left optic

nerve (CN II; afferent limb) or by a lesion of the left oculomotor nerve (CN III; efferent limb).

Inability to abduct the right eye (**choice C**) could be caused by a lesion of the right abducens nerve (CN VI), which innervates the lateral rectus muscle.

Loss of pain and temperature of the left face (**choice D**) could be caused by a lesion of the spinal nucleus of V. This nucleus is located in the medulla and receives pain and temperature information from the face via the trigeminal nerve (CN V).

Loss of taste from the anterior two thirds of the right tongue (**choice E**) could result from a lesion of the right CN VII.

9. **The correct answer is A.** Graves disease is the most common cause of hyperthyroidism in a young female and is the only one that causes exophthalmos ("bulging of both eyes"). Graves disease is an autoimmune disorder in which a thyroid-stimulating IgG immunoglobulin (TSI) binds to the thyroid-stimulating hormone (TSH) receptors, causing increased release of thyroid hormone. The exophthalmos is caused by lymphocytic infiltration of the extraocular muscles.

Hashimoto thyroiditis (**choice B**) results in hypothyroidism and is associated with a diffusely enlarged thyroid gland and antimicrosomal antibodies against the thyroid parenchyma.

Multinodular toxic goiter (**choice C**) causes hyperthyroidism but does not result in exophthalmos.

Papillary carcinoma (**choice D**) will only very rarely present as a hypersecreting nodule. Most cases will be nonsecreting, cold nodules. There is no exophthalmos. This is the most common thyroid cancer and has the best prognosis of all thyroid cancers.

Subacute thyroiditis (**choice E**) is an uncommon form of thyroiditis that lasts approximately 8 months and is self-limited. Early on, with destruction of thyroid tissue, there may be release of thyroid hormone and symptoms of hyperthyroidism, but exophthalmos is generally absent.

10. **The correct answer is C.** Conditions that produce microcytic anemia include iron deficiency, thalassemia minor, anemia of chronic disease, and the anemia produced by erythrocyte fragmentation.

Folate deficiency (**choice A**) and vitamin B_{12} deficiency (**choice E**) usually produce a macrocytic anemia.

Hereditary spherocytosis (**choice B**) and sickle cell anemia (**choice D**) usually produce an anemia with cells of normal volume.

11. **The correct answer is E.** Weight loss of more than 5% of body weight is considered a very adverse prognostic feature in cancer since it usually indicates the presence of widespread disease. (Uncommonly, a relatively small primary lesion that has not yet metastasized can cause cachexia.) Both tumor necrosis factor (TNF) and interleukin 1-beta have been implicated in the production of cachexia with weight loss, loss of appetite, and alteration in taste. Large tumor burdens may additionally alter protein and energy balance, often with negative nitrogen balance. Therapy, in whatever form (surgery, radiation, chemotherapy), may also contribute to cachexia late in the course secondary to effects on the digestive system.

Clathrin (**choice A**) is a protein that helps to form pinocytotic vesicles.

Histamine (**choice B**) is released by mast cells and basophils and contributes to allergic responses.

Interferon (**choice C**) is important in the body's response to viral infection.

Interleukin 1-beta, not 2 (**choice D**), is produced by activated monocytes and macrophages and has been implicated in cachexia. Interleukin 2 is released by helper T cells and augments B-cell growth as well as antibody production.

12. **The correct answer is C.** The patient most likely has acute pancreatitis, which is commonly caused by either alcoholism or impaction of a small gallstone in the common bile duct. Acute pancreatitis causes the release of many digestive enzyme precursors, which are then converted to the active form in the damaged tissues. These enzymes degrade the adipose tissue around the pancreatic lobules, producing enzymatic fat necrosis. As part of this process, many free fatty acids are produced that can bind as soaps with extracellular calcium in chemical equilibrium with serum calcium. This will often cause a significant decrease in serum calcium levels.

Caseous necrosis (**choice A**) is seen in granulomata produced by infection with *Mycobacterium tuberculosis*.

Coagulative necrosis (**choice B**) preserves the outlines of cells in affected tissue. This common type of necrosis is seen in the heart following an infarct.

Gangrenous necrosis (**choice D**) is massive necrosis associated with loss of vascular supply and is generally accompanied by bacterial infection.

Liquefactive necrosis (**choice E**) results in liquefaction of tissues due to the release of lysosomal enzymes. Cellular outlines are not preserved. This type of necrosis characterizes bacterial infections and CNS infarcts.

13. **The correct answer is C.** This woman has all the classic findings of Cushing syndrome: obesity, hypertension, hirsutism, acne, striae, glucose intolerance, and osteoporosis. Cushing syndrome may be caused by excess production of cortisol due to bilateral adrenal hyperplasia or an adrenal neoplasm; by excess production of corticotropin (ACTH) by a pituitary adenoma; or by ectopic production of ACTH by a tumor, most commonly a small cell lung carcinoma (major clue in the question stem!).

Destruction of the adrenal glands bilaterally (**choice A**) or of the anterior pituitary by metastases (**choice B**) would cause a deficiency of cortisol and ACTH, respectively, and would lead to a syndrome of cortisol deficiency with orthostatic hypotension, malaise, nausea, and weight loss.

Ectopic production of gastrin (**choice D**), as seen in Zollinger-Ellison syndrome, causes severe refractory peptic ulcer disease.

Ectopic production of parathyroid hormone (PTH; **choice E**), which can be seen in squamous cell lung carcinoma, would result in hypercalcemia.

14. **The correct answer is E.** The patient has a left cervical rib. This anatomic variant, which is typically bilateral but can occur on only one side, is due to formation of an extra rib at the C7 level. Cervical ribs, while often asymptomatic, can cause thoracic outlet obstruction. This results in pain due to distortion of blood vessels; pain or paresthesias related to brachial plexus impingement (notably sensory disturbances in the distribution of the ulnar nerve); and palpable abnormalities in the greater supraclavicular fossa.

Horner syndrome (ptosis, anhidrosis, and miosis; **choice A**) occurs with Pancoast tumors (**choice C**) at the apex of the lung, as well as with certain brainstem or spinal cord lesions.

Osteopetrosis (**choice B**) is a hereditary disease characterized by increased density and thickening of bone cortex with narrowing of medullary cavities. Bones are brittle and fracture easily.

Shoulder dislocation (**choice D**) does not present with a supraclavicular bony structure.

15. **The correct answer is D.** This patient has thoracic outlet syndrome; one of the main diagnostic tests for this condition is the Adson test.

Choice A is associated with carpal tunnel syndrome.

Choice B is associated with bicipital tendonitis.

Choice C is used to assess shoulder range of motion and is helpful with the diagnosis of all shoulder problems.

Choice E is useful in detecting tears in the rotator cuff.

16. **The correct answer is D.** Noncommunicating hydrocephalus is caused by a block in cerebrospinal fluid (CSF) circulation in the ventricles or in the foramina of Luschka and Magendie, by which the fourth ventricle communicates with the subarachnoid space. Tumor compression of the fourth ventricle is a good example of acquired noncommunicating hydrocephalus.

Arnold Chiari malformation (**choice A**) is a congenital form of noncommunicating hydrocephalus in which an elongated medulla oblongata blocks passage of CSF through the subarachnoid space at the level of the foramen magnum.

In communicating hydrocephalus (**choice B**), the block occurs outside the brain proper. The arachnoid villi (which resorb CSF in the subarachnoid space) are often dysfunctional.

Dandy-Walker syndrome (**choice C**) is a congenital, noncommunicating hydrocephalus in which a failure of development of the cerebellar vermis leads to obstruction of the foramina of Luschka and Magendie.

Syringomyelia (**choice E**) is a cystic dilatation of the spinal cord (usually cervical) that may extend into the brainstem.

17. **The correct answer is D.** Malignant tumors of the larynx are relatively uncommon, except for those arising from surface epithelium. Most occur on the vocal cords, although they can occur anywhere. 95% of laryngeal cancers are squamous cell carcinomas, which can cause hoarseness, difficulty swallowing, pain, hemoptysis, and, eventually, respiratory compromise (by obstructing the airway). Ulceration can lead to superinfection. Complications arise because of direct extension, metastases, and infection. Risk factors include smoking, alcohol abuse, and chronic irritation (as might occur in singers).

Adenocarcinomas (**choice A**), anaplastic carcinomas (**choice B**), and transitional cell carcinomas (**choice E**) usually occur in the nasopharynx.

A papilloma (**choice C**) is usually a soft, friable nodule on the true vocal cords. It frequently ulcerates and bleeds with manipulation. It appears as multiple finger-like projections composed of fibrous tissue covered with squamous epithelium. It rarely undergoes malignant transformation.

18. **The correct answer is C.** Diverticulitis commonly produces a steady, aching pain, localized to the left lower quadrant of the abdomen, with referral to the back in some cases. In addition, a mass (due to inflammation) may be appreciated on abdominal examination, and the patient may be febrile with an increased white count.

Remember, if a patient presents with symptoms and signs similar to appendicitis, but the complaints concern the left rather than the right side of the abdomen, think of diverticulitis as a likely diagnosis. Also, take note that diverticulosis, not diverticulitis, is the most common cause of massive lower gastrointestinal bleeding in adults.

Burning substernal pain after meals (**choice A**) is suggestive of reflux esophagitis. The pain may be referred to the left arm.

A severe, diffuse ache in the periumbilical region (**choice B**) is suggestive of bowel infarction, although it must be distinguished from the early pain of appendicitis. The pain of bowel infarction is often aching and severe, whereas appendicitis can (but doesn't always) produce crampy pain.

Steady, boring epigastric pain with referral to the back at the T5-T9 spinal level (**choice D**) and little relation to meals may indicate pancreatitis. Nausea and vomiting frequently accompany the pain.

Sudden, severe, left lower quadrant pain that the patient describes as "tearing" or "ripping," with referral to the flank (**choice E**), may indicate a distal dissecting aortic aneurysm. The pain may also be periumbilical.

19. **The correct answer is D.** Dilated cardiomyopathy can be caused by ethanol abuse. Malnourishment often accompanies severe alcoholism and implies thiamine deficiency, which can lead to heart disease (wet beriberi). Suspect this diagnosis in any alcoholic presenting with symptoms and signs of congestive heart failure. In this patient, an echocardiogram would be expected to reveal bilateral ventricular dilatation with impaired contraction throughout both chambers.

A carotid pulse tracing with spike and dome configuration (**choice A**) and left ventricular hypertrophy with asymmetric septal hypertrophy (**choice E**) are both associated with hypertrophic cardiomyopathy, also known as idiopathic hypertrophic subaortic stenosis.

Bilateral atrial enlargement and ventricular thickening (**choice B**) is associated with restrictive cardiomyopathy. Common causes of this condition are amyloidosis (in the elderly) and sarcoidosis (in the young).

Depressed left ventricular function with pericardial effusion (**choice C**) would be consistent with myocarditis accompanied by pericarditis.

20. **The correct answer is D.** Before starting any lymphatic techniques, you must open the thoracic inlet fascia with an indirect or direct technique.

Choices A, B, C, and E cannot be done first because they would cause fluid to build up at the unopened thoracic inlet.

21. **The correct answer is C.** This patient's low hematocrit and hemoglobin indicate that he has an anemia. It useful to divide anemias into three categories: low mean corpuscular volume (MCV), normal MCV, and high MCV (these are referred to as micro-, normo-, and macrocytic anemias). The only anemia associated with these neurologic symptoms is a megaloblastic anemia caused by a cobalamin (vitamin B$_{12}$) deficiency. This is a macrocytic anemia characterized by hypersegmented neutrophils, leukopenia, and a normal-to-low reticulocyte count. This makes sense, since B$_{12}$ is required for DNA synthesis. Without it, RBC precursors cannot divide as often and consequently produce larger RBCs in fewer numbers, hence the high MCV and normal-to-low reticulocyte count (compare with **choices A, D, and E**). Similarly, fewer WBCs can be made. The array of neurologic symptoms is characteristic of subacute combined degeneration, caused by demyelination of the dorsal and lateral columns of the spinal cord and peripheral sensory nerves.

Although folate deficiency (**choice B**) can also cause a megaloblastic anemia, it does not cause neurologic symptoms. Also, the MCV here was too low to qualify as megaloblastic anemia.

Target cells (**choice E**) are associated with impaired hemoglobin production, as in thalassemia, and are found in micro- to normocytic anemias, not in macrocytic anemia as in this distracter.

Remember that a good way to approach questions like these is to isolate one lab value, such as MCV, in order to eliminate incorrect distracters. This will greatly facilitate solving the problem and will save you precious time.

22. **The correct answer is E.** This patient has Wernicke aphasia, which is caused by a lesion of Wernicke's area, located in the posterior part of the superior temporal gyrus (area 22) of the language-dominant hemisphere.

Lesions of the basal ganglia (**choice A**) produce extrapyramidal motor symptoms.

Lesions of the frontal lobe (**choice B**) can produce spastic paralysis, Broca's aphasia (expressive, nonfluent aphasia), disorders of higher order thinking, and deviation of the eyes. (Mnemonic: Broca's aphasia is associated with broken speech).

Lesions of the occipital lobe (**choice C**) can produce visual disturbances.

Lesions of the parietal lobe (**choice D**) can produce a variety of higher cortical dysfunctions and a loss of sensation, but would not produce the type of language problem seen in this patient.

23. **The correct answer is C.** A small percentage of patients (5% to 10%) develop a nonoliguric form of acute renal failure when treated with aminoglycosides such as gentamicin. Gentamicin can accumulate in the kidneys to produce a delayed form of acute renal failure with elevation of the serum creatinine level. The nonoliguric form of renal failure seen in this patient is the typical presentation for gentamicin nephrotoxicity.

Acute glomerulonephritis (**choice A**) is typically associated with hypertension and the appearance of an active urinary sediment containing casts and red blood cells.

Cephalothin (**choice B**) is a first-generation cephalosporin commonly used in the treatment of severe infection of the genitourinary tract, gastrointestinal tract, and respiratory tract, as well as skin infections. This antibiotic can produce an acute interstitial nephritis; however, the patient's presentation is consistent with gentamicin nephrotoxicity. Interstitial nephritis is associated with acute renal failure, fever, rash, and eosinophilia.

Renal artery occlusion (**choice D**) is commonly caused by thrombosis or embolism. The clinical features of acute renal artery occlusion are hematuria, flank pain, fever, nausea, elevated LDH, elevated AST, and acute renal failure.

Since the patient has normal vital signs and no history of hypotension, a diagnosis of sepsis (**choice E**) is unlikely.

24. **The correct answer is B.** The posterior cerebral arteries supply the cortical surfaces of the occipital and medial temporal lobes. Damage to one occipital lobe (e.g., by trauma or by ischemia/infarction due to stroke) usually produces a contralateral homonymous hemianopia. Occlusion of the right posterior cerebral artery would therefore result in a left homonymous hemianopia—blindness in the left half of the visual field in both eyes. In addition, involvement of the medial temporal lobe might give rise to peduncular hallucinosis—visual illusions or elementary (unformed) hallucinations. Bilateral lesions would cause "cortical" blindness, which does not affect the pupillary reflexes.

Bitemporal hemianopia (**choice A**) is a loss of vision in the temporal quadrants of the visual field. (It is also termed heteronymous hemianopia). This occurs in lesions of the optic chiasm, which may occur with pituitary tumors.

Superior quadrantanopia (**choices C and E**) is caused by lesions in the upper portion of the contralateral temporal lobe.

Right homonymous hemianopia (**choice D**) would result from left posterior cerebral artery occlusion.

25. **The correct answer is C.** This brief histologic description refers to *brown tumors*, which develop in association with hyperparathyroidism. These lesions result from repeated microfractures, with subsequent accumulation of hemosiderin-laden macrophages and reactive osteoclastic and fibroblastic proliferation. The brown color is due to hemosiderin deposition.

Cushing syndrome (**choice A**) is caused by excess of cortisol from endogenous or exogenous sources. Administration of glucocorticoids for therapeutic purposes is the most common form. Osteoporosis is the most significant effect of excess glucocorticoids.

Graves disease (**choice B**) is due to a hyperfunctioning thyroid, stimulated by autoantibodies to TSH-receptors. Excessive production of thyroid hormone results in a complex clinical picture, in which bone changes are not seen.

Hypoparathyroidism (**choice D**) is an uncommon disorder most often due to surgical removal of the parathyroids. The most characteristic manifestation is *tetany*, resulting from decreased calcemia and consequent neuromuscular hyperexcitability.

Hypothyroidism (**choice E**) is a disorder of diminished thyroid function, most commonly due to previous Hashimoto thyroiditis. If hypothyroidism is present *in utero*, infancy, or early childhood, short stature, mental retardation, and other abnormalities develop (*cretinism*).

26. **The correct answer is D.** The patient has a stag-horn calculus. These very large calculi are almost always principally composed of magnesium ammonium phosphate (often with enough calcium to be radio-opaque) and form in the setting of infection by urea-splitting bacteria, such as *Proteus*.

Increased urine ammonia concentrations are a byproduct of the bacterial metabolism of urea and tend to increase urine pH (compare with **choice A**).

Hypercalciuria, with or without hypercalcemia (**choice B**), is a cause of calcium oxalate stones.

Uric acid stones can be seen in patients with hyperuricemia (**choice C**) secondary to gout, or in conditions in which a very rapid cell turnover occurs (e.g., leukemias).

Genetically determined defects in the renal transport of amino acids are associated with cystine stones (**choice E**).

27. **The correct answer is D.** The left kidney has a sympathetic referral to the left paraspinal musculature at levels T11-L1.

Choice A is the sympathetic reflex for the liver and gallbladder.

Choice B is the sympathetic reflex for the stomach and spleen.

Choice C is the sympathetic reflex for the right kidney.

There is no sympathetic innervation at this level (**choice E**).

28. **The correct answer is C.** The presence of blood in the spinal tap indicates bleeding within the subarachnoid space, and rupture of berry aneurysms represents the most frequent cause leading to this form of intracranial bleed. Berry aneurysms develop as outpouchings of the arterial wall in the circle of Willis and consist of intima and adventitia; the media is absent. Congenital weakness at branching points is thought to be the underlying pathogenetic mechanism, but hypertension plays a facilitating role in their development and rupture.

Amyloid angiopathy (**choice A**) usually leads to hemorrhages occurring in the neocortex in a "lobar" distribution. The amyloid depositing in the vessel walls is Aβ, the same type as the amyloid in senile plaques of Alzheimer disease. Blood is usually absent in a spinal tap.

Hypertensive vascular changes (**choice B**) affect intraparenchymal arterioles and small arteries. These changes constitute the predisposing condition for the development of hypertensive bleeding, which is intraparenchymal and often involves the basal ganglia, cerebellum, or pons. The subarachnoid space is free of blood, unless the bleeding extends into the subarachnoid space.

Tearing of bridging veins (**choice D**) is the most frequent mechanism of *subdural hemorrhage*, occurring most commonly in people with cerebral atrophy. In this setting, such veins become stretched and thus more vulnerable to trauma.

Tearing of the middle meningeal artery (**choice E**) is the most common cause of epidural hemorrhage, usually resulting from trauma and often associated with calvarial fracture. Blood collects rapidly between the dura and the overlying bone, leading to increased intracranial pressure and impending danger of cerebral herniation.

29. **The correct answer is E.** This patient is diagnosed with bleeding within the subarachnoid space. Cranial treatment is contraindicated in any patient with intracranial bleeding, increased intracranial pressure, or skull fracture.

Choices A, B, C, and D are all cranial treatments and are therefore incorrect.

30. **The correct answer is E.** This child has neonatal respiratory distress syndrome (hyaline membrane disease), which is caused by the inability of the immature lungs to synthesize adequate amounts of surfactant. Surfactant, which reduces surface tension, helps keep alveoli dry,

and aids in expansion of the lungs, is synthesized by type II pneumocytes.

Alveolar capillary endothelial cells (**choice A**) are important in maintaining the capillary structure and permitting flow of gases into and out of the blood stream.

Bronchial mucous cells (**choice B**) produce the usually thin (in healthy individuals) coat of mucus that lines the bronchi.

The ciliated bronchial respiratory epithelium (**choice C**) is responsible for moving the dust-coated mucus layer out of the bronchi.

Type I pneumocytes (**choice D**) are the squamous cells that line alveoli and permit easy gas exchange. These cells tend to be immature (and thick) in premature infants but do not produce surfactant.

31. **The correct answer is D.** The clinical picture of confusion, ataxia, and variable disturbances of eye movements (e.g., nystagmus and ophthalmoplegia) is due to *Wernicke encephalopathy*, which results from thiamine deficiency. Hemorrhage and necrosis in the abovementioned areas are the underlying pathologic changes. Alcoholics are particularly prone to this condition.

Axonal degeneration of posterior and lateral columns of spinal cord (**choice A**), or *subacute combined degeneration,* results from two different etiologies: vitamin B_{12} deficiency and HIV myelopathy. Ataxia, numbness, and spastic paresis of the lower extremities are the clinical manifestations.

Demyelination affecting the central region of the basis pontis (**choice B**) is known as *central pontine myelinolysis*. This complication is most commonly encountered in severely malnourished and dehydrated alcoholics. Rapid correction of hyponatremia triggers this condition.

Demyelination involving the corpus callosum and anterior commissure (**choice C**), or *Marchiafava-Bignami disease,* is a rare disorder associated with chronic alcoholism. It is probably related to some dietary deficiency.

Loss of neurons in the neocortex, cerebellar Purkinje cells, and hippocampal pyramidal neurons (**choice E**) results from hypoxia or hypoglycemia-related necrosis. These neurons are the most vulnerable to hypoxic or hypoglycemic injury.

32. **The correct answer is B.** Infectious mononucleosis is caused by the Epstein-Barr virus (EBV), although most EBV infections do not result in acute disease. In patients with the African form of Burkitt lymphoma, and in some AIDS patients with B-cell lymphomas, there is evidence of EBV infection. In these patients, leukemic cells contain multiple copies of the EBV genome. A translocation between the cellular proto-oncogene *myc* on chromosome 8 and immunoglobulin chains on chromosomes 2, 14, or 22 is a typical finding in these cells. Evidence of EBV infection is therefore relevant (but not required) for the diagnosis of B-cell lymphoma.

Severely elevated levels of IgM (**choice A**) are found in patients with Waldenström macroglobulinemia. Levels of IgM are high enough to cause hyperviscosity syndrome and to interfere with blood clotting. Waldenström macroglobulinemia can eventually lead to an aggressive B-cell lymphoma.

Bence-Jones proteins (**choice C**) are immunoglobulin light chains that have "spilled" into the urine. This is seen primarily in patients with multiple myeloma or its advanced stages, known as plasma cell leukemia. These cells overproduce antibodies and their building blocks, such as light chains, which are then excreted in the urine.

The diagnostic marker of Hodgkin disease is the presence of Reed-Sternberg cells (**choice D**) in lymph node biopsies. Reed-Sternberg cells are multinucleated, often with mirror-image nuclei, and contain giant nucleoli.

More than 95% of patients with CML have a translocation between chromosomes 9 and 22 in their leukemic cells (**choice E**). The "new" chromosome that is generated by this event is referred to as the Philadelphia chromosome. Different translocations are responsible for other hematologic malignancies. For example, Burkitt lymphoma often shows a translocation between chromosomes 8 and 14.

33. **The correct answer is B.** A little knowledge, such as the "knee-jerk" association between asbestos exposure and malignant mesothelioma (**choice D**), can get you into trouble on this type of COMLEX question. Malignant mesothelioma is a very rare tumor that is much more common in individuals with a history of asbestos exposure. However, bronchogenic carcinoma is more common than malignant mesothelioma in asbestos-exposed individuals, as well as in the population at large. Asbestos exposure is also associated with pulmonary interstitial fibrosis and pleural reactions.

Bladder carcinoma (**choice A**) is associated with cigarette smoking and exposure to naphthalene dyes.

Lymphomas (**choice C**) and leukemias are often associated with chromosomal rearrangements (e.g., translocations) that alter the locations of proto-oncogenes (e.g., *c-myc, c-abl, bcl-1, bcl-2*).

The association between scrotal carcinoma (**choice E**) and hydrocarbon exposure was first noted by Percival Pott, who noticed an increased incidence of scrotal cancer in chimney sweeps in London.

34. **The correct answer is B.** This patient has an autonomous neurogenic bladder, which is a type of "lower motor neuron" bladder. There are three types of lower motor neuron bladders: an autonomous neurogenic bladder (lesion to the sacral spinal cord centers involved in bladder function), a motor neurogenic bladder (**choice C**; lesion of motor and visceral efferents to the bladder), and a sensory neurogenic bladder (**choice D**; lesion of sensory afferents from the bladder). All these conditions are associated with a flaccid bladder that fills to capacity. Whereas a normal bladder typically empties at 300 mL, these bladders fill to about 1000 mL. These patients have overflow incontinence, which means the bladder expands completely. Because they cannot void, these patients dribble urine. These are the most dangerous neurogenic bladders, because urinary stasis predisposes patients to lower urinary tract infections, which may ascend to the kidneys, producing pyelonephritis.

An automatic neurogenic bladder (**choice A**) is a type of "upper motor neuron" bladder. This condition is caused by a lesion that disconnects the pontine micturition center (the center that is responsible for producing coordinated voiding) from the sacral spinal cord centers. The bladder is still able to void to some degree, but functions "on its own" without input from the brainstem center. As a result, the urethral sphincter does not relax when the detrusor muscle contracts, leading to urinary retention.

An uninhibited neurogenic bladder (**choice E**) is another type of "upper motor neuron" bladder. Normal adults have cortical control over their pontine micturition center, but when the corticopontine pathways are not functioning properly, the patient develops an uninhibited neurogenic bladder. In these patients, the act of voiding is well coordinated, but not under conscious control. This is seen in patients with frontal lobe lesions and in normal children prior to toilet training.

35. **The correct answer is B.** Osteoarthritis is characterized by mechanical, rather than inflammatory, damage to the joint. The damage usually begins as multiple small fractures of the cartilage tips of the involved bones, which can lead to wearing down of the cartilage to expose the underlying bone. In long-standing cases, the articular ends of the bones may develop a mushroom-like or flattened deformation.

Synovial proliferation with pannus formation (**choice A**) suggests chronic inflammatory joint disease, such as rheumatoid arthritis.

White flecks (**choice C**) in a joint suggest the crystals of gout or pseudogout.

The presence of pus (**choice E**) suggests an acute inflammatory (possibly infectious) etiology.

36. **The correct answer is E.** After any surgery you must maintain a high degree of suspicion for pulmonary embolism (PE). In this case, the patient is 70 years old with a hip replacement and is immobilized, which increases the chance of clot formation. The presentation is classic for PE: dyspnea, tachypnea, and tachycardia, with neck vein distension. Many times the patient complains only of anxiousness and a cough.

Choice A is unlikely because the chest x-ray was normal.

Choice B is unlikely because there were no diminished heart sounds.

Choice C usually presents in a different manner. It is usually preceded by a low-grade fever, dullness to percussion, and decreased breath sounds at the bases of the lungs.

Choice D is an unlikely choice because the patient did not complain of chest pain and no EKG results were given; it would not be incorrect to order an EKG at this point.

37. **The correct answer is E.** $\dot{V}/\dot{Q}$ scan is the gold standard for detection of a pulmonary embolism.

Choices A and C would be used in the workup of a suspected myocardial infarction.

Choice B is used to relieve cardiac tamponade.

Choice D is used in the workup of pneumonia.

38. **The correct answer is E.** The tumor described is the linitis plastica form of gastric adenocarcinoma, in which individual mucin-producing tumor cells diffusely infiltrate the mucosa and muscularis propria to produce a rigid, thickened, "leather-bottle" gastric wall. This tumor is poorly differentiated and has a poor prognosis.

Keratohyalin granules (**choice A**) are a feature of squamous cell carcinoma, which does not usually occur in the stomach.

Melanosomes and premelanosomes (**choice B**) are observed with electron microscopy in melanocytic lesions, including melanoma.

Positive immunostaining for gastrin (**choice C**) would be a feature of gastrin-secreting carcinoids, which typically form small, yellow nodules composed of nests or cords of small cells with centrally located, round-to-oval, stippled nuclei.

Positive immunostaining for leukocyte common antigen (**choice D**) is associated with lymphoma, which can also affect the stomach, appearing similar to linitis plastica grossly. Microscopically, however, the individual malignant lymphocytes usually have centrally located nuclei and lack the large, clear, cytoplasmic vacuoles described in this question.

39. **The correct answer is C.** Cervical intraepithelial neoplasia (CIN) is associated with human papilloma virus

(HPV) infection, particularly types 16 or 18. These papillomaviruses produce E6 and E7 proteins, which induce the expression of cellular p53 and p110^{Rb} oncogenes, respectively.

EBNA proteins (**choice A**) are produced by the Epstein-Barr virus and are associated with hepatocellular carcinoma, Burkitt lymphoma, and carcinoma of the nasopharynx.

E1A and E1B proteins (**choice B**) are produced by adenoviruses 12, 18, and 31. They also bind to the p53 and p110^{Rb} oncogenes, respectively.

Large tumor antigen (**choice D**) is produced by simian virus 40 (SV40), a papovavirus found in monkeys that is known to produce sarcoma in laboratory hamsters.

40. **The correct answer is E.** The testicular changes described are those observed in Klinefelter syndrome, most often due to 47,XXY genetics.

Testicular feminization syndrome (**choice A**) is due to a genetically determined unresponsiveness to testosterone that produces a phenotypic female in an individual with 46,XY chromosomes.

Trisomy 18 (**choice B**) is Edwards syndrome, characterized by facial features that are small and delicate.

Trisomy 21 (**choice C**) is Down syndrome, the most common trisomy. Characteristics include oblique palpebral fissures, epicanthal folds, endocardial cushion defects, simian creases, and a high-arched palate, among other anomalies.

Turner syndrome, 45,XO (**choice D**), produces a sterile but phenotypic female of short stature with webbing of the neck.

41. **The correct answer is E.** Congenital hypertrophic pyloric stenosis typically presents as described in the question stem and is more frequent in male infants. Physical examination reveals a palpable ovoid mass in the epigastrium; surgical splitting of the hypertrophic pyloric muscle is curative. The etiology is not well understood.

Caroli disease (**choice A**) is a malformation that causes segmental dilatation of the intrahepatic biliary tree. Vomiting is not a prominent feature.

Cystic fibrosis (**choice B**) presents with malabsorption and/or pulmonary infection due to a global defect in chloride secretion.

Diaphragmatic hernia (**choice C**) is characterized by respiratory insufficiency at birth.

Gastric ulcers (**choice D**) would be quite unusual in an infant.

42. **The correct answer is B.** This is the finding for a pyloric stenosis.

Choice A is the finding for diverticulitis.

Choice C is the finding for abdominal aortic aneurysm.

Choice D is the finding for intussusception in a child.

Choice E is the finding in Hirschsprung disease.

43. **The correct answer is A.** On barium study, the string sign is the finding for pyloric stenosis.

Choice B is an x-ray sign that usually indicates an abdominal mass or an abdominal aortic aneurysm.

Choice C is Curschmann spirals, which are associated with cystic fibrosis.

Choice D in barium study is a sign for hiatal hernia.

Choice E is the barium study sign for intussusception.

44. **The correct answer is D.** Hemosiderosis is due to increased total body iron content and is associated with the intracellular storage of excess iron as ferritin and hemosiderin. Iron may be found not only in the organs in which it is usually found but also in the pancreas, heart, kidneys, endocrine organs, and skin. This iron excess may be due to high levels of dietary iron or blood transfusion. Hemosiderin, a denatured form of ferritin, appears microscopically as yellow-brown granules in cytoplasm.

Although cells contain excess iron in hemosiderosis, they are not damaged by the accumulation. In contrast, hepatocytes are damaged by intracellular iron accumulation (**choice A**) in hemochromatosis, a much more severe form of iron overload than hemosiderosis. Hemochromatosis results from a hereditary abnormality of iron absorption.

Cells would exhibit intense staining with Prussian blue, not with methylene blue (**choice B**).

Storage of excess copper in hepatocytes (**choice C**) occurs in Wilson disease, not in hemosiderosis.

Hemosiderin-laden macrophages (**choice E**), also called heart-failure cells, are associated with pulmonary edema and are seen in bronchial lavage.

45. **The correct answer is B.** The patient has palmar fibromatosis, also known as Dupuytren contracture. This is a benign condition that may stabilize spontaneously or may require surgical excision. Incidence is highest in patients older than 40 who have chronic diseases (including diabetes and liver disease).

Desmoids (aggressive fibromatosis; **choice A**) are proliferations of fibrous tissue that biologically lie somewhere between exuberant reactive fibroproliferations and low-grade fibrosarcomas. They are often found in or near the abdomen.

Neurofibromas (**choice C**) produce tumors involving peripheral nerves.

Peyronie disease (**choice D**) is similar to Dupuytren contracture, but involves the penis.

Plantar fibromatosis (**choice E**) is similar to this patient's condition, but involves the foot.

46. **The correct answer is E.** This is the only one commonly associated with Dupuytren contracture.

    Choices A, B, C, and D have no known associations.

47. **The correct answer is B.** These findings are characteristic of Conn syndrome (primary hyperaldosteronism), in which increased aldosterone secretion causes sodium retention, increased total plasma volume, increased renal artery pressure, and inhibition of renin secretion.

    Bartter syndrome (**choice A**), or secondary hyperaldosteronism, is associated with juxtaglomerular hyperplasia and failure to thrive.

    Kimmelstiel-Wilson syndrome (**choice C**) is a late complication of diabetes in which intercapillary glomerulosclerosis, hypertension, and edema occurs, accompanied by proteinuria. The syndrome develops approximately 20 years after the onset of diabetes.

    Sheehan syndrome (**choice D**) is due to hemorrhagic or ischemic infarction of the pituitary following postpartum hemorrhage with excessive bleeding or shock. It may be present with failure to lactate in the postpartum period.

    Waterhouse-Friderichsen syndrome (**choice E**) is characterized by adrenal apoplexy resulting from a massive, sudden adrenal hemorrhage, usually associated with meningococcal septicemia.

48. **The correct answer is D.** Three pieces of information are needed to answer this question. First, a lesion of the right motor cortex leads to a left paresis or paralysis (immediately narrowing the choices to **D, E, or F**). Second, the leg is represented in the part of the motor cortex that is adjacent to the interhemispheric fissure. Third, the anterior cerebral artery supplies the medial surface of the hemisphere extending from the frontal pole to the parieto-occipital sulcus; this would include the motor and somatosensory cortices.

    Blockade of the left anterior cerebral artery (**choice A**) would lead to a right leg paresis or paralysis and diminished sensation over the right leg.

    The left middle cerebral artery (**choice B**) supplies the lateral convexity of the right hemisphere. Blockade would lead to a paresis or paralysis of the right face and

arm. The middle cerebral artery is the most common location for stroke.

Blockade of the left posterior cerebral artery (**choice C**), which supplies the left occipital lobe, would lead to a right hemianopia with macular sparing.

The right middle cerebral artery (**choice E**) supplies the lateral convexity of the right hemisphere. Blockade would lead to paresis or paralysis of the left face and arm.

49. **The correct answer is B.** Chronic nonspecific lymphadenitis is a reactive lymph node hyperplasia that can take three distinct forms, seen in different clinical settings. In chronic bacterial infections, such as this patient's chronic tonsillitis, there is a stimulation of B cells that leads to prominence of germinal centers.

    Acute nonspecific lymphadenitis (**choice A**), characterized by necrotic debris, prominent follicles, and, sometimes, a neutrophilic infiltrate, is seen as a response to acute, rather than chronic, infection.

    This patient has a reactive, rather than neoplastic, etiology for lymph node enlargement (**choice C**).

    Immunologic reactions induced by drugs such as phenytoin (Dilantin) produce reactive changes in the paracortical T cells, leading to expansion of cells outside the germinal centers (paracortical lymphoid hyperplasia; **choice D**).

    Sinus histiocytosis (**choice E**) is seen in lymph nodes draining cancers (notably breast) and consists of lymphatic sinusoids packed with histiocytes.

50. **The correct answer is C.** Hospital-acquired pneumonia (or *nosocomial* pneumonia) is defined as a pneumonia that manifests more than 48 hours after admission to the hospital. It more commonly affects patients who are in the ICU or are mechanically ventilated. The most frequent causative microorganisms are *Pseudomonas aeruginosa*, *Staphylococcus aureus*, *Klebsiella pneumoniae*, *Escherichia coli*, and Enterobacter. Pathologic features are those of acute bronchopneumonia, but the mortality rate is high, around 50%.

    Anaerobic pneumonia (**choice A**) occurs in individuals predisposed to aspiration, i.e., those with depressed levels of consciousness, impaired deglutition, or tracheal/nasogastric tubes. Periodontal disease is an additional risk factor, as it leads to increased numbers of anaerobic bacteria in aspirated material. Necrotizing pneumonia, lung abscess, and pleural empyema are the most common pathologic lesions.

    Community-acquired pneumonia (**choice B**) is usually caused by pneumococcus (*Streptococcus pneumoniae*) and results in homogeneous consolidation of an entire lobe. Microscopically, a fibrinopurulent exudate fills the alveolar spaces.

Lipid pneumonia (**choice D**) is characterized histologically by large numbers of lipid-laden macrophages. This form of pneumonia occurs in association with obstructive bronchial lesions or aspiration of mineral oils.

In primary atypical pneumonia (**choice E**) there is a lymphomonocytic infiltrate confined to interalveolar septa and interstitium. *Mycoplasma pneumoniae* is the most frequent etiologic agent.

Pathology and Pathophysiology

1. A 45-year-old woman presents with complaints of easy fatigability, anorexia, and weight loss. Blood tests reveal striking leukocytosis, with 100,000 leukocytes/mL, of which most are immature granulocytic precursors with less than 5% blasts. Cytogenetic studies demonstrate the presence of a reciprocal translocation between the long arms of chromosomes 9 and 22, giving rise to the Philadelphia chromosome. Which of the following is the most likely diagnosis?

   (A) Acute myelogenous leukemia (AML)

   (B) Chronic lymphocytic leukemia (CLL)

   (C) Chronic myelogenous leukemia (CML)

   (D) Leukemoid reaction

   (E) Myelofibrosis

2. Biopsy of the right femur in a 50-year-old man demonstrates irregularly shaped, thick, well-calcified, bony spicules with an abnormal arrangement of cement lines forming a mosaic pattern. This biopsy is most consistent with which of the following conditions?

   (A) Aneurysmal bone cyst

   (B) Chondrosarcoma

   (C) Osteomalacia

   (D) Osteoporosis

   (E) Paget disease

3. A 4-year-old girl with a history of a viral upper respiratory infection 3 weeks ago presents with mucous membrane bleeding. Physical examination is significant for petechiae. Structural examination reveals acute tissue-texture changes at T2-T8 bilaterally. Laboratory studies reveal a platelet count of 15,000/mm³. BUN and creatinine are normal. A peripheral blood smear exhibits large platelets. Which of the following is the most likely diagnosis?

   (A) Disseminated intravascular coagulation

   (B) Hemolytic uremic syndrome

   (C) Idiopathic thrombocytopenic purpura (ITP)

   (D) Thrombotic thrombocytopenic purpura (TTP)

   (E) Unable to discern with information given

4. Neurologic examination of a 34-year-old man reveals a direct and a consensual light reflex in his left eye, but neither a direct nor a consensual light reflex in his right eye. Which of the following signs is also likely to be found during his examination?

   (A) Abducted right eye

   (B) Absence of the right corneal reflex

   (C) Hyperacusis of the right ear

   (D) Inability to close the right eye

   (E) Visual field defect of the right eye

5. A 30-year-old, otherwise healthy woman presents to her physician with complaints of fatigue and dyspnea. Physical examination reveals normal breath sounds and the presence of third and fourth heart sounds. Structural examination reveals chronic somatic dysfunction at T1-T4. A chest x-ray film shows clear lung fields but right ventricular enlargement, main pulmonary artery enlargement, and "pruning" of the peripheral vasculature. An electrocardiogram shows right axis deviation and right ventricular hypertrophy. Left ventricular function appears normal on echocardiography. Serologic studies show antinuclear antibodies. Which of the following pathologic findings would this patient also show, either at autopsy or if an appropriate biopsy were taken?

   (A) Mural thrombus of the right atrium

   (B) Necrosis and scarring of the left ventricle

   (C) Plexogenic pulmonary vasculopathy

   (D) Pulmonary artery stenosis

   (E) Severe pulmonary fibrosis

6. Patient A has carbon monoxide (CO) poisoning, and patient B has iron deficiency anemia. Assume that CO is binding 50% of the available O_2-binding sites on the hemoglobin, and that the anemic patient has 50% of the normal amount of hemoglobin. Patient A is more at risk of tissue hypoxia because CO causes

   (A) arterial hypoxemia, while anemia does not

   (B) a decrease in diffusing capacity

   (C) a decrease in the P_{50} of Hb for O_2

   (D) a greater decrease in the concentration of arterial oxygen

   (E) a reduced rate of O_2 binding to available Hb

7. A 27-year-old woman complains that she is constantly thirsty and has to urinate every 2 hours. An osteopathic structural examination reveals ropy, fibrotic tissues bilaterally at the T5-T9 spinal levels. Her plasma osmolality is 295 mOsmol/kg, and her urine osmolality is 100 mOsmol/kg. Her urine is negative for glucose. As part of a diagnostic workup, the patient is deprived of fluids for 3 hours. Her urine osmolality remains 100 mOsmol/kg. One hour after injection of arginine vasopressin (AVP), her urine osmolality becomes 400 mOsmol/kg. Which of the following is the most likely diagnosis?

   (A) Diabetes mellitus

   (B) Nephrogenic diabetes insipidus

   (C) Neurogenic diabetes insipidus

   (D) Primary polydipsia

   (E) SIADH (syndrome of inappropriate antidiuretic hormone)

8. A 64-year-old man presents to his physician with vague complaints of fatigue. Physical examination is remarkable for splenomegaly without lymphadenopathy. Structural examination reveals T5-T9 NS_LR_R. The patient's hematocrit is 30%, his platelet count is 80,000/mm^3, and his leukocyte count is 2500/mm^3. Bone marrow biopsy shows "fried egg" cells expressing pan B-cell markers CD19 and CD20. Which of the following is the most likely diagnosis?

   (A) Aplastic anemia

   (B) Hairy cell leukemia

   (C) Hereditary spherocytosis

   (D) Hodgkin disease

   (E) Sézary syndrome

9. A sports announcer reports that an older athlete will not be playing because he has a "ruptured" disc. Which of the following correctly describes the gross pathology of this condition?

   (A) The anulus fibrosus protrudes anteriorly through a weakened nucleus pulposus

   (B) The anulus fibrosus protrudes anteromedially through a weakened nucleus pulposus

   (C) The anulus fibrosus protrudes posteriorly through a weakened nucleus pulposus

   (D) The nucleus pulposus protrudes anteriorly through a weakened anulus fibrosus

   (E) The nucleus pulposus protrudes posterolaterally through a weakened anulus fibrosus

10. A 4-year-old child develops a soft tissue mass in the orbit of his left eye, which on biopsy demonstrates a variety of cell geometries, including "strap" and "tadpole" eosinophilic cells. Bizarre mitotic figures are seen. This child most likely has which of the following conditions?

    (A) Leiomyoma

    (B) Leiomyosarcoma

    (C) Lipoma

    (D) Malignant fibrous histiocytoma

    (E) Rhabdomyosarcoma

11. A 32-year-old man was revived after having been submerged underwater for 15 minutes. His physicians were concerned that he sustained hypoxic damage to his brain. Which of the following structures would most likely be damaged?

    (A) Claustrum

    (B) Layer 2 of the cerebral cortex

    (C) Mammillary bodies

    (D) Purkinje layer of the cerebellum

    (E) Subiculum

12. A 24-year-old male has just been in a car accident. After several hours in the emergency department, he has not produced a urine output. Which of the following is an example of a prerenal cause of oliguria?

    (A) Acute glomerulonephritis

    (B) Bladder tumor

    (C) Prostatic hyperplasia

    (D) Shock

    (E) Transplant rejection

13. A 50-year-old woman reports a sensation of "the room spinning" when she lies down from a sitting position. Her hearing is unaffected, and she is able to walk a straight line with her eyes closed. Her symptoms are caused by damage to the

    (A) frontal bone

    (B) posterior inferior cerebellar artery

    (C) semicircular canals

    (D) utricle and saccule

    (E) vestibulocochlear nerve

14. A 70-year-old hypertensive man arrives at the emergency department complaining of shortness of breath. His history is significant for chronic hypertension, paroxysmal nocturnal dyspnea, and nocturia. Physical examination reveals evidence of pulmonary and peripheral edema. Structural examination reveals somatic dysfunction at T1-T4. The tissues are cool, ropy, and fibrotic. The patient is admitted, and furosemide is administered. A low-sodium diet is ordered. The purpose of this dietary restriction is to

    (A) decrease tubular reabsorption of sodium

    (B) increase extracellular water

    (C) increase intracellular water

    (D) reduce extracellular water

    (E) reduce intracellular water

15. A 14-year-old girl with a high fever and sore throat presents to the emergency department. Physical examination reveals acute changes at T1-T3. A complete blood count with differential implies the presence of a viral infection. Which of the following best describes the cells that indicate a viral etiology to her illness?

    (A) They are basophilic with spherical dark-stained nuclei

    (B) They are precursors of osteoclasts and liver Kupffer cells

    (C) They contain a peripheral hyalomere and central granulomere

    (D) They have azurophilic granules and multilobed nuclei

    (E) They remain in the circulation approximately 120 days

16. A bronchial biopsy from a long-term smoker demonstrates focal areas where the normal respiratory epithelium is replaced by keratinizing squamous epithelium. The same change may occur as a pathologic response to deficiency of which of the following vitamins?

    (A) Vitamin A

    (B) Vitamin B_{12}

    (C) Vitamin C

    (D) Vitamin D

    (E) Vitamin E

17. A 65-year-old, fair-skinned man develops scaly erythematous papules that have a sandpaper texture on his forehead. A biopsy shows nuclear crowding, hyperchromasia, and pleomorphism of the basal keratinocytes, with alteration of the normal epidermal maturation. Hyperkeratosis is also present. Which of the following neoplasms may arise from this lesion?

    (A) Basal cell carcinoma

    (B) Melanoma

    (C) Merkel cell carcinoma

    (D) Mycosis fungoides

    (E) Squamous cell carcinoma

18. A 38-year-old woman comes to clinical attention because of chest pain of recent onset. Her blood pressure is 150/60 mm Hg, and auscultation reveals a diastolic murmur along the left sternal border. Her structural examination revealed that T2-T4 had chronic tissue-texture changes. Laboratory studies are significant for a positive fluorescent treponemal antibody absorption test (FTA-ABS). Which of the following pathologic alterations is most likely associated with this clinical presentation?

    (A) Calcification of aortic cusps with stenosis of the aortic orifice

    (B) Fibrous thickening of mitral leaflets with commissural fusion

    (C) Intrachordal ballooning of mitral valve leaflets

    (D) Scarring of the ascending aorta with tree-barking appearance

    (E) Severe atherosclerosis of coronary arteries

19. A 60-year-old man presents with progressive weakness, recurrent fever, and night sweats. Physical examination reveals multiple enlarged lymph nodes in the lateral cervical region. A biopsy of one of these nodes demonstrates diffuse effacement of the nodal architecture by uniform sheets of large atypical lymphoid cells with frequent mitoses. Which of the following is the most likely diagnosis?

    (A) High-grade non-Hodgkin lymphoma

    (B) Hodgkin lymphoma

    (C) Low-grade non-Hodgkin lymphoma

    (D) Paracortical lymphoid hyperplasia

    (E) Reactive follicular hyperplasia

20. A 50-year-old man presents with renal colic. Physical examination revealed somatic dysfunction at T11-L1. An IV pyelogram demonstrates "clumps" of contrast medium limited to the medulla, as well as multiple small stones. Blood chemistries are all within normal limits. Which of the following is the most likely explanation for these findings?

    (A) Adult polycystic renal disease

    (B) Horseshoe kidney

    (C) Infantile polycystic renal disease

    (D) Medullary sponge kidney

    (E) Renal dysplasia

21. A 30-year-old man presents to the dermatologist with silvery, scaling plaques on his elbows and knees. His mother had been afflicted with the same condition in the past. Which of the following is the most likely diagnosis?

    (A) Acne rosacea

    (B) Acne vulgaris

    (C) Pemphigus vulgaris

    (D) Pityriasis rosea

    (E) Psoriasis vulgaris

22. Testicular biopsy of an infertile man demonstrates a complete absence of sperm or sperm precursors in spermatic tubules that have a regular, round cross-section and are closely packed together. Which of the following is the most likely etiology of this condition?

    (A) Diabetes mellitus

    (B) Maturation arrest

    (C) Seminoma

    (D) Sertoli-only syndrome

    (E) Tuberculosis

23. When watching a routine immunization injection being given to her 2-year-old brother, a teenage girl suddenly complains of feeling faint and starts hyperventilating. A nurse has her sit on the floor and gives her a paper bag. What is the rationale for this therapy?

    (A) The higher CO_2 content of the bag will correct the patient's compensated respiratory acidosis

    (B) The higher CO_2 content of the bag will correct the patient's compensated respiratory alkalosis

    (C) The higher CO_2 content of the bag will correct the patient's uncompensated respiratory acidosis

    (D) The higher CO_2 content of the bag will correct the patient's uncompensated respiratory alkalosis

    (E) The paper bag is a placebo

24. A 30-year-old football player lacerates his face in a fall during practice. He is taken to a surgeon, who finds a clean wound with well-approximated edges. There is little surrounding tissue damage. Which of the following stages of wound healing will occur first?

    (A) A thin, continuous epithelial cover will appear

    (B) Fibroblasts will lay down collagen fibers

    (C) Granulation tissue will fill the wound

    (D) Macrophages will appear

    (E) Neutrophils will line the wound edge

25. The presence of the Philadelphia chromosome is associated with a more favorable prognosis in patients with which of the following diseases?

    (A) Acute lymphoblastic leukemia

    (B) Acute myelogenous leukemia

    (C) Chronic lymphocytic leukemia

    (D) Chronic myelogenous leukemia

    (E) Hairy cell leukemia

26. A 65-year-old man with hyperlucent lung fields develops extreme shortness of breath over a period of about 15 minutes. A quick osteopathic examination reveals acute tissue changes at T2-T7 on the right side. A chest x-ray film shows shift of the mediastinum to the right, and the lung field on the left appears even more hyperlucent than before, with the exception of a white shadow near the heart border. Which of the following is the most probable cause of the patient's current problem?

    (A) Bronchogenic carcinoma

    (B) Pleural effusion

    (C) Pulmonary embolism

    (D) Rupture of an emphysematous bulla

    (E) Tuberculosis

27. Two bone marrow aspirates are studied under the microscope. One is taken from an adult with Hemoglobin SS disease (sickle cell anemia), and the other is from an adult with normal Hemoglobin A. The marrow aspirate from the patient with sickle cell anemia could be identified because of its increased

    (A) fat

    (B) iron stores

    (C) medullary bone

    (D) megakaryocytes

    (E) myeloid:erythroid ratio

28. After a complete cardiac workup, you order a biopsy. Microscopic examination of this biopsy obtained from a heart shows ventricular hypertrophy with asymmetric septal thickening. Which of the following findings would be expected?

    (A) Aschoff bodies

    (B) Disorganization of myofibrils

    (C) Infiltration by inflammatory cells

    (D) Localized fibrous scarring

    (E) Structures resembling poorly formed vessels

29. An 18-year-old girl whose grandmother was recently diagnosed with breast cancer discovers a large, round, moveable nodule in her left breast. An osteopathic examination reveals no dysfunction. Concerned, she visits her primary care physician. Which of the following diagnoses is most likely?

    (A) Cystosarcoma phyllodes

    (B) Fibroadenoma

    (C) Fibrocystic breast disease

    (D) Infiltrating ductal carcinoma

    (E) Intraductal papilloma

30. A 38-year-old man has paroxysmal hypertension. He is subsequently found to have medullary carcinoma of the thyroid, pheochromocytoma, and mucosal neuromas. Parathyroid involvement is not noted. Which of the following is the most likely diagnosis?

    (A) Multiple endocrine neoplasia (MEN) type I

    (B) MEN type II

    (C) MEN type III

    (D) Sipple syndrome

    (E) Wermer syndrome

31. On a routine physical examination of a patient, you find somatic dysfunction at T1-T4 and a very large neck mass. A biopsy of this mass shows a benign thyroid lesion composed of colloid-filled follicles separated by fibrous scars. Which of the following is the most likely diagnosis?

    (A) Diffuse nontoxic goiter

    (B) Multinodular goiter

    (C) Subacute thyroiditis

    (D) Thyroid adenoma

    (E) Thyroid cyst

32. A 30-year-old woman presents to her physician with fever, night sweats, and weight loss. Physical examination reveals supraclavicular and lower cervical adenopathy. Lymph node biopsy reveals the presence of Reed-Sternberg cells with lacunae surrounding the nuclei of the cells. Which of the following variants of Hodgkin disease is most likely present?

    (A) Lymphocyte depletion

    (B) Lymphocyte predominance

    (C) Mixed cellularity

    (D) Nodular sclerosis

    (E) Hairy cell

33. A patient presents with secondary amenorrhea. She reports that "things smell odd now." During the physical examination, papilledema is noted in one eye, and careful tests reveal loss of vision in some parts of the visual field. This patient should be carefully evaluated for a tumor in which of the following sites?

(A) Falx cerebri

(B) Hippocampus

(C) Posterior fossa

(D) Sphenoidal ridge

(E) Suprasellar region

34. A 20-year-old African American woman with a history of multiple small bowel resections for Crohn disease presents complaining of fatigue and dyspnea on exertion. Her physical examination is notable for pallor and a wide-based, unsteady gait. An osteopathic examination reveals chronic hypersympathetic tone at T9-T12. Her lab studies reveal a hemoglobin of 10.0 g/dL, with a mean corpuscular volume of 120 μm^3. Examination of the peripheral blood smear shows macrocytosis, anisocytosis, poikilocytosis, and neutrophils with 6-8 nuclear lobulations. Which of the following is the most likely cause of this patient's anemia?

(A) Beta-thalassemia trait

(B) Folate deficiency

(C) Iron deficiency

(D) Sickle cell trait

(E) Vitamin B_{12} deficiency

35. A 5-year-old boy with a 1-month history of fevers and lassitude is found to have severe anemia, moderate thrombocytopenia, and a white blood count of 12,000 cells per mm^3. A bone marrow biopsy would most likely reveal

(A) acute lymphoblastic leukemia (ALL)

(B) acute myeloblastic leukemia (AML)

(C) chronic lymphocytic leukemia

(D) chronic myeloid leukemia

(E) hairy cell leukemia

36. A 12-year-old girl, with history of a streptococcal sore throat that occurred several weeks ago, presents to her physician with an erythematous macular skin rash in a "bathing suit" distribution. Which of the following signs would be necessary to make the diagnosis of rheumatic fever?

(A) Elevated erythrocyte sedimentation rate

(B) Leukocytosis

(C) Migratory polyarthritis

(D) Prolonged PR interval on EKG

(E) Temperature greater than 100.4 F

37. A 53-year-old woman presents with a 6-month history of dysphagia, substernal pain, and melena. Her substernal pain is exacerbated when she eats large meals or goes to bed for the evening. Physical examination reveals chronic tissue changes at T2-T8 on the left paraspinal musculature. Her symptoms are due to dysfunction of which of the following sphincters?

(A) Ileocecal

(B) Lower esophageal

(C) Pyloric

(D) Sphincter of Oddi

(E) Upper esophageal

38. A patient with a pulmonary thromboembolism has blockage of the anterior branch of the right superior pulmonary artery, causing an infarct in the corresponding region of the right lung. Along with breathlessness, rapid respiration, and increased heart rate, the patient complains of chest pain, which is attributed to lack of blood supply to the pleura overlying the affected bronchopulmonary segment. Physical examination reveals acute tissue-texture changes on the right paraspinal musculature at the T2-T7 spinal level. Which nerve transmits pain sensation from the affected area of pleura?

(A) Greater splanchnic nerve

(B) Intercostal nerve

(C) Phrenic nerve

(D) Pulmonary plexus

(E) Vagus nerve

39. A 65-year-old woman with a long-standing disease has bone marrow fibrosis and increased bone remodeling, with bone resorption exceeding bone formation. She has a history of passing calcium-oxalate kidney stones. Structural examination reveals chronic tissue changes at T1-T4 and T11-L2. Which of the following laboratory result profiles would be expected in the serum of this patient?

	Ca^{2+}	PO_4^{3-}	PTH
(A)	↓	↓	↑
(B)	↓	↑	↓
(C)	↓	↑	↑
(D)	↑	↓	↑
(E)	↑	↑	↑

40. A 24-year-old man has progressive, painless enlargement of neck lymph nodes. Physical examination reveals a decrease in all range of motion in the cervical region. A routine chest film followed by CT scan demonstrates marked enlargement of mediastinal nodes. No nodules are seen in the liver or lungs. When evaluating the biopsy of one of the involved nodes, the pathologist should specifically look for which of the following?

(A) Abnormal plasma cells

(B) Giant platelets

(C) Immature neutrophil precursors

(D) Melanin pigment

(E) Reed-Sternberg cells

41. A 47-year-old man presents with a small, red, plaque-like lesion on the glans of his penis. A diagnosis of Bowen disease is made on biopsy examination. Which of the following changes of the uterine cervix is histopathologically equivalent to this patient's disease?

(A) Carcinoma *in situ*

(B) Chronic cervicitis

(C) Invasive squamous cell carcinoma

(D) Mild cervical dysplasia

(E) Nabothian cyst

42. A 25-year-old man presents with bilateral hearing loss. MRI reveals bilateral tumors within the cerebellopontine angles. Surgery is performed, and the tumors are removed. Both are found to be neurilemomas ("schwannoma"). Which of the following is the most likely diagnosis?

(A) Metastatic disease

(B) Multiple sclerosis

(C) Neurofibromatosis type 1

(D) Neurofibromatosis type 2

(E) Tuberous sclerosis

43. A 62-year-old man with a long history of cigarette smoking develops high blood pressure, a moon face, and central obesity. Physical examination reveals chronic somatic dysfunction at T2-T8 bilaterally. Serum ACTH is increased, but MRI studies of the pituitary and hypothalamus fail to demonstrate any tumors. A chest x-ray film reveals a small tumor in the right upper lobe, and a biopsy is performed. Histologically, the tumor is composed of sheets of anaplastic cells with a high nuclear/cytoplasmic ratio. The tumor is immunoreactive to antibodies directed against ACTH. Which of the following is the most likely diagnosis?

(A) Adenocarcinoma

(B) Carcinoid tumor

(C) Hamartoma

(D) Small cell carcinoma

(E) Squamous cell carcinoma

44. A 35-year-old, obese, former football player complains of joint stiffness of the knees and distal interphalangeal joints of the fingers. Physical examination reveals decreased range of motion of the affected joints, crepitus, and bony swelling. Structural examination reveals bilaterally chronic tissue changes at T10-L2. X-ray films display narrowing of the affected joint spaces. Which of the following is the most likely etiology of this patient's disorder?

(A) Accumulation of calcium pyrophosphate in joint fluid

(B) Antibodies against the Fc fragment of IgG

(C) Chondrocyte injury and abnormal collagen activity

(D) Hematogenous seeding of joints during bacteremia

(E) Inborn error of purine metabolism

45. A 15-year-old boy who very recently immigrated to the U.S. presents to the physician with fever, headache, and stiff neck. Examination is remarkable for asymmetric weakness and hyporeflexia. He has a poor immunization history, and poliomyelitis is diagnosed. What is the primary mechanism by which poliovirus causes paralytic disease?

    (A) Demyelination of lower motor neuron axons

    (B) Demyelination of upper motor neuron axons

    (C) Destruction of cell bodies of lower motor neurons

    (D) Destruction of muscle cells

    (E) Destruction of synapses between the axon and the muscle

46. A severely ill patient in shock develops acute renal failure with oliguria and azotemia. Physical examination reveals acute somatic dysfunction at T10 and T11 bilaterally. The urine osmolality approaches that of the glomerular ultrafiltrate (specific gravity 1.010). A renal biopsy would most likely show which of the following?

    (A) Acute pyelonephritis

    (B) Acute tubular necrosis

    (C) Chronic pyelonephritis

    (D) Crescentic glomerulonephritis

    (E) Renal cell carcinoma

Questions 47-50

<u>SET A</u>

Directions: For each numbered item (**patient presentation**), select the one lettered heading (**etiology**) most closely associated with it. Each lettered heading may be selected once, more than once, or not at all.

    (A) cholecystitis

    (B) pancreatitis

    (C) ectopic pregnancy

    (D) splenic rupture

    (E) nephrolithiasis

    (F) appendicitis

    (G) obturator hernia

47. An 18-year-old woman presents with abdominal pain and has ecchymosis periumbilically.

48. A 42-year-old man presents with pain down the medial aspect of the left thigh radiating to the knee.

49. A 22-year-old man complains of severe left shoulder pain after playing in a football game in which he received a hit to the left lower ribcage by the helmet of an opposing player.

50. A 56-year-old man presents with severe abdominal pain the day after Thanksgiving and has a bluish discoloration around the umbilicus.

Pathology and Pathophysiology

ANSWERS AND EXPLANATIONS

1.	C	26.	D
2.	E	27.	B
3.	C	28.	B
4.	A	29.	B
5.	C	30.	C
6.	C	31.	B
7.	C	32.	D
8.	B	33.	E
9.	E	34.	E
10.	E	35.	A
11.	D	36.	C
12.	D	37.	B
13.	C	38.	B
14.	D	39.	D
15.	A	40.	E
16.	A	41.	A
17.	E	42.	D
18.	D	43.	D
19.	A	44.	C
20.	D	45.	C
21.	E	46.	B
22.	D	47.	C
23.	D	48.	G
24.	E	49.	D
25.	D	50.	B

1. **The correct answer is C.** Chronic myelogenous leukemia (CML) is one of the chronic myeloproliferative disorders, which develop from neoplastic transformation of a stem cell that may differentiate along erythrocytic, megakaryocytic, granulocytic, or monocytic lines. CML is characterized by the presence of the Philadelphia chromosome, arising from a balanced translocation involving 9q and 22q. This results in the formation of a bcr/abl fusion gene encoding a protein with tyrosine kinase activity.

   Acute myelogenous leukemia (AML; **choice A**) is usually associated with a large number of blasts in peripheral blood, as well as in the bone marrow. Although the Philadelphia chromosome is absent, other chromosomal and genetic abnormalities define the various subtypes of AML. The most frequent form (with full myeloid maturation) is associated with t(8;21).

   Chronic lymphocytic leukemia (CLL; **choice B**) and its lymphomatous counterpart—small lymphocytic lymphoma—derive from neoplastic proliferation of small well-differentiated lymphocytes. CLL is often associated with absolute lymphocytosis (up to 200,000/mL) in peripheral blood.

   A leukemoid reaction (**choice D**) is an exuberant form of leukocytosis (with leukocyte counts up to 50,000/mL) that may follow infections. Sometimes it is difficult to distinguish between true leukemia and a leukemoid reaction, but the presence of the Philadelphia chromosome rules out the latter.

   Myelofibrosis (**choice E**) is a chronic myeloproliferative disorder characterized by marrow fibrosis and widespread extramedullary hematopoiesis, resulting in massive splenomegaly. The Philadelphia chromosome is absent.

2. **The correct answer is E.** This is the microscopic pattern seen in Paget disease. This disorder is characterized by excessive bone resorption coupled with excessive formation of highly vascular bone with a rubbery consistency and increased susceptibility to fracture. Early on, osteolytic activity is greatest; later, osteoblastic activity becomes more marked. Eventually, the bone becomes sclerotic. The etiology of this condition is unknown. It usually occurs in adults older than 40, and may involve either a single site on one bone or many sites on multiple bones (particularly bones with marrow). Many cases are asymptomatic. In about 1% of the cases, osteosarcoma or other sarcomas may develop in the affected bone.

   Aneurysmal bone cyst (**choice A**) produces a solitary, large, cystic space filled with blood, typically in the shaft of a long bone or vertebral body in children or adolescents.

   Chondrosarcoma (**choice B**) is a malignant, cartilage-forming tumor composed of cells (sometimes with a bizarre appearance) that form variable amounts of poorly-to-well-formed neoplastic cartilage.

   There is a decreased amount of well-calcified bone in both osteomalacia (**choice C**) and osteoporosis (**choice D**). In osteomalacia, the problem is a failure to calcify the bony matrix; in osteoporosis, active bone resorption produces thin bony spicules.

3. **The correct answer is C.** Idiopathic thrombocytopenic purpura (ITP) classically occurs acutely in children several weeks after a viral infection (a viral exanthem or upper respiratory infection in 70% of cases) and is the most common thrombocytopenic purpura of childhood. Physical examination findings usually include easy bruisability, mucous membrane bleeding, gastrointestinal or genitourinary bleeding, and petechiae. CNS bleeding may occur. The peripheral smear typically shows a few, large, young platelets. The other cell lines are normal.

   Disseminated intravascular coagulation (**choice A**) is an acquired consumption deficiency of clotting factors and platelets, often resulting in fatal thrombosis and hemorrhage.

   Hemolytic uremic syndrome (**choice B**) generally occurs in children following diarrhea due to *Shigella*, *Salmonella*, *Escherichia coli* O157:H7, or a virus. Patients typically present with renal failure (BUN and creatinine would be abnormal) along with bleeding and anemia. The disease is similar to thrombotic thrombocytopenic purpura (TTP; **choice D**).

   TTP (**choice D**) is associated with fever, renal failure, neurologic changes, and microangiopathic hemolytic anemia. Platelet aggregation leads to the development of microthrombi throughout the vasculature. The peripheral smear shows few platelets, fragmented red blood cells (schistocytes), and helmet cells.

4. **The correct answer is A.** Two pieces of information are necessary to answer this question. First, you need to determine which nerve is involved. Second, you need to know what other effects a lesion of that nerve would produce. The pupillary light reflex is assessed by shining a light in one eye and observing pupillary constriction in the same eye (direct response) and in the other eye (consensual response). The afferent limb of this reflex is the optic nerve (CN II), and the efferent limb is the oculomotor nerve (CN III). Clearly, the left CN II and left CN III are working because a direct response is seen in the left eye. Also, the right CN II must be working to produce a consensual response in the left eye. However, there must be a lesion of the right CN

III because pupillary constriction is not observed under any circumstance in the right eye. CN III also innervates the medial rectus muscle of the eye. Absence of innervation of this muscle would result in unopposed action of the lateral rectus muscle, causing an outward deviation of the eye.

Absence of the right corneal reflex (**choice B**) would result from a lesion of the right trigeminal nerve (CN V; afferent limb) or the right facial nerve (CN VII; efferent limb).

Hyperacusis of the right ear (**choice C**) could result from a lesion of the right CN V (which innervates the tensor tympani muscle) or the right CN VII (which innervates the stapedius muscle). Both of these muscles dampen sound through the middle ear.

Inability to close the right eye (**choice D**) would be produced by a lesion of the right CN VII. In fact, a CN III lesion would cause the eyelid to droop because the levator palpebrae muscle would be denervated.

A visual field defect of the right eye (**choice E**) would occur if the right CN II was lesioned, but because a consensual light response was elicited in the left eye, the right CN II must be functional.

5. **The correct answer is C.** The presentation described is classic for pulmonary hypertension and, more specifically, the primary idiopathic form of pulmonary hypertension. This rare condition is thought to be related to the collagen vascular diseases, since up to 50% of patients have antinuclear antibodies (despite the absence of frank presentation of other autoimmune disease). Also, a similar, known secondary form of pulmonary hypertension is sometimes seen in patients with a wide variety of collagen vascular diseases, including systemic lupus erythematosus, polymyositis, dermatomyositis, systemic sclerosis, and adult and juvenile forms of rheumatoid arthritis. A wide variety of other conditions have also been associated with secondary pulmonary hypertension, including shunts, left atrial hypertension, chronic hypoxia, pulmonary embolism, drug reaction, hepatic cirrhosis, and sickle cell disease. Both primary and secondary forms of pulmonary hypertension are associated with prominent changes in the pulmonary vasculature, which can include muscularization of smaller arterioles, concentric hypertrophy of the intima ("onion skinning"), and a distinctive plexiform lesion (plexogenic pulmonary vasculopathy) in which the smallest arterioles become markedly dilated with lumens partially occluded by endothelial (or possibly mesenchymal) cells and sometimes thrombus. The prognosis of untreated pulmonary hypertension is poor. However, the use of the vasodilator hydralazine with anticoagulation can slow the course (fatal in about

3 years in untreated patients). If the pulmonary hypertension is secondary, therapy of the primary disease can be helpful.

Unlike cor pulmonale, atrial fibrillation with mural thrombus formation (**choice A**) is uncommon in primary pulmonary hypertension.

The absence of left ventricular findings on echocardiography tends to exclude myocardial infarction as the source of the patient's findings (**choice B**).

The presence of enlargement of the main pulmonary artery excludes pulmonary artery stenosis (**choice D**).

The clear lung fields exclude severe pulmonary fibrosis (**choice E**).

6. **The correct answer is C.** The P_{50} is defined as the partial pressure of oxygen necessary to bind 50% of available hemoglobin. CO will decrease the P_{50} of Hb for O_2. Another way of stating this is that CO left-shifts the oxygen-hemoglobin dissociation curve. CO is deadly because it not only binds hemoglobin with a greater affinity than does O_2 (240 times better), it also left-shifts the curve, thereby making it more difficult to unload O_2 in peripheral tissues.

Neither of these conditions will cause arterial hypoxemia (**choice A**).

CO will not diminish the diffusing capacity of the lung (**choice B**); in fact, it is routinely used to measure diffusing capacity.

The concentration of oxygen in arterial blood will be approximately the same for both cases (**choice D**). If anything, the concentration will be slightly greater in the patient with CO poisoning because CO left-shifts the curve; therefore, the available binding sites of Hb for O_2 will be slightly more saturated.

CO does not change the rate of O_2 binding to Hb (**choice E**). It does, however, bind to hemoglobin with 240 times the affinity of oxygen.

7. **The correct answer is C.** ADH (antidiuretic hormone, vasopressin) is normally released from the posterior pituitary in response to hypovolemia and increased osmotic pressure. It acts on the collecting duct of the nephron, increasing its permeability to water. This concentrates the urine and conserves water. Diabetes insipidus (DI) is a condition in which ADH function is absent.

Two forms of DI exist: neurogenic and nephrogenic. Neurogenic DI (**choice C**) is due to absence of ADH secretion from the posterior pituitary; thus, serum ADH levels are always low, even in states of serious volume depletion. Nephrogenic DI (**choice B**) is due to complete or partial resistance to ADH; therefore, even though ADH levels are high, the hormone has no effect on renal water regulation.

You are told in the question that the patient's urine did not concentrate on a water deprivation test. This immediately suggests DI. (Normally, when an individual is deprived of fluids for 3 hours, her kidneys respond by concentrating the urine and conserving water). Your task then becomes determining which type of DI the patient has. This is achieved by evaluating the results of the arginine vasopressin (AVP) suppression test. Patients with neurogenic DI readily respond to AVP by producing more concentrated urine. Patients with nephrogenic DI do not concentrate urine in response to AVP because of continued renal resistance.

Although thirst is a common symptom of diabetes mellitus (**choice A**), the absence of glucosuria argues against this diagnosis.

Primary polydipsia (**choice D**) usually occurs in patients taking antipsychotic drugs that cause dry mouth (e.g., phenothiazines), promoting the sensation of thirst. As a result, these patients drink large quantities of water. They excrete dilute urine, and eventually may dilute their serum as well, to the point of electrolyte imbalance. On water deprivation, however, their urine will concentrate normally.

SIADH (syndrome of inappropriate antidiuretic hormone; **choice E**) occurs when there is oversecretion of ADH, for example by a small cell carcinoma of the lung or other ADH-producing neoplasm. One would expect test results opposite to those in this patient. In contrast to DI, the diagnosis of SIADH is usually made with a water-load test.

8. **The correct answer is B.** Hairy cell leukemia is characterized by pancytopenia, often with massive splenomegaly. Lymphadenopathy is unusual. The proliferating cells express the pan B-cell markers CD19 and CD20 as well as monocyte markers. Histologically, the cells display fine, hairlike projections. A "fried-egg" appearance of bone marrow biopsies arises because of the fixation artifacts from the hairlike projections on many of the cells. Tartrate-resistant acid phosphatase (not mentioned in this question) is virtually diagnostic of hairy cell leukemia. Interferon-alfa is used for treatment.

    Aplastic anemia (**choice A**), or marrow aplasia, is also characterized by pancytopenia; however, the marrow would be hypocellular, with fatty replacement of hematopoietic cells.

    Hereditary spherocytosis (**choice C**) is due to a defect in the membrane of the red cells and would be accompanied by abnormal red cell morphology. Splenomegaly is

typical, but other cell lines (white blood cells, platelets) are not affected. Remember that spherocytes exhibit increased osmotic fragility.

Hodgkin disease (**choice D**) is a lymphoma characterized by the presence of Reed-Sternberg cells in a variable lymphocytic infiltrate.

Sézary syndrome (**choice E**) is related to mycosis fungoides, a cutaneous T-cell (not B-cell) lymphoma. In both disorders, there is a characteristic "cerebriform" cell, which circulates in the blood in Sézary syndrome but remains confined to the skin in most cases of mycosis fungoides.

9. **The correct answer is E.** Herniated intervertebral discs, often called "slipped" or "ruptured" discs by lay people, occur when the weakened outer anulus fibrosus of the disc permits herniation of the centrally located nucleus pulposus. The defect typically occurs in a posterolateral direction, where it may compress an adjacent spinal nerve root, causing severe low back or leg pain.

    Hint on strategy: This was a question in which formulating your answer before looking at the choices would have prevented a lot of confusion and saved time.

10. **The correct answer is E.** The child has a rhabdomyosarcoma, which is the most common form of malignant soft-tissue tumor seen in infants and children. The characteristic strap and tadpole cells are immature forms of rhabdomyoblasts (and may be hard to find among many poorly differentiated cells). This child probably has embryonal rhabdomyosarcoma, which can also be seen in the genital urinary tract (where it may form "bunches of grapes"). Despite the prevalence in textbooks of dramatic photographs of genitourinary rhabdomyosarcomas in young children, these tumors actually occur more frequently in the head and neck region, particularly the orbit, nasopharynx, and middle ear.

    The presence of abnormal mitotic figures excludes the possibility of a benign tumor (**choices A and C**).

    Leiomyosarcoma (**choice B**) and malignant fibrous histiocytoma (**choice D**) are both malignant tumors, but would not be expected to contain strap and tadpole cells.

11. **The correct answer is D.** The Purkinje cell layer of the cerebellar cortex, pyramidal cells in the CA1 subfield of the hippocampus, and pyramidal cells in layers 3 and 5 of the cerebral cortex are all very sensitive to the effects of cerebral hypoxia and ischemia. The basis for this selective vulnerability may be NMDA-receptor mediated excitotoxic injury of these specific populations of neurons.

The claustrum (**choice A**) is a thin sheet of gray matter located between the external capsule and the extreme capsule. It is not selectively targeted by hypoxic/ischemic injury to the brain.

Layer 2 of the cerebral cortex (**choice B**) is the external granular layer, populated by closely packed granule cells. This layer is not affected by ischemia to the same extent as layers 3 and 5, the external and internal pyramidal cell layers.

The mammillary bodies (**choice C**) are hypothalamic structures located at the base of the brain. They are damaged in Wernicke-Korsakoff syndrome, which is due to thiamine deficiency.

The subiculum (**choice E**) lies medial and inferior to the hippocampus. The subiculum is not selectively vulnerable to hypoxia, in contrast to the nearby CA1 subfield of the hippocampus.

12. **The correct answer is D.** It is important to remember that not all oliguria is caused by intrinsic renal disease. Shock, of any etiology, is an example of a prerenal cause of oliguria in which poor renal perfusion leads to inadequate urine output. Other examples of prerenal causes include hepatorenal syndrome, postoperative oliguria, and dehydration. Postrenal causes of oliguria usually involve bilateral obstruction and may be due to disease of the ureters, bladder neck, or urethra.

Acute glomerulonephritis (**choice A**) and transplant rejection (**choice E**) are examples of renal causes of oliguria.

Bladder tumor (**choice B**) and prostatic hyperplasia (**choice C**) are examples of postrenal causes of oliguria.

13. **The correct answer is C.** Each semicircular canal contains sensory areas that respond to movements of endolymph caused by motion of the head in the same plane as the duct. The posterior canal is implicated in backward motion of the head, as in the change from a sitting to a reclining position.

Insufficient blood flow to the posterior inferior cerebellar artery (**choice B**) would result in cerebellar symptoms, which include the inability to walk a straight line with the eyes closed.

The utricle and saccule (**choice D**) react to acceleration and deceleration of the head rather than to rotary movement.

Damage to the vestibulocochlear nerve (**choice E**) would result in disturbances of both equilibrium and hearing.

14. **The correct answer is D.** This hypertensive patient has symptoms and signs of congestive heart failure (paroxysmal nocturnal dyspnea, nocturia, and pulmonary and peripheral edema), for which dietary sodium restriction is recommended to reduce water retention. Most of the sodium in the body exists in locations outside cells, such as plasma, interstitial fluid, cerebrospinal fluid, intraocular fluid, semen, peritoneal fluid, and pleural fluid. The concentration of sodium in these fluids is tightly regulated by the kidney's action on blood plasma. When dietary sodium is severely restricted, the losses in the kidney (and small losses in sweat) exceed the intake, and the total body sodium is decreased. The body then tries to maintain serum sodium concentration by excreting more water via the kidneys. Most of the water comes from the extracellular fluid rather than the intracellular fluid (**choice E**), since sodium ion is not a quantitatively important component of intracellular fluid. Decreased dietary sodium will increase tubular reabsorption of sodium rather than decreasing it (**choice A**).

15. **The correct answer is A.** This question is really asking you two things. First, it tests whether you know that lymphocytosis is associated with viral infection. Second, it tests your knowledge of the lymphocytes' histologic appearance. Note that these cells are generally small and normally constitute 25% to 33% of leukocytes. Two types of lymphocytes have been distinguished: T cells (involved in cell-mediated immunity) and B cells (involved in humoral immunity).

Monocytes are precursors of osteoclasts and liver Kupffer cells (**choice B**) and also give rise to tissue macrophages and alveolar macrophages.

Platelets contain a peripheral hyalomere and central granulomere (**choice C**).

Neutrophils have azurophilic granules and multilobed nuclei (**choice D**). They increase in number in response to bacterial infection.

Erythrocytes remain in the circulation for about 120 days (**choice E**).

16. **The correct answer is A.** The histopathologic change described here is *squamous metaplasia*, which may be induced by vitamin A deficiency in different types of epithelial membranes, including conjunctiva, respiratory airways, and urinary tract. This change is probably related to the fact that vitamin A and retinoids play an important role in regulating epithelial differentiation.

Vitamin B_{12} deficiency (**choice B**) results in megaloblastic anemia and degeneration of the posterolateral tracts of the spinal cord.

Vitamin C deficiency (**choice C**) causes scurvy, a syndrome characterized by vascular fragility and bleeding diathesis, with resultant recurrent hemorrhage in the gums, skin, and joints.

Vitamin D deficiency (**choice D**) results in two different clinical pictures depending on the patient's age, i.e., rickets in children and osteomalacia in adults.

Vitamin E (**choice E**) is a major free radical scavenger. For obscure reasons, deficiency of vitamin E results in degeneration of the ascending axons in the posterior spinal column and spinocerebellar tract.

17. **The correct answer is E.** The lesion described is *actinic keratosis*, which is frequent on sun-exposed areas of people of fair complexion. It is related to progressive dysplastic changes triggered by the carcinogenic action of ultraviolet light. Actinic keratosis is a premalignant change, but only a small number of untreated lesions will eventually progress to invasive squamous cell carcinoma.

Basal cell carcinoma (**choice A**) is a common skin neoplasm with minimal metastatic potential. It is also most frequent on sun-exposed areas, but actinic keratosis is not a precursor.

As with squamous cell and basal cell carcinomas, sunlight is an important predisposing condition for the development of skin melanomas (**choice B**), but actinic keratosis is not. Besides sunlight, preexisting nevi, genetic factors, and possibly chemical carcinogens play a pathogenetic role.

Merkel cell carcinoma (**choice C**) is a rare neoplasm that is morphologically identical to small cell carcinoma of the lung. It originates from the epidermal Merkel cells. No premalignant precursor is known for this cancer.

Mycosis fungoides (**choice D**) is a malignant T-cell lymphoma that arises from the skin manifesting with scaly patches, plaques, and nodules. Malignant lymphocytes accumulate underneath the epidermis and infiltrate the overlying epidermis.

18. **The correct answer is D.** This patient has syphilis. In its tertiary stage, syphilis may affect the ascending aorta causing an *obliterative endarteritis* of the vasa vasorum. This results in scarring of the media with wrinkling of the intima, producing the characteristic tree-barking appearance. The aortic ring becomes dilated and the coronary ostia narrowed, leading to aortic regurgitation and myocardial ischemia. Hence, the murmur and the chest pain. Note the typically high systolic pressure and low diastolic pressure accompanying aortic insufficiency.

Calcification of aortic cusps with stenosis of the aortic orifice (**choice A**) is found in elderly patients with clinically evident aortic stenosis. This would lead to an ejection systolic murmur.

Fibrous thickening of mitral leaflets with commissural fusion (**choice B**) is characteristic of chronic rheumatic heart disease and is associated with mitral stenosis. A diastolic murmur is heard at the apex, but this is not associated with a wide difference between systolic and diastolic pressure.

Intrachordal ballooning of mitral valve leaflets (**choice C**) refers to the ballooning of mitral valve leaflets secondary to mitral valve prolapse. This condition may cause mitral valve regurgitation with a systolic murmur.

Severe atherosclerosis of coronary arteries (**choice E**) would be highly unusual in a young patient and would not explain signs of aortic insufficiency. However, cardiovascular syphilis leads to development of secondary atherosclerosis of the ascending aorta.

19. **The correct answer is A.** The presence of atypical lymphocytes, frequent mitoses, and effacement of the lymph node architecture clearly indicates that this is a highly malignant neoplastic process. High-grade non-Hodgkin lymphomas are characterized by markedly atypical cells with usually brisk mitotic activity. The large size of the cells and diffuse pattern of growth suggest *diffuse large cell lymphoma*, the most frequent aggressive non-Hodgkin lymphomas affecting adult patients.

Hodgkin lymphoma (**choice B**) also leads to effacement of the nodal architecture, but it is characterized by the presence of *Reed-Sternberg cells* within a polymorphic cellular background including small lymphocytes, histiocytes, plasma cells, and eosinophils.

Low-grade non-Hodgkin lymphoma (**choice C**) may present with a follicular pattern that mimics the normal follicular architecture of lymph nodes or a diffuse pattern. In both cases, neoplastic lymphocytes are well-differentiated (i.e., similar to their normal counterpart), and mitotic activity is scanty.

Paracortical lymphoid hyperplasia (**choice D**) and follicular reactive hyperplasia (**choice E**) represent normal reactive patterns of the T-cell and B-cell dependent areas, respectively. In both forms, the lymph node architecture is preserved.

20. **The correct answer is D.** This is a classic presentation for medullary sponge kidney, which has a male predominance and typically presents at 40-60 years of age. Histologically, medullary sponge kidney shows multiple small cysts lined by columnar or cuboidal epithelium localized to the medullary collecting tubules. The cysts can contain laminated concretions of calcium phosphates. Renal failure is rare in patients with medullary sponge kidney, and the pathogenesis for the lesion has not been clarified. The rare uremic medul-

lary sponge kidney, unlike the more common form, occurs in 20- to 30-year-olds, is associated with salt-losing nephropathy, and progresses to renal failure.

The kidney of adult polycystic disease (**choice A**) is massively enlarged and filled throughout with round cysts of varying sizes. Adult polycystic kidney disease often presents with hypertension rather than renal failure or stones.

Horseshoe kidney (**choice B**) involves fusion of the upper or lower (most common) pole of the kidney. It is fairly common (as high as 1:500) and is typically an incidental finding at autopsy.

Infantile polycystic kidney (**choice C**) produces a small kidney with round medullary cysts and "radiating" linear cortical cysts.

Renal dysplasia (**choice E**) can also cause cystic change in a kidney but typically involves only the medulla and cortex of part of the kidney.

21. **The correct answer is E.** Psoriasis vulgaris usually appears on the nails, knees, elbows, and scalp. It does not generally affect the mucous membranes. Lesions are well-demarcated, coral-colored plaques with a white or silvery scale (classic clue). Histologically, epidermal hyperplasia causing thickening and lengthening of the rete ridges is apparent, as is thinning of the epidermis over the dermal papillae. There is a recognized genetic component to this condition. Peak incidence is at age 30.

Acne rosacea (**choice A**) affects the central face. Erythema, telangiectasias, acneform lesions (papules, cysts, pustules), and rhinophyma (telangiectasias and hyperplasia of nasal soft tissue) are found in various combinations. It is common from ages 30 to 50. Women are affected three times more frequently than men, but the syndrome is more severe in the latter.

Acne vulgaris (**choice B**) causes comedones, papules, and cysts. It may be related to hormones, drugs, diet, irritants, and genetic factors. Allergy to *Propionibacterium acnes* has been found to contribute to this condition.

Pemphigus vulgaris (**choice C**) starts with small vesicles, usually on the oral or nasal mucosa, then spreads to other parts of the body. Bullae are delicate and flaccid. The condition is due to autoantibodies to intercellular junctions between keratinocytes. Nikolsky's sign (production of blistering by light stroking or rubbing of the skin) is positive. Pemphigus is most common from ages 40 to 60.

Pityriasis rosea (**choice D**) presents first with a red, scaling, "herald patch" approximately 4 cm in diameter. It is followed within days by eruption in a "short-sleeve turtleneck" distribution. The classic clue to the diagnosis is the appearance of crops of small, pink, oval patches in a "fir tree configuration" on the flexural lines.

22. **The correct answer is D.** All of the conditions listed can cause infertility because of a low or absent sperm count. Only in Sertoli-only syndrome is there a complete absence of sperm precursors in an undamaged tubule. There is no known method to correct Sertoli-only syndrome (or maturation arrest) that is not due to a treatable chronic disease.

Chronic diseases, such as diabetes mellitus (**choice A**) or tuberculosis (**choice E**), can arrest the maturation of sperm but do not usually show a complete absence of sperm precursors.

In maturation arrest (**choice B**), mature sperm are absent, but precursors are found.

Tumors such as seminomas (**choice C**) cause infertility by occluding the flow of semen or by replacing the seminiferous tubules. Sampling of a seminiferous tubule not replaced by tumor would probably still demonstrate sperm.

23. **The correct answer is D.** Hyperventilation can be triggered by emotional stress, and the resulting rapid breathing tends to "blow off" more CO_2 from the lung than usual. Since CO_2 is carried in the serum principally as bicarbonate plus hydrogen ion, blowing off CO_2 shifts the balance so that less bicarbonate and less hydrogen ion are present in the blood. Less hydrogen ion translates to higher blood pH, i.e., alkalosis, which in this case is of respiratory origin. It is an uncompensated respiratory alkalosis, since renal compensation takes several days to occur. Re-breathing air, which is easily accomplished by breathing into a paper bag, will slow the rate of CO_2 loss and quickly correct the alkalosis. The manifestations of the type of mild respiratory alkalosis seen in emotional hyperventilation include light headaches, paresthesias, and sometimes syncope. Severe respiratory alkalosis (not seen in this setting) can also cause cramps, tetany, seizures, and cardiac arrhythmias.

24. **The correct answer is E.** Neutrophils line the wound edge within 24 hours of injury.

A thin, continuous epithelial cover appears (**choice A**) 24-48 hours after injury. Soon after, macrophages replace the neutrophils (**choice D**), while granulation tissue fills the wound (**choice C**). By day 5, fibroblasts lay down collagen fibers (**choice B**) along fibrin and fibronectin matrices formed across the site of incision. Full maturation of the scar requires up to 1 year.

25. **The correct answer is D.** The presence of the Philadelphia chromosome, a translocation from the long arm of chromosome 22 to chromosome 9 [t(9;22)], is associ-

ated with a more favorable prognosis in patients with chronic myelogenous leukemia.

Acute lymphoblastic leukemia (ALL; **choice A**) is the most common cause of leukemia in children. The presence of the Philadelphia chromosome is associated with a worse prognosis for the patient. This form of leukemia is also associated with a B-ALL translocation of the c-*myc* proto-oncogene of chromosome 8 to chromosome 14 [t(8;14)(q24;q32)].

Acute myelogenous leukemia (AML; **choice B**) is the most common acute leukemia in adults. The M2 subtype is associated with the t(8;21) translocation, and the M3 subtype is associated with the t(15;17) translocation.

More than half the patients with chronic lymphocytic leukemia (**choice C**) display one of several chromosomal abnormalities. This includes trisomy 12 (involves the h-*ras* proto-oncogene), translocation t(11;14) (involves k-*ras* and *bcl-1* proto-oncogenes), and deletion (14q-) or inversion (14q) (involves immunoglobulin heavy chain gene).

Hairy cell leukemia (**choice E**) is associated with the expression of tartrate-resistant acid phosphatase (TRAP) on the surface of B cells.

26. **The correct answer is D.** The patient's initially hyperlucent lung fields strongly suggest the presence of emphysema. The radiologic findings after the increase in shortness of breath are consistent with free air in the chest, which has collapsed the left lung and caused a shift in the location of the mediastinum. Such air might have been introduced by rupture of a bulla. Small pneumothoraces are usually well tolerated, but larger ones may require decompression (the needle from a syringe is sometimes used), or even surgical correction if bullae continue to leak air.

Bronchogenic carcinoma (**choice A**) would be expected to produce a mass lesion.

Pleural effusion (**choice B**) usually develops slowly and causes a whitening of lung fields when fluid is present.

Pulmonary embolism (**choice C**) can cause sudden shortness of breath but would not cause an increase in the lucency of the lung fields.

Tuberculosis (**choice E**) would be expected to produce a mass lesion in the lung.

27. **The correct answer is B.** Adults with sickle cell disease have undergone decades of accelerated RBC formation and destruction, leading to accelerated erythropoiesis in the bone marrow. Consequently, the bone marrow becomes hyperplastic, with marked increases in the number of normoblasts (erythroblasts) at the expense of marrow fat and marrow bone (**choices A and C**).

Although the white cell and megakaryocyte lines are undiminished (**choices D and E**), there is a marked increase in RBC precursors and iron stores. Iron storage increases as a consequence of both chronic transfusions and increased dietary absorption; these increased iron stores can be appreciated with a Prussian blue stain.

28. **The correct answer is B.** Microscopic examination of heart muscle from a patient with hypertrophic cardiomyopathy would reveal short, thick myofibrils arranged in circular patterns admixed with normal tissue. On electron microscopy, myofibrils and myofilaments appear disarrayed.

Aschoff bodies (**choice A**) appear in rheumatic myocarditis and consist of degenerating material and leukocytes. These occur along with Anitschkow myocytes, which contain "ribbon-like" nuclei and eosinophilic cytoplasm.

Infiltration by inflammatory cells (**choice C**) would be expected in association with an infectious process, such as acute bacterial endocarditis.

Localized fibrous scarring (**choice D**) is associated with myocardial healing after infarction.

Structures resembling poorly formed vessels (**choice E**) are found in cardiac myxoma, the most common primary tumor of the heart. The tumor cells are derived from primitive multipotent mesenchymal cells. They may be sessile or pedunculated masses.

29. **The correct answer is B.** Fibroadenoma is the most common benign breast tumor. It occurs in women of reproductive age, generally before age 30, and may be related to increased estrogen sensitivity. It presents as a single, movable breast nodule, not fixed to the skin. Surgical excision is required for definitive diagnosis.

Cystosarcoma phyllodes (**choice A**) is a fibroadenoma-like tumor that has become large, cystic, and lobulated. It may contain malignant elements.

Fibrocystic breast disease (**choice C**) is the most common breast disorder. It usually affects women older than 35. It involves a distortion of the normal breast changes associated with the menstrual cycle. Patients often have lumpy, tender breasts, especially during the several days prior to menstruation.

Infiltrating ductal carcinoma (**choice D**) is the most common type of breast cancer. It occurs most frequently after age 40. Other risk factors include nulliparity, family history, early menarche, late menopause, previous history of breast cancer, obesity, and high-fat diet.

Intraductal papilloma (**choice E**) is associated with bloody or serous nipple discharge. It is most common in women aged 20–50.

30. **The correct answer is C.** Multiple endocrine neoplasia type III (MEN III), also known as MEN IIb, is characterized by medullary thyroid carcinoma, pheochromocytoma, and mucosal neuromas.

    Wermer syndrome, also called MEN type I (**choices A and E**), is characterized by pancreatic (insulinoma), pituitary, and parathyroid involvement.

    Sipple syndrome, or MEN type II (**choices B and D**), is similar to MEN III, but it has parathyroid involvement (tumor or adenoma) as opposed to neuromas.

31. **The correct answer is B.** Multinodular goiters can produce the most extreme enlargements of any of the benign thyroid diseases. The multinodular goiters are composed of nodules created by colloid-filled or hyperplastic follicles separated by fibrous scars. Focal hemorrhage, hemosiderin deposition, calcifications, and microcyst formation may also be present. Multinodular goiters often arise from smaller simple goiters, but the trigger for development of multinodularity is poorly understood. Like simple goiters, most cases in endemic areas are related to iodine deficiency, whereas sporadic cases may have multifactorial causes.

    The other conditions listed in the answers can also cause thyroid enlargement, but the degree of enlargement is usually much less.

32. **The correct answer is D.** The nodular sclerosis variant of Hodgkin disease is more common in women and is associated with the presence of lacunar cells [Reed-Sternberg (RS) cells with nuclei surrounded by a clear space] and fibrous bands in the lymph nodes. It has a good prognosis.

    Lymphocyte depletion (**choice A**) is associated with scarcity of lymphocytes, multiple RS cells, fibrosis, and necrosis. It has a poor prognosis.

    Lymphocyte predominance (**choice B**) is the least common form of Hodgkin disease. It is associated with an abundance of lymphocytes and histiocytes and scant RS cells.

    Mixed cellularity (**choice C**) is the most common form of Hodgkin disease. It is associated with the presence of neutrophils, lymphocytes, eosinophils, plasma cells, and histiocytes. Many classic RS cells may be identified.

    Hairy cell (**choice E**) is a B-cell leukemia.

33. **The correct answer is E.** A large tumor involving the suprasellar region and adjacent base of the brain can produce the deficits noted. Examples of such tumors include craniopharyngiomas and large pituitary adenomas that have outgrown the pituitary fossa. The patient's amenorrhea is due to pituitary destruction. The loss of vision is due to involvement of the optic nerve or chiasm, and the optic disc changes are related to pressure from behind pressing on the optic nerve and disc. The olfactory changes are related to involvement of cranial nerve I.

    A tumor of the falx (**choice A**) or the parasagittal meninges typically produces sensory or motor dysfunction of the leg.

    A tumor of the hippocampus (**choice B**) might produce memory problems or seizures.

    A tumor of the posterior fossa (**choice C**) produces unilateral deafness, tinnitus, vertigo, and, sometimes, sensory loss in the distribution of cranial nerves V or VII.

    A tumor of the sphenoidal ridge (**choice D**) can cause cranial nerve palsies involving III, IV, V, or VI.

34. **The correct answer is E.** The patient has a macrocytic anemia with hypersegmented neutrophils. This picture is consistent with either folate or vitamin B_{12} deficiency. The history of small bowel resections and the presence of neurologic signs on physical examination tip the diagnosis to B_{12} deficiency.

    Beta-thalassemia trait (**choice A**) and iron deficiency (**choice C**) cause a microcytic, not a macrocytic, anemia.

    Folate deficiency (**choice B**) causes a similar picture on peripheral blood smear but is not associated with neurologic signs and symptoms.

    Sickle cell trait (**choice D**) does not cause anemia and is associated with a normal peripheral blood smear under usual physiologic conditions.

35. **The correct answer is A.** Acute lymphoblastic leukemia (ALL) is primarily a disease of children, with peak incidence at 4 years of age. Approximately 80% of childhood leukemias are of the ALL type. Other features in this scenario that further support an acute leukemia are fevers and anemia without marked elevations of the white blood cell count.

    Acute myeloblastic leukemia (AML; **choice B**) would present in a similar fashion—acute symptoms and anemia with thrombocytopenia. Bone marrow biopsy is needed to definitively differentiate ALL and AML, but AML represents only 20% of childhood leukemias. AML is primarily a disease of adolescents and young adults.

    The chronic leukemias (**choices C and D**) are diseases of adulthood that present with nonspecific symptoms and are typically diagnosed when white counts are markedly elevated. Chronic myeloid leukemia (**choice D**), a neoplasm of a pluripotent stem cell, also may present with thrombocytosis, rather than thrombocytopenia.

    Hairy cell leukemia (**choice E**) is a relatively rare leukemia of older men. It infiltrates the spleen early in its course and tends to present with pancytopenia due to bone marrow failure and splenic sequestration.

36. **The correct answer is C.** This patient's macular skin rash in a "bathing suit" distribution is also known as erythema marginatum, one of the five major Jones criteria for diagnosing rheumatic fever. The other four major criteria are migratory polyarthritis, Sydenham chorea, subcutaneous nodules, and pancarditis. In context of prior streptococcal infection, the presence of two of five major criteria or one major plus two minor criteria (**choices A, B, C, D**) is sufficient to establish the diagnosis. Other minor criteria include previous rheumatic fever and elevated C-reactive protein.

A mnemonic for the major criteria is "CANCER" (not pleasant, but easy to remember): Chorea, Arthritis, Nodules, Carditis, Erythema marginatum, Rheumatic fever diagnosis.

37. **The correct answer is B.** This patient has reflux esophagitis due to an incompetent lower esophageal sphincter (which separates the esophagus from the stomach). Her symptoms arise from the reflux of gastric contents back into the esophagus, leading to inflammation of the esophageal mucosa. Her symptoms are exacerbated by large meals, which lead to increased gastric acid secretion, and lying in bed, a position that allows more of the gastric contents to pass back through the incompetent lower esophageal sphincter.

The ileocecal sphincter (**choice A**), also called the ileocecal valve, separates the small intestine from the large intestine. Relaxation of this sphincter is modulated by the presence of food within the stomach (gastroileal reflex), which increases peristalsis and facilitates the transfer of the contents of the small intestine to the large intestine.

The pyloric sphincter (**choice C**) separates the stomach from the duodenum. Pyloric stenosis results in a palpable mass that obstructs gastric outflow and leads to projectile vomiting. Congenital pyloric stenosis is 3 to 4 times more prevalent in males than in females.

The sphincter of Oddi (**choice D**) is a band of circular muscle fibers that envelops the openings of the bile duct and the main pancreatic duct into the duodenum. Relaxation of this sphincter is stimulated by cholecystokinin.

The upper esophageal sphincter (**choice E**) separates the pharynx from the esophagus. It is voluntarily relaxed at the time of swallowing to allow passage of the food bolus from the pharynx to the esophagus.

38. **The correct answer is B.** The costal parietal pleura is supplied by intercostal nerves. Visceral pleuritic pain is referred to the area of skin representing the cutaneous distribution of the intercostal nerves over the affected bronchopulmonary segment.

The greater splanchnic nerve (**choice A**) is composed of the preganglionic sympathetic fibers from the sympathetic trunk that bypass the sympathetic chain ganglia, run in the thorax against the bodies of thoracic vertebrae, pierce the diaphragm, and innervate sympathetic ganglia in the abdomen.

The phrenic nerve (**choice C**) provides motor innervation to the diaphragm. Although it does carry sensory fibers from the diaphragm, pericardium, and mediastinal pleura, it would not be involved with the pleura adjacent to the anterior bronchopulmonary segment.

The pulmonary plexus (**choice D**) is where the vagal preganglionics synapse with the parasympathetic postganglionics to the smooth constrictor muscles of the bronchial tree.

The vagus nerve (**choice E**) in the chest carries only preganglionic parasympathetic fibers, which are visceral motor in function.

39. **The correct answer is D.** This is one of those questions for which having a good idea of what you are looking for before exploring the answer choices will certainly save you valuable time. The answers all look alike, and you could have been easily confused if you were not confident of the answer before approaching the choices.

This patient has long-standing hyperparathyroidism (*elevated PTH*), which predisposes to the development of osteitis fibrosa, her bone disease. PTH acts initially on osteocytes of bone tissue (osteocytic osteolysis) and subsequently on osteoclasts (osteoclastic resorption) to resorb calcium from bone matrix and make it available to the circulation. This *increases plasma calcium* levels. PTH also causes decreased phosphate reabsorption in the proximal renal tubule, yielding *hypophosphatemia*. Hypercalciuria is another sequela of excess PTH production, which predisposes the patient to the formation of calcium oxalate stones.

Choices A and E correspond to neither hyper- nor hypoparathyroid states.

Choice B is the profile of hypoparathyroidism. You should have quickly eliminated this choice since the PTH was decreased, and you were looking for a profile consistent with *hyper*parathyroidism.

Choice C is the profile of secondary hyperparathyroidism. This occurs when the parathyroid overproduction is due to a nonparathyroid cause. By far, the most common cause is chronic renal failure. In such cases, there is decreased calcium absorption, since the kidneys are involved in the conversion of $25(OH)D_3$ to the active form $1,25(OH)D_3$. The decreased calcium ion level stimulates the parathyroid, leading to elevated PTH levels. Hyperphosphatemia results from diminished renal synthesis of 1,25 dihydroxyvitamin D_3, creating further calcium-phosphate imbalance and enhanced PTH production.

40. **The correct answer is E.** This is a classic presentation of Hodgkin disease, which is a form of lymphoma characterized by neoplastic proliferation of Reed-Sternberg cells admixed with variable numbers of reactive lymphocytes, neutrophils, and eosinophils. The cell of origin of the Reed-Sternberg cells is still disputed. These cells have a distinctive appearance with a large double nucleus that contains paired, large, nucleoli that are often red in hematoxylin and eosin stains, producing an "owl's eye" effect.

Abnormal plasma cells (**choice A**) would be a feature of multiple myeloma or some B-cell leukemias and lymphomas, which are not as likely in this patient.

Giant platelets (**choice B**) are a feature seen in several myeloproliferative disorders (notably essential thrombocytopenia), which do not cause lymphadenopathy.

Immature neutrophil precursors (**choice C**) would most likely be a feature of a myeloid leukemia, which would not cause a lymphadenopathy.

Melanin pigment (**choice D**) would be a feature of malignant melanoma, which would probably have caused lung or liver metastases if it were at such an advanced stage as to have caused massive lymphadenopathy.

41. **The correct answer is A.** Bowen disease is one of three different clinical designations that produce the same histopathologic change of the penis, i.e., carcinoma *in situ*. Erythroplasia of Queyrat and bowenoid papulosis are the other two forms of carcinoma *in situ* of the penis. All these conditions are strongly associated with human papillomavirus (HPV), especially type 16. Carcinoma *in situ* refers to a malignant epithelial neoplasm confined within the basement membrane, without invasion of the underlying stroma. Once carcinoma *in situ* breaks through the basement membrane, invasive carcinoma (**choice C**) is diagnosed. Both carcinoma *in situ* of the penis and carcinoma *in situ* of the cervix have a strong propensity to invade the underlying stroma and transform into invasive squamous cell carcinoma.

Chronic cervicitis (**choice B**) is a very common chronic condition characterized by lymphocytic and, to a lesser extent, neutrophilic infiltration of the cervix. Some degree of chronic cervicitis can be found in any woman. Unless associated with infectious agents, such as *Chlamydia*, gonococcus, *Mycoplasma*, or herpesvirus, chronic cervicitis does not have clinical importance and **is not** associated with an increased frequency of dysplasia.

Mild cervical dysplasia (**choice D**) refers to the presence of dysplasia involving the lower third of the squamous epithelium of the cervix. Most cases spontaneously regress, but some progress to more severe degrees of dysplasia and, eventually, carcinoma.

Nabothian cysts (**choice E**) derive their name from the surgeon Martin Naboth (Leipzig, 1675-1721), who first described these small, mucus-containing cysts in the lower cervix. Nabothian cysts represent a normal effect of the *transformation zone*. After menarche, the simple columnar epithelium of the exposed endocervical epithelium is replaced by squamous epithelium advancing from the ectocervix. This process leads to obstruction of the endocervical crypts, with subsequent accumulation of mucus and formation of cystlike spaces. Nabothian cysts are therefore **normal** histologic features.

42. **The correct answer is D.** Neurofibromatosis type 2 is an autosomal dominant condition caused by mutations of a gene on chromosome 22 coding for a cytoskeleton-related protein called *merlin*. Much less common than neurofibromatosis type 1, it manifests with multiple CNS tumors, the most frequent of which are schwannomas of the 8th cranial nerve and meningiomas. Bilateral schwannomas are virtually pathognomonic (i.e., diagnostic) of neurofibromatosis type 2.

Metastases to the CNS (**choice A**) are often multiple and usually involve the gray-white matter junction. Besides the unusual location, the young age would make this diagnosis highly improbable.

Multiple sclerosis (**choice B**) is a chronic remitting/relapsing demyelinating disease. It manifests with focal neurologic deficits caused by well-circumscribed areas of myelin loss in the white matter of the brain (usually periventricular), brainstem, spinal cord, or optic nerves. It is not associated with an increased incidence of any type of brain tumor.

Neurofibromatosis type 1 (**choice C**) is also autosomal dominant and is caused by mutations of a gene on chromosome 17 coding for *neurofibromin*, a protein involved in signal transduction. The most characteristic clinical features include café-au-lait spots, neurofibromas (tumors of peripheral nerves different from schwannomas), Lisch nodules (pigmented nodules of the iris), and CNS tumors, but not schwannomas.

Tuberous sclerosis (**choice E**), like neurofibromatosis, is a "neurocutaneous syndrome," i.e., a condition characterized by concomitant neurologic and skin lesions. Tuberous sclerosis is caused by mutations in two loci, either TS1 or TS2. Multiple hamartomas of the brain (cortical "tubers") and other organs, shagreen patches, ash-leaf patches, and other skin lesions constitute the clinical findings in this disorder.

43. **The correct answer is D.** Small cell carcinoma of the lung is composed of extremely undifferentiated (i.e., anaplastic) cells, with high nuclear/cytoplasmic ratio. This neoplasm is very aggressive and tends to metastasize so early in its course that even small tumors are considered inoperable by the time of clinical diagnosis. One of the most interesting characteristics of this type of tumor is the frequent association with paraneoplastic syndromes, the most common of which is due to ectopic production of ACTH. Paraneoplastic syndromes also occur with other types of lung tumors.

Adenocarcinomas of the lung (**choice A**) are composed of mucin-producing neoplastic cells arranged in a glandular pattern. Its histologic features make this tumor easily distinguishable from small cell carcinoma.

Carcinoid tumors of the lung (**choice B**) are histologically similar to carcinoid tumors of the gastrointestinal tract. They are composed of cords and islands of uniform cuboidal cells. Carcinoid syndrome may be produced because of the ability of the tumor to produce and release serotonin.

A hamartoma (**choice C**) is not a true neoplasm, but rather a malformative lesion consisting of normal lung tissues arranged in haphazard manner. Hamartomas are often discovered incidentally on chest x-ray films as "coin lesions" and contain cartilage, smooth muscle, and cystlike spaces lined by bronchial epithelium.

Squamous cell carcinomas (**choice E**) are characterized by neoplastic squamous epithelium with evidence of extracellular and/or intracellular keratin production. The most frequent paraneoplastic syndrome accompanying pulmonary squamous cell carcinomas is hypercalcemia.

Finally, remember that cigarette smoking is a strong risk factor for all types of lung cancer, especially squamous cell carcinoma and small cell carcinoma.

44. **The correct answer is C.** This patient has osteoarthritis, a degenerative joint disease that is very common in the elderly and in those with a history of "wear and tear" or overuse of the joints (as found in football players). Chondrocyte injury occurs along with abnormal collagen activity. Predisposing factors include obesity, previous joint injury, and synovial disease. Clinically, patients have joint stiffness, decreased range of motion, effusions, crepitus, and bony swelling. The most commonly affected joints include the vertebrae, hips, knees, and distal interphalangeal (DIP) joints of the fingers. [Note that Heberden's nodes (terminal phalanx) and Bouchard's nodes (proximal phalanx) are characteristic

of this disease.] Symptoms of nerve compression may occur secondary to compression by osteophytes and bone spur development. A classic finding on x-ray is joint space narrowing. Joint fluid shows few cells and normal mucin.

Accumulation of calcium pyrophosphate in joint fluid (**choice A**) is associated with pseudogout [which is also known as calcium pyrophosphate dihydrate (CPPD) crystal deposition disease].

Antibodies against the F_c fragment of IgG (**choice B**) are associated with rheumatoid arthritis (RA).

Hematogenous seeding of joints during bacteremia (**choice D**) is the etiology of suppurative arthritis (septic).

An inborn error of purine metabolism (**choice E**) results in the development of gout.

Be careful not to confuse your crystals! Remember:

Gout = negatively birefringent urate crystals

*P*seudogout = *p*ositively birefringent calcium pyrophosphate crystals

Don't confuse your nodules either!

Gout = tophi

Osteoarthritis = Heberden's and Bouchard's nodes

Rheumatoid arthritis = subcutaneous nodules on extensor surfaces

45. **The correct answer is C.** The poliovirus kills alpha motor neurons present in the ventral horns of the spinal cord. These lower motor neurons are the cells whose axons form the motor nerves that innervate the muscles of the body.

Guillain-Barré syndrome is an acute, inflammatory, demyelinating disease of peripheral nerves, including the axons of lower motor neurons (**choice A**).

Multiple sclerosis can cause demyelination of upper motor neurons (**choice B**).

Trauma, including extremely strenuous exercise, is an example of a process that can directly damage muscle (**choice D**).

Selective destruction of synapses between the muscle and the lower motor neurons (**choice E**) is not directly involved in the pathology of poliomyelitis.

46. **The correct answer is B.** This is the typical clinical scenario in which acute tubular necrosis develops secondary to shock, and further destabilizes an already desperately ill patient. Acute tubular necrosis can also occur following exposure to nephrotoxins or as a manifestation of acute rejection in a transplanted kidney. The prognosis depends on the patient's overall health. In patients who

recover, the initial oliguric phase (lasting 1–2 weeks) is followed by a diuretic phase (weeks to months) before eventual restoration of tubular function.

Acute pyelonephritis (**choice A**) is not typically a cause of renal failure with loss of concentrating ability.

Chronic pyelonephritis (**choice C**) actually refers to chronic interstitial nephritis, which usually does not produce loss of concentrating ability (except in rare cases in which the reaction is so severe that acute tubular necrosis ensues).

Crescentic glomerulonephritis (**choice D**) is associated with rapidly progressive renal failure, characterized by hypertension, hematuria, proteinuria, and an active urinary sediment.

Renal cell carcinoma (**choice E**) is not a typical cause of renal failure with loss of concentrating ability. Hematuria is the most common presenting symptom.

47. **The correct answer is C.** The ecchymosis around the umbilicus (also known as Cullen sign) is associated with ectopic pregnancy and rupture, causing intraperitoneal bleeding.

48. **The correct answer is G.** Pain down the medial aspect of the thigh to the knee (also known as Romberg-Howship sign) is caused by the obturator hernia putting pressure on the obturator nerve.

49. **The correct answer is D.** This patient sustained trauma to the left lower ribcage and may have a ruptured spleen, which refers pain to the left shoulder (also known as Kehr sign).

50. **The correct answer is B.** This patient has post-holiday hemorrhagic pancreatitis, which can occur after eating large fatty meals for several days (also known as Cullen sign).

Pharmacology

1. A 67-year-old man presents to the emergency department with shaking chills and a temperature of 101 F. Physical examination reveals T2 FRS_L, T4 FRS_L, and there are chronic tissue changes. Laboratory examination reveals a hematocrit of 23%, and urine tests are positive for blood. The patient states that he is taking only one medication for his "irregular heartbeat." Which of the following drugs most likely caused the appearance of these signs and symptoms in this patient?

    (A) Digoxin

    (B) Hydralazine

    (C) Propranolol

    (D) Quinidine

    (E) Verapamil

2. A 41-year-old diabetic woman presents to her physician complaining of gastrointestinal distress and bloating, particularly after meals. Physical examination reveals acute and chronic somatic dysfunction at T5-T9 primarily in the right paraspinal musculature. Which of the following drugs should her physician prescribe to relieve her symptoms?

    (A) Cisapride

    (B) Diphenoxylate

    (C) Famotidine

    (D) Prochlorperazine

    (E) Sucralfate

3. A 58-year-old woman arrives at her physician's office complaining of moderate anxiety. On physical examination, extreme muscle tension was palpated in cervical and upper thoracic areas. Which of the following drugs will help relieve her anxiety, with a minimum of unwanted sedative side effects?

    (A) Buspirone

    (B) Chlordiazepoxide

    (C) Lorazepam

    (D) Trazodone

    (E) Zolpidem

4. A 55-year-old woman is receiving chemotherapy for non-Hodgkin lymphoma. Several days after a treatment, she notices blood in her urine. An osteopathic structural examination reveals warm, erythematous tissues paraspinally at T11-L2. Which of the following antineoplastic drugs is most likely responsible for this side effect?

    (A) Bleomycin

    (B) Cisplatin

    (C) Cyclophosphamide

    (D) Doxorubicin

    (E) Plicamycin

5. The pharmacokinetic properties of a new drug are being studied in normal volunteers during phase I clinical trials. The volume of distribution and clearance determined in the first subject are 80 L and 4 L/hr, respectively. The half-life of the drug in this subject is approximately

    (A) 0.03 hours

    (B) 14 hours

    (C) 78 hours

    (D) 139 hours

    (E) 222 hours

6. A 45-year-old man presents to the emergency department with severe pneumonia. He recently returned from a business trip, and has a history of smoking and alcohol use. Physical examination reveals chronic somatic dysfunction at T2-T8 bilaterally. An x-ray film shows extensive consolidation affecting portions of each lung lobe. Culture on charcoal yeast extract medium grows out a small gram-negative bacterium. Which of the following antibiotics is the most appropriate treatment for this patient?

(A) Ceftriaxone

(B) Chloramphenicol

(C) Clindamycin

(D) Erythromycin

(E) Metronidazole

7. A 46-year-old woman visits her podiatrist to have several bunions removed from her right foot. She chooses conscious sedation rather than general anesthesia for this procedure. She is given IV midazolam to supplement the local anesthetics that are injected into her foot. Midway through the surgery, she suddenly becomes agitated and combative and exhibits involuntary movements. The anesthesiologist determines that she is having a paradoxical reaction to the midazolam and immediately administers

(A) flumazenil

(B) glucagon

(C) naloxone

(D) nitrite

(E) protamine

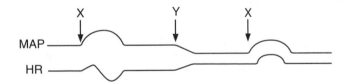

8. Mean arterial blood pressure (MAP) and heart rate (HR) measurements were recorded during the IV administration of two different drugs (see above figure). Select the most likely drugs given at the indicated points.

	X	Y
(A)	Epinephrine	hexamethonium
(B)	Isoproterenol	propranolol
(C)	Metaproterenol	propranolol
(D)	Norepinephrine	hexamethonium
(E)	Phenylephrine	phentolamine

9. A 55-year-old diabetic man is brought to the emergency department in an unresponsive state. The following laboratory values are obtained:

PCO_2: 19 mm Hg

Bicarbonate: 11 mEq/L

pH: 6.9

Which of following is the most appropriate immediate treatment for this patient?

(A) Administration of bicarbonate

(B) Administration of insulin

(C) Administration of an oral hypoglycemic agent

(D) Close observation only

(E) Indiscernible because of information given

10. A 62-year-old woman is being prepared for cardiac bypass surgery. Before she is intubated, she is given a skeletal muscle relaxant that causes her to have muscle fasciculations prior to muscle relaxation. Which of the following drugs was most likely administered?

(A) Atracurium

(B) Decamethonium

(C) Pancuronium

(D) Rocuronium

(E) Vecuronium

11. A 62-year-old white man complains of left thigh and leg pain and swelling that are exacerbated by walking. One week earlier, the patient underwent cardiac catheterization. The patient is currently vacationing and has spent the past 28 hours in a car. Physical examination reveals warmth, erythema, and sharp pain on palpation of the left lower extremity, as well as at T10-L2. Which of the following drugs, which might be prescribed in this instance, works by inhibiting the enzyme epoxide reductase?

(A) Acetylsalicylic acid

(B) Dipyridamole

(C) Heparin

(D) Streptokinase

(E) Warfarin

12. A 58-year-old man presents with difficulty initiating movements and a resting tremor. On physical examination, his face appears expressionless and he has a slow shuffling gait. He is started on amantadine. Which of the following is the mechanism of action of this drug?

    (A) It inhibits degradation of dopamine by MAO type B

    (B) It inhibits dopa decarboxylase

    (C) It is an agonist at dopamine receptors

    (D) It is a precursor of dopamine

    (E) It stimulates dopamine release

13. A 34-year-old man with a long history of asthma is referred to a pulmonologist. Physical examination reveals chronic somatic dysfunction bilaterally at T2-T7. The physician decides to prescribe zileuton. The mechanism of action of this drug is to

    (A) antagonize LTD_4 receptors

    (B) inhibit 5-lipoxygenase

    (C) inhibit phosphodiesterase

    (D) inhibit phospholipase A_2

    (E) stimulate beta$_2$ receptors

14. A 60-year-old hypertensive woman presents to her physician with visual changes. Structural examination reveals chronic somatic dysfunction at T1-T4. Transient ischemic attack is ruled out. She is then referred to an ophthalmologist, who prescribes a medication that subsequently causes drowsiness and tingling in her arms. Laboratory evaluation reveals hyperchloremic metabolic acidosis. Which of the following drugs was most likely prescribed?

    (A) Acetazolamide

    (B) Demeclocycline

    (C) Ethacrynic acid

    (D) Furosemide

    (E) Hydrochlorothiazide

15. A patient was administered trimethaphan during surgery. This drug will most likely cause which of the following responses?

    (A) Accommodation

    (B) Hypertension

    (C) Peristalsis

    (D) Pupillary constriction

    (E) Tachycardia

16. A 70-year-old man complains of chronic heartburn. It is painful for him to bend over, and he sleeps on a wedge-shaped pillow to try to reduce the burning sensation. Physical examination reveals chronic somatic dysfunction in the left paraspinal tissues at T5-T9. Which of the following agents would be the most efficacious in reducing his symptoms?

    (A) Bisacodyl

    (B) Cimetidine

    (C) Magnesium hydroxide

    (D) Omeprazole

    (E) Promethazine

17. An 82-year-old woman presents to her physician complaining of difficulty sleeping and problems coping throughout the day since the recent death of her husband. An osteopathic craniosacral examination reveals a decreased amplitude in her cranial rythm. She requests a medication that will help her through this time of her life. Her physician prescribes oxazepam. The most likely rationale behind prescribing this drug is that oxazepam

    (A) does not deplete liver glutathione

    (B) does not have first pass metabolism

    (C) does not require phase I metabolism

    (D) does not require phase II metabolism

    (E) induces cytochrome P450

18. A continuous IV infusion of lidocaine is given to a 70-kg patient with cardiac arrhythmias. The pharmacokinetic parameters for lidocaine are as follows: clearance (CL) = 9 mL/min/kg, volume of distribution (V_d) = 70 L, half-life = 2 hours. How long will it take for drug levels to reach 87.5% of steady state?

    (A) 1.75 hours

    (B) 3.5 hours

    (C) 5.5 hours

    (D) 6.0 hours

    (E) 8.0 hours

19. A 5-year-old boy with no previous medical history is brought to the emergency department by his mother because he accidentally ingested a large dose of rat poison. He is conscious but appears quite agitated. On physical examination, his blood pressure is 110/70 mm Hg and pulse is 90/min. Laboratory results are significant for an elevated prothrombin time (PT) but a normal partial prothrombin time (PTT). Which of the following is the most appropriate pharmacotherapy?

    (A) Atropine

    (B) Flumazenil

    (C) N-acetylcysteine

    (D) Protamine

    (E) Vitamin K

20. A patient is given a drug that produces vasodilatation by increasing cGMP in the smooth muscle cells of arterioles. Which of the following drugs has this mechanism of action?

    (A) Bethanechol

    (B) Isoproterenol

    (C) Metaproterenol

    (D) Nifedipine

    (E) Phentolamine

21. A 74-year-old woman with multiple myeloma is being treated with high doses of doxorubicin (Adriamycin). She has also received cyclophosphamide and prednisone recently. During an examination, the physician should check the patient for which of the following?

    (A) Abdominal tenderness

    (B) Bladder distention

    (C) Limitation of movement

    (D) Papilledema

    (E) Pulmonary rales

22. A 48-year-old smoker with deep venous thrombosis is given heparin. An osteopathic examination reveals chronic changes at T2-T7 bilaterally and acute somatic dysfunction at T10-L2. Heparin achieves its anticoagulant activity by binding to which of the following substances?

    (A) Alpha$_2$ antiplasmin

    (B) Alpha$_2$ macroglobulin

    (C) Antithrombin III

    (D) Factor VIII

    (E) Factor IX

23. An elderly man presents with complaints of ringing in his ears, blurred vision, and upset stomach. He is taking multiple medications. His wife states that he has had a few episodes of confused, delirious behavior over the past few weeks. Which of the following agents might be responsible for this man's symptoms?

    (A) Allopurinol

    (B) Hydralazine

    (C) Niacin

    (D) Quinidine

    (E) Spironolactone

24. A patient is administered a skeletal muscle relaxant prior to abdominal surgery. The patient soon begins to exhibit hypotension, bronchospasm, and excessive bronchial and salivary secretions. Which of the following skeletal muscle relaxants did this patient most likely receive?

    (A) Atracurium

    (B) Baclofen

    (C) Dantrolene

    (D) Tubocurarine

    (E) Vecuronium

25. Genetic analysis of a female infant with a broad, enlarged neck demonstrates an XO karyotype. When the child reaches puberty, hormone replacement therapy should be started with which of the following agents?

    (A) Estrogen only

    (B) Estrogen and progestin

    (C) Insulin

    (D) Progestin only

    (E) Thyroid hormone

26. A former drug abuser visits his physician to ask for pain medication for a legitimate back pain. Physical examination reveals muscle spasm and L5 ERS$_L$ with a left on right sacral torsion. The physician takes the history of drug abuse into account. Which of the following medications has the greatest potential for abuse?

    (A) Codeine

    (B) Loperamide

    (C) Meperidine

    (D) Nalbuphine

    (E) Pentazocine

27. A 48-year-old type 2 diabetic patient on daily extended-release glipizide presents with complaints of polyuria and polydipsia. Physical examination reveals somatic dysfunction at T1-T3 and T6-T8. Laboratory evaluation reveals a blood glucose of 192 mg/dL. She states that her diabetes had been well controlled and that she had been symptom-free for the past 8 years. Recently, however, she began taking medication for hypertension. Which of the following antihypertensive drugs is she most likely taking?

    (A) Diltiazem

    (B) Enalapril

    (C) Hydrochlorothiazide

    (D) Methyldopa

    (E) Terazosin

28. A 33-year-old with a history of asthma is being treated for symptoms of hyperthyroidism. Physical examination is significant for T1-T4 chronic somatic dysfunction. Which of the following beta-blockers would be an appropriate therapy for this patient?

    (A) Isoproterenol

    (B) Labetalol

    (C) Metoprolol

    (D) Propranolol

    (E) Timolol

29. A patient with essential hypertension is starting diuretic therapy. He has a history of calcium oxalate renal stones. His structural examination shows chronic somatic dysfunction at T1-T4 and T11-L1. Which of the following diuretics would be most appropriate for this patient?

    (A) Acetazolamide

    (B) Furosemide

    (C) Hydrochlorothiazide

    (D) Spironolactone

    (E) Triamterene

30. A 64-year-old man presents to his family physician complaining of difficulty urinating and "dribbling" at the end of urination. Physical examination reveals a grade III prostate with chronic somatic dysfunction at T11-L2. The physician diagnoses benign prostatic hyperplasia. Which of the following drugs would be most appropriate for treating this man's condition?

    (A) Finasteride

    (B) Leuprolide

    (C) Mifepristone

    (D) Pergolide

    (E) Tamoxifen

31. A 15-year-old girl admits that she had been abusing laxatives in an effort to lose weight. Physical examination reveals chronic somatic dysfunction at T12-L2. Her physician diagnoses an atonic colon. Assuming that she has been taking only one type of laxative, which of the following drugs was she most likely abusing?

    (A) Docusate sodium

    (B) Domperidone

    (C) Lactulose

    (D) Methylcellulose

    (E) Phenolphthalein

32. A 30-year-old woman with a history of tonic-clonic seizures complains of double vision, thickened gums, and growth of facial hair since starting a new medication. Which of the following anticonvulsant medications is most likely responsible for her symptoms?

    (A) Carbamazepine

    (B) Ethosuximide

    (C) Phenobarbital

    (D) Phenytoin

    (E) Valproic acid

33. A 32-year-old woman who is 36 weeks pregnant is told during a prenatal appointment that her fetus is in a breech presentation. An external cephalic version is scheduled for the following week. For this procedure, the uterus must be relaxed. Which of the following drugs would be most appropriate for achieving this result?

    (A) Clomiphene

    (B) Phenylephrine

    (C) Progesterone

    (D) Propranolol

    (E) Ritodrine

34. A 26-year-old woman undergoing surgery is given an inhalant anesthetic. She is also given an IV dose of succinylcholine. Within minutes, she develops a heart rate of 124/min and increasing core body temperature. Which of the following is the mechanism of action of the drug of choice for this patient's condition?

    (A) It interferes with the release of Ca^{2+} from the sarcoplasmic reticulum

    (B) It is a competitive antagonist of ACh at the motor end plate

    (C) It is a GABA receptor agonist that enhances inhibition of nerve impulses

    (D) It uncouples oxidative phosphorylation, thereby preventing heat formation

    (E) There is no known mechanism of action

35. A neurophysiologist is studying the consequences of diminished brain perfusion in an experimental animal. The carotid artery is occluded, and brain function is monitored by positron emission tomography. Which of the following drugs would be most effective in reversing the change in heart rate produced by the experimental occlusion?

    (A) Atropine

    (B) Metaproterenol

    (C) Neostigmine

    (D) Phenoxybenzamine

    (E) Propranolol

36. A 33-year-old man receiving chemotherapy for testicular carcinoma develops signs of renal tubular damage. Osteopathic structural examination confirms your diagnosis with acute somatic dysfunction at T11-L1 bilaterally. Which of the following drugs is most likely responsible for this nephrotoxicity?

    (A) Bleomycin

    (B) Cisplatin

    (C) Cyclophosphamide

    (D) Vinblastine

    (E) Vincristine

37. A new antibiotic is being tested in clinical trials. The following pharmacokinetic parameters have previously been determined:

    > Clearance = 100 mL/min
    >
    > Volume of distribution (V_d) = 50 L
    >
    > Half-life = 3 hours

    Assuming that the drug is being administered intravenously, what loading dose (LD) should be given to a patient to quickly obtain a plasma concentration of 10 mg/L?

    (A) 5 mg

    (B) 25 mg

    (C) 100 mg

    (D) 500 mg

    (E) 1,000 mg

38. A 24-year-old migrant farm worker is rushed to a nearby emergency department after an accidental exposure to parathion. He is in respiratory distress and is bradycardic. Which of the following drugs can be given to increase the activity of his acetylcholinesterase?

    (A) Atropine

    (B) Deferoxamine

    (C) Dimercaprol

    (D) Physostigmine

    (E) Pralidoxime

39. A 48-year-old vagrant with a history of alcoholism ingests a bottle of antifreeze and presents to the emergency department obtunded but with intact vision. Which of the following is the most appropriate pharmacotherapy?

    (A) Amyl nitrite

    (B) Atropine

    (C) Ethanol

    (D) Glucagon

    (E) Naloxone

40. A 47-year-old man presents with acute pain in his big toe. Laboratory tests reveal a uric acid level of 10 mg/dL. He is started on medication (Drug 1). Several days after the resolution of the acute attack, he is started on a second medication (Drug 2). Drug 2 decreases both the serum and urine levels of uric acid. Which of the following is Drug 2?

    (A) Allopurinol

    (B) Colchicine

    (C) Indomethacin

    (D) Probenecid

    (E) Sulfinpyrazone

41. A 57-year-old smoker with a long history of chronic obstructive lung disease presents to the physician with a blood pressure of 150/95 mm Hg. Physical examination reveals fibrotic, cool, and stiff tissues at T2-T7 bilaterally. Which of the following antihypertensives could possibly worsen this patient's COPD?

    (A) Acebutolol

    (B) Atenolol

    (C) Esmolol

    (D) Metoprolol

    (E) Nadolol

42. Ethacrynic acid acts at which of the above areas of the nephron?

    (A) A

    (B) B

    (C) C

    (D) D

    (E) E

43. A worried mother complains to her pediatrician that both she and her 6-year-old son's teacher have noticed that the child has become inattentive. She states that her son frequently stops what he is doing and "stares blankly into space" before resuming his activities. Electroencephalography reveals a 3/second spike and slow wave pattern of discharges. Which of the following agents would most effectively treat this child's disorder?

    (A) Carbamazepine

    (B) Diazepam

    (C) Ethosuximide

    (D) Methylphenidate

    (E) Phenytoin

44. Two alpha-adrenergic antagonists (Drugs A and B) decrease blood pressure by the same amount following IV administration to a patient at the following doses:

    Drug A: 120 mg

    Drug B: 15 mg

    This information implies that Drug A

    (A) has a higher therapeutic index than Drug B

    (B) has a lower bioavailability than Drug B

    (C) has a shorter half-life than Drug B

    (D) is less efficacious than Drug B

    (E) is less potent than Drug B

45. While performing osteopathic manipulation on your patient, you see a suspicious skin lesion and decide to biopsy it. Which of the following drugs is a long-duration ester local anesthetic?

    (A) Bupivacaine

    (B) Cocaine

    (C) Lidocaine

    (D) Procaine

    (E) Tetracaine

46. A 24-year-old woman attempts suicide by ingesting 50 acetaminophen tablets. She is rushed to the emergency department. Which of the following treatments would the attending physician most likely order?

    (A) Alkalinization of urine

    (B) Ca^{2+}/EDTA chelation

    (C) Deferoxamine

    (D) N-acetylcysteine

    (E) Protamine sulfate

47. A 52-year-old man with peptic ulcer disease has been on drug therapy for 3 months and has noticed changes in his bowel habits, increasing headaches, dizziness, skin rashes, loss of libido, and gynecomastia. His physical examination reveals a group dysfunction at T5-T9 NS_LR. Which of the following drugs is most likely responsible for these side effects?

    (A) Cimetidine

    (B) Famotidine

    (C) Metronidazole

    (D) Omeprazole

    (E) Sucralfate

48. A 72-year-old hypertensive man complains of a cold. Structural examination reveals chronic tissue changes at T1-T4. The patient is currently taking reserpine for his hypertension. After treating his structural finding, he wants to know what over-the-counter medication he could take for his cold. Which of the following drugs will cause an increase in blood pressure after chronic administration of reserpine?

    (A) Amphetamine

    (B) Bethanechol

    (C) Cocaine

    (D) Guanethidine

    (E) Phenylephrine

Questions 49-50

SET A

For each numbered item (**patient presentation**), select the one heading (**treatment**) most closely associated with it. Each lettered heading maybe used once, more than once, or not at all.

    (A) Permethrin 5% cream

    (B) Mupirocin 2% ointment

    (C) Penciclovir 1% cream

    (D) Diflorasone diacetate 0.05% ointment

    (E) Tretinoin 0.025% cream

    (F) Calcipotriene 0.005% ointment

    (G) Hydrocortisone acetate 1% cream

49. A 38-year-old woman complains of a pruritic, erythematous, sharply demarcated, rounded, scaly plaque that appears on her knees. She has never before sought treatment.

50. A 5-year-old woman presents with a pruritic lesion that has a yellowish brown crust and which started as a pustule.

Pharmacology

ANSWERS AND EXPLANATIONS

1.	D		26.	C
2.	A		27.	C
3.	A		28.	C
4.	C		29.	C
5.	B		30.	A
6.	D		31.	E
7.	A		32.	D
8.	D		33.	E
9.	B		34.	A
10.	B		35.	E
11.	E		36.	B
12.	E		37.	D
13.	B		38.	E
14.	A		39.	C
15.	E		40.	A
16.	D		41.	E
17.	C		42.	C
18.	D		43.	C
19.	E		44.	E
20.	A		45.	E
21.	E		46.	D
22.	C		47.	A
23.	D		48.	E
24.	D		49.	D
25.	B		50.	B

1. **The correct answer is D.** Hemolytic anemia is a disorder in which red blood cell survival is decreased, either episodically or continuously. Although the bone marrow has the ability to increase erythroid production, this type of anemia is typically seen when the bone marrow is unable to compensate for the marked hemolysis of red blood cells. Since red blood cells typically survive for 120 days, the hematocrit will fall at a rate of 1% per day, in the absence of red blood cell production. The mechanism for the hemolytic anemia in this patient is related to the formation of an immune complex between a circulating red blood cell and quinidine, a medication used in the treatment of premature atrial, AV-junctional, and ventricular contractions, as well as various other arrhythmias. Since the immune complex is viewed as foreign, the red blood cell in this complex is lysed by the complement system. The quinidine molecule then dissociates from the lysed red blood cell and binds to another red blood cell to repeat the process. This recycling of drug-antibody complex accounts for the dramatic decrease in the hematocrit.

   Digoxin (**choice A**) is typically used to treat atrial fibrillation, atrial flutter, and paroxysmal atrial tachycardia. Digoxin is not associated with the development of hemolytic anemia.

   Hydralazine (**choice B**) is a vasodilator used in the treatment of essential hypertension. Although it is not associated with the development of hemolytic anemia, it has been known to cause a lupus-like syndrome.

   Neither propranolol (**choice C**), a beta-blocker, nor verapamil (**choice E**), a calcium channel blocker, is associated with the development of hemolytic anemia.

2. **The correct answer is A.** Patients with diabetes may have damage to the nerves innervating their viscera, resulting in gastroparesis (loss of motility of the esophagus and stomach). This loss of motility causes delayed gastric emptying, bloating, and nausea. Therefore, an appropriate drug to prescribe is one that stimulates gastrointestinal motility. Cisapride is such a prokinetic agent, probably acting via serotonin receptors to enhance the release of myenteric acetylcholine. In addition to its ability to improve gastric emptying, cisapride also enhances lower esophageal tone and esophageal peristalsis, and is thus useful in the therapy of gastroesophageal reflux disease.

   Diphenoxylate (**choice B**), which is structurally related to meperidine, is an antidiarrheal agent. By diminishing gastric motility even further, diphenoxylate would likely exacerbate this woman's symptoms.

   Famotidine (**choice C**) is an H_2-receptor antagonist that inhibits histamine-induced gastric acid secretions.

Excessive gastric acid secretion does not underlie this patient's problems.

   Prochlorperazine (**choice D**) is an antiemetic agent that acts as a D_2-receptor antagonist at the chemoreceptor trigger zone in the medulla. Although this woman's bloating may cause her to feel nauseous, this symptom would be relieved by treating the underlying motility problem.

   Sucralfate (**choice E**), or aluminum sucrose sulfate, is a poorly soluble agent that polymerizes in the acid environment of the stomach. The polymer then binds to ulcerated tissue and protects it from pepsin-mediated protein hydrolysis and damage by acid. It also binds bile salts, which are thought to play a role in the pathogenesis of gastric ulcers. However, there is no indication that this woman has gastric ulcer disease.

3. **The correct answer is A.** Buspirone is a nonbenzodiazepine anxiolytic that is devoid of the sedative (or anticonvulsive and muscle relaxant) properties typically associated with the benzodiazepines. It is a partial agonist at 5-HT_{1A} receptors.

   Chlordiazepoxide (**choice B**) and lorazepam (**choice C**) are benzodiazepines. Although they are useful anxiolytics, they produce sedation.

   Trazodone (**choice D**) is a very sedating atypical antidepressant.

   Zolpidem (**choice E**) is a nonbenzodiazepine hypnotic used for the treatment of insomnia.

4. **The correct answer is C.** Step 1 questions related to antineoplastic agents are most likely going to ask you about mechanism of action, cell cycle specificity, or side effects. Bone marrow suppression, nausea, vomiting, ulcers, and alopecia are common side effects; however, you are probably more likely to be asked about the unique side effects of certain drugs. In this case, cyclophosphamide has the unique side effect of hemorrhagic cystitis, which could cause hematuria. Note that cyclophosphamide is also consistent with the fact that the patient is being treated for non-Hodgkin lymphoma.

   All the other answer choices have unique, COMLEX-worthy side effects:

   Bleomycin (**choice A**) is notable for its pulmonary toxicity. Although bleomycin can be used to treat lymphoma, you are more likely to see it as part of the treatment regimen (with vinblastine and cisplatin) for testicular tumors.

   Cisplatin (**choice B**) is notable for its nephrotoxicity and ototoxicity. It is used in the treatment of testicular and lung cancers. It would not be used in a patient with lymphoma.

Doxorubicin (**choice D**) is also called Adriamycin. It is an antibiotic agent used in the treatment of many cancers, including lymphomas, sarcomas, and many carcinomas. Its unique side effect is its cardiotoxicity.

You might have been tempted by plicamycin (**choice E**) if you recalled that it can cause a hemorrhagic diathesis. You could have eliminated this answer, however, because plicamycin is not used in the treatment of lymphoma. It is used in the treatment of testicular cancer and cases of hypercalcemia.

5. **The correct answer is B.** The half-life of a drug can be determined using the following equation:

$$t_{1/2} = \frac{(0.693 \times V_d)}{CL}$$

Therefore,

$$t_{1/2} = \frac{(0.693 \times 80\ L)}{4\ L/hour}$$

$$t_{1/2} \approx 14\ hours$$

6. **The correct answer is D.** This patient has Legionnaires disease, an acute, and sometimes fatal, pneumonia. It is caused by *Legionella pneumophila*, a facultative intracellular parasite that can be grown on charcoal yeast agar; erythromycin is the treatment of choice. *Legionella* is acquired from inhaling an infectious aerosol produced from sources such as air conditioning systems of large buildings (e.g., hotels) or respiratory therapy equipment. Legionnaires disease affects men more often than women, and is more common in individuals older than 40. The disease is more severe in smokers, alcoholics, diabetics, and immunosuppressed patients.

Ceftriaxone (**choice A**) is a third-generation cephalosporin. It is a broad-spectrum antibiotic and is the drug of choice for *Neisseria gonorrhoeae* infections.

Chloramphenicol (**choice B**) is a broad-spectrum antibiotic that is rarely used in the U.S. because of the risk of aplastic anemia, a rare but fatal side effect. In developing nations, it is the drug of choice for typhoid fever.

Clindamycin (**choice C**) is broad-spectrum antibiotic active against gram-positive cocci and anaerobic bacteria. It is the most common agent associated with antibiotic-induced pseudomembranous colitis due to *Clostridium difficile*.

Metronidazole (**choice E**) is active against many obligate anaerobes, certain protozoa, and *Helicobacter pylori*.

7. **The correct answer is A.** Flumazenil is a benzodiazepine antagonist and has been approved to hasten the recovery from benzodiazepines used in anesthetic and diagnostic settings and to reverse the CNS depressant effects following an overdose with benzodiazepines. Flumazenil can be used only for benzodiazepines; it is not useful in reversing the effects of other CNS depressants, such as barbiturates and ethanol.

Glucagon (**choice B**) is an antidote for beta-blocker overdose.

Naloxone (**choice C**), an opioid receptor antagonist, is an antidote for opioid overdose.

Nitrite (**choice D**), or sodium nitrite, is an antidote for cyanide poisoning.

Protamine (**choice E**) is an antidote for heparin overdose.

8. **The correct answer is D.** Several strategies are useful in solving drug tracing problems: 1) *Always* look at blood pressure first and heart rate second. Blood pressure changes will be the direct result of the administered drug; heart rate changes may be a direct effect or they may result from a baroreceptor reflex. 2) Assume that when an agonist effect is gone, so is the agonist; however, also assume that an antagonist stays on board for the entire trace. 3) Eliminate as many options as possible by examining the initial agonist effect.

The only two agonists that would be expected to raise blood pressure to this degree are norepinephrine (alpha$_1$, alpha$_2$, and beta$_1$ agonist) and phenylephrine (alpha$_1$ agonist). Thus, **choices A, B, and C** can be eliminated immediately.

Drug Y lowers blood pressure and raises heart rate. Hexamethonium (ganglionic blocker) would lower blood pressure and increase heart rate by blocking the predominant tone of the arterioles (sympathetic) and the heart (parasympathetic). Phentolamine (alpha antagonist) would lower blood pressure by blocking arteriolar alpha$_1$ receptors. The increase in heart rate would be a baroreceptor reflex.

The second administration of Drug X causes an increase in both blood pressure and heart rate. Only the combination of norepinephrine and hexamethonium could do this. Norepinephrine would still increase blood pressure by stimulating end organ receptors; however, the baroreceptor reflex would be blocked by hexamethonium. The ability of norepinephrine to increase heart rate by stimulating cardiac beta$_1$ receptors is now revealed.

Choice A: Epinephrine would cause a small increase in mean blood pressure, but not enough to elicit a baroreceptor reflex. So, an increase in heart rate would be seen as a result of beta$_1$ stimulation of the heart. Hexamethonium would cause a decrease in blood pressure and an increase in heart rate. Hexamethonium should not affect subsequent epinephrine administration because a baroreceptor reflex was not initially produced.

Choice B: Isoproterenol (beta$_1$ and beta$_2$ agonist) would cause a decrease in blood pressure (by stimulating arteriolar beta$_2$ receptors) and an increase in heart rate (a combination of cardiac beta$_1$ receptor stimulation and baroreceptor reflex). Phenoxybenzamine (alpha antagonist) would cause a decrease in blood pressure and increase in heart rate (baroreceptor reflex). Phenoxybenzamine should not have an effect on subsequent administration of isoproterenol.

Choice C: Metaproterenol (beta$_2$ agonist) would decrease blood pressure (by stimulating arteriolar beta$_2$ receptors) and increase heart rate (baroreceptor reflex). Propranolol (beta$_1$ and beta$_2$ antagonist) would decrease blood pressure and increase heart rate. It would completely block subsequent administration of metaproterenol.

Choice E: Phenylephrine would increase blood pressure and decrease heart rate (baroreceptor reflex). Phentolamine would decrease blood pressure and increase heart rate (baroreceptor reflex). Phentolamine would completely block subsequent administration of phenylephrine.

9. **The correct answer is B.** This patient is in a diabetic ketoacidotic coma. The goals in treating such a patient are to increase the rate of glucose utilization by insulin-dependent tissues, to reverse ketonemia and acidosis, and to replenish fluids.

Treatment with bicarbonate (**choice A**) would result in only a transient elevation of pH.

Oral hypoglycemic agents (**choice C**) are commonly prescribed for the maintenance of patients with type 2 diabetes and would not be appropriate in an acute setting.

Because this is a life-threatening condition, monitoring the patient without treatment (**choices D and E**) are unacceptable.

10. **The correct answer is B.** This patient was given decamethonium, a depolarizing neuromuscular blocker. It initially causes fasciculations because it stimulates the nicotinic acetylcholine receptors on skeletal muscle (N$_M$) and causes depolarization of the skeletal muscle. Muscle fasciculations can be observed before the muscle goes into depolarization block, at which time the patient will have flaccid paralysis. Note that succinylcholine, also a depolarizing blocker, produces similar effects.

All the other drugs listed are nondepolarizing, or competitive, skeletal muscle relaxants. These drugs act by competitively blocking the N$_M$ receptors. Patients receiving these drugs would exhibit flaccid paralysis immediately.

11. **The correct answer is E.** This patient has deep venous thrombi (DVT). He has several risk factors for the development of DVT, including a recent hospitalization that likely included catheterization in the femoral region and a recent period of prolonged stasis. The enzyme epoxide reductase is responsible for converting vitamin K into its active quinone form. The drugs that inhibit epoxide reductase are the vitamin K antagonists such as warfarin. Clotting factors II, VII, IX, and X and proteins C and S are all dependent on vitamin K, which acts as a cofactor for carboxylation reactions. Carboxylation makes factors II, VII, IX, and X better able to interact with calcium, and thus better able to form clots.

Acetylsalicylic acid (**choice A**) acts as a platelet aggregation inhibitor by decreasing thromboxane A$_2$ production, which under normal circumstances causes platelet aggregation.

Dipyridamole (**choice B**) is also a platelet aggregation inhibitor that increases cAMP levels by inhibiting cyclic nucleotide phosphodiesterase. This causes inhibition of thromboxane A$_2$ production in platelets and may potentiate the effects of prostacyclin, causing decreased platelet adhesion to thrombogenic surfaces. Dipyridamole may be used in combination with warfarin, in contrast to acetylsalicylic acid, which may cause an unpredictable potentiation of warfarin anticoagulation.

Heparin (**choice C**) is used in cases of DVT but is limited to parenteral use because it does not readily cross membranes. It acts by potentiating the activity of antithrombin III, which is a suicide inhibitor of thrombin and factors IXa, Xa, XIa, and XIIa.

Streptokinase (**choice D**) is also used in cases of DVT but it is limited to IV, intra-arterial, and intracoronary use. It is a protein produced by beta hemolytic streptococci that converts plasminogen to plasmin, which is involved in digesting fibrin clots.

12. **The correct answer is E.** This question allows us to review the various mechanisms of action of the antiparkinsonian drugs. Although amantadine was developed as an antiviral agent (influenza A), it was noted to have antiparkinsonian effects. Amantadine stimulates the release of dopamine from presynaptic nerve terminals.

Selegiline inhibits the degradation of dopamine by MAO type B (**choice A**).

Carbidopa works by inhibiting dopa decarboxylase (**choice B**). Carbidopa is unable to cross the blood-brain barrier; therefore, it prevents the conversion of levodopa (L-dopa) to dopamine in the periphery, but this conversion still occurs in the brain. This significantly reduces the dosage of L-dopa required to achieve an effect and is generally used in combination with L-dopa.

Bromocriptine and pergolide are dopaminergic receptor agonists (**choice C**). Bromocriptine is typically administered in combination with levodopa. It is also useful in end-stage Parkinson disease, when L-dopa loses its effectiveness because of progressive degeneration of the nigrostriatal neurons.

L-dopa is a precursor of dopamine (**choice D**). At higher doses, it has many side effects and is therefore often used in combination with carbidopa or bromocriptine (see above).

Note that muscarinic antagonists (e.g., benztropine, biperiden, procyclidine, trihexyphenidyl) are also used as adjuncts to the dopaminergic agents in the treatment of parkinsonism. Recall that dopaminergic neurons have an inhibitory effect on striatal cholinergic interneurons. So, if there is a decrease in dopaminergic activity (e.g., as in Parkinson disease), there will be an increase in striatal ACh. Therefore, administration of these anticholinergics aids in maintaining a dopamine/acetylcholine balance in the striatum.

13. **The correct answer is B.** Zileuton is a recently approved oral inhibitor of 5-lipoxygenase, the first enzyme in the pathway from arachidonic acid to leukotrienes. Leukotrienes are synthesized in many inflammatory cells in the airways, such as mast cells, macrophages, eosinophils, and basophils. LTC_4 and LTD_4 are thought to be responsible for many of the symptoms of asthma, including bronchoconstriction, increased bronchial reactivity, hypersecretion of mucus, and mucosal edema. In addition, LTB_4 is a potent chemotactic agent for neutrophils. Zileuton and similar agents are efficacious in the treatment of asthma because they inhibit leukotriene production.

Zafirlukast is another drug that is used to interrupt the leukotriene pathway. This drug acts as an LTD_4 antagonist (**choice A**); it is taken orally.

Methylxanthines, such as theophylline, inhibit phosphodiesterase (**choice C**), thus increasing intracellular levels of cAMP and resulting in smooth muscle relaxation. At therapeutic doses, methylxanthines also block adenosine receptors.

Corticosteroids prevent the release of arachidonic acid from cell membranes by inhibiting phospholipase A_2 (**choice D**). This reduces the production of both leukotrienes and prostaglandins. Corticosteroids also inhibit the production of cytokines, which are thought to play an important role in initiating the inflammatory cascade provoked by antigen inhalation and viral infection. Examples of corticosteroids include beclomethasone, budesonide, flunisolide, fluticasone, and triamcinolone.

Beta$_2$ agonists (**choice E**), such as albuterol, terbutaline, metaproterenol, and bitolterol, cause smooth muscle relaxation by increasing intracellular levels of cAMP.

14. **The correct answer is A.** This patient's visual changes may be attributed to glaucoma, for which she was given acetazolamide. Side effects of acetazolamide (a carbonic anhydrase-inhibiting diuretic used primarily for treating glaucoma) include paresthesias and drowsiness. The drug can cause a hyperchloremic metabolic acidosis, with decreased serum bicarbonate, increased serum chloride, and decreased serum pH. Renal stones may also occur. Hepatic encephalopathy may appear in patients with hepatic impairment.

Demeclocycline (**choice B**), an antidiuretic hormone (ADH) antagonist and a tetracycline, causes bone and teeth abnormalities in children younger than 8 years. Demeclocycline can be used in the treatment of SIADH.

Ethacrynic acid (**choice C**) and furosemide (**choice D**) are loop diuretics that can cause hypovolemia and cardiovascular complications. They can also induce a hypokalemic metabolic alkalosis and ototoxicity. Furosemide, a sulfonamide, may also cause sulfonamide allergy.

Hydrochlorothiazide (**choice E**), a thiazide diuretic, can cause hyponatremia, an uncommon but potentially dangerous early side effect. Potassium wasting can occur with chronic use. Thiazides are sulfonamides and can cause sulfonamide allergy.

15. **The correct answer is E.** Trimethaphan is a ganglionic blocker that is sometimes administered during surgery to maintain controlled hypotension and to minimize blood loss. The trick to determining the effect of a ganglionic blocker is to first know the predominant tone of the end organ in question. The blocker will produce the opposite effect of the predominant tone. The vessels, arterioles, and veins are predominantly under sympathetic tone. Most everything else is under parasympathetic tone. The heart is under predominantly parasympathetic control. Parasympathetic stimulation of the heart causes bradycardia. Removal of this tone with trimethaphan would result in tachycardia.

The eye is predominantly under parasympathetic control. Parasympathetic stimulation causes the eye to accommodate (focus for near vision, **choice A**). Removal of this tone with trimethaphan would produce focusing for far vision.

Arterioles are predominantly under sympathetic control. Sympathetic stimulation produces vasoconstriction and possibly hypertension (**choice B**). Removal of this tone with trimethaphan would produce vasodilatation and hypotension.

The gut is predominantly under parasympathetic control, which increases gut motility (**choice C**). Removal of parasympathetic tone with trimethaphan would diminish gut motility.

The eye is predominantly under parasympathetic control. Parasympathetic stimulation causes the pupil to constrict (**choice D**). Removal of this tone with trimethaphan would produce mydriasis.

16. **The correct answer is D.** Omeprazole is an irreversible inhibitor of H$^+$/K$^+$/ATPase of the parietal cell. It is used in the treatment of peptic ulcer disease, reflux esophagitis, and Zollinger-Ellison syndrome. Omeprazole can reduce daily gastric acid secretion by more than 95%. This drug is of particular value to patients who do not respond sufficiently to H$_2$ antagonists. Because of the profound reduction in gastric acid secretion, patients can develop modest hypergastrinemia. In laboratory rats, the increased gastrin causes hyperplasia of oxyntic mucosal cells and carcinoid tumors. Although there has been concern that the hyperplasia could also occur in humans, this has not been substantiated to date.

Bisacodyl (**choice A**) is a stimulant laxative.

Cimetidine (**choice B**) is an H$_2$-receptor antagonist that would block histamine-induced acid secretion. It is not as efficacious as omeprazole.

Magnesium hydroxide (**choice C**) is an antacid. It would help relieve the heartburn but would not be as efficacious as omeprazole.

Promethazine (**choice E**), a dopamine-receptor antagonist, is an antiemetic.

17. **The correct answer is C.** Phase I metabolism, which is accomplished largely by cytochrome P450, becomes less efficient with age. Phase II metabolism, which conjugates drugs to yield polar, inactive metabolites, is not generally affected by age. Oxazepam is a benzodiazepine that does not require phase I metabolism; it simply undergoes conjugation, making it a useful drug for elderly individuals. Lorazepam is the other benzodiazepine that undergoes only phase II metabolism. These two drugs are also useful for patients with liver failure; phase I metabolism can be severely affected by liver failure.

18. **The correct answer is D.** It takes one half-life to reach 50% of steady state, two half-lives to reach 75% of steady state, three half-lives to reach 87.5% of steady state, and four half-lives to reach 93.75% of steady state. Each successive half-life brings the level of the drug closer to 100%, but by a smaller amount (half of the previous increase) in each case. In this case, it should take three half-lives to reach 87.5% of steady state, or $2 \times 3 = 6$ hours. Note: The clearance and volume of distribution were not necessary to answer this question!

19. **The correct answer is E.** As you might have guessed from his elevated PT, the active ingredient in rat poison is warfarin. It acts as an anticoagulant by interfering with the normal hepatic synthesis of the vitamin K–dependent clotting factors II, VII, IX, and X. The most important adverse effect of warfarin is bleeding. The action of warfarin can be reversed with vitamin K.

Atropine (**choice A**) is used as an antidote for anticholinesterase toxicity (e.g., ingestion of organophosphates).

Flumazenil (**choice B**) is used as an antidote for benzodiazepine toxicity (e.g., Valium).

N-acetylcysteine (**choice C**) is used as an antidote for acetaminophen toxicity.

Protamine (**choice D**) is used as an antidote for heparin overdose. Note that heparin enhances the activity of antithrombin III, augmenting its anticoagulant effect. Heparin toxicity would have resulted in an elevated PTT.

20. **The correct answer is A.** Muscarinic agonists stimulate noninnervated muscarinic (M3) receptors located on the endothelium of blood vessels. These receptors activate phospholipase C (via G$_q$), thereby raising levels of inositol triphosphate (IP$_3$) and diacylglycerol (DAG). IP$_3$ produces an increase in intracellular calcium, which activates nitric oxide synthase and thus produces nitric oxide. Nitric oxide, in turn, diffuses to the smooth muscle cells of arterioles and raises cGMP by activating guanylate cyclase. cGMP causes vasodilatation, possibly by dephosphorylating myosin light chain, thus preventing the interaction of myosin with actin.

Isoproterenol (**choice B**), a nonselective beta agonist, causes vasodilatation by activating beta$_2$ receptors located in the smooth muscle of arterioles. Beta$_2$ receptors activate adenylate cyclase, thus raising levels of cAMP. cAMP activates cAMP-dependent protein kinase (protein kinase A), which phosphorylates myosin light chain kinase (MLCK), rendering this enzyme inactive. MLCK can no longer phosphorylate the myosin light chain, an essential step in smooth muscle contraction.

Metaproterenol (**choice C**), a beta$_2$ agonist, causes vasodilatation by the same mechanism as isoproterenol.

Nifedipine (**choice D**) blocks L-type calcium channels in both smooth and cardiac muscle. Increased blocking of calcium channels in the smooth muscle cells of arterioles prevents the activation of MLCK. MLCK can no longer phosphorylate the myosin light chain, an essential step in smooth muscle contraction.

Phentolamine (**choice E**) causes vasodilatation by blocking alpha receptors on arteriolar smooth muscle cells. Alpha$_1$ receptors cause constriction by IP$_3$-induced increases in intracellular calcium. Phentolamine therefore decreases intracellular calcium, thereby causing less activation of MLCK.

21. **The correct answer is E.** Doxorubicin (Adriamycin) is an anthracycline antibiotic. When given in high doses (>550 mg/m^2), it can produce cardiomyopathy leading to congestive heart failure, accompanied by pulmonary edema and rales. This complication is especially likely if the patient is older than 70 years of age, has received cardiac irradiation, has underlying heart disease or hypertension, or has received cyclophosphamide.

    Abdominal tenderness (**choice A**), bladder distention (**choice B**), limitation of movement (**choice C**), and papilledema (**choice D**) are not typically associated with administration of doxorubicin. Doxorubicin does, however, cause alopecia and suppress the bone marrow.

22. **The correct answer is C.** Heparin, a highly negatively charged molecule, binds to the coagulation inhibitor antithrombin III, increasing its activity 100 to 1000 times.

    Alpha$_2$-antiplasmin (**choice A**) binds plasmin. Plasmin functions to break down clots, and the binding of alpha$_2$-antiplasmin to plasmin acts to inhibit clot lysis.

    Alpha$_2$-macroglobulin (**choice B**) is a circulating antiprotease macromolecule that assists in preventing blood clotting by inhibiting the action of proteolytic coagulation factors.

    The remaining answer choices (**choices D and E**) are clotting factors. They do not interact with heparin.

23. **The correct answer is D.** The collection of symptoms described above—tinnitus, blurred vision, gastrointestinal upset, and delirium—is known as cinchonism, a side effect of quinidine toxicity. EKG changes, such as prolongation of the QT and QRS intervals, may also occur. Quinidine is an antiarrhythmic used for the treatment of ventricular arrhythmias and atrial fibrillation.

    Allopurinol (**choice A**) is used in the treatment of gout. Its side effects include rash and fever.

Hydralazine (**choice B**) is a vasodilator used for the treatment of hypertension. Side effects include tachycardia, headache, nausea, and a lupus-like syndrome.

Niacin (**choice C**) is used in the treatment of hyperlipidemia. Its side effects include cutaneous flushing and pruritus.

Spironolactone (**choice E**) is a potassium-sparing diuretic that blocks the effect of aldosterone at its receptor. Side effects include hyperkalemia and gynecomastia.

24. **The correct answer is D.** The symptoms described were caused by drug-induced histamine release. Of all the drugs listed, only tubocurarine produces a substantial amount of histamine release.

    Atracurium (**choice A**) would also be appropriate for this procedure. However, it results in much less histamine release than tubocurarine.

    Baclofen (**choice B**) is an antispasmodic but would not be used for this procedure. In addition, it does not cause histamine release.

    Dantrolene (**choice C**) is a skeletal muscle relaxant but would not be used for this procedure; it is instead used in the treatment of malignant hyperthermia. In addition, it does not cause histamine release.

    Vecuronium (**choice E**) would also be appropriate for this procedure. However, it does not cause histamine release.

25. **The correct answer is B.** The infant has Turner syndrome, in which only one sex chromosome, the X chromosome, is present as a result of chromosomal loss early after fertilization of the egg. The chromosome loss can occur either in all cells, or only in part of the body, because of random X-chromosome inactivation, producing the variant known as a Turner mosaic. Affected infants often have a prominent "webbed" neck related to lymphatic stasis in the neck, sometimes producing a frank cystic hygroma (large cystic mass composed of dilated lymphatic channels). Edema of the dorsum of the hands and feet caused by similar mechanisms is also seen in these infants. An infant with these clinical features should have a chromosomal analysis. Affected infants should also be carefully checked for cardiac anomalies (notably preductal coarctation of the aorta and aortic stenosis with endocardial fibroelastosis), since congenital heart disease can cause early death. By puberty, the neck and extremity edema generally has resolved, but careful physical examination often reveals residual redundant skin of the neck and shoulders, producing the mature form of webbed neck. Mosaic patients and patients with partial deletions of one X

chromosome may present only at puberty with the combination of short stature and primary amenorrhea. The ovaries (usually not biopsied in obvious cases) lose all their oocytes by 2 years of age ("menopause before menarche") and become atrophic fibrous strands without ova or follicles ("streak ovaries"). Hormonal replacement in Turner patients should include both estrogens and progestins, since unopposed estrogens (**choice A**) can cause atypical adenomatous hyperplasia of the endometrium.

Insulin (**choice C**) replacement is not required in these patients.

Replacement of progestin alone (**choice D**) is not recommended.

Thyroid hormone (**choice E**) replacement is not required in these patients.

26. **The correct answer is C.** The drug that is most likely to be abused is that which causes the greatest euphoric effect. Euphoria is mediated by mu opioid receptors, and meperidine is the only drug listed that is a full mu agonist.

    Codeine (**choice A**) is a moderately effective agonist at the mu receptor and therefore has less abuse potential than meperidine.

    Loperamide (**choice B**) is an over-the-counter antidiarrheal agent with very limited abuse potential.

    Nalbuphine (**choice D**) is a mixed agonist/antagonist (also called a kappa-sigma agonist) with antagonist actions at the mu receptor. As a result, it has less abuse potential than meperidine.

    Pentazocine (**choice E**) is a mixed agonist/antagonist (also called a kappa-sigma agonist). It is either a weak agonist or an antagonist at the mu receptor. As a result, it has less abuse potential than meperidine.

27. **The correct answer is C.** The fact that the patient had well-controlled diabetes until the addition of an anti-hypertensive medication suggests that the new agent is responsible for increasing the blood glucose level. Hydrochlorothiazide is a thiazide diuretic that is known to increase fasting blood glucose in diabetic patients. Dosage adjustments of both oral hypoglycemic agents, like glipizide, and insulin may be required to maintain euglycemia. None of the other agents would directly increase the blood glucose level in this patient. Thus, all these agents are considered to be safe and effective for the treatment of hypertension in diabetic patients.

    Diltiazem (**choice A**), a calcium channel blocker, and enalapril (**choice B**), an ACE inhibitor, can both be used in the treatment of hypertension in diabetic patients. Since these agents have favorable side effect

profiles, their use in the initial treatment of hypertension would be recommended.

Both methyldopa (**choice D**), a centrally acting alpha receptor agonist, and terazosin (**choice E**), a peripherally acting alpha receptor blocking agent, can be used to treat hypertension in diabetic patients. Because of their side effect profiles, however, these agents should be used after other more tolerable agents have been attempted.

28. **The correct answer is C.** Symptoms related to hyperthyroidism include palpitations and tachycardia. If the patient also has asthma, you should select a drug that blocks beta$_1$-receptors without affecting the beta$_2$-receptors found in the respiratory smooth muscle. Therefore, a selective beta$_1$-blocker (such as metoprolol) would be appropriate.

    Isoproterenol (**choice A**) is a (nonselective) beta agonist, not antagonist.

    Labetalol (**choice B**) is a mixed alpha and nonselective beta antagonist used for chronic hypertension and hypertensive emergencies.

    Propranolol (**choice D**) is a nonselective beta antagonist. It would block both beta$_1$ and beta$_2$ receptors and would therefore be contraindicated in a patient with asthma.

    Timolol (**choice E**) is also a nonselective beta-antagonist that is used topically in the treatment of glaucoma.

29. **The correct answer is C.** A thiazide diuretic would be the drug of choice for this patient because it is the only class of diuretic that decreases urinary secretion of calcium. Thiazide diuretics, like hydrochlorothiazide, inhibit the Na^+/Cl^- cotransporter in the distal convoluted tubule and promote the reabsorption of calcium.

    Acetazolamide (**choice A**), a carbonic anhydrase inhibitor, and furosemide (**choice B**), a loop diuretic, induce diuresis at the expense of all three major cationic electrolytes (Na^+, K^+, and Ca^{2+}), which are secreted in increased amounts.

    Spironolactone (**choice D**) and triamterene (**choice E**), so-called potassium-sparing diuretics, block Na^+/K^+ exchange in the collecting duct. Although they decrease K^+ secretion, they elevate Na^+ and Ca^{2+} secretion.

30. **The correct answer is A.** Finasteride, an inhibitor of 5-alpha-reductase, prevents the conversion of testosterone to dihydrotestosterone (DHT). Since dihydrotestosterone is essential for the normal growth and development of the prostate gland, finasteride is an effective treatment for benign prostatic hyperplasia, which is a DHT-dependent process.

    Leuprolide (**choice B**) is a gonadotropin-releasing hormone (GnRH) analog. It is used at times for the palliative treatment of advanced prostate carcinoma.

Mifepristone (**choice C**), also known as RU486, is a competitive inhibitor at progesterone receptors. It has been used as a contraceptive or as an abortifacient to terminate early pregnancy.

Pergolide (**choice D**), a synthetic ergoline, is a direct agonist at dopamine D_1 and D_2 receptors. It has been used in association with levodopa in the therapy of Parkinson disease.

Tamoxifen (**choice E**) is a competitive antagonist at estrogen receptors located in the breast. This drug is used in reducing the recurrence of estrogen-receptor-positive breast cancer, particularly in postmenopausal women.

31. **The correct answer is E.** Phenolphthalein is a stimulant laxative that normally promotes the accumulation of water and electrolytes in the lumen of the colon and stimulates peristalsis. Stimulant laxatives can cause abdominal cramping. With prolonged use, however, there can be deterioration of intestinal functioning, leading to an atonic colon.

    Docusate sodium (**choice A**) is a surfactant laxative that acts like a detergent to soften stool. Docusate sodium can produce mild cramping, rashes, and nausea. Since it increases the intestinal absorption of mineral oil, phenolphthalein, and quinidine, concurrent administration with any of these drugs is ill-advised.

    Domperidone (**choice B**) is a dopamine antagonist that acts at D_2 receptors. It is used as an antiemetic and as a prokinetic agent. Its primary adverse effect is hyperprolactinemia.

    Lactulose (**choice C**), a disaccharide of fructose and galactose, is an osmotic laxative. Adverse effects include cramps, diarrhea, flatulence, and electrolyte disturbances.

    Methylcellulose (**choice D**), a bulk laxative, is a polysaccharide polymer that is not broken down by digestion in the upper part of the gastrointestinal tract. It retains water in the lumen of the gut and promotes peristalsis. Bulk-forming laxatives have few side effects, though flatulence and borborygmi (abdominal gurgling) may occur.

32. **The correct answer is D.** Diplopia, gingival hyperplasia, and hirsutism are classic side effects of phenytoin. Other side effects include nystagmus, sedation, ataxia, and enzyme induction. Phenytoin is used in the treatment of grand mal and tonic-clonic seizures. It is not used for absence seizures.

    Carbamazepine (**choice A**) does produce diplopia, but not the other symptoms in this vignette. It can also produce ataxia, enzyme induction, and blood dyscrasias. It is useful in tonic-clonic and partial seizures and in tic douloureux.

Ethosuximide (**choice B**) causes gastrointestinal distress, headache, and lethargy. It is used exclusively for absence seizures.

Phenobarbital (**choice C**) is used for grand mal and partial seizures. It causes sedation, enzyme induction, and dependence.

Valproic acid (**choice E**) causes gastrointestinal distress, hepatotoxicity, and inhibition of drug metabolism. It can be used for all seizure types but is particularly useful in myoclonic and petit mal seizures.

33. **The correct answer is E.** Stimulation of beta$_2$ receptors causes uterine relaxation. Ritodrine is a beta$_2$ agonist. Terbutaline is also sometimes used.

    Clomiphene (**choice A**) is a nonsteroidal estrogen used in the treatment of infertility. In women, it can improve follicular development and induce ovulation. In men, it can improve spermatogenesis.

    Phenylephrine (**choice B**) is an alpha$_1$ agonist; alpha$_1$ stimulation causes contraction in the pregnant uterus.

    Progesterone (**choice C**) is used in oral contraceptives and in the treatment of dysmenorrhea, dysfunctional uterine bleeding, and endometriosis.

    Beta$_2$ stimulation causes uterine relaxation; propranolol (**choice D**) is a nonspecific beta antagonist.

34. **The correct answer is A.** This is a three-step question. First you need to figure out the diagnosis, then you need to determine the drug of choice for this condition, and, finally, you need to remember the mechanism of action of that drug. The clinical picture presented suggests malignant hyperthermia. The treatment for this condition (a COMLEX favorite) is dantrolene. Dantrolene prevents the release of Ca^{2+} from the sarcoplasmic reticulum, thereby reducing skeletal muscle contractions. Side effects include muscle weakness and hepatotoxicity (if used chronically). Other uses include spasticity, multiple sclerosis, and cerebral palsy.

    Nondepolarizing blockers competitively inhibit the activity of acetylcholine at the neuromuscular junction (**choice B**). Examples include curare, atracurium, and vecuronium.

    Baclofen is a GABA$_B$ receptor agonist that is inhibitory at synapses in the spinal cord (**choice C**).

    Uncouplers of oxidative phosphorylation (**choice D**) include dinitrophenol and thermogenin.

35. **The correct answer is E.** The first thing that you have to know is the effect that carotid occlusion will have on this animal. A carotid occlusion blocks blood flow to the carotid baroreceptors, thereby simulating a low blood pressure. The animal's response will be to initi-

ate a baroreceptor response, which will increase sympathetic output and decrease parasympathetic output. The net result will be an increase in blood pressure and heart rate. The second thing to determine is which drug will oppose this increase in heart rate. Propranolol, a nonspecific beta antagonist, will prevent norepinephrine from acting on the beta$_1$ receptors on the heart following an increase in sympathetic output, thus opposing the reflex increase in heart rate.

Atropine (**choice A**), a muscarinic antagonist, might further increase heart rate. However, because part of the baroreceptor reflex involves withdrawing parasympathetic output, the effect of atropine would be negligible.

Metaproterenol (**choice B**), a beta$_2$ agonist, does not have much of a direct effect on heart rate because the predominant adrenergic receptor on the heart is beta$_1$. Metaproterenol decreases blood pressure by producing vasodilatation in the skeletal muscle vasculature, which is sensed at the aortic arch baroreceptors. This in itself elicits a baroreceptor reflex that is additive to the reflex produced by the carotid occlusion.

Neostigmine (**choice C**), a carbamylating acetylcholinesterase inhibitor, may slow the heart slightly. However, because parasympathetic output is withdrawn during a carotid occlusion, there is not a sufficient amount of acetylcholine present even if its metabolism is prevented by a cholinesterase inhibitor.

Phenoxybenzamine (**choice D**), an alpha-adrenergic antagonist, does not affect heart rate directly because there are no alpha-adrenergic receptors in the heart. It acts to decrease blood pressure by blocking alpha receptors in the vasculature. This true decrease in blood pressure is sensed by the aortic arch baroreceptors, contributing further to the baroreceptor reflex initiated by the carotid occlusion and further increasing heart rate.

36. **The correct answer is B.** Cisplatin is an antineoplastic drug used in the treatment of carcinoma of the testes (along with bleomycin and vinblastine), ovaries, bladder, and lung (especially small cell). Along with the typical side effects of nausea, vomiting, and bone marrow suppression, cisplatin is notable for its dose-limiting nephrotoxicity and ototoxicity.

The other answer choices also have unique, COMLEX test-worthy side effects:

Bleomycin (**choice A**) is very effective against testicular tumors and is used in combination with cisplatin and vinblastine. The most noteworthy side effect of bleomycin is pulmonary toxicity that can progress to pulmonary fibrosis.

Cyclophosphamide (**choice C**) is a commonly used chemotherapeutic that is effective in the treatment of lymphomas, multiple myeloma, lymphoblastic leukemias, carcinomas (e.g., breast, ovary, lung, cervix), mycosis fungoides, and neuroblastoma. Note that it is not used in the treatment of testicular cancer. In addition, its most notable side effect is hemorrhagic cystitis (not nephrotoxicity).

Vinblastine (**choice D**) is used for the treatment of testicular tumors. It is also used for Hodgkin disease, lymphomas, and Kaposi sarcoma. Vinblastine is notable for its dose-limiting bone marrow suppression.

Vincristine, also known as Oncovin (**choice E**), is used as part of the MOPP (mechlorethamine, Oncovin, procarbazine and prednisone) regimen for the treatment of Hodgkin disease. It is also used in the treatment of acute lymphocytic leukemia (ALL), sarcoma, CNS tumors, and Wilms tumor. Vincristine's noteworthy side effect is its dose-limiting neurotoxicity.

37. **The correct answer is D.** The object of a loading dose (LD) is to "load up" the volume of distribution in order to quickly achieve the desired plasma concentration. You can calculate it by the following equation:

$$LD = V_d \times C_p$$

(V_d = volume of distribution; C_p = plasma concentration)

In this case, LD = (50 L) × (10 mg/L) = 500 mg

38. **The correct answer is E.** Pralidoxime (2-PAM) is an acetylcholinesterase (AChE) reactivating agent. It is useful only for counteracting AChE inhibitors that act by phosphorylating the enzyme (organophosphates). Pralidoxime can remove the phosphate group from AChE, thus regenerating the enzyme. This must be done in a timely fashion because normally after the phosphate group is bound to the enzyme, it undergoes a chemical reaction known as "aging." Once this bond ages, pralidoxime will no longer be effective.

Atropine (**choice A**) is a nonselective muscarinic antagonist. Although atropine would be an appropriate agent for this patient, it acts by preventing the excess ACh from stimulating muscarinic receptors rather than altering the activity of AChE.

Deferoxamine (**choice B**) is a chelator used for iron poisoning.

Dimercaprol (**choice C**) is a chelator used alone for arsenic, mercury, and gold poisoning. It is also used in conjunction with edetate calcium disodium (EDTA) to treat severe lead poisoning.

Physostigmine (**choice D**) is a carbamylating acetylcholinesterase inhibitor that can be used to treat antimuscarinic overdose. This drug would certainly exacerbate this patient's symptoms.

39. **The correct answer is C.** Ethanol is the appropriate treatment for patients who have ingested methanol or ethylene glycol. This therapy is effective because ethanol competes for the same enzyme (alcohol dehydrogenase) that is required for methanol/ethylene glycol breakdown. Methanol can cause blindness; ethylene glycol (a component of antifreeze) does not. Therefore, the patient probably ingested ethylene glycol. Ethylene glycol is a CNS depressant; ingestion produces obtundation and unresponsiveness to painful stimuli.

Amyl nitrite (**choice A**) is the appropriate antidote for cyanide poisoning; sodium nitrite is also used.

Atropine (**choice B**) is the appropriate antidote for carbamate-type or organophosphate-type acetylcholinesterase insecticide poisoning. It acts by blocking muscarinic receptors. 2-Pyridine aldoxime methiodide (2-PAM, pralidoxime) can also be given early in the course of organophosphate poisoning to help regenerate the enzyme.

Glucagon (**choice D**) is the approved therapy for treating beta-adrenergic blocker overdose, helping to restore blood glucose levels.

Naloxone (**choice E**) is the approved treatment for overdose of opioids. It is an antagonist at opioid receptors.

40. **The correct answer is A.** This is a simple drug mechanism question made somewhat more difficult by the additional information presented in the stem. First, the diagnosis of gout should have been easily made. (Other "classic clues" for gout include negatively birefringent needle-shaped crystals and the presence of tophi.) The only crucial information in the question is that Drug 2 decreases uric acid in both the serum and the urine. Allopurinol inhibits the formation of uric acid by blocking the conversion of hypoxanthine to xanthine and xanthine to uric acid by xanthine oxidase (allopurinol is an analog of hypoxanthine). If uric acid synthesis is decreased, you would expect to see a decrease in both the serum and urine levels. Note that allopurinol is used in the treatment of severe hyperuricemia, whether or not it is related to gout. Also note that in acute attacks of gout, therapy with allopurinol should be delayed until after the acute episode has resolved and the patient is on maintenance doses of colchicine (probably Drug 1 in this vignette).

Colchicine (**choice B**) works by interfering with microtubule polymerization, thereby preventing granulocyte migration to the inflammatory site and decreasing metabolic and phagocytic activity of granulocytes. Colchicine has no effect on uric acid levels and is not an analgesic. Colchicine is used to treat acute attacks of gout and is also given prophylactically to prevent recurrent episodes.

Indomethacin (**choice C**) is a nonsteroidal antiinflammatory drug (NSAID) that works by inhibiting both cyclooxygenase and the motility of polymorphonuclear leukocytes. Although indomethacin can be used in the treatment of acute gout, it affects neither the serum nor the urine levels of uric acid.

Both probenecid (**choice D**) and sulfinpyrazone (**choice E**) increase urinary excretion of uric acid (uricosuric). As such, you would expect increased, not decreased, urine levels of uric acid in patients taking either drug (serum levels would be decreased).

41. **The correct answer is E.** The point of this question is that nonselective beta-blockers are contraindicated in patients with lung disease. These agents will cause bronchoconstriction by blocking the $beta_2$ receptors responsible for promoting bronchial smooth muscle relaxation (recall that $beta_2$ agonists are a mainstay of asthma therapy). Acebutolol (**choice A**), atenolol (**choice B**), esmolol (**choice C**), and metoprolol (**choice D**) are all cardioselective $beta_1$ blockers that could be used in a patient with lung/airway disease. Another cardioselective blocker that is not listed is betaxolol. As for nadolol (**choice E**), it is a nonselective beta-blocker and should NOT be used in a patient with lung disease.

42. **The correct answer is C.** Ethacrynic acid is a loop diuretic and acts by inhibiting the $Na^+/K^+/2Cl^-$ transporter located in the ascending loop of Henle.

No known diuretics act at the glomerulus (**choice A**).

Carbonic anhydrase inhibitors, such as acetazolamide, inhibit sodium bicarbonate reabsorption from the proximal tubule (**choice B**).

Thiazide diuretics inhibit the Na^+/Cl^- transporter in the early segment of the distal convoluted tubule (**choice D**).

Potassium-sparing diuretics act as antagonists of the intracellular aldosterone receptor located in the collecting tubule (**choice E**). By doing so, they decrease the expression of the genes for sodium channels and the Na^+/K^+ ATPase.

43. **The correct answer is C.** The child has absence (petit mal) seizures. The age of onset is typically from 3 to 7 years; seizures may continue into adolescence, but generally subside before adulthood. These seizures have been known to occur up to 100 times a day. Ethosuximide is indicated for this type (but no other type) of seizure.

Other drugs used in the treatment of absence seizures are valproic acid, clonazepam, and lamotrigine.

Carbamazepine (**choice A**) is used in the treatment of tonic-clonic (grand mal) and partial (focal) seizures.

Diazepam (**choice B**) has long been the drug of choice for status epilepticus. Recently, lorazepam (a shorter acting benzodiazepine) has also been accepted as a drug for this condition. IV phenytoin is used if prolonged therapy is required. Phenobarbital has also been used, especially in children. If the status epilepticus is very severe and does not respond to these measures, general anesthesia may be used.

Methylphenidate (Ritalin; **choice D**) is a stimulant used to treat children with attention deficit disorder. This child has no history of hyperactivity, and the underlying cause of his "inattentiveness" is his seizure disorder.

Phenytoin (**choice E**) is effective in all seizure types except for the one in this question (absence). Note that phenytoin has some idiosyncratic, test-worthy side effects, including hirsutism and gingival hyperplasia.

44. **The correct answer is E.** Both drugs produce exactly the same effect, but Drug B achieved the blood pressure response with one-eighth the dosage of Drug A. This means that Drug A is 8 times less potent than Drug B.

A high therapeutic index (**choice A**) means that the drug is relatively safe. However, the safety of a drug is not necessarily related to its potency.

Differences in bioavailability (**choice B**) between these two drugs cannot be determined because both of these drugs were administered intravenously. Bioavailability is the fraction of a (typically orally administered) drug that reaches the systemic circulation. Bioavailability is by definition 1 (100%) when drugs are administered intravenously.

The half-life (**choice C**) is the amount of time it takes for the concentration of a drug to fall to 50% of a previous measurement. There is no information provided to determine the half-lives of these drugs.

Efficacy (**choice D**), which is a measurement of the drug's maximal response, is given by the maximal height of the dose-response curve. At these doses, each drug produced the same effect, but there is no information provided to determine what the maximal effect of each drug would be. In addition, potency and efficacy are not necessarily related.

45. **The correct answer is E.** Tetracaine is a long-duration ester local anesthetic.

Bupivacaine (**choice A**) is a long-duration amide.

Cocaine (**choice B**) is a medium-duration ester and an uptake blocker.

Lidocaine (**choice C**) is a medium-duration amide and an antiarrhythmic.

Procaine (**choice D**) is a short-duration ester.

46. **The correct answer is D.** N-acetylcysteine is the drug of choice for treatment of overdose of acetaminophen, the active ingredient in Tylenol.

Alkalinization of urine (**choice A**) is a reasonable strategy for salicylate poisoning, e.g., due to aspirin overdose, or for other poisonings that produce metabolic acidosis.

Ca^{2+}/EDTA (**choice B**) and/or dimercaprol are chelators used in cases of lead poisoning.

Deferoxamine (**choice C**) is an effective chelator for poisoning with iron salts.

Protamine sulfate (**choice E**) is administered to reverse the anticoagulant effects of heparin overdose.

47. **The correct choice is A.** Cimetidine, an H_2-receptor antagonist, can produce all the side effects exhibited when taken in high doses over a long period of time. In addition, cimetidine can alter the hepatic metabolism of several drugs.

Famotidine (**choice B**) is also an H_2-receptor antagonist, but it does not have the side effects of cimetidine.

Metronidazole (**choice C**) is an antibacterial and anti-protozoal drug that may present with the adverse effects of headaches, dizziness, diarrhea, and rashes, but not gynecomastia.

Omeprazole (**choice D**) is a proton-pump inhibitor, and sucralfate (**choice E**) is a physical barrier to gastric acid. Neither has been associated with effects on sexual function or breast development.

48. **The correct answer is E.** Reserpine acts by blocking vesicular uptake of monoamine neurotransmitters (norepinephrine, dopamine, serotonin), thus making the neurotransmitter vulnerable to the catabolic effects of monoamine oxidase (MAO) present in the nerve terminal. High doses of reserpine can even destroy synaptic vesicles. Chronic administration of reserpine causes depletion of norepinephrine. Therefore, for a drug to raise blood pressure after norepinephrine depletion, it must act directly on the alpha$_1$ adrenergic receptors present on arterioles. Phenylephrine, a direct alpha$_1$ agonist, is such a drug.

Amphetamine (**choice A**) is an indirect-acting sympathomimetic. It raises blood pressure by causing the release of endogenous norepinephrine.

Bethanechol (**choice B**), a muscarinic agonist, decreases blood pressure by stimulating the noninnervated muscarinic receptors present on arterioles.

Cocaine (**choice C**) is an indirect-acting sympathomimetic that raises blood pressure by blocking the reuptake of norepinephrine.

Guanethidine (**choice D**) is an adrenergic neuron blocker that acts by blocking the release of norepinephrine.

49. **The correct answer is D.** This patient has psoriasis. Psoriasis can be pruritic papules and/or plaques with silvery scales. It commonly occurs on the elbows, knees, scalp, low back, nails, and any traumatized area (Koebner or isomorphic phenomenon). First-line treatment is a high or highest strength ointment, such as diflorasone diacetate. Calcipotriene (**choice F**) is a second-line treatment for psoriasis, especially in patients who have failed steroid treatment.

50. **The correct answer is B.** This patient has impetigo. Impetigo can occur anywhere, but in children it tends to occur around the nose and mouth. It is described as papules, vesicles, or pustules, often with honey-colored crusts. Because this patient has one small lesion, treatment would be with topical mupirocin ointment; the patient does not warrant systemic antibiotics because he does not have a large infected area, fever, or toxicity.

Pharmacology

1. A 74-year-old man has not been able to pass urine today, but had been able to do so normally the previous 2 days. Physical examination is remarkable for a blood pressure of 175/90 mm Hg. Structural examination shows chronic somatic dysfunction at T11-L1. Laboratory examination reveals a serum creatinine of 4.5 mg/dL and a blood urea nitrogen of 115 mg/dL. Urinalysis reveals a specific gravity of 1.01 mg/dL and an occasional white blood cell per high-powered field. Which of the following could be used to ameliorate the patient's symptoms?

    (A) Benazepril
    (B) Doxazosin
    (C) Furosemide
    (D) Hyoscyamine
    (E) Phenazopyridine

2. A female patient is thinking about terminating her pregnancy at home. Which of the following eicosanoids is available as a vaginal suppository to induce abortion?

    (A) LTA_4
    (B) PGD_2
    (C) PGE_2
    (D) PGF_2
    (E) PGG_2

3. Several hospitals are participating in a study to test the efficacy of a newly developed drug prior to its release. This drug is designed to lower cholesterol levels. Of the 1,000 patients who are involved in this study, half receive the drug and half receive a placebo. Neither the physicians in charge of the study nor the patients are permitted to know what the patients have received. Which of the following steps in the drug development process does this scenario most closely describe?

    (A) Investigational New Drug (IND) Application
    (B) Phase I
    (C) Phase II
    (D) Phase III
    (E) Phase IV

4. A patient has been given an anticoagulant for thrombosis. Which of the following findings suggests that she was given warfarin, not heparin?

    (A) Anticoagulation is being monitored by measuring the prothrombin time (PT)
    (B) Anticoagulation was achieved within 1 hour of drug administration
    (C) The anticoagulant's effects are reversed by administering protamine sulfate
    (D) The anticoagulant was administered intravenously
    (E) The anticoagulant can be used in pregnancy

5. A 64-year-old man presents to his physician with aching, burning pain after meals. He had been self-medicating with antacids for several months but has found this to be increasingly ineffective. Physical examination reveals ropy tissue at T5-T9 on the left. His physician decides to take him off the antacids and instead places him on a combination of ranitidine and sucralfate. Why is this combination a bad idea?

(A) Ranitidine increases the toxicity of sucralfate

(B) Ranitidine inhibits the action of sucralfate

(C) Sucralfate and ranitidine coprecipitate

(D) Sucralfate increases the toxicity of ranitidine

(E) Sucralfate inhibits the action of ranitidine

6. A young woman has recurrent bladder infections related to sexual intercourse. Physical examination reveals somatic dysfunction at T11-L2. Which of the following antibiotic regimens would be most appropriate for prophylaxis?

(A) Ampicillin given orally daily

(B) Ampicillin given orally following coitus

(C) Chloramphenicol given orally following coitus

(D) Trimethoprim-sulfamethoxazole given orally daily

(E) Trimethoprim-sulfamethoxazole given orally following coitus

7. A 55-year-old man with hypertension and a past medical history of myocardial infarction is prescribed atenolol. This medication will lower his blood pressure by

(A) blocking catecholamine release

(B) blocking the conversion of angiotensin I to angiotensin II

(C) decreasing cardiac output

(D) decreasing intravascular volume

(E) increasing renin release from the kidney

8. A 24-year-old woman presents to her physician with a rasping cough. Physical examination reveals no rales or rhonchi with warm, erythmatous tissues at T2-T7 paraspinally. The physician gives her a sample of an antitussive drug that is neither addicting nor constipating. Which of the following drugs was she mostly likely given?

(A) Codeine

(B) Dextromethorphan

(C) Diphenoxylate

(D) Levorphanol

(E) Oxycodone

9. A 68-year-old man presents with complaints of chronic fatigue, exertional and nocturnal dyspnea, orthopnea, and a chronic nonproductive cough. On examination, respiratory wheezing and rhonchi are noted. Cardiac examination reveals a diminished first heart sound and an S3 gallop. Structural examination reveals T2 FRS_L and T4 FRS_L. The patient indicates that he was recently treated for hypertension and vasospastic angina. On the basis of his initial presentation, which of the following agents was most likely prescribed?

(A) Amlodipine

(B) Captopril

(C) Furosemide

(D) Hydralazine

(E) Verapamil

10. A patient with Graves disease is scheduled for a subtotal thyroidectomy. Propylthiouracil is used to control her hyperthyroidism until surgery. The enzyme inhibited by this drug is involved in which of the following reactions?

(A) Conversion of iodide to iodine at the apex of the follicular cell

(B) Iodide uptake at the base of the follicular cell

(C) Iodination of thyroglobulin in the colloid

(D) Proteolysis of iodinated thyroglobulin into monoiodotyrosine (MIT) and diiodotyrosine (DIT)

(E) Reuptake of iodinated thyroglobulin from the follicular lumen

11. A 48-year-old woman is being treated for breast carcinoma. Over the past few days, she has been complaining of dysuria and frequency. Physical examination reveals acute somatic dysfunction at T11-L2. Laboratory examination reveals the presence of microscopic hematuria. The next day the patient develops gross hematuria. Which of the following agents most likely caused the development of these signs and symptoms?

(A) Cyclophosphamide

(B) Mitomycin

(C) Paclitaxel

(D) Tamoxifen

(E) Vincristine

12. A 24-year-old man underwent treatment for Hodgkin lymphoma 1 year ago. He presents with increasing dyspnea and cough. Physical exam is remarkable for rales bilaterally. Structural examination reveals warm, swollen tissue bilaterally at T2-T8. Arterial blood gases show hypoxia, and bilateral pulmonary infiltrates are seen on chest x-ray. Which of the following chemotherapeutic agents most likely produced these side effects?

    (A) Bleomycin

    (B) Cyclophosphamide

    (C) Doxorubicin

    (D) Etoposide

    (E) 5-Fluorouracil

13. A 27-year-old drug abuser ingested 15 10-mg dextroamphetamine tablets 5 hours ago, and is brought to the emergency department in an agitated state. Which of the following agents can hasten the elimination of the drug from this patient?

    (A) Acetazolamide

    (B) Ammonium chloride

    (C) Penicillamine

    (D) Probenecid

    (E) Sodium bicarbonate

14. A 70-year-old man with a history of atrial fibrillation is started on an oral anticoagulant. His prothrombin time (PT) is monitored on a regular basis. A few months into therapy, he begins treatment for a duodenal ulcer and develops symptoms of a bleeding diathesis. Physical examination now reveals acute tissue changes at T5-T9. Which of the following ulcer medications is most likely responsible for this change in his hemostatic status?

    (A) Cimetidine

    (B) Famotidine

    (C) Misoprostol

    (D) Omeprazole

    (E) Ranitidine

15. A 65-year-old patient has experienced several transient ischemic attacks over the past few months. Because his general health is poor, he is not considered an appropriate candidate for carotid endarterectomy. The decision is made to treat him medically. Which of the following agents would be most appropriate for his therapy?

    (A) Aspirin

    (B) Coumadin

    (C) Dipyridamole

    (D) Heparin

    (E) Sulfinpyrazone

16. A 24-year-old man presents to the emergency department with hypertension, tachycardia, an elevated body temperature, diaphoresis, mydriasis, and severe agitation. His mother reports that he uses illicit drugs, although she is not sure which kind. Which of the following agents is the most appropriate therapy for this patient?

    (A) Atropine

    (B) Flumazenil

    (C) Labetalol

    (D) Naloxone

    (E) Physostigmine

17. A 59-year-old man with a history of myocardial infarction presents to his physician complaining of shortness of breath. On examination, his heart rate is 110/min and respiratory rate is 22/min. He has rales in both lung fields, a normal sinus rhythm with an S3 gallop, and 2+ pitting ankle edema. Osteopathic structural examination reveals T4 FRS$_L$ with fibrotic tissues surrounding it. A chest x-ray film reveals cardiomegaly, and his ejection fraction on echocardiogram is calculated at 37%. Which of the following medications would alleviate this patient's symptoms by significantly reducing both the preload and afterload on the heart without affecting its inotropic state?

    (A) Digoxin

    (B) Diltiazem

    (C) Enalapril

    (D) Furosemide

    (E) Propranolol

18. A patient needs chemotherapy to treat his recently diagnosed cancer. Which of the following chemotherapeutic agents is specific for the M phase of the cell cycle?

    (A) Cytarabine
    (B) Daunorubicin
    (C) Hydroxyurea
    (D) Mechlorethamine
    (E) Vincristine

19. A 35-year-old woman with systemic lupus erythematosus abruptly stops taking her glucocorticoids because "she is well now and does not want to get fat." Several days later, the woman goes to the emergency department because she "feels terrible." If serum studies are performed on this patient, which of the following findings would be expected?

    (A) Elevated ACTH
    (B) Elevated cortisol
    (C) Hypernatremia
    (D) Hypoglycemia
    (E) Hypokalemia

20. A 33-year-old newlywed presents to her physician with a sharp, burning epigastric pain. She had recently begun a regimen of nonsteroidal antiinflammatory drugs (NSAIDs) to help relieve pain caused by rheumatoid arthritis. A physical examination confirms acute somatic dysfunction at T5–T9. Her physician recommends misoprostol to relieve her gastric distress. Before prescribing this drug, the physician should first obtain the results of a(n)

    (A) antinuclear antibody test
    (B) barium swallow
    (C) esophageal manometry
    (D) osmotic fragility test
    (E) pregnancy test

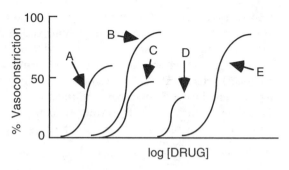

21. Which of the above curves would be obtained from the combination of the agonist represented in curve B and a noncompetitive antagonist?

    (A) A
    (B) B
    (C) C
    (D) D
    (E) E

22. A 19-year-old girl accompanies her 21-year-old boyfriend into the emergency department after a party. He is agitated and diaphoretic, and has dilated pupils. He resists efforts to subdue him, stating, "there are ants crawling up my arm." The girl recalls seeing her boyfriend and others at the party heating "something on aluminum foil" with a cigarette lighter and inhaling the fumes. Which of the following substances did he most likely inhale?

    (A) Heroin
    (B) Jimson weed
    (C) Lysergic acid diethylamide (LSD)
    (D) Methamphetamine
    (E) Model airplane glue

23. A 54-year-old man comes to the office complaining of upper back pain. There is a chronic somatic dysfunction at T1–T4, which resolves after manipulation. Because of the location of his dysfunction, you check his blood pressure and find that he his severely hypertensive. You decide to prescribe a diuretic for initial treatment. Which of the following diuretics acts at the distal tubule of the nephron?

    (A) Ethacrynic acid
    (B) Furosemide
    (C) Hydrochlorothiazide
    (D) Mannitol
    (E) Spironolactone

24. A 10-year-old asthmatic is prescribed a cromolyn sodium inhaler to be administered prior to vigorous activity to prevent an attack. Which of the following is the mechanism of action of this drug?

    (A) It blocks muscarinic receptors
    (B) It inhibits the degranulation of mast cells
    (C) It reduces bronchial inflammation and edema
    (D) It selectively stimulates beta$_2$ receptors
    (E) It stimulates all beta receptors

25. A 49-year-old alcoholic businessman complains of 2 days of severe worsening pain with redness and swelling of his first metatarsophalangeal joint. He has no history of injury or trauma. He is afebrile with no constitutional symptoms. Which of the following drugs is the most appropriate pharmacotherapy?

    (A) Allopurinol
    (B) Colchicine
    (C) Colestipol
    (D) Pravastatin
    (E) Probenecid

26. A 32-year-old man is spraying malathion on the plum trees in his backyard. While taking a break, he reaches down to grab his drink and accidentally takes a swig of malathion instead. His girlfriend immediately takes him to a nearby emergency department. Which of the following drugs could be given to induce emesis?

    (A) Apomorphine
    (B) Loperamide
    (C) Metoclopramide
    (D) Ondansetron
    (E) Ranitidine

27. An airplane pilot working for a major commercial airline suffers from hay fever. The patient has chronic somatic dysfunction at T1-T4. Which of the following drugs would be most suitable for the pilot during working hours?

    (A) Chlorpheniramine
    (B) Diphenhydramine
    (C) Fexofenadine
    (D) Meclizine
    (E) Pyrilamine

28. A patient who is being treated for a myocardial infarction that occurred 2 hours ago is medicated with IV nitroprusside. Which of the following is the expected action of this drug?

    (A) Constriction of arterioles alone
    (B) Constriction of both arterioles and venules
    (C) Constriction of venules alone
    (D) Dilatation of arterioles alone
    (E) Dilatation of arterioles and venules

29. A 72-year-old man with prostate cancer is treated with leuprolide. Which of the following is the mechanism of action of this drug?

    (A) It inhibits 5α-reductase
    (B) It is a competitive antagonist at androgen receptors
    (C) It is a competitive inhibitor of LH
    (D) It is a synthetic analog of GnRH
    (E) It is a testosterone agonist

30. A 50-year-old man with moderate familial hypertriglyceridemia is treated with gemfibrozil. Which of the following is the primary mechanism of action of this drug?

    (A) Binding of bile acids in the intestine
    (B) Inhibition of hepatic VLDL secretion
    (C) Inhibition of HMG-CoA reductase
    (D) Stimulation of HDL production
    (E) Stimulation of lipoprotein lipase

31. A 58-year-old man with a history of atrial fibrillation is prescribed warfarin to prevent clot and embolism formation. His prothrombin time (PT) is regularly monitored. Administration of which of the following drugs would result in an increase in his PT and require readjustment of his warfarin dosage?

    (A) Amobarbital
    (B) Carbamazepine
    (C) Ketoconazole
    (D) Phenytoin
    (E) Rifampin

32. In retinitis pigmentosa, "night-blindness" is an early symptom of visual loss. Which of the following explains this phenomenon?

    (A) Cones are relatively preserved compared with ganglion cells

    (B) Cones are relatively preserved compared with rods

    (C) Ganglion cells are relatively preserved compared with cones

    (D) Ganglion cells are relatively preserved compared with rods

    (E) Rods are relatively preserved compared with cones

33. A patient admitted to the emergency department with chest pain is diagnosed with myocardial infarction. On discharge, the patient is prescribed aspirin but develops an allergic hypersensitivity reaction. Ticlopidine is prescribed instead as a maintenance anticoagulant. Which of the following is the mechanism of action of this drug?

    (A) It binds to the active site of cyclooxygenase via acetylation

    (B) It blocks the binding of plasmin to fibrin

    (C) It hinders the production of thromboxane A_2

    (D) It prevents fibrinogen from binding to platelets

    (E) It stimulates platelet adenylyl cyclase

34. A patient with severe systemic lupus erythematosus is receiving long-term glucocorticoid therapy. She should consequently receive supplemental therapy with which of the following?

    (A) Calcium

    (B) Carotene

    (C) Folate

    (D) Iron

    (E) Vitamin B_{12}

35. A 72-year-old woman who has had recurrent urinary tract infections comes to the office complaining that the last drug prescribed for her didn't work. Physical examination reveals a chronic somatic dysfunction at T11-L1 and suprapubic tenderness. You repeat the urine culture, which reveals the same causative organism. You choose imipenem as her next medication. The antimicrobial imipenem is usually administered in combination with which of the following drugs?

    (A) Cilastatin

    (B) Clavulanic acid

    (C) Para-aminobenzoic acid (PABA)

    (D) Sulbactam

    (E) Trimethoprim

36. A 24-year-old woman on her honeymoon presents to the cruise ship physician with a dilated right eye and complains that she could not read the lunch menu with the same eye. Which of the following drugs is most likely responsible for her symptoms?

    (A) Phenylephrine

    (B) Physostigmine

    (C) Pilocarpine

    (D) Scopolamine

    (E) Tetrahydrozoline

37. A hypertensive patient with elevated serum potassium levels needs diuresis. Which of the following diuretic agents is most likely to cause hyperkalemia?

    (A) Acetazolamide

    (B) Furosemide

    (C) Hydrochlorothiazide

    (D) Metolazone

    (E) Triamterene

38. A 50-year-old woman with urinary incontinence is diagnosed with detrusor instability on urodynamic evaluation. Physical examination reveals chronic somatic dysfunction at T11-L2. Stimulation of which of the following results in contraction of this muscle?

    (A) Alpha-adrenergic receptors

    (B) Beta-adrenergic receptors

    (C) Muscarinic receptors

    (D) Nicotinic receptors

    (E) GABA receptors

39. A 20-year-old female college athlete develops irregular menstrual cycles, acne, a deepening voice, and recent growth of facial hair. Lab values are significant for elevated liver transaminases. She is not on oral contraceptives. Which of the following drugs could be responsible for her presentation?

    (A) Ethinyl estradiol

    (B) Flutamide

    (C) Medroxyprogesterone

    (D) Megestrol acetate

    (E) Nandrolone

40. The reflex change in heart rate in response to IV isoproterenol administered to a patient would be enhanced by which of the following drugs?

    (A) Dobutamine

    (B) Esmolol

    (C) Hexamethonium

    (D) Phenylephrine

    (E) Pirenzepine

41. A patient with an acute myocardial infarction meets the criteria for thrombolytic therapy. Which of the following is an advantage of tissue plasminogen activator (tPA) over streptokinase for fibrinolytic therapy?

    (A) It can be used in the setting of acute myocardial infarction

    (B) It cannot cause hemorrhage

    (C) It is less expensive

    (D) It is not likely to produce an allergic reaction

    (E) It results in the activation of plasminogen

42. A 42-year-old patient has had recurrent nocturnal attacks of acute arthritis involving the right first metatarsophalangeal joint, with serum uric acid levels greater than 7.5 mg/dL. He develops slowly growing subcutaneous nodules in his feet and olecranon. Aspiration of a nodule reveals crystals of sodium urate. Which of the following drugs will most likely shrink, and possibly eliminate, these nodules?

    (A) Allopurinol

    (B) Aspirin

    (C) Colchicine

    (D) Indomethacin

    (E) Thiazide diuretics

43. A 22-year-old woman develops secondary amenorrhea and galactorrhea, and MRI of the head reveals a small intrasellar tumor. Which of the following is the most appropriate pharmacologic treatment for this patient's condition?

    (A) Cholinesterase inhibitors

    (B) Dopamine agonists

    (C) Dopamine antagonists

    (D) Drugs enhancing GABAergic transmission

    (E) Serotonin reuptake inhibitors

44. A 32-year-old man, infected with HIV, is diagnosed with Hodgkin lymphoma. If the patient's CD4 count is 505/mm^3, which of the following agents would be suitable for the treatment of this patient's lymphoma without further compromising his immune system?

    (A) Busulfan

    (B) Cisplatin

    (C) Cyclophosphamide

    (D) Paclitaxel

    (E) Vincristine

45. A patient with uncontrolled diabetes has chronic somatic dysfunction at T5-T9 and complains of severe attacks of hypoglycemia after taking his current medication. Which of the following drugs used in the treatment of type 2 diabetes mellitus has no effect on the secretion of insulin?

   (A) Acetohexamide

   (B) Chlorpropamide

   (C) Glyburide

   (D) Metformin

   (E) Tolbutamide

Questions 46-50

SET A

Directions: For each numbered item (**patient presentation**), select the one lettered heading (**treatment**) most closely associated with it. Each lettered heading may be selected once, more than once, or not at all.

   (A) physostigmine

   (B) naloxone

   (C) ethanol

   (D) oxygen

   (E) flumazenil

   (F) acetylcysteine

   (G) deferoxamine

46. A 22-year-old man has been found unresponsive. During your examination you note that his vitals are: blood pressure 60/40, pulse 40 beats/min, and respirations 5-6/min. He also has constricted pupils.

47. A 5-year-old girl was found drinking ethylene glycol.

48. A 54-year-old woman who has fibromyalgia ran out of her normal pain medication. Her physician was out of town so she took four tablets of 500-mg acetaminophen every 4 hours to stop the pain for the last 24 hours.

49. A 3-year-old child is known to have ingested an entire bottle of multivitamins.

50. A 54-year-old woman who has been anxious recently was given oxazepam 30 mg. One day later, the patient was found in a stupor after having ingested the whole bottle.

Pharmacology

ANSWERS AND EXPLANATIONS

1.	B	26.	A
2.	C	27.	C
3.	D	28.	E
4.	A	29.	D
5.	B	30.	E
6.	E	31.	C
7.	C	32.	B
8.	B	33.	D
9.	E	34.	A
10.	A	35.	A
11.	A	36.	D
12.	A	37.	E
13.	B	38.	C
14.	A	39.	E
15.	A	40.	A
16.	C	41.	D
17.	C	42.	A
18.	E	43.	B
19.	D	44.	E
20.	E	45.	D
21.	C	46.	B
22.	D	47.	C
23.	C	48.	F
24.	B	49.	G
25.	B	50.	E

1. **The correct answer is B.** Prostatic hypertrophy in elderly men is very common; therefore, it should be considered as a primary cause of renal insufficiency until proven otherwise. The patient's signs and symptoms are consistent with obstructive uropathy; there is a history of high urine output followed by periods of almost no urine output. This pattern leads to the accumulation of urine in the collecting system, which creates a high pressure system. The high pressure is then "transmitted" back to the kidney and results in renal insufficiency. Since the patient's obstructive uropathy is most likely caused by prostatic hypertrophy, doxazosin should be used to treat the cause of these signs and symptoms. Doxazosin is a peripherally acting alpha1-adrenergic blocking agent indicated for the treatment of urinary outflow obstruction secondary to benign prostatic hyperplasia (BPH). It is also indicated for the treatment of hypertension, especially in men with BPH. Therefore, the use of this agent will correct the obstructive uropathy and treat his hypertension.

Benazepril (**choice A**) is an ACE inhibitor used in the treatment of hypertension; however, it is known to cause azotemia and oliguria, especially in those with renal insufficiency. Therefore, this agent would be contraindicated.

Furosemide (**choice C**) is a loop diuretic used to increase urine output in patients without a urinary tract obstruction.

Hyoscyamine (**choice D**) is used in the treatment of gastrointestinal disorders caused by spasm and hypermotility. Since this agent is a potent anticholinergic, it would not be recommended in a patient with urinary obstruction. Remember, anticholinergic agents cause urinary retention.

Phenazopyridine (**choice E**) is a urinary tract analgesic used to decrease the dysuria associated with urinary tract infections. The use of this agent in patients with renal insufficiency is not recommended because phenazopyridine can accumulate, resulting in renal stones and transient renal failure.

2. **The correct answer is C.** PGE_2 is available clinically as dinoprostone. It can be used to induce abortion, evacuate a missed abortion, or treat a benign hydatidiform mole.

LTA_4 (**choice A**) is the first leukotriene produced by the lipoxygenase pathway. (Note that 5-HPETE is produced by the direct action of lipoxygenase on arachidonic acid; 5-HPETE is then converted to either 5-HETE or LTA_4.) On Step 1, you might be asked about LTC_4 or LTD_4

since they form the slow-reacting substance of anaphylaxis (SRS-A) and are potent bronchoconstrictors.

PGD_2 (**choice B**) causes both vasodilatation and vasoconstriction, depending on the vascular bed.

PGF_2 (**choice D**), which is also vasoactive, increases cardiac output, constricts bronchial smooth muscle, initiates uterine contractions, and causes contraction of gastrointestinal longitudinal muscle.

PGG_2 (**choice E**) is unstable and isomerized to form PGD_2 (**choice B**), PGE_2 (**choice C**), or PGF_2 (**choice D**). Note that PGG_2 does not have any known physiologic effects of importance.

3. **The correct answer is D.** Phase III trials consist of large, double-blind, controlled studies using patients for whom the drug is targeted. Typically, 500–5,000 patients participate in the study, which is designed to determine whether the drug is more efficacious than placebo and to compare it with older therapies. Drug toxicity is also monitored; infrequent toxicities have a greater likelihood of appearing in this phase (because of the greater number of subjects) than the previous two phases.

For human testing to commence, an IND Application (**choice A**) must be submitted by the manufacturer to the Food and Drug Administration (FDA). This application includes chemical and manufacturing information about the drug, data from animal testing, and designs for clinical testing.

Phase I trials (**choice B**) are the first phase of clinical testing. Approximately 20–30 normal volunteers are used to determine the safety and pharmacokinetic properties of a new drug. Occasionally, patients are used in this phase (e.g., cancer patients who are tested with new chemotherapeutic agents).

Phase II trials (**choice C**) test a new drug on a small group of selected patients (100-300) with regard to therapeutic efficacy, dose range, kinetics, and metabolism.

Phase IV (**choice E**) is the post-marketing surveillance phase, which is not regulated by the FDA and essentially consists of physicians reporting toxic side effects to the FDA. This phase hopefully detects drugs with infrequent side effects that could not be determined with the limited number of subjects used in clinical testing. If it is determined that a drug does exhibit toxic side effects, and that its benefits do not outweigh its costs, the drug can be pulled from the market. (Incidentally, this is how the diet drug fenfluramine was removed from the market.)

4. **The correct answer is A.** The following chart summarizes the differences between heparin and warfarin:

Heparin	Warfarin
Increased effect of antithrombin III on thrombin	Interferes with synthesis of vitamin K clotting factors
Monitored by PTT	Monitored by PT
Given IV or SQ	Given orally
Toxicity treated with protamine sulfate	Toxicity treated with vitamin K and fresh frozen plasma
Rapid anticoagulation	2-3 days before anticoagulation
Can be used in pregnancy	Can't be used in pregnancy

5. **The correct answer is B.** Sucralfate is a promising drug that is not currently in widespread use because it is incompatible with H$_2$ antagonists, such as cimetidine, ranitidine, famotidine, and nizatidine. Sucralfate is aluminum sucrose sulfate, a sulfated disaccharide, which polymerizes and binds to ulcerated tissue. It forms a protective coating against acid, pepsin, and bile, giving the tissue a chance to heal. Unfortunately, a low gastric pH is required for polymerization, meaning that sucralfate is incompatible with drugs that reduce gastric acidity, such as H$_2$ blockers and antacids. The moral of the story is that you cannot assume that two medications that are individually helpful in a medical condition will be synergistic. Learning the mechanisms by which the drugs work will help you spot potential interactions and earn you points on the COMLEX.

6. **The correct answer is E.** Trimethoprim-sulfamethoxazole is a good choice for prophylaxis of lower urinary tract infections, and the combination can be given after an event, such as sexual intercourse, that has previously triggered a recurrent infection. Since trimethoprim-sulfamethoxazole is concentrated in the urine, a single dose can quickly produce effective levels in the bladder, preventing the growth of bacteria introduced into the bladder during coitus. If a specific inciting event, such as sexual intercourse, is known to trigger the infections, daily prophylaxis of trimethoprim-sulfamethoxazole (**choice D**) is not needed.

Ampicillin and chloramphenicol (**choices A, B, and** C) are not used for prophylaxis of urinary tract infections.

7. **The correct answer is C.** Atenolol is a beta-adrenergic receptor blocking agent used in the treatment of hypertension. Medications in this drug class lower blood pressure by reducing both cardiac output and decreasing renin release from the kidney (to a lesser extent).

Blocking catecholamine release from peripheral sympathetic nerves (**choice A**) is the antihypertensive effect seen with peripherally acting adrenergic neuron blockers (e.g., guanethidine and bretylium).

Angiotensin converting enzyme (ACE) inhibitors block the conversion of angiotensin I to angiotensin II (**choice B**).

Diuretics decrease intravascular volume (**choice D**), which ultimately leads to a reduction in blood pressure.

Increasing renin release from the kidney (**choice E**) would increase, not decrease, blood pressure.

8. **The correct answer is B.** Dextromethorphan is a synthetic morphine derivative that acts centrally to suppress coughing by an opioid receptor-independent mechanism. It does not produce significant addiction, constipation, analgesia, respiratory depression, or euphoria. It is therefore available as an over-the-counter medication (e.g., Robitussin DM).

Codeine (**choice A**), or methylmorphine, is a more effective antitussive than dextromethorphan, but it has abuse liability and is constipating.

Diphenoxylate (**choice C**) is an oral antidiarrheal agent that is a derivative of meperidine. This drug exhibits typical opioid effects at high doses and is prescribed only in combination with atropine.

Levorphanol (**choice D**) is a potent analgesic used for severe pain and has the typical side effects of opioids: euphoria, respiratory depression, and constipation. It has substantial abuse liability. Although levorphanol would suppress cough, it is not prescribed for this purpose.

Oxycodone (**choice E**) is a morphine derivative used for moderate-to-severe pain. It produces typical opioid effects, including constipation and dependence. Although oxycodone would suppress cough, it is not prescribed for this purpose.

9. **The correct answer is E.** The patient is presenting with classic signs and symptoms of congestive heart failure: chronic fatigue, exertional and nocturnal dyspnea, orthopnea, a chronic nonproductive cough, respiratory wheezing, and rhonchi, as well as a diminished first heart sound and an S3 gallop. Verapamil is a calcium channel blocker used to treat both hypertension and vasospastic angina. However, it has a strong negative inotropic effect on the heart that can cause signs and

symptoms of heart failure. Furthermore, some clinical studies have shown that congestive heart failure can develop in a small percentage of individuals taking verapamil.

Amlodipine (**choice A**) is also a calcium channel blocker used in the treatment of both hypertension and vasospastic angina. However, it does not have a negative inotropic effect on the heart and does not cause signs and symptoms of heart failure. Furthermore, amlodipine is generally well tolerated in heart failure patients.

Captopril (**choice B**) is an ACE inhibitor used in the treatment of both hypertension and congestive heart failure. Therefore, this agent would not potentiate signs and symptoms of congestive heart failure.

Furosemide (**choice C**) is a diuretic commonly used to treat the congestion and edema associated with heart failure. It can also be used to treat hypertension.

Hydralazine (**choice D**) is a vasodilator used primarily to treat signs and symptoms associated with heart failure. The use of this agent in patients with angina is not recommended because it can potentiate the angina.

10. **The correct answer is A.** Propylthiouracil inhibits thyroid peroxidase, the enzyme that allows the iodide taken up at the base of the thyroid follicular cell to be oxidized to iodine at the apex of the cell. Thyroid peroxidase also catalyzes the oxidative coupling of two diiodotyrosine (DIT) molecules into T_4 and of one DIT and one monoiodotyrosine (MIT) into T_3. Note: if you knew that thyroid peroxidase was involved in oxidations, then you probably could have arrived at choice A by the process of elimination.

Iodide uptake at the base of the follicular cell (**choice B**) occurs via an active transport mechanism; thyroid peroxidase is not involved.

Iodination of thyroglobulin in the colloid (**choice C**) into DIT and MIT does not involve thyroid peroxidase.

Proteolysis of the iodinated thyroglobulin into MIT and DIT (**choice D**) occurs in the follicular cell and is catalyzed by lysosomal enzymes, not by thyroid peroxidase.

Reuptake of iodinated thyroglobulin from the follicular lumen (**choice E**) occurs via endocytosis and does not involve thyroid peroxidase.

11. **The correct answer is A.** Cyclophosphamide is metabolized to acrolein, which is excreted in the urine. If the patient's urine is concentrated, this toxic metabolite may cause severe bladder damage. Early symptoms of bladder toxicity include dysuria and frequency. This can be distinguished from a urinary tract infection, since there is no bacteriuria with cyclophosphamide-induced bladder toxicity. However, microscopic hematuria is often pres-

ent on urinalysis. In severe hemorrhagic cystitis, large segments of the bladder mucosa may be shed, which can lead to prolonged, gross hematuria. The incidence of cyclophosphamide-induced hemorrhagic cystitis can be decreased by ensuring that the patient maintains a high fluid intake. Cyclophosphamide is an alkylating agent used in the treatment of breast carcinoma, malignant lymphoma, multiple myeloma, and adenocarcinoma of the ovary, as well as various other forms of cancer. The major toxic reactions commonly seen with this agent include mucositis, nausea, hepatotoxicity, sterile hemorrhagic and non-hemorrhagic cystitis, leukopenia, neutropenia, and interstitial pulmonary fibrosis.

Mitomycin (**choice B**) is an antibiotic, antineoplastic agent used in the treatment of breast carcinoma and adenocarcinoma of the pancreas and stomach, as well as various other forms of cancer. The major toxic reactions commonly seen with this agent include bone marrow depression, nausea, hepatotoxicity, acute bronchospasm, thrombocytopenia, and interstitial pneumonitis.

Paclitaxel (**choice C**) is an antineoplastic agent primarily used in the treatment of ovarian and breast cancer. The major toxic reactions commonly seen with this agent include bone marrow depression, nausea, hepatotoxicity, bronchospasm, thrombocytopenia, and neutropenia.

Tamoxifen (**choice D**) is an antineoplastic hormone primarily used in the palliative treatment of estrogen-receptor positive breast cancer patients. The major toxic reactions commonly seen with this agent include depression, dizziness, thrombosis, mild leukopenia, and thrombocytopenia.

Vincristine (**choice E**) is a mitotic inhibitor antineoplastic agent used in the treatment of breast cancer, Hodgkin disease, non-Hodgkin lymphoma, advanced testicular cancer, and various other types of cancer. The major toxic reactions commonly seen with this agent include mental depression, hemorrhagic enterocolitis, bone marrow depression, nausea, thrombocytopenia, and leukopenia.

12. **The correct answer is A.** Pulmonary toxicity (characterized by interstitial pneumonitis that may progress to pulmonary fibrosis) is a dose-related complication seen with the administration of bleomycin, an antibiotic chemotherapeutic agent. Other agents associated with pulmonary toxicity include methotrexate and busulfan.

Cyclophosphamide (**choice B**) is an alkylating agent used in the treatment of numerous cancers (e.g., breast, testicular), leukemia, and Hodgkin lymphoma. It is also used as a conditioning agent for bone marrow transplant. Hemorrhagic cystitis, which can be severe and even fatal, can develop. The mechanism is thought to be secondary to irritation from the toxic cyclophosphamide metabolite acrolein.

Doxorubicin (**choice C**) is an antibiotic chemotherapeutic that acts by intercalating between DNA and inducing DNA strand breaks via topoisomerase II. Irreversible cardiotoxicity is an important adverse reaction. This includes EKG changes and congestive heart failure.

Etoposide (**choice D**) interferes with topoisomerase, inducing DNA strand breaks, and is used to treat testicular and lung cancers. Adverse reactions include stomatitis, erythema, and bone marrow suppression.

5-Fluorouracil (**choice E**) is an S/G_1 phase-specific antimetabolite that is a widely used antineoplastic agent used systemically to treat solid tumors and topically to treat skin cancers. Adverse reactions include alopecia, bone marrow suppression, dermatitis, stomatitis, and gastrointestinal distress.

13. **The correct answer is B.** Ammonium chloride acidifies the urine (ascorbic acid could also be used) and hastens the elimination of weak bases, such as amphetamine. This occurs because basic drugs are not charged in their nonionized, free base form, and can easily diffuse out of the urine across tubular epithelial cells, back into the bloodstream. Ionizing the drug (in this case by lowering the urine pH) prevents it from leaving the filtrate, and the drug is excreted in the urine.

Acetazolamide (**choice A**) is a carbonic anhydrase inhibitor. It is used to alkalinize the urine in patients with hyperuricemia to increase the solubility of uric acid in the urine. It would tend to delay the elimination of the ingested amphetamine.

Penicillamine (**choice C**) is effective in chelating lead in cases of poisoning by that metal. It also chelates copper and is used in treatment of Wilson disease.

Probenecid (**choice D**) blocks renal tubular acid transport. It is used as a uricosuric.

Sodium bicarbonate (**choice E**) would alkalinize the urine, thus delaying the elimination of the ingested amphetamine.

14. **The correct answer is A.** Warfarin is the oral anticoagulant the patient was most likely taking. This drug is commonly prescribed to patients with atrial fibrillation to prevent the formation of atrial thrombi. Warfarin increases the PT because it interferes with the synthesis of the vitamin K clotting factors of the liver (II, VII, IX, and X); therefore, regular monitoring of the PT is necessary. Cimetidine is an H_2-blocker that inhibits hepatic enzymes, including those that metabolize warfarin.

Consequently, coadministration of warfarin and cimetidine results in enhanced warfarin activity, producing pronounced anticoagulation and the bleeding diathesis seen in this patient. Cimetidine has one of the worst side effect profiles of all the H_2-blockers and may also result in gynecomastia in men.

Famotidine (**choice B**) is an H_2-blocker that does not affect liver metabolism.

Misoprostol (**choice C**) is a prostaglandin E_1 analog used in peptic ulcer disease. It does not affect hepatic metabolism.

Omeprazole (**choice D**) is a proton-pump inhibitor used to decrease acid production in patients with peptic ulcer disease or reflux. It does not affect drug metabolism by the liver.

Ranitidine (**choice E**) is another H_2-blocker. It does not inhibit liver enzymes as strongly as cimetidine does.

15. **The correct answer is A.** Although treatment of transient ischemic attacks (actually prophylaxis against stroke) remains a controversial area, you should be aware of current recommendations. Daily aspirin therapy has been shown in prospective, randomized studies to reduce the incidence of stroke and death in patients with transient ischemic attacks. If alternative therapy is needed, either because the patient cannot tolerate aspirin or because aspirin therapy has failed, the antiplatelet agent ticlopidine can be used.

Anticoagulation with Coumadin (**choice B**) does not decrease the risk of stroke and death but does increase the risk of intracerebral hemorrhage.

Despite the antiplatelet activity of dipyridamole (**choice C**), therapeutic trials have not shown efficacy in the prophylaxis of stroke.

Anticoagulation with heparin (**choice D**) does not decrease the risk of stroke and death but does increase the risk of intracerebral hemorrhage.

Despite the antiplatelet activity of sulfinpyrazone (**choice E**), therapeutic trials have not shown efficacy in the prophylaxis of stroke.

16. **The correct answer is C.** The patient described above is probably under the influence of a CNS stimulant, such as methamphetamine. Labetalol is a nonselective alpha- and beta-antagonist that blocks many of the dangerous peripheral side effects of CNS stimulants, such as hypertension and cardiac stimulation. Other appropriate medications include antipsychotic agents (to control the agitation and psychotic symptoms) and diazepam (to control possible seizures). Supportive care should be given as needed to control the hyperthermia and to maintain respiration.

Atropine (**choice A**), which is a muscarinic antagonist, would be an appropriate therapy for an acetylcholinesterase inhibitor overdose. Patients presenting with an acetylcholinesterase inhibitor overdose would not be expected to have an elevated body temperature or hypertension. Their eyes would be miotic, not mydriatic. Bradycardia, not tachycardia, would be expected. They would, however, have diaphoresis because of increased cholinergic tone at the sweat glands, which are innervated by sympathetic cholinergics.

Flumazenil (**choice B**) is a benzodiazepine receptor antagonist. It is specifically useful in the case of a benzodiazepine overdose.

Naloxone (**choice D**), which is an opioid receptor antagonist, would be an appropriate therapy for an opiate (e.g., heroin or morphine) overdose. A patient would appear sleepy, lethargic, or comatose, depending on the degree of overdose. Pupils would be miotic, not mydriatic. Blood pressure and heart rate would usually be decreased. Respiration would be depressed.

Physostigmine (**choice E**), which is an acetylcholinesterase inhibitor, might be used for overdose of an antimuscarinic drug, such as atropine, scopolamine, or Jimson weed. An antimuscarinic overdose can look similar to a CNS stimulant overdose, with at least one important exception. The hyperthermia seen with an antimuscarinic overdose is accompanied by *hot and dry skin* (because of blockade of the sympathetic cholinergics to the sweat glands). Stimulant overdose is often characterized by *profuse sweating*. Tachycardia, hypertension, hyperthermia, mental changes, and mydriasis are common to both.

17. **The correct answer is C.** Everything in this case points to congestive heart failure (CHF): dyspnea, elevated heart rate, S3, peripheral edema, and reduced ejection fraction. A drug that will alleviate the symptoms by decreasing both preload and afterload is necessary.

    Enalapril is an angiotensin-converting enzyme (ACE) inhibitor. ACE inhibitors (captopril, enalapril, lisinopril) work by blocking the conversion of angiotensin I to angiotensin II in the lungs. Angiotensin II is both a potent vasoconstrictor and a stimulator of aldosterone production. Aldosterone acts by promoting sodium (and thus water) reabsorption by the kidney. An ACE inhibitor will therefore promote vasodilatation (reducing afterload), as well as reduce intravascular volume (decreasing preload). It does not affect the heart's inotropic state.

    Although digoxin (**choice A**) is a mainstay in the therapy of CHF, it has no effect on either preload or afterload. Instead, it works by having a positive inotropic effect on the heart. The mechanism involves inhibition of Na^+/K^+ ATPase and a consequent increase in intracellular calcium, which, in turn, increases the heart's contractile force.

    Diltiazem (**choice B**) is a calcium-channel blocker. As their name implies, calcium-channel blockers block the influx of calcium (via specific calcium channels) into the cell from the extracellular fluid; this interferes with excitation-contraction coupling in cardiac muscle, producing a negative inotropic effect. Although these drugs can be used in the treatment of hypertension and angina (they inhibit the contraction of the vascular smooth muscle and thereby decrease peripheral vascular resistance/afterload), they are contraindicated in patients with CHF because of their negative inotropic effect.

    Furosemide (**choice D**) is a loop diuretic. It decreases intravascular volume (and hence, preload), but at typical doses has no significant effect on either afterload or inotropic state. Diuretics are often used in the treatment of CHF, and furosemide is used for the immediate relief of pulmonary congestion.

    Propranolol (**choice E**) is a beta-blocker. It has a negative inotropic effect on the heart and is therefore contraindicated in patients with CHF.

18. **The correct answer is E.** Vincristine (and vinblastine) are Vinca alkaloids that bind to tubulin, a component of cellular microtubules. This leads to disruption of the mitotic spindle apparatus and results in metaphase arrest because the chromosomes are unable to segregate. Since these drugs interfere with mitosis, they are considered cell-cycle specific for the M phase.

    Cytarabine (**choice A**) belongs to the class of antineoplastics that are antimetabolites. This drug class interferes with normal metabolic pathways by competing for enzymatic sites. Specifically, cytarabine (Ara-C) is a pyrimidine nucleoside analog. It interrupts DNA synthesis and function by inhibiting DNA polymerase and incorporating into the DNA or RNA of the cell. As you would expect, this drug is cell-cycle specific for the S phase.

    Daunorubicin (**choice B**) is one of the antibiotic antineoplastic agents (others include dactinomycin, doxorubicin, bleomycin, plicamycin, and mitomycin). These agents work by disrupting DNA functioning. Daunorubicin binds to DNA between base pairs on adjacent strands, resulting in uncoiling of the helix and destruction of the DNA template. Although this drug has its maximal effect during the S phase, it is not cell-cycle specific. (Note: the only antibiotic that is cell-cycle specific is bleomycin.)

    Hydroxyurea (**choice C**) works by interfering with ribonucleoside diphosphate reductase, the enzyme responsible for generating the deoxyribonucleotides needed for DNA synthesis. It is S-phase specific.

Mechlorethamine (**choice D**) is a nitrogen mustard. The nitrogen mustards (mechlorethamine, cyclophosphamide, melphalan, chlorambucil) belong to the larger class of alkylating agents. These agents work by alkylating DNA (along with RNA and proteins). The alkylating agents are generally *not* cell-cycle specific.

19. **The correct answer is D.** Long-term, particularly daily, use of exogenous systemic corticosteroids causes pituitary/adrenal suppression, and abrupt cessation may induce an Addison-like crisis characterized by hypotension, hypoglycemia, and sometimes (if mineralocorticoid function is suppressed as well) hyponatremia (opposite of **choice C**) and hyperkalemia (opposite of **choice E**). Decreased ACTH (opposite of **choice A**) and low cortisol (opposite of **choice B**) would also be expected. Treatment is with IV steroids, and, if the patient is in shock, IV saline. The patient should also be examined for other conditions (such as infection) that may have contributed to the acute adrenal crisis.

20. **The correct answer is E.** Misoprostol, a methyl analog of prostaglandin E_1, is approved for the prevention of ulcers caused by the administration of NSAIDs. Because this drug is a potential abortifacient, it should not be given to pregnant women, or to women who are attempting to conceive.

Antinuclear antibodies (**choice A**) are associated with autoimmune diseases, such as systemic lupus erythematosus, scleroderma, Sjögren syndrome, and inflammatory myopathies. The test would be of no value in this case.

A barium swallow (**choice B**) is not indicated prior to the administration of misoprostol.

Esophageal manometry (**choice C**) is used to evaluate the competency of the lower esophageal sphincter and to assess esophageal motor activity.

The osmotic fragility test (**choice D**) is performed by placing erythrocytes into a low-salt solution. An increased susceptibility to osmotic lysis is found in hereditary spherocytosis.

21. **The correct answer is C.** Noncompetitive, or irreversible, antagonists block receptors in several different ways. They can bind covalently at the active site, or can bind either covalently or noncovalently at other sites on the receptor. Either way, adding more agonist does not reverse the effects of the antagonist. Noncompetitive antagonists essentially decrease the number of working receptors by binding to them. Any receptors that do not bind the noncompetitive antagonist behave normally. This can be depicted graphically by a downward shift in the dose-response curve. The efficacy is decreased, but

the potency remains the same. In this example, **curve B** is the original agonist dose-response curve, and **curve C** is the same agonist in the presence of a noncompetitive antagonist.

Competitive antagonists bind reversibly to the agonist binding site of a receptor, and their effects can be surmounted if a sufficient amount of agonist is present. This is graphically depicted as a parallel right shift of the curve. In this example, **curve B** represents the agonist alone. **Curve E** represents the agonist in the presence of a competitive antagonist. Thus, one can achieve the same response, but a greater concentration of agonist is required.

The other curves represent drugs with greater and lesser efficacy and potency than Drug B:

Curves A and D represent drugs that have a lower efficacy than Drug B.

Curve A represents a drug that is more potent than Drug B; **Curve D** represents a drug that is less potent than Drug B.

22. **The correct answer is D.** The patient was probably smoking methamphetamine hydrochloride from aluminum foil. This practice can swiftly produce very high blood levels of the drug, since the vaporized methamphetamine is absorbed efficiently from the lungs and goes directly into the systemic circulation. The symptoms are classic for psychostimulant toxicity (agitation, diaphoresis, dilated pupils), including the delusional perception of insects crawling on or in the skin ("formication").

Heroin (**choice A**) could be smoked from aluminum foil but would produce miosis, respiratory depression, and sedation.

Jimson weed (from Datura species; **choice B**) contains potent antimuscarinic agents, such as atropine and scopolamine. It might produce delirium and agitation but would not produce diaphoresis (instead, the skin would be dry and warm). Also, Jimson weed is typically brewed as a tea, rather than smoked.

LSD (**choice C**) generally produces brightly colored hallucinations with a clear sensorium, and is unlikely to produce a sensation of bugs crawling on the skin. LSD is ingested, rather than smoked.

Model airplane glue (**choice E**) contains toluene and/or ketones that produce a narcotic-like "high" if inhaled, rather than symptoms of stimulant overdose. These agents are not typically heated on aluminum foil, as they are very flammable and are sufficiently volatile to be inhaled at room temperature.

23. **The correct answer is C.** The thiazide diuretics (e.g., hydrochlorothiazide, chlorothiazide, benzthiazide) promote diuresis by inhibiting reabsorption of NaCl, primarily in the early distal tubule.

Ethacrynic acid (**choice A**) and furosemide (**choice B**) are loop diuretics. They act by inhibiting electrolyte reabsorption in the thick ascending loop of Henle. If you didn't know where these agents act, but did know that they both belong to the same class of diuretics, you could have eliminated them as possibilities since there can't be more than one correct answer choice.

Mannitol (**choice D**) is an osmotic diuretic. It is freely filtered at the glomerulus and is not reabsorbed. Its primary action occurs at the proximal tubule.

Spironolactone (**choice E**) is a potassium-sparing diuretic. It acts on the collecting tubule to inhibit the reabsorption of Na^+ and the secretion of K^+. Spironolactone is a structural analog of aldosterone that binds to its receptor. (Triamterene and amiloride are also potassium-sparing diuretics but are not aldosterone antagonists.)

24. **The correct answer is B.** Cromolyn sodium inhibits the degranulation of mast cells, thereby preventing the release of histamine and other bronchoconstrictive autacoids. It is administered by inhalation and is used prophylactically to prevent an asthma attack (especially in children). It has no direct bronchodilator, adrenergic, antihistaminic, or antiinflammatory actions.

The remaining answer choices relate to some of the other major categories of drugs available for the treatment of asthma:

Muscarinic antagonists (**choice A**) work by inhibiting acetylcholine-induced bronchoconstriction. Atropine and other belladonna alkaloids used to be first-line drugs for the treatment of asthma, but with little success. The newer agent, ipratropium, is a quaternary amine designed for aerosol use. It is a much more successful agent than the earlier muscarinic blockers and has limited side effects because it is minimally absorbed.

Corticosteroids are useful in asthma because they reduce inflammation and edema (**choice C**). They also potentiate the bronchodilating effects of the adrenergic agonists. Their use is limited by their many systemic side effects, and they are typically used only in cases of severe or acute bronchospasm or in the treatment of status asthmaticus. Fewer systemic side effects occur in aerosolized preparations such as beclomethasone dipropionate.

Selective $beta_2$ agonists (**choice D**) include metaproterenol, albuterol, and terbutaline. These drugs are the mainstay in the treatment of acute asthma. They work by stimulating $beta_2$-mediated bronchodilation (bronchial smooth muscle relaxation) without the cardiac side effects of nonselective beta agonists (**choice E**), such as isoproterenol. Note that new long-acting beta agonists have been developed (salmeterol and formoterol) for prophylactic use.

25. **The correct answer is B.** This patient is experiencing an acute attack of gout. The association of gout with alcoholism is well documented. Gout is caused by overproduction or underexcretion of uric acid. Precipitation of sodium urate (uric acid is ionized at body pH) in joint fluid causes an acute inflammatory synovitis with synovial edema and leukocytic infiltrate. It usually affects the joints of the lower extremity, most commonly, the large toe. Formation of tophi (urate deposits surrounded by inflammatory cells, including foreign body giant cells) is pathognomonic.

Colchicine is an anti-gout drug that binds to microtubule proteins and interferes with microtubule assembly. In this way, it impairs leukocyte chemotaxis, thus preventing the migration of granulocytes to the inflammatory site. Colchicine is the drug of choice for attacks of acute gout. Note that non-steroidal antiinflammatory drugs (NSAIDs) can also be used in the treatment of acute gout. They are as efficacious as colchicine; however, symptomatic improvement takes longer.

Allopurinol (**choice A**) is an anti-gout drug indicated for the treatment of chronic gout. Allopurinol functions to inhibit the enzyme xanthine oxidase, which results in decreased production of uric acid from its immediate precursor, xanthine. It lowers both serum and urinary concentrations of uric acid.

Colestipol (**choice C**) is a bile acid sequestrant that is useful in lowering cholesterol levels in familial hyperlipidemias. It is not used for the treatment of gout.

Pravastatin (**choice D**) is a hydroxymethylglutaryl-CoA (HMG-CoA) reductase inhibitor useful in the treatment of familial hyperlipidemias. It is not used for the treatment of gout.

Probenecid (**choice E**) is indicated for the treatment of chronic gout. Probenecid inhibits uric acid reabsorption and therefore increases the urinary excretion of uric acid.

26. **The correct answer is A.** Apomorphine is a dopamine and opioid agonist that stimulates the chemoreceptor trigger zone in the medulla of the brainstem to induce vomiting. It must be administered parenterally and, because it is a respiratory depressant, it should not be given to patients with compromised respiration. If necessary, the apomorphine-induced respiratory depression can be reversed by naloxone.

Loperamide (**choice B**) is an over-the-counter antidiarrheal.

Metoclopramide (**choice C**) is a dopamine receptor antagonist used to stimulate upper gastrointestinal motility. Because it is a dopamine antagonist, it also acts as an antiemetic.

Ondansetron (**choice D**), a 5HT$_3$ antagonist, is an antiemetic.

Ranitidine (**choice E**), an H$_2$ antagonist, reduces histamine-induced gastric acid release.

27. **The correct answer is C.** Fexofenadine, which belongs to the piperidine drug class, is the only drug listed that does not cross the blood-brain barrier and therefore does not cause sedation (a bad thing for someone flying an airplane). Other drugs from the same class include cetirizine and levocabastine. Terfenadine and astemizole were also members of this second generation of antihistamines but have since been removed from the U.S. market becasue their metabolism was easily inhibited (by Ketoconazole, itraconazole, macrolide antibiotics, and even by grapefruit juice), resulting in high concentrations that could lead to a lethal arrhythmia (torsade de pointes).

All the other choices have some degree of sedation as a side effect and therefore would not be recommended for someone who is flying an airplane or operating any kind of machinery.

28. **The correct answer is E.** Nitroprusside is somewhat tricky to use, but is a very useful IV agent that causes dilatation of both arterioles and venules. It has a very rapid onset of action and is typically used in an emergency department or intensive care unit situation. The typical setting is a patient with acute or chronic low cardiac output and high ventricular filling pressures due to poor systolic left ventricular function. Underlying causes for the poor ventricular function may be diverse: dilated cardiomyopathy, acute myocardial infarction, chronic coronary heart disease, or aortic or mitral incompetence. Nitroprusside can improve perfusion of vital organs and reduce the workload of the heart. Problems sometimes encountered with this drug include hypotension (best avoided by starting with a low dose and continuously monitoring systemic arterial and pulmonary capillary wedge pressures) and accumulation of toxic metabolites of cyanide in patients with liver or renal failure. Many physicians prefer to use IV nitrate rather than nitroprusside because of its lesser toxicity.

29. **The correct answer is D.** Leuprolide is a GnRH analog. Given long-term in a continuous fashion, it will inhibit FSH and LH release, thereby decreasing testosterone

production and exacting a chemical castration in men. It can be used in the treatment of prostate cancer, polycystic ovary syndrome, uterine fibroids, and endometriosis.

Inhibition of 5α-reductase (**choice A**) is the mechanism of action of finasteride. It thereby inhibits the production of dihydrotestosterone. It is used in the treatment of benign prostatic hyperplasia (BPH).

Flutamide is another drug used in the treatment of prostate cancer. It is a competitive antagonist at androgen receptors (**choice B**).

Since LH activates interstitial cells to secrete testosterone, a synthetic analog of LH (**choice C**) would not be appropriate treatment for prostatic cancer. The same goes for a testosterone analog (**choice E**).

Here is a brief chart that will aid you in remembering the actions of these similar sounding drugs:

Drug	Action	Indication
Leuprolide	GnRH analog	Prostate CA
Flutamide	Competitive androgen antagonist	Prostate CA
Finasteride	5α-reductase inhibitor	BPH

Remember, "loo"-prolide and "floo"-tamide are both used for prostate cancer. Finasteride is used for BPH.

30. **The correct answer is E.** Gemfibrozil (as well as clofibrate) works by increasing the activity of lipoprotein lipase, leading to increased clearance of VLDLs, which are elevated in familial hypertriglyceridemia. This question gives us the opportunity to review the mechanisms of action of the drugs used in the treatment of hyperlipidemia:

Binding of bile acids (**choice A**) is the mechanism of action of resins such as cholestyramine. They cause the liver to use cholesterol for the synthesis of new bile acids.

Inhibition of hepatic VLDL secretion (**choice B**) is the mechanism of action of niacin.

Inhibition of HMG-CoA reductase (**choice C**) is the mechanism of action of lovastatin and simvastatin.

Stimulation of HDL production (**choice D**) may occur with both gemfibrozil and niacin, but it is not the main mechanism of action.

31. **The correct answer is C.** This question is testing a favorite COMLEX concept—the relationship between the hepatic cytochrome P-450 system and the metabolism of drugs. Certain drugs can affect the metabolism of other drugs by either inducing or inhibiting hepatic microsomal enzyme

activity. In this case, you are told that the PT of this patient increases with the administration of the second drug. This means that the amount of circulating warfarin increased and that you are looking for a drug that inhibits the P-450 system (thereby decreasing warfarin metabolism). Of the drugs listed, only ketoconazole inhibits the P-450 system. Other important inhibitors include cimetidine and isoniazid.

You should study all the other choices in this question because they are all inducers of the P-450 system and would require an increased dose of warfarin to achieve the same level of anticoagulation.

32. **The correct answer is B.** Retinitis pigmentosa is a familial degenerative disease of the retina that most often has recessive genetics. The initial problem appears to be alterations in the pigmented epithelium below the retina, particularly in the most anterior portions of the retina. The pigmented epithelial cells become disrupted and leak pigment, which accumulates along the attenuated blood vessels (and can be seen with an ophthalmoscope). A consequence of this damage is that the rod cells that are normally nutritionally supported and "groomed" by the pigment epithelium also undergo degenerative changes. Since the cones are relatively preserved, day vision is preserved. However, night vision, which is highly dependent on rods, begins to decay. With disease progression, vision is completely or nearly completely lost, and the retina becomes so distorted that a single row of cone nuclei with scattered stumpy cone remnants is all that remains of the photoreceptor layer.

33. **The correct answer is D.** Ticlopidine is an antiplatelet drug that interacts with platelet glycoprotein IIb/IIIa, a fibrinogen receptor that links platelets together and leads to plug formation. Thus, the drug prevents fibrinogen from binding to platelets. The drug is useful both for patients with coronary disease and for those with cerebrovascular disease such as stroke. Of course, hemorrhagic stroke should first be ruled out before it is deemed safe to use any anticoagulant. Ticlopidine is particularly indicated for stroke prophylaxis after a transient ischemic attack.

Aspirin acetylates cyclooxygenase at or near the active site (**choice A**) and thus hinders the production of thromboxane A$_2$ (**choice C**).

Aminocaproic acid strongly inhibits fibrinolysis. It blocks the binding of plasmin to fibrin (**choice B**) by attaching to lysine binding sites on plasmin and plasminogen.

Dipyridamole is a phosphodiesterase inhibitor that also blocks the reuptake of adenosine, which acts on the platelets to stimulate adenylyl cyclase (**choice E**).

34. **The correct answer is A.** Long-term corticosteroid use can cause osteopenia with vertebral compression factors. This can be minimized with oral calcium supplementation. If the patient is a post-menopausal woman, estrogen therapy is also useful. More controversial is the use of vitamin D, thiazide diuretics, calcitonin, and diphosphonates. Exercise, in moderation, may stimulate bone formation.

Carotene (**choice B**) is an antioxidant and has no role in the amelioration of bone loss due to long-term corticosteroid treatment.

Some patients with lupus develop hemolytic anemia, and extra-nutritional support with folate (**choice C**) or iron (**choice D**) may be helpful. However, the anemia is a feature of the disease itself, rather than of the steroid therapy.

Supplementation with vitamin B$_{12}$ (cobalamin; **choice E**) is not indicated with glucocorticoid therapy.

35. **The correct answer is A.** Imipenem is a broad-spectrum (including activity against *Pseudomonas*), synthetic, beta-lactam antibiotic that is currently the most potent and broadest spectrum beta-lactam available. It is given in combination with cilastatin, which limits imipenem's toxicity by blocking renal dipeptidase, thereby minimizing accumulation of nephrotoxic metabolites.

Clavulanic acid (**choice B**) covalently reacts with bacterial penicillinase (beta-lactamase), thereby inhibiting the enzyme that cleaves the beta-lactam ring of penicillins, such as amoxicillin and ticarcillin.

Para-aminobenzoic acid (PABA; **choice C**) is a folic acid precursor. Sulfonamides are structural analogs of PABA, and thus interfere with folate synthesis in bacteria.

Sulbactam (**choice D**) is a penicillinase (beta-lactamase) inhibitor used with parenteral ampicillin.

Trimethoprim (**choice E**) is an antibiotic that is usually given in conjunction with sulfamethoxazole, because the two drugs block sequential steps in bacterial folate synthesis.

36. **The correct answer is D.** The question is asking for a drug that dilates the pupil (mydriasis) and prevents accommodation by paralyzing the ciliary muscle (cycloplegia). Scopolamine would produce both of these actions by blocking muscarinic acetylcholine receptors on the pupillary constrictor muscle (leading to mydriasis) and on the ciliary muscle (producing cycloplegia). An additional hint to arrive at this answer is the fact that she is on a cruise ship. Scopolamine patches are used to prevent motion sickness. The woman most likely applied the patch and subsequently rubbed her eye.

Phenylephrine (**choice A**), an alpha$_1$-adrenergic agonist, could produce mydriasis by acting on receptors present on the radial dilator muscle. This would constrict the radial dilator muscles without affecting the ciliary muscles, which have muscarinic receptors (and a few beta-adrenergic receptors).

Physostigmine (**choice B**) is an intermediate-acting carbamylating inhibitor of acetylcholinesterase; it would increase cholinergic tone to the pupillary constrictor muscle, producing miosis, and cause ciliary muscle contraction to focus for near vision. It is used in the treatment of glaucoma.

Pilocarpine (**choice C**) is a nonspecific muscarinic agonist and would therefore produce miosis and contraction of the ciliary muscle to focus for near vision. It is used in the treatment of glaucoma.

Tetrahydrozoline (**choice E**) is an alpha$_1$-adrenergic agonist and is the active ingredient in Visine. It "gets the red out" by vasoconstricting vessels of the eye. It could cause some mydriasis by acting on alpha-receptors on the radial dilator muscle; however, it would not have an effect on the ciliary muscle.

37. **The correct answer is E.** Triamterene is grouped in the category of potassium-sparing diuretics. Along with spironolactone and amiloride, these diuretic agents may cause excess renal retention of potassium. In this manner, use of these drugs may increase potassium levels and cause hyperkalemia.

Acetazolamide (**choice A**) is a carbonic anhydrase inhibitor that initially causes a moderate amount of potassium loss. This would predispose the patient to hypokalemia.

Furosemide (**choice B**) is a loop diuretic that causes a moderate to severe loss of potassium.

Hydrochlorothiazide and metolazone (**choices C and D**) are thiazide diuretics that cause moderate amounts of potassium loss.

38. **The correct answer is C.** Stimulation of muscarinic receptors (cholinergic parasympathetic) causes contraction of the detrusor muscle, which is located in the wall of the bladder and is responsible for bladder emptying. Detrusor instability, resulting in incontinence, can therefore be effectively treated with anticholinergic medications, such as oxybutynin (Ditropan). Note that this is also why drugs with anticholinergic activity (e.g., tricyclic antidepressants) can result in urinary retention.

Alpha-adrenergic stimulation, specifically alpha$_1$ (**choice A**), causes contraction of the trigone of the bladder and smooth muscle of the urethra (including the internal urethral sphincter). Alpha agonists are therefore useful for treating stress incontinence, which results from an incompetent sphincter. Alpha antagonists, which relax the sphincter, are useful for treating overflow incontinence resulting from bladder outlet obstruction.

Beta-adrenergic stimulation, specifically beta$_2$ (**choice B**), of the detrusor muscle causes relaxation, not contraction, of the structure.

Stimulation of nicotinic cholinergic receptors (**choice D**) causes contraction of the external urethral sphincter, which consists of skeletal muscle.

Stimulation of GABA receptors (**choice E**) produces inhibitory postsynaptic potentials limited to the brain and spinal cord.

39. **The correct answer is E.** Nandrolone is an anabolic steroid. The clue in this question is that the woman competes in athletic events. The other signs (facial hair, menstrual irregularity, and acne) support the supposition that this woman is taking androgenic steroids.

Ethinyl estradiol (**choice A**) is a synthetic steroidal estrogen used for oral contraception.

Flutamide (**choice B**) is a nonsteroidal anti-androgen used in the treatment of prostate carcinoma.

Medroxyprogesterone and megestrol acetate (**choices C and D**) are synthetic progestins. They are also used in oral contraception, in combination with estrogens.

40. **The correct answer is A.** The first thing you need to know to answer this question is what effect isoproterenol has on blood pressure. Isoproterenol, a nonselective beta agonist, decreases blood pressure primarily because of beta$_2$-induced vasodilatation. This would lead to a reflex increase in heart rate by stimulating the sympathetic nervous system and inhibiting the parasympathetic nervous system. The next step is to determine which drug would enhance this increase in heart rate. Of all the drugs listed, only dobutamine would increase heart rate. Dobutamine is a beta$_1$ agonist that increases heart rate by stimulating cardiac receptors; it is typically given intravenously in a hospital setting.

Esmolol (**choice B**) is a beta$_1$ antagonist. This would prevent some of the reflex increase in heart rate by blocking beta$_1$ receptors on the heart.

Hexamethonium (**choice C**) is a ganglionic blocker that acts by blocking nicotinic receptors at peripheral ganglia. This would prevent any baroreceptor reflexes by blocking all sympathetic and parasympathetic outflow.

Phenylephrine (**choice D**) is an alpha$_1$-selective agonist. This would not have a direct effect on the heart and, if anything, would diminish the isoproterenol-induced baroreceptor reflex because it would cause peripheral vasoconstriction.

Pirenzepine (**choice E**) is a selective muscarinic$_1$ (M$_1$) antagonist. This would not have an effect on the heart because M$_2$ receptors are the subtype of muscarinic receptor that reside on the heart. Atropine, a nonselective muscarinic antagonist, would enhance the reflex increase in heart rate.

41. **The correct answer is D.** Tissue plasminogen activator is produced by and secreted from endothelial cells. Since it is not a foreign protein like streptokinase (derived from hemolytic streptococci), tPA is not allergenic.

Both drugs can be used in the setting of acute myocardial infarction (**choice A**).

Both drugs can result in hemorrhage (**choice B**), especially during prolonged therapy for treatment of pulmonary embolism or venous thrombosis.

tPA is as much as 10 times more expensive (**choice C**) than streptokinase.

Both drugs result in the activation of plasminogen (**choice E**).

42. **The correct answer is A.** This patient has gouty arthritis, which most frequently affects the first metatarsophalangeal joint and manifests with acute pain and swelling, often at night. Elevated serum urate levels and the presence of urate crystals within subcutaneous nodules are confirmatory. These subcutaneous nodules, called *tophi*, regress with appropriate treatment aimed at decreasing urate levels. Allopurinol inhibits xanthine oxidase, thus preventing formation of uric acid. In contrast, aspirin (**choice B**) and thiazide diuretics (**choice E**) inhibit uric acid excretion and cause hyperuricemia. These drugs are contraindicated in patients with gout.

Colchicine (**choice C**) and indomethacin (**choice D**) are both used in the treatment of acute gout, but these drugs do not have any effect on uric acid formation. Colchicine acts as an antiinflammatory drug by inhibiting cell movement and chemotaxis of leukocytes, whereas indomethacin blocks synthesis of prostaglandins by cyclooxygenase.

43. **The correct answer is B.** Whenever secondary amenorrhea develops in association with galactorrhea, hyperprolactinemia should be suspected. A prolactin-secreting pituitary adenoma is the most frequent cause of this condition, which can be treated either pharmacologically or surgically. Prolactin secretion (as any anterior pituitary hormone) is regulated by factors released by the hypothalamus. In this case, prolactin secretion is inhibited by *dopamine*. Thus, drugs such as bromocriptine, which act as agonists on dopamine receptors, will inhibit prolactin release. In contrast, dopamine antagonists (**choice C**), such as most antip-

sychotic drugs, may increase prolactin secretion and cause amenorrhea-galactorrhea syndrome.

Cholinesterase inhibitors (**choice A**) that cross the blood-brain barrier, such as tacrine, are used to enhance cholinergic neurotransmission in Alzheimer disease, but they have no effect on pituitary physiology.

Drugs enhancing GABAergic transmission (**choice D**) include compounds such as benzodiazepines, valproic acid, and gabapentin, which potentiate GABA inhibitory action through different mechanisms. These drugs are used in the treatment of epilepsy.

Serotonin reuptake inhibitors (**choice E**) are used to treat mental depression (see, for example, fluoxetine and sertraline). They prolong the action of serotonin in serotoninergic pathways, which are involved in mood regulation.

44. **The correct answer is E.** Bone marrow suppression, diarrhea, and alopecia are the most common side effects seen with cancer chemotherapy regimens. Vincristine, a mitotic inhibitor, is a chemotherapeutic agent that is not associated with the development of bone marrow suppression and would be the most appropriate agent to use in this patient. Vincristine is effective in the treatment of acute lymphoblastic leukemia and other leukemias, Hodgkin disease, lymphosarcoma, neuroblastoma, and various other types of cancer. Bleomycin is another antineoplastic agent that does not cause bone marrow suppression.

Busulfan (**choice A**) is an alkylating agent primarily used in the palliative treatment of chronic myelogenous leukemia; it is known to cause severe bone marrow suppression. As a general rule, the alkylating agents typically produce severe immunosuppressive effects.

Cisplatin (**choice B**) is another alkylating agent indicated for the treatment of metastatic testicular and ovarian tumors in combination with other agents. This agent can also cause profound bone marrow suppression.

Cyclophosphamide (**choice C**) is classified as a nitrogen mustard, a subcategory of the alkylating agents. It is primarily used to treat breast, testicular, and other solid tumors, as well as leukemia and lymphoma. This drug suppresses bone marrow.

Paclitaxel (**choice D**) is an antimicrotubule agent typically used in the treatment of ovarian and breast cancer. Profound neutropenia is typically seen with this agent.

45. **The correct answer is D.** Metformin is often used in conjunction with oral hypoglycemic agents for the treatment of type 2 diabetes. Its mechanism of action is twofold: (*1*) it decreases the production of glucose in the liver; and (*2*) it increases the uptake of glucose in

the liver. Metformin has no effect on the secretion of pancreatic insulin.

Acetohexamide (**choice A**), chlorpropamide (**choice B**), glyburide (**choice C**), and tolbutamide (**choice E**) are oral hypoglycemic agents that are sulfonylurea derivatives. These agents stimulate secretion of insulin from the pancreas.

46. **The correct answer is B.** This patient has all the classic signs of opioid toxicity and requires naloxone.

47. **The correct answer is C.** This patient has ingested antifreeze and needs ethanol to block the formation of glycolic and oxalic acid by competing for alcohol dehydrogenase.

48. **The correct answer is F.** This patient has acetaminophen toxicity and would require acetylcysteine.

49. **The correct answer is G.** This child mostly has iron toxicity because it is a component of most multivitamin preparations. The danger is depression of the myocardium, gastric erosion, or decrease of peripheral vascular resistance and disruption of the Krebs cycle enzymes. Deferoxamine is used because it is a selective iron chelator.

50. **The correct answer is E.** This patient has overdosed on a benzodiazepine and needs flumazenil.

Behavioral Science and Biostatistics

1. A 48-year-old man is brought to the psychiatric emergency department after an attempted suicide. He claims to hear voices telling him to kill himself. The patient's family notes that he has been on several different kinds of antipsychotic medications, with no improvement of his symptoms. The attending psychiatrist places the patient on a new medication and admits him. One week after therapy has begun, a routine blood test reveals profound depletion of polymorphonuclear leukocytes. Which of the following drugs is most likely responsible for these symptoms?

    (A) Chlorpromazine
    (B) Clozapine
    (C) Fluoxetine
    (D) Haloperidol
    (E) Imipramine

2. After a bout of aseptic meningitis, a patient is unable to recall a surgical procedure he underwent before the infection. He is, however, able to register and recall present events. The patient most likely has which of the following conditions?

    (A) Anterograde amnesia
    (B) Proactive inhibition
    (C) Retroactive inhibition
    (D) Retrograde amnesia
    (E) Transient global amnesia

3. A 9-year-old boy has been caught stealing the lunches of his classmates on three separate occasions. He sleeps in class and usually does not participate in the educational process. The boy is small for his age and generally does not interact with his classmates except when they hit him. When his 4th-grade teacher tries to contact the parents for a conference, she discovers that they have no telephone and the address given to the school is a post office box. Which of the following is most likely cause of this child's behavior?

    (A) Antisocial personality
    (B) Child abuse
    (C) Mental retardation
    (D) Oppositional defiant disorder
    (E) Thyroid dysfunction

4. A city has a population of 250,000. Of these, 10,000 have disease X, which is incurable. There are 1000 new cases and 400 deaths each year from this disease. There are 2500 deaths per year from all causes. The prevalence of this disease is given by

    (A) 400/250,000
    (B) 600/250,000
    (C) 1,000/250,000
    (D) 2,500/250,000
    (E) 10,000/250,000

5. In the evaluation of a psychiatric patient, which of the following disorders is most likely to be missed even by a trained observer?

    (A) Delirium
    (B) Dementia
    (C) Fugue
    (D) Somnambulism
    (E) Stupor

6. A 30-year-old heterosexual man repeatedly cross-dresses to achieve sexual excitement but is content with his biologic gender. Which of the following is the most likely diagnosis?

(A) Exhibitionism

(B) Transsexualism

(C) Transvestic fetishism

(D) Voyeurism

(E) Frotteurism

7. In which of the following statistical distributions are the mean, median, and mode all the same?

(A) Bimodal

(B) Negatively skewed

(C) Normal

(D) Population

(E) Positively skewed

8. A 27-year-old man believes that he lives on a planet circling the star Alpha Centauri. His speech is rambling, he giggles frequently at inappropriate times, and he does not make sense when talking with others, He exhibits purposeful behaviors that do not accomplish an end and often "hears voices." The first episode of this behavior occurred when he was 18 years old. Which of the following is the most likely diagnosis?

(A) Catatonic schizophrenia

(B) Disorganized schizophrenia

(C) Paranoid schizophrenia

(D) Residual schizophrenia

(E) Undifferentiated schizophrenia

9. A 5-year-old boy is taken to a dermatologist to remove a suspicious-looking lesion from his back. He is extremely afraid of receiving an injection and of the procedure in general. The best way to alter his pain perception threshold would be to

(A) allow his parents to be present during the procedure

(B) divert his attention away from the procedure

(C) encourage him to vent his emotions

(D) explain sensory pain pathways to him

(E) have him focus on and examine the nature of the pain

10. A 64-year-old woman is hospitalized for an acute exacerbation of schizophrenia. The medications that she is prescribed cause some immediate adverse effects, but she tolerates them and continues to be compliant. A few years pass and she begins to develop neurologic abnormalities. These include involuntary, repetitive movement of the lips and tongue, as well as of her trunk and extremities. Which of the following medications should now be prescribed to this patient?

(A) Chlorpromazine

(B) Clozapine

(C) Fluphenazine

(D) Haloperidol

(E) Metoclopramide

11. A 27-year-old woman reveals to her gynecologist that her last three miscarriages were caused by spousal abuse while she was pregnant. Her husband also abuses her at times when she is not pregnant. When the husband is confronted with this report, he does not deny it. The husband's behavior is most likely explained by which of the following?

(A) Being the first-born child

(B) Concern about financial security

(C) Dislike of children

(D) Feelings of inadequacy

(E) Wanting out of the marriage

12. A 25-year-old actress tends to behave seductively and with exaggerated charm to obtain continuous attention. She often puts on an overdramatized display of emotion but lacks genuine deep feelings. She craves control in her interpersonal relationships, often causing them to disintegrate. This patient most likely has which of the following personality disorders?

(A) Histrionic

(B) Narcissistic

(C) Paranoid

(D) Passive-aggressive

(E) Schizotypal

13. A 72-year-old woman has just been told that her husband died. Kubler-Ross's stages of dying are listed below:

    1. Acceptance
    2. Anger
    3. Bargaining
    4. Denial
    5. Sadness/depression

    Which of the following correctly expresses the order of these stages?

    (A) 1-2-4-5-3
    (B) 2-5-3-1-4
    (C) 3-2-4-1-5
    (D) 4-2-3-5-1
    (E) 5-3-4-1-2

14. A 32-year-old man reports difficulty maintaining an erection during intercourse with his wife. This has developed gradually over the past 3 years. He had experienced no such difficulty prior to marriage. He reports full morning erections with wakening. He had a sexual experience on a recent business trip and noted no difficulty on that occasion. He looks embarrassed as he gives his history. Although there is no evidence for anger when speaking about his wife, evidence of anxiety is prominent. Which of the following is the most likely diagnosis?

    (A) Adjustment disorder with anxious mood
    (B) Hypoactive sexual desire disorder, psychogenic
    (C) Inhibited male orgasm, psychogenic
    (D) Latent ego-dystonic homosexuality
    (E) Male erectile disorder, psychogenic

15. An 88-year-old man complaining of abdominal pain enters the emergency department with his wife. A mini-mental status exam reveals pronounced forgetfulness and confusion. The patient is discovered to have acute appendicitis requiring immediate surgery. He is unable to understand the situation and cannot provide informed consent. Which of the following further actions must the physician take?

    (A) Do not perform surgery
    (B) Have another physician confirm the necessity of surgery
    (C) Obtain a court order to perform surgery
    (D) Obtain consent from his wife to perform surgery
    (E) Try to persuade the patient to consent to surgery

16. A 37-year-old man is referred to a psychiatrist for evaluation for sexual reassignment. He states that from as early as he can remember, he has been sexually attracted only to other men. However, he always feels enormous guilt after a sexual liaison with a man. While he has functioned adequately with women, he has no emotional or physical affinity for them. He is requesting sexual reassignment because he wants to have a husband and a normal heterosexual life. Which of the following is the most likely diagnosis?

    (A) Ego-dystonic gender identity disorder
    (B) Ego-dystonic homosexuality
    (C) Ego-syntonic gender identity disorder
    (D) Ego-syntonic homosexuality
    (E) Paraphilia

17. An 18-month-old child is brought to a pediatrician by his 17-year-old mother because the child weighs only 14 lb. His birth weight was 7.25 lb. The mother states the infant never "ate right." Observation reveals a hypokinetic child who is dull and listless with a poverty of spontaneous activity. He appears sad and miserable but visually tracks the physician. Examination suggests malnourishment. His muscle tone is poor, and his skin is cool and more mottled than expected. There are no signs of physical trauma. The mother spends a great deal of time talking to the pediatrician about her own problems. Which of the following is the most likely diagnosis?

    (A) Autistic disorder
    (B) Möbius syndrome
    (C) Reactive attachment disorder of infancy
    (D) Rett syndrome
    (E) Tay-Sachs disease

18. A 43-year-old man is sitting on the examining table with his shoulders slumped. His head and eyes are downcast. His eyes are red. He looks up slowly and, after a deep sigh, says "I am sorry to bother you, Doctor, but I have to talk to someone. I have been so discouraged and so depressed for over 2 years, and I can't take it anymore." Which of the following is the most likely diagnosis?

    (A) Dysthymic disorder
    (B) Major depressive disorder
    (C) Organic affective syndrome
    (D) Schizoaffective disorder
    (E) Uncomplicated bereavement

19. The grief and bereavement process would take the longest to resolve after the death of which of the following individuals?

    (A) Child
    (B) Grandparent
    (C) Parent
    (D) Sibling
    (E) Spouse

20. A 73-year-old woman has difficulty concentrating and demonstrates some mild immediate-memory problems. She has a poor appetite and has lost 24 lb in 6 weeks. She resists participation in recreational activities, and she wakes up at 4:00 AM everyday and is unable to get back to sleep. Her condition is worsening on a daily basis. Which of the following is the most likely diagnosis?

    (A) Alcohol-related delirium
    (B) Dementia of the Alzheimer type
    (C) Hypothyroidism
    (D) Normal pressure hydrocephalus
    (E) Pseudodementia

21. A 29-year-old man reveals to his psychiatrist that he has been hearing voices telling him to kill his girlfriend. Which of the following principles requires that the physician inform the girlfriend that she is in danger?

    (A) Good Samaritan law
    (B) Irresistible Impulse rule
    (C) McNaughten rule
    (D) Tarasoff I decision
    (E) Tarasoff II decision

22. A disgruntled surgical technician who is being treated for depression with phenelzine takes an analgesic he found on the drug cart in the surgical suite. Several hours later, he arrives at the emergency department in a delirious state and has a temperature of 105 F. Soon after his arrival, he begins having convulsions. Which of the following analgesics did he most likely take?

    (A) Buprenorphine
    (B) Codeine
    (C) Meperidine
    (D) Pentazocine
    (E) Propoxyphene

23. The parents of a 7-year-old boy divorce. The boy lives with the mother and sees his father every-other weekend. During these visits, the boy is alternately sullen and angry with the father, but when it is time to return home, he clings to the father and cries in a desperate manner while saying "I'm sorry! I want you and mom to live together again." Which of the following is the most helpful statement that the father can make to the son?

    (A) "Big boys don't cry."
    (B) "I left your mother, I didn't leave you."
    (C) "I'll see you in two weeks."
    (D) "You're the man of the house now."
    (E) "Your mother was too hard to live with."

24. At the Academy Awards ceremony, a very successful movie star becomes loud and agitated when she does not win in the category in which she had been nominated. She states to those around her that her performance was superior to that of the winner, that the Academy clearly does not appreciate her genius and acting skills and that there should be a separate category for persons of her extraordinary abilities. She further states that she did not win because the Academy members are envious of her skills. This person most likely has which of the following disorders?

    (A) Antisocial personality disorder
    (B) Histrionic personality disorder
    (C) Narcissistic personality disorder
    (D) Paranoid personality disorder
    (E) Schizophrenia, paranoid type

25. A group of patients with lung cancer is matched to a group of patients without lung cancer. Their smoking habits over the course of their lives is compared. On the basis of this information, researchers compute the rate of lung cancer in patients who smoke versus those who never smoked. This is an example of a

    (A) case-control study
    (B) cohort study
    (C) cross-sectional study
    (D) longitudinal study
    (E) randomized control study

26. A research study investigating the effects of three variables (age, sex, and ethnicity) on the efficacy of a new malaria vaccine reports a significant ($p < 0.001$) analysis of variance (ANOVA) result. There is a significant two-way interaction. Regarding these variables, which of the following is the best interpretation of these results?

    (A) Any of the three variables alone affects the vaccine's efficacy

    (B) The interaction suggests the vaccine has no efficacy

    (C) The three variables all work together to produce the vaccine's efficacy

    (D) The three variables interact together and have no affect on the vaccine's efficacy

    (E) Two of the three variables affect the vaccine's efficacy

27. A 42-year-old man has just been informed that he has poorly differentiated small cell carcinoma of the lung. When asked whether he understands the serious nature of his illness, the patient proceeds to tell his physician how excited he is about renovating his home. Which of the following defense mechanisms is this patient exhibiting?

    (A) denial

    (B) displacement

    (C) projection

    (D) rationalization

    (E) reaction formation

28. A 72-year-old woman is brought to the emergency department with bruises all over her body. Physical abuse is suspected. Which of the following best describes the attributes of individuals who commit elder abuse?

    (A) They are concerned caretakers of the abused person

    (B) They expect nothing in return from the abused person

    (C) They have lived with the abused person for a long period of time

    (D) They have no history of being abused

    (E) They occasionally use alcohol/drugs in a recreational manner

29. A 44-year-old man has completed college, has had a good work history, and has never had difficulty with the authorities. However, he has few friends and attends meetings of persons who share telepathic interests and "abilities." When his coworkers attempt to talk to him about these meetings, he is quiet and vague regarding what is done at the meetings and where they are held. His only close associations are with his relatives. He is more likely than the average person to have a relative with a diagnosis of

    (A) anxiety disorder

    (B) bipolar disorder, type II

    (C) factitious disorder

    (D) major depressive disorder

    (E) schizophrenia

30. A 52-year-old white man who had been found wandering the streets is brought into the hospital by police. On initial physical examination, his motor behavior is notable for bradykinesia and a 4- to 6-Hz hand tremor at rest. He is kept under observation in the psychiatric ward but is not medicated. Over the next few days, his motor symptoms start to abate, but he becomes increasingly paranoid and confused and insists that he is the President of the United States. Which of the following conditions best describes the patient at the time of admission?

    (A) Alcoholic experiencing acute symptoms of withdrawal

    (B) Chronic amphetamine user experiencing drug-induced psychosis

    (C) Chronic schizophrenic experiencing tardive dyskinesia

    (D) Parkinsonian patient overmedicated with L-dopa

    (E) Schizophrenic overmedicated with haloperidol

31. A 60-year-old man has had difficulty falling asleep for the past several weeks and asks his physician for advice. The patient has no underlying psychopathology. Which of the following is the most appropriate nonpharmaceutical treatment for this patient?

    (A) Increasing fluid intake during the 3 hours prior to sleep

    (B) Retiring for sleep at the same time each day

    (C) "Sleeping in" if the time of retiring has been delayed

    (D) Staying in bed until sleep is attained

    (E) Strenuous exercise 1 hour before retiring

32. Medical students at a major teaching hospital are routinely assigned to observe obstetric patients and to assist during delivery. When a male medical student introduces himself to an obstetric patient, the patient becomes agitated and requests that no students be present during her delivery. The patient had been informed, prior to admission, that this was a teaching hospital and that a student would be assigned to her case. When informed of the patient's refusal, the attending physician in charge should

(A) ask the patient's husband for his consent

(B) do not allow any medical students to observe this patient

(C) have the student approach the patient again and explain the necessity for student observation

(D) have the student observe in the background as a part of the health care team

(E) meet with the patient and discuss the value of observation in medical training

33. Eight research scientists are brought into the hospital by paramedics. The scientists are experiencing diaphoresis, blurred vision, palpitations, and hallucinations with brilliant colors. Police suspect that the coffee at their lab meeting was laced with a psychoactive substance. Which of the following substances is most likely to be found in the coffee pot?

(A) Lysergic acid diethylamide (LSD)

(B) Methadone

(C) Phencyclidine (PCP)

(D) Phenobarbital

(E) Tetrahydrocannabinol (THC)

34. A 15-year-old woman presents to your office seeking counseling on HIV. Which of the following individuals is at the lowest risk to contract HIV during unprotected sex?

(A) Female heterosexual

(B) Female homosexual

(C) Male heterosexual

(D) Male homosexual

(E) Male transsexual

35. A 27-year-old, rather plain-appearing woman, fabricates a story that she was raped in the restroom at her child's school. She inflicts wounds on her body with a pair of scissors, gives herself a mild concussion by hitting her head on the sink, and describes the attacker and the episode in great detail when the emergency care persons arrive and take her to the hospital. Later she admits that there was no attack and that she produced the signs and symptoms herself. She states that she did it to get more attention from her husband. If she has a personality disorder, the most likely diagnosis would be

(A) antisocial personality disorder

(B) borderline personality disorder

(C) dependent personality disorder

(D) histrionic personality disorder

(E) narcissistic personality disorder

36. A child is in psychotherapy that is financially supported by the parents. Which of the following is the best way to avoid breaching the child's confidentiality while the parents are legally responsible for the child's welfare?

(A) Give parents information only after they agree not to discuss the information with the child

(B) Give parents information only if it has been so ordered by the court

(C) Inform the child that parents have the right to any and all information since they are the responsible party

(D) Invite the child to attend all parent meetings in which the child is discussed

(E) Make a blanket rule to hold all information coming from the child as off-limits to the parents

37. A second-year medical student falls asleep during a lecture. The instructor observes that the instant the student falls asleep, his eyes make rapid lateral movements under his closed eyelids. Which of the following is the most likely diagnosis?

(A) Dysthymic disorder

(B) Major depressive disorder

(C) Narcolepsy disorder

(D) Sleep-deprived hypersomnia disorder

(E) Substance-induced sleep disorder

38. Cognitive therapy for the treatment of a depressed patient is based on the theory that the disorder is caused by

    (A) anger toward others that is turned on the self
    (B) distorted negative beliefs and self-talk that reinforces those beliefs
    (C) fluctuating neurotransmitter levels
    (D) genetic predisposition
    (E) significant object loss in the first 3 years of life

39. In a study, a group of people are exposed to an environmental toxin but are not treated. Instead, they are observed over time on a standard set of measures to ascertain the potential effects of the toxin. This type of study design is called

    (A) Clinical trial
    (B) Double-blind
    (C) Longitudinal
    (D) Prospective
    (E) Retrospective

40. Which of the following is the most common reason for an individual of higher socioeconomic status to "move downward" into a significantly lower socioeconomic group?

    (A) Disabling physical problems
    (B) Disabling psychiatric problems
    (C) Inability to defer gratification
    (D) Lack of education
    (E) Unwillingness to work

41. A husband comes to the family physician to discuss his wife's sleep behavior. During the past 2 months, she has been kicking and hitting him in her sleep. She does not remember these occurrences the next morning or if he wakens her in the night. He is concerned that she has developed some anger toward him, which she is unwilling or unable to discuss. Which of the following is the most likely diagnosis?

    (A) Narcolepsy
    (B) Night terrors
    (C) Non-REM sleep disorder
    (D) Rapid eye movement (REM) sleep disorder
    (E) Sleep apnea disorder

42. A 60-year-old man hospitalized with metastatic colon cancer signs a DNR order. This means that the medical staff treating him is required to

    (A) discontinue narcotic pain medication
    (B) not attempt CPR in case of cardiac arrest
    (C) refrain from prescribing future medications
    (D) withhold parenteral nutrition and IV fluid hydration
    (E) withhold osteopathic manipulation

43. A patient presents to the office because he thinks he may have a sexual problem. Which of the following sexual dysfunctions may be effectively treated by surgical intervention?

    (A) Dyspareunia
    (B) Premature ejaculation
    (C) Primary impotence
    (D) Secondary orgasmic dysfunction in females
    (E) Vaginismus

44. A group of researchers mistakenly concludes from a poorly designed experiment that acetaminophen cures the common cold. These researchers have committed which of the following types of error?

    (A) $1-\beta$
    (B) Alpha
    (C) Beta
    (D) Type 1
    (E) Type 2

Questions 45-50

<u>SET A</u>

Directions: For each numbered item (**scenario**), select the one lettered heading (**legal term**) most closely associated with it. Each lettered heading may be selected once, more than once, or not at all.

(A) breach of warranty

(B) causation

(C) negligence

(D) vicarious liability

(E) battery

(F) assault

(G) competency

(H) lack of informed consent

(I) assumption of risk

45. A patient needs sutures removed. Your nurse removes them for you. If she makes a mistake, you could be sued on this legal principle.

46. A patient who has just had a surgery complains of severe pain. On a postoperative x-ray, a sponge is found. This finding is which element of a tort?

47. A surgeon promises his patient he will be able to walk after the surgeon performs a special surgery. The patient recovers from the surgery with no complications but cannot walk. The patient can sue the doctor according to this legal principle.

48. A patient goes to a dermatologist to have a lesion examined. The doctor, without any explanation, removes the lesion.

49. The aforementioned patient is so angry he makes verbal threats against the doctor's life. The patient shoves a chair at the doctor but misses him.

50. A Mexican migrant worker who doesn't speak English well and cannot read signed a surgical release form for a surgery. After the surgery the patient sues.

Behavioral Science and Biostatistics

ANSWERS AND EXPLANATIONS

1.	B	26.	E
2.	D	27.	A
3.	B	28.	C
4.	E	29.	E
5.	C	30.	E
6.	C	31.	B
7.	C	32.	B
8.	B	33.	A
9.	B	34.	B
10.	B	35.	B
11.	D	36.	D
12.	A	37.	C
13.	D	38.	B
14.	E	39.	C
15.	D	40.	A
16.	B	41.	D
17.	C	42.	B
18.	A	43.	A
19.	A	44.	D
20.	E	45.	D
21.	D	46.	B
22.	C	47.	A
23.	B	48.	E
24.	C	49.	F
25.	A	50.	H

1. **The correct answer is B.** The antipsychotic drug clozapine has been shown to cause agranulocytosis, an acute condition characterized by profound leukopenia, with marked reduction in polymorphonuclear leukocytes (<500 cells/mm³). Infected ulcers are likely to form in the throat, intestinal tract, and other mucous membranes, as well as on the skin. Other side effects caused by clozapine include orthostatic hypotension, sinus tachycardia, hypersalivation, temperature elevation, lowered seizure threshold, and constipation. Clozapine is generally prescribed only after several other alternative neuroleptic medications have failed, because of the possibility of agranulocytosis and the drug's prohibitive cost.

   Chlorpromazine (**choice A**) is an antipsychotic drug that has antimuscarinic side effects, such as dry mouth and constipation. It can also cause orthostatic hypotension, sedation, and tardive dyskinesia. It does not cause agranulocytosis.

   Fluoxetine (**choice C**) is a selective serotonin reuptake inhibitor (SSRI), an antidepressant drug that can cause anxiety and insomnia, altered appetite and weight loss, activation of mania or hypomania, seizures, and cognitive motor impairment.

   Haloperidol (**choice D**) is an antipsychotic drug that has less antimuscarinic side effects than does chlorpromazine, but has more extrapyramidal effects, such as acute dystonia (face, neck, and back spasms, and abnormal posture), parkinsonism, neuroleptic malignant syndrome (catatonia, rigidity, stupor, fever, dysarthria, fluctuating BP), and akathisia (restlessness). It can also cause tardive dyskinesia. It does not cause agranulocytosis.

   Imipramine (**choice E**) is a tricyclic antidepressant drug that can cause orthostatic hypotension, anticholinergic effects, antihistamine effects, and hypomania. It does not cause agranulocytosis.

2. **The correct answer is D.** Retrograde amnesia is characterized by an inability to remember events prior to the onset of disease, with preservation of the ability to form new memories.

   Anterograde amnesia (**choice A**) is characterized by an inability to register and form lasting memories of new or present events.

   Proactive inhibition (**choice B**) is when something newly learned interferes with previously learned information. New material inhibits old material.

   Retroactive inhibition (**choice C**) is when previously learned material interferes with the ability to acquire new information. Old material inhibits new material.

   Transient global amnesia (**choice E**) is characterized by confusion and impairment of recent memory. It often occurs in elderly people and resolves without sequelae.

3. **The correct answer is B.** This is a case of child abuse of the neglect type. The family fits the pattern of social isolation often found in child abuse. The boy's sleepiness in class suggests lack of appropriate rest at home, often caused by turmoil in the home or unsupervised late night activity, or lack of appropriate nutrition in the morning.

   Antisocial personality disorder (**choice A**) is not correct because a person must be 18 years of age to be so classified.

   Mental retardation (**choice C**) is not correct because this boy is advancing appropriately in school. He is 9 years old and in the 4th grade.

   Oppositional defiant disorder (**choice D**) is not correct since these children usually act out in a defiant and rebellious manner to authority figures.

   Thyroid dysfunction (**choice E**) is not correct because these conditions usually produce agitated behavior of some type along with cognitive-emotional dysfunction, regardless of whether there is hypo- or hyperthyroidism.

4. **The correct answer is E.** The prevalence of a disease is defined as the number of cases of the disease at a given time divided by the total population. In this case, it would be 10,000/250,000.

   The disease-specific mortality rate is the number of deaths per year from a specific disease divided by the population; in this case, 400/250,000 (**choice A**).

   The rate of increase of a disease is given by the number of new cases per year, minus the number of deaths (or cures) per year, divided by the total population. In this case, (1000–400)/250,000 = 600/250,000 (**choice B**).

   The incidence of a disease is given by the number of new cases in a given period divided by the total population. This gives 1000/250,000 (**choice C**).

   The crude mortality rate is given by the number of deaths from all causes, divided by the population; in this case, 2500/250,000 (**choice D**).

5. **The correct answer is C.** In fugue, the person has an abrupt change of geographic location or identity without alterations in consciousness or memory changes.

   In delirium (**choice A**), the patient has an altered state of consciousness that is easily recognized.

   In dementia (**choice B**), a trained observer can ask questions related to memory to establish that cognitive functioning is impaired.

   In somnambulism (**choice D**), the patient walks while asleep. These patients are unresponsive to outside persons or questions, for example.

In stupor (**choice E**), there is a clear alteration in the level of consciousness such that even an untrained person can recognize that something is wrong.

6. **The correct answer is C.** Do not confuse transvestic fetishism with transsexualism (**choice B**). Transsexuals might cross-dress, but they do so because of persistent discomfort with their anatomic sex. Transvestic fetishism involves no such discomfort.

Exhibitionism (**choice A**) refers to exposing one's genitals to unsuspecting strangers for sexual excitement.

Voyeurism (**choice D**) refers to observing unsuspecting people, generally strangers, who are naked, undressing, or engaged in sexual activity, for sexual excitement.

Frotteurism (**choice E**) refers to a man rubbing his genitals against a fully clothed woman to achieve orgasm; usually occurs on subways and buses.

7. **The correct answer is C.** In a normal (also called a binomial or "bell-shaped") distribution, the mean (arithmetic average), median (midpoint), and mode (most common score) all coincide.

A bimodal distribution (**choice A**) has two distinct clusters of scores. This type of distribution may have two modal scores.

A negatively (**choice B**) or positively (**choice E**) skewed distribution can have different values for the measures of central tendency, because extreme scores tend to influence the mean.

Population distribution (**choice D**) is a general term that refers to the underlying characteristics of the total distribution of all scores. The distribution can be bimodal, skewed, or normal.

8. **The correct answer is B.** The disorganized type of schizophrenia is characterized by disorganized speech, disorganized behavior, and an inappropriate affect. This patient's rambling speech, inappropriate giggling, and purposeful behavior illustrate these issues.

Catatonic schizophrenia (**choice A**) is characterized by movement disorders, peculiarities like posturing or stereotyped behaviors, and echolalia.

Paranoid schizophrenia (**choice C**) is characterized by manifest delusions and hallucinations involving persecution or grandeur.

Residual schizophrenia (**choice D**) is diagnosed when there is a clear schizophrenic problem; however there are no prominent delusions or hallucinations, and the person's behavior and speech are not disorganized (as seen in this patient).

Undifferentiated schizophrenia (**choice E**) has characteristics of all the above types; however, they are too fluid to place into a specific diagnostic category.

9. **The correct answer is B.** Diverting the child's attention with such things as talk, games, television, and virtual reality is a very effective mechanism for pain control.

Allowing parents to be present (**choice A**) will often only intensify the child's reaction because parents might display their own fears and concerns.

Encouraging the child to vent his emotions (**choice C**) can be of some assistance. However, because of the child's limited cognitive structures, this is not a recommended procedure.

The young child does not yet have the cognitive structures to control pain mentally; therefore, neither explaining sensory pathways (**choice D**) nor having the child focus on and examine pain sensations (**choice E**) will be effective.

10. **The correct answer is B.** A serious side effect of the antipsychotics is tardive dyskinesia, which has been seen with virtually every neuroleptic [e.g., chlorpromazine (**choice A**), fluphenazine (**choice C**), and haloperidol (**choice D**)]. Usually, the symptoms of tardive dyskinesia appear late in treatment and consist of involuntary, repetitive movements of the lips, tongue (e.g., tongue thrusting, lip smacking), and, not infrequently, the extremities and trunk. Patients older than 60 and those with pre-existing CNS pathology are at a higher risk for this disorder (up to 70%), but other risk factors have not been confirmed. Clozapine is called an atypical antipsychotic medication because of its lack of extrapyramidal side effects, including tardive dyskinesia, and would be an appropriate medication for a patient who is developing tardive dyskinesia. Metoclopramide (**choice E**) is a centrally acting antiemetic that has been shown to cause tardive dyskinesia as well.

11. **The correct answer is D.** Abusive husbands usually use the abuse to bully and humiliate their wives in order to build up their own self-esteem. They often view their behavior as an attempt to communicate.

Being the first-born child (**choice A**) is incorrect because there has never been a birth-order effect established in spousal abuse.

Concern about financial security (**choice B**) is incorrect because spousal abuse occurs in all socioeconomic groups, and fiscal concerns have not been demonstrated to be etiologic.

A dislike of children (**choice C**) is incorrect because it is the spouse who is being abused, not a child. Disliking children would be more likely to result in some permanent form of birth control.

Wanting out of the marriage (**choice E**) is incorrect because the abuse itself is an attempt to pull the spouse closer and control her, not to separate from the spouse and give her freedom.

12. **The correct answer is A.** This is a typical description of histrionic personality disorder. Clues are seductive behavior, exaggerated charm, need for attention, overdramatized emotions, shallowness of feelings, and craving control.

Narcissistic personality disorder (**choice B**) is characterized by the word "entitlement." These individuals have a grandiose but unstable sense of self-importance that often alternates with feelings of unworthiness.

Paranoid personality disorder (**choice C**) is characterized by suspiciousness, excessive vigilance toward the environment, mistrust of others, and a concern with hidden meanings or motivations.

Passive-aggressive personality disorder (**choice D**) is associated with difficulties in assertiveness and the appropriate expression of anger. People with this disorder may act out their anger indirectly, presenting a resistant stance in situations involving social or occupational functioning.

People with schizotypal personality disorder (**choice E**) are emotionally cold and aloof like schizoids, but display magical thinking as well (e.g., beliefs that others can sense their thoughts or feelings). They may have ideas of reference, recurrent perceptual illusions, depersonalization, or suspiciousness.

13. **The correct answer is D.** If you understand the thought process behind these stages, you are unlikely to forget the progression. Patients first experience denial that they are dying. Once aware, they become angry at their lot and proceed to "bargain" for a more favorable outcome. When this proves futile, they become depressed. Then, they finally accept the truth. The mnemonic is DABSA.

14. **The correct answer E.** This patient has male erectile disorder, psychogenic. It is defined by the DSM IV as the persistent inability to attain or maintain adequate erection for completion of sexual activity. It causes distress and interpersonal difficulties. The disorder may be due to psychologic factors if it occurs only with specific partners or during certain situations. This patient's dysfunction occurs only with his wife, implying no physiologic etiology to his problem.

An adjustment disorder (**choice A**) requires there be a stressor as the etiologic factor; no such event is noted in the history.

Since the patient can attain an erection and is emotionally distressed by the situation with his wife, he does not have hypoactive sexual desire disorder (**choice B**).

There is no mention of orgasmic problems, and erection is not necessary for orgasm. Therefore, inhibited male orgasm, psychogenic (**choice C**) is unlikely.

There is nothing in the history to suggest a homosexual orientation; therefore, latent ego-dystonic homosexuality (**choice D**) is not the best diagnosis.

15. **The correct answer is D.** In cases in which an emergency exists, the patient is incompetent to give consent, and the withholding of treatment would be potentially life-threatening, the physician must obtain consent from a close relative of the patient. The physician should proceed with treatment, assuming the patient would concur had he or she understood the situation.

Not performing surgery (**choice A**) could cost the patient's life.

Having another physician confirm the necessity of surgery (**choice B**) is favorable (if done immediately) but not mandatory and does not change the patient's consent status.

Obtaining a court order (**choice C**) is not necessary with the patient's wife immediately accessible.

Trying to persuade the patient to consent to surgery (**choice E**) would not only waste time and prove futile but might agitate the patient as well.

16. **The correct answer is B.** This man is basically homosexual; however, his homosexuality causes him to experience feelings of guilt if he participates in homosexual physical activity (therefore, his homosexuality is ego-dystonic, rather than ego-syntonic, **choice D**).

The man does not have a gender identity disorder (syntonic, **choice C** or dystonic, **choice A**) because he does not have a female gender identity and has not described any feelings of abhorrence regarding his genitalia.

He does not have a paraphilia (**choice E**), which is the general term for a diagnosable sexual disorder in which the person conceals the behaviors from others, the behaviors exclude or harm others, and the behaviors disrupt the potential for bonding between persons.

17. **The correct answer is C.** Reactive attachment disorder of infancy is caused by severe interruption in the parent-child bond, with the parent being unable to supply the nurturing needed for adequate development of the infant. The description of this child is classic, and unless the underlying pathologic bonding process is addressed, the child may die. Sometimes this syndrome is seen in children who have had multiple care takers

(e.g., orphanages and foster homes) or, as in the case described here, a young, immature, and inadequate mother (and/or father).

This is not autistic disorder (**choice A**) because the child visually tracks the pediatrician. Children with autistic disorder do not interact socially with others.

In Möbius syndrome (**choice B**), or congenital facial diplegia, the face is expressionless, and ocular palsy may be present. Frequently, this is accompanied by clubfoot and syndactyly, and patients may be mentally retarded. None of these symptoms are described in this patient.

Rett syndrome (**choice D**) is characterized by normal development in the first 6 months of life followed by a precipitous deterioration. This child's development has never been normal.

Tay-Sachs disease (**choice E**) is an autosomal-recessive inborn error of metabolism that results in mental retardation, macular changes, seizures, and spasticity. None of these are described in this child.

18. **The correct answer A.** Dysthymic disorder is the most likely diagnosis. The patient is severely depressed by his own assessment; however, it is not of psychotic proportion. The patient has recognized the severity of his symptoms and taken appropriate action by going to the doctor. He has also indicated that this is not a new event for him (supporting the diagnosis of dysthymic disorder, which tends to be chronic, lasting longer than 2 years). Note that dysthymic patients tend to cry a lot, explaining this patient's red eyes.

Major depressive disorders (**choice B**) are characterized by depressed mood, diminished interest in activities, weight loss without change in diet or exercise, sleep disturbances, fatigue, feelings of worthlessness, decreased ability to concentrate, and thoughts about death. This patient does not report such concrete symptoms and therefore does not qualify for the diagnosis of major depressive disorder.

Organic affective syndrome (**choice C**) and uncomplicated bereavement (**choice E**) require trigger etiologies that are not implied in this case.

There is no thought disorder or other psychotic symptoms, ruling out the diagnosis of schizoaffective disorder (**choice D**).

19. **The correct answer is A.** The natural order in which one comes to expect losses (through social learning) is chronologic. That is, grandparents (**choice B**) die first, parents (**choice C**) die next, then siblings (**choice D**) and spouses (**choice E**), and finally one's children. When this natural order is inverted, there is a much more severe and protracted grief reaction than for the loss of an older relative.

20. **The correct answer is E.** Pseudodementia is more appropriately described as major depression in an elderly person. She has all the symptoms of depressive disorder (sleep difficulties, appetite and weight problems, concentration problems, lack of interest in pleasurable activities) but none of the hallmarks of an organic condition.

Delirium (**choice A**) is associated with fluctuation of consciousness. This patient's memory problems are mild and confined to immediate memory difficulties. If she were demented, she would demonstrate more recent and long-term memory problems.

Alzheimer disease (**choice B**) is associated with more recent and long-term memory impairment.

Hypothyroidism (**choice C**) is associated with wider mood swings, from depressive affect to manic-like episodes, as well as with more indices of psychotic level disturbance (e.g., hallucinations and paranoia).

Normal pressure hydrocephalus (**choice D**) is associated with depressive symptomatology; however, it is also characterized by the diagnostic triad of progressive dementia, gait disturbance, and urinary incontinence, none of which is present in this woman.

21. **The correct answer is D.** The Tarasoff I decision requires that physicians warn a potential victim if they truly believe the patient will cause harm to that person. The Tarasoff II decision (**choice E**) states that even though physicians must warn a potential victim, they must also protect the patient from harm from that person.

The Good Samaritan law (**choice A**) states that stopping at the scene of an accident to render care is not required but that once physicians initiate such care they must practice within their confidence and may not abandon the patient.

The Irresistible Impulse rule (**choice B**) is involved in insanity defenses in criminal prosecution. It considers whether a person's actions were under voluntary control or resulted from an uncontrollable passion.

The McNaughten rule (**choice C**) is also involved in insanity defenses. It acknowledges that people may not realize the nature and consequences of their actions because of mental illness.

22. **The correct answer is C.** The combination of an MAO inhibitor (such as phenelzine) and meperidine produces a severe drug reaction. Many types of reactions have been reported, including delirium, hyperpyrexia, convulsions, and hypertension. Other patients react as if they have had an overdose of meperidine and present with severe respiratory depression, cyanosis, hypotension, and coma. Meperidine is contraindicated

in patients who have taken MAO inhibitors during the previous 14 days.

Interactions with MAO inhibitors and other opioid analgesics, such as buprenorphine (**choice A**), codeine (**choice B**), pentazocine (**choice D**), and propoxyphene (**choice E**), have not been observed.

23. **The correct answer is B.** This statement from the father would reflect his understanding of the egocentric nature of school-aged children. That is, the child is assuming that he is responsible for the divorce between his parents. The anger and withdrawal reflect the child's frustration with the situation, but the tears and apology suggest the child's fear and assumed responsibility for the breakup.

"Big boys don't cry" (**choice A**) is a demeaning and belittling statement.

"I'll see you in 2 weeks" (**choice C**) ignores the child's felt responsibility for the divorce.

"You're the man of the house now" (**choice D**) places too much responsibility on a 7-year-old child.

"Your mother was too hard to live with" (**choice E**) places all the blame and responsibility for the divorce on the parent with whom the boy lives on a daily basis. It ignores the reality that divorce is usually due to difficulties that both parents have with each other.

24. **The correct answer is C.** In narcissistic personality disorder, the person feels "entitled" to recognition, admiration, and privileges. In addition, they often believe they are so special that others are envious of their talents. They do not tolerate perceived rejection well.

People with antisocial personality disorder (**choice A**) commit behaviors that are against societal rules. They commit criminal offenses against others and property.

People with histrionic personality disorder (**choice B**) are overly dramatic and exhibit seductive behavior.

People with paranoid personality disorder (**choice D**) believe others are out to harm them. They tend to be secretive in their thoughts, fearing that others will use information against them, and they are concerned with fidelity in intimate relations with others. Although this patient displays thoughts of envy from others, this is secondary to the non-recognition of her "specialness" rather than a malevolent intent.

There is no evidence of a psychotic level thought disorder such as schizophrenia (**choice E**); there are no hallucinations or disorganized emotions or behaviors.

25. **The correct answer is A.** Case-control studies are retrospective and are as described in the question stem. Case-control studies allow researchers to compute an odds ratio.

In cohort studies (**choice B**), subjects are assembled on the basis of some common experience (such as attending medical school) and are then monitored for a specified amount of time at regular intervals (e.g., taking COMLEX Levels 1, 2, and 3; see also longitudinal studies below), until they develop the outcome of interest (they become practicing physicians) or the follow-up time ends. The cohort study minimizes many of the biases evident in case-control designs and is the definitive observational clinical study. Cohort studies allow researchers to compute a relative risk.

Cross-sectional studies (**choice C**) usually have more modest goals than those of case-control and cohort studies. A variable or group of variables is measured in a sample of a larger population to get an idea of the distribution and interrelationships of those variables in that population.

Longitudinal studies (**choice D**) identify individual subjects and follow them over a given period of time. For example, the study of cholesterol-lowering drugs on cardiovascular events requires that the same subject is observed over a significant period of time (e.g., 10 years).

A randomized controlled trial (**choice E**) is considered the most rigorous and powerful approach to answering a clinical question in which two treatments, strategies, or therapies are compared or when one therapy is compared with placebo. In this type of study, subjects are assigned treatments on a randomized basis.

26. **The correct answer is E.** The term "two-way interaction" indicates that two of the three variables in the study affect the efficacy of the vaccine. For example, persons of a given sex and age group benefit the most from the vaccine, regardless of ethnic group.

A one-way interaction (**choice A**) indicates that any of the three variables in isolation can affect the vaccine's efficacy.

The vaccine has efficacy (compare with **choice B**), as evidenced by the positive results ($p < 0.001$) in the study.

A three-way interaction (**choice C**) indicates that only people of a given ethnic group, age, and sex benefit from the vaccine.

The three variables would have no effect on the efficacy (**choice D**) only if there were no interaction effect at all.

27. **The correct answer is A.** This patient is in denial about his serious illness. By talking about something totally unrelated, he is trying to avoid the bad news he has just received.

Displacement (**choice B**) involves the transferring of feelings to an inappropriate person, situation, or object (e.g., a man who has been yelled at by his boss takes out his anger on his wife).

Projection (**choice C**) is the attribution of one's own traits to someone else (e.g., a philandering husband accuses his wife of having an affair).

Rationalization (**choice D**) involves creating explanations for an action or thought, usually to avoid self-blame.

Reaction formation (**choice E**) is the unconscious changing of a feeling or idea to its opposite (e.g., a man acts very friendly toward a coworker when in fact he is unconsciously jealous).

28. **The correct answer is C.** Persons who abuse elderly people usually have lived with the elderly person for some time. There has been opportunity for idiosyncratic behavior on the part of the elderly person to create resentment in the caretaker. Elder abuse is usually not the expression of a momentary impulse; rather, it develops over some time.

Abusers tend to want their needs to be met by the abused person (unlike **choice B**), have a history of having been abused themselves (the opposite of **choice D**), are unwilling caretakers (often fiscal conditions necessitate the living arrangement; the opposite of **choice A**), and usually abuse drugs, not just use them occasionally (**choice E**).

29. **The correct answer is E.** The description of this man is consistent with the diagnosis of schizotypal personality disorder. Persons with this condition have a higher incidence of schizophrenia among their biologic relatives. There is also a higher incidence of the disorder in monozygotic vs. dizygotic twins, suggesting an underlying biologic foundation in which there is significant impairment in the social interaction skills.

No such correlation exists between schizotypal personality disorder and anxiety disorder (**choice A**), bipolar disorder, type II (**choice B**), factitious disorder (**choice C**), or major depressive disorder (**choice D**).

30. **The correct answer is E.** The patient is a schizophrenic overmedicated with haloperidol. When the patient was first brought into the hospital, he was experiencing parkinsonian motor symptoms that are a significant side effect of many neuroleptics (particularly haloperidol). Over the next few days, he remained unmedicated, and the effects of haloperidol began to wear off, which relieved his motor symptoms but led to the reappearance of his psychotic symptoms.

Although alcohol withdrawal (**choice A**) can produce delirium tremens, it would not explain the initial presentation with parkinsonian symptoms.

Chronic amphetamine use (**choice B**) can result in an amphetamine-induced psychosis that resembles an acute schizophrenic attack. However, these attacks abate within a few days after drug use ceases. This patient's psychosis surfaced after a few days without medication.

Chronic schizophrenics (**choice C**) with an extensive history of neuroleptic use can develop tardive dyskinesia, which is characterized by involuntary jaw and tongue movements.

A parkinsonian patient overmedicated with L-dopa (**choice D**) may have visual and auditory hallucinations, as well as involuntary movements. These symptoms are the result of increased activity in the dopamine system and would be expected to abate after several days without treatment. Parkinsonian motor symptoms suppressed by L-dopa would be expected to reemerge as the drug is cleared from the system.

31. **The correct answer is B.** In the treatment of "normal" insomnia (the patient has no underlying psychopathology), it is important to establish a routine that does not vary. Therefore, the person should retire and rise at the same time each day.

While some may think that increasing fluid intake (**choice A**) will assist sleep by precluding awakening from thirst, it actually encourages sleep interruption by pressure from a full bladder.

One should not sleep in (**choice C**), since it disrupts the routine.

Since it is important not to classically condition the bed to wakefulness, if one does not fall asleep within 20 minutes, one should arise and perform a nonstimulating activity, such as reading a book, rather than staying in bed until sleep is attained (**choice D**).

Strenuous exercise before retiring (**choice E**) does not "wear the person out." Instead, it stimulates the autonomic nervous system and drives wakefulness. Exercise should not be done during the 2-3 hours before sleep.

32. **The correct answer is B.** The patient has the right to decide who will or will not be present during her care. This includes the right to refuse to be a part of a student's educational experience. The desires of the patient, not the physician or training facility, come first. If the patient does not want a medical student present during the delivery, respect the patient's wishes.

Choice A is incorrect because the patient's consent, not her husband's, is required. The husband cannot give consent for an alert, competent patient.

Choice C is incorrect because the patient has already refused. Having the student go back and ask again will only make the student uncomfortable and may make the patient angry.

Choice D is incorrect because sneaking the student in to observe in the background is a direct contradiction of the patient's wishes.

Choice E is incorrect because meeting with the patient to discuss the value of teaching encounters suggests putting pressure on the patient to change her mind. The purpose of the medical encounter is to seek the greatest benefit for the patient, not seek the best educational experience for the student. The patient's wishes predominate here.

33. **The correct answer is A.** These eight researchers are probably under the influence of LSD, which causes hallucinations notable for their brilliant colors. LSD also shows activity at serotonin receptors and can activate the sympathetic nervous system, resulting in symptoms such as diaphoresis, blurred vision (due to pupil dilation), and palpitations.

    Methadone (**choice B**) is a synthetic opiate used to treat heroin addiction. It has analgesic properties but does not ordinarily induce hallucinations.

    PCP (**choice C**) can cause hallucinations marked by alterations of body image and distortions of space and time. PCP can also cause a dissociative anesthesia and analgesia. Common side effects of PCP use include hypersalivation, muscular rigidity, hypertension, and nystagmus. Highly colored visual hallucinations are not as commonly seen with PCP intoxication as with LSD intoxication.

    Phenobarbital (**choice D**) is a long-acting barbiturate that acts as a CNS depressant. It is used in the long-term management of seizure disorders.

    THC (**choice E**) is found in marijuana and produces a euphoric high followed by subsequent relaxation and sleepiness. Marijuana use can result in visual hallucinations, delusions, and a toxic psychosis, but generally only at extremely high doses.

34. **The correct answer is B.** The key to this question rests on the basic fact that HIV transmission occurs through the exchange of bodily fluids. Lesbian sexual activity mainly involves oral and digital contact and body friction. The likelihood of contaminated bodily fluid transmission is minimal with these practices.

    Female heterosexual transmission (**choice A**) is very high, as is male homosexual (**choice D**) and male transsexual (**choice E**) transmission, because transference of seminal fluid during receptive intercourse is common.

    Male heterosexuals (**choice C**) have the second lowest risk of acquiring HIV since they are not routinely exposed to contaminated fluids for an extended period of time after intercourse.

35. **The correct answer is B.** The lives of persons with borderline personality disorder are filled with very unstable interpersonal relations. They usually demand a great deal of attention and care from others. They frequently mutilate themselves, with the motivation being to elicit caring and closer relations with the other persons in their lives.

    Individuals with antisocial personality disorder (**choice A**) tend to hurt others, not themselves, and they do not have interest in closer relations with anyone.

    People with dependent personality disorder (**choice C**) characteristically subjugate themselves to others in order to get their dependency needs met. They would not report an attack; rather, they would try to cling to the attacker.

    The central feature of histrionic personality disorder (**choice D**) is a flamboyant, overly dramatic presentation of everything, including physical appearance. However, these individuals tend to not sexualize actual physical relations. They are seductive everywhere except the bedroom.

    The central issue in narcissistic personality disorder (**choice E**) is "entitlement" and self-importance. These individuals would not mutilate themselves, because they perceive themselves as too important to self-inflict bodily injury.

36. **The correct answer is D.** This is a difficult situation since the parents do have a legal responsibility for the child, and the child needs to trust the therapist to respect his or her innermost thoughts and feelings. Generally the parents know most of the child's behaviors and worries; however, they may not know the child's extensive and deep rooted concerns. The best way to approach this is to invite the child to attend all parent meetings in which the child is discussed. Given this scenario, the parents are unlikely to request extremely personal data, and the child can build a trust in the therapist to not violate intimate details.

    Choice A aligns the therapist in a conspiracy of silence with the parents and is not recommended.

    Choice B is not recommended because it sets up a comparable but opposite scenario as **choice A**. That is, it aligns the therapist with the child against the parents.

    Choice C will reliably result in the child withholding sensitive information with which he or she is struggling.

    Choice E can place the therapist in an untenable position if the child is self-destructive and needs parental intervention. Remember, only parents and courts can legally detain a child; a physician cannot. This choice also works against the therapist-patient-parent alliance, which is necessary for good outcomes in psychotherapy with a child.

37. **The correct answer is C.** Narcolepsy is defined as recurrent intrusions of elements of rapid eye movement (REM) sleep into the transition between sleep and wakefulness.

Although affective disorders (**choices A and B**) are associated with sleep abnormalities, they are not characterized by sudden onset of REM.

Likewise, sleep deprivation hypersomnia (**choice D**) and substance-induced sleep disorders (**choice E**) do not present with sudden onset of REM.

38. **The correct answer is B.** Cognitive therapy is based on the theory that depressed persons have acquired negative cognitions about themselves, reinforcing these cognitions with self-talk that is often not verbalized. The goal of therapy is to identify the negative cognitions, question the validity of the beliefs, and substitute more positively reinforcing self-talk for the aversive self-criticism.

Internalized anger (**choice A**) and early loss of significant love objects (**choice E**) are psychodynamic explanations for depression.

Neurotransmitter (**choice C**) and genetic (**choice D**) underpinnings are biologic explanations for depression.

39. **The correct answer is C.** In a longitudinal study, the same group is followed over a long period of time. Generally, no active intervention is instituted after the initial event. Note that the event may be either negative or positive.

Clinical trials (**choice A**) are predicated on some treatment being administered to the persons in the study. In the described situation, nothing is done to this group except observation and evaluation.

In a double-blind study (**choice B**), neither the subject nor the experimenter knows whether the subject is getting a treatment or a placebo.

In a prospective study (**choice D**), subjects are identified and followed over time; the outcome has not yet occurred when the study begins.

A retrospective study (**choice E**) looks backward in subjects' histories to see whether a particular event or events occurred.

40. **The correct answer is A.** Contrary to popular impressions, the most common reason for a significant downward shift in socioeconomic status (SES) is the presence of serious health problems, which both use up financial resources and prevent a person from working full-time at a high-paying job, or from working at all in some cases.

Significant psychiatric illness (**choice B**) is a cause of decline in SES, but is quantitatively less important than physical problems.

Inability to defer gratification (**choice C**), lack of education (**choice D**), and unwillingness to work (**choice E**) can all contribute to a decline in SES, but are not numerically as important as disabling physical problems.

41. **The correct answer is D.** In rapid eye movement (REM) sleep disorder, the normal paralysis of muscles during REM sleep is not present, and the person "acts out" the dream they are experiencing. This often results in injury to oneself or to others with whom the person is sleeping. In addition, the content of the dreams associated with this sleep problem is often violent or aggressive.

Night terrors (**choice B**) typically have their onset in childhood; in some persons, however, they persist into adulthood. During night terrors, the person exhibits terrified behavior, such as screaming during sleep. They do not involve an organized attack on another person.

Narcolepsy (**choice A**) is characterized by the sudden onset of REM sleep at inappropriate times (e.g., while driving), during which there is loss of muscle tone.

Non-REM sleep disorder (**choice C**) encompasses both night terrors and sleepwalking. People do not act out dreams in either of these conditions. Rather, their behavior is autonomous and not aggressive toward others.

Sleep apnea disorder (**choice E**) is a breathing problem during sleep in which the person stops regular breathing. It is not associated with acting out behavior.

42. **The correct answer is B.** The DNR (do not resuscitate) order means that the patient asks that his or her life not be prolonged by artificial means. It does not mean that the patient wishes to forgo palliative therapy, such as current narcotic pain medication (**choice A**), future medications (**choice C**), and nutrition and hydration (**choice D**). Limitations on such interventions might be specified on living wills or advance directives, however.

Withholding osteopathic manipulation (**choice E**) would not prolong his life, but it would help to relieve his pain.

43. **The correct answer is A.** Relaxation of uterine ligaments or endometriosis can produce dyspareunia. These conditions can be corrected by surgical intervention.

Premature ejaculation (**choice B**) is addressed by behavior modification techniques such as the "squeeze" technique to teach the male how to voluntarily control the ejaculatory response.

Primary impotence (**choice C**) is diagnosed in a patient who has always had difficulty attaining and maintaining an erection. That is, the problem has existed ever since the male became sexually active.

Secondary orgasmic dysfunction (**choice D**) is addressed by resolving the traumatic issue that precipitated the symptoms.

Graduated dilators are the treatment for vaginismus (**choice E**).

44. **The correct answer is D.** Type 1 errors occur when researchers reject the null hypothesis when they should not have. In other words, they conclude a significant result when in actuality it does not exist. This is a particularly dangerous error to make, as it could lead to the administration of an ineffective drug to patients in need of life-preserving treatment.

The term "1-β error" (**choice A**) is not used, but 1-β does correspond to a meaningful value. It reflects the power of a study, which equals the probability of rejecting the null hypothesis when it is false, or in other words, the probability of discovering a true relationship (e.g., concluding that acetaminophen has antipyretic action).

The term "alpha error" (**choice B**) is not used, but alpha values do correspond to a meaningful concept. Alpha is the probability of committing a type 1 error (explained above). Alpha corresponds to the p value (< 0.05) commonly used in statistical analysis.

The term "beta error" (**choice C**) is not used, but beta values do correspond to a meaningful concept. Beta is the probability of committing a type 2 error. Type 2 errors (**choice E**) occur when researchers accept the null hypothesis when it is false, thereby failing to detect a true relationship (e.g., concluding that acetaminophen has no antipyretic action).

A good mnemonic for distinguishing type 1 and type 2 errors is as follows: Type 1 kills everyone. Type 2 makes professors blue (because they can't publish their statistically insignificant results).

45. **The correct answer is D.** This is the principle of vicarious liability. This is the liability that a supervisory party (such as the doctor) bears for the actionable conduct of a subordinate (such as the nurse) because of the employer/employee relationship that exists between the two.

46. **The correct answer is B.** Causation is part of a tort (lawsuit). The other three parts are duty, negligence, and injury. The finding of the sponge is considered the causation of the lawsuit by the doctrine of *Res ipsa loquitur* (Latin: the object speaks for itself). The most minimum standard is the one used for physicians to infer negligence.

47. **The correct answer is A.** Breach of warranty occurs when the physician promises that the patient will be able to walk after surgery. Even though the surgeon made no mistakes and was not negligent in any way, he implied or expressed a warranty and did not keep it.

48. **The correct answer is E.** Battery is unlawful beating of another. It includes every willful, angry, and violent or negligent touching of another person without their consent. The doctor willfully touched with the scalpel a patient who had not given consent to be touched. The removal of the lesion would then be considered an injury to the patient.

49. **The correct answer is F.** The patient has committed assault, which is defined as an apparent violent attempt (verbal threats, shoving the chair) or willful offer with force or violence to do harm to another, without the actual doing of the harm threatened.

50. **The correct answer is H.** The doctor didn't check to see if the patient could read the surgical release. Therefore, the patient didn't understand what he signed. Lack of informed consent is the principle for which the doctor would be sued. The doctor has a duty to explain verbally or in writing the surgical procedure and its complications, being sure that the patient is able to understand what was explained. Clearly, if the patient can't read and the consent form was not read to him by a translator, he failed to obtain proper consent. (Always have the translator sign the form as well, with the date and time included.)

Behavioral Science and Biostatistics

1. A 25-year-old man is brought to the psychiatric emergency department by his wife, who reports that he has been acting strangely. He recently has spent thousands of dollars on a new sports car, has become uncharacteristically promiscuous, and has been working and speaking at a frantic pace. History is significant for an episode of major depression last year. Urine toxicology screen is negative. He is prescribed a medication that effectively alleviates his symptoms. Which of the following is a well-established side effect of the drug of choice for his condition?

    (A) Agranulocytosis

    (B) Akathisia

    (C) Diabetes insipidus

    (D) Hyperprolactinemia

    (E) Urinary retention

2. A 55-year-old woman was diagnosed with schizophrenic disorder, paranoid type at age 23. She has been on neuroleptic medications for the majority of time since diagnosis. Which of the following conditions would be most likely to appear at this time as a consequence of her treatment?

    (A) Akathisia

    (B) Anticholinergic symptoms

    (C) Dystonia of the laryngeal muscles

    (D) Neuroleptic malignant syndrome

    (E) Tardive dyskinesia

3. A 34-year-old man presents to the hospital complaining of weight loss, nausea, vomiting, and lethargy. There is no evidence of edema, orthostatic hypotension, or dehydration. Blood samples show hyponatremia, but his urine is highly concentrated. A water-load test is performed, in which the patient is instructed to drink a large volume of water and 5 hourly samples of urine are analyzed. All samples show concentrated urine. Which of the following drugs could have caused this condition?

    (A) Baclofen

    (B) Carbamazepine

    (C) Dantrolene

    (D) Phenelzine

    (E) Phenytoin

4. A 22-year-old model worries about her job security when a more experienced model is hired. She begins to throw temper tantrums and continuously makes negative statements about the new employee behind her back to her boss. Which of the following defense mechanisms is the model exhibiting?

    (A) Reaction formation

    (B) Regression

    (C) Repression

    (D) Splitting

    (E) Sublimation

5. A 15-year-old boy presents at his family physician's office with a chief complaint of burning on urination. A purulent urethral discharge is noted on physical examination; a Gram stain of the smear is consistent with gonorrhea. The patient explains that he had sexual intercourse with a female friend about 7 days earlier. The physician may treat the patient

   (A) but must have both parents' consent
   (B) but must inform the parents
   (C) with one parent's consent
   (D) without a parent's consent or informing the parents
   (E) without informing parents, but must inform the court

6. A businessman whose work entails much traveling complains to his physician that he has sleep difficulties after returning home from long trips. His lack of sleep has affected his productivity on the job. Which of the following drugs would be most appropriate for treating this patient's jet lag?

   (A) Alprazolam
   (B) Diazepam
   (C) Flurazepam
   (D) Prazepam
   (E) Triazolam

7. The mother of a newborn infant wants to know what is the earliest age at which toilet training is likely to be successful?

   (A) 10 months
   (B) 13 months
   (C) 16 months
   (D) 19 months
   (E) 22 months

8. An experimental serologic test is developed to detect the presence of HIV antibody. Epidemiologic analysis reveals the results shown below.

	People with HIV antibody	People without HIV antibody
Positive test	100	50
Negative test	20	950

Which of the following is the sensitivity of this test?

   (A) 11%
   (B) 67%
   (C) 83%
   (D) 95%
   (E) 98%

9. A 10-year-old boy is sent home from school for hitting younger children and taking things from them by force. The parents meet with the school principal. During the conference, the father says to the principal, "Just wait till I get home. He's going to get his butt whipped." The father's disciplinary technique, with the resultant behavior in the son, is an example of which type of learning?

   (A) Classical conditioning
   (B) Cognitive learning
   (C) Imprinting
   (D) Operant conditioning
   (E) Social learning

10. A 35-year-old night watchman has few close relationships with family or friends because they find him cold and aloof. He has no particularly odd behaviors except for his preference for being alone. This patient most likely has which of the following personality disorders?

   (A) Antisocial
   (B) Avoidant
   (C) Borderline
   (D) Dependent
   (E) Schizoid

11. A 16-year-old girl is pregnant and seeking an abortion. She does not want her parents to know either that she is pregnant or that she wants an abortion. The physician may perform the abortion

    (A) but must have at least one parent's consent

    (B) but must have both parents' consent

    (C) but must inform the parents

    (D) without parental consent only in certain states

    (E) without telling the parents

12. A trial comparing coronary bypass surgery with medical treatment for coronary artery disease is conducted at a hospital specializing in cardiothoracic surgery. Which of the following types of biases should be considered in evaluating the results of this trial?

    (A) Ascertainment bias

    (B) Detection bias

    (C) Proficiency bias

    (D) Recall bias

    (E) Referral bias

13. Which of the following epidemiologic parameters would directly affect the positive predictive value of a test?

    (A) Incidence of the disease

    (B) Odds ratio for contracting this disease

    (C) Prevalence of the disease

    (D) Relative risk for contracting the disease

    (E) Duration of the disease

14. A 23-year-old woman visits a primary care physician complaining of recurrent nausea and generalized abdominal pain, which has distressed her and compromised her functioning for the past several months. Thorough evaluations by a gynecologist and gastroenterologist have revealed no abnormalities. She was referred to a neurologist for headaches and has been taking acetaminophen for her "joint pains." The osteopathic primary care physician completes a thorough structural and physical exam, and the results are normal. Which of the following is the most likely diagnosis?

    (A) Body dysmorphic disorder

    (B) Conversion disorder

    (C) Factitious disorder

    (D) Malingering

    (E) Somatization disorder

15. A 19-year-old man describes episodes in which he feels as if he's "floating out of his body" and observing himself from a place about 2 feet over his head. He is aware of everything going on around him and can respond to others. Which of the following terms most accurately describes what this patient is experiencing?

    (A) Delirium tremens

    (B) Delusion

    (C) Dementia

    (D) Depersonalization

    (E) Derealization

16. A physician enters an examination room where a 31-year-old woman is sitting on a chair with tears running down her face. After the physician introduces herself, which of the following is the most appropriate first statement to get the most correct information from the patient in the least amount of time?

    (A) "Are you depressed?"

    (B) "How are you feeling?"

    (C) "What is scaring you?"

    (D) "You seem to be sad."

    (E) "You seem to be upset."

17. Of the following reflexes present in a neonate, which is most critical to its immediate survival?

    (A) Grasp
    (B) Plantar
    (C) Rooting
    (D) Startle
    (E) Tonic neck

18. A researcher publishes new results on the efficacy of a procedure using transplanted embryonic cells to correct a diabetic condition induced in experimental animals by chemical ablation of pancreatic beta cells. At another institution, a different researcher attempts to reproduce the findings, but cannot. This disparate finding calls into question the first study's

    (A) accuracy
    (B) power
    (C) reliability
    (D) sensitivity
    (E) validity

19. In a patient with sexual dysfunction, which type would be the most difficult to treat?

    (A) Dyspareunia
    (B) Premature ejaculation
    (C) Primary ejaculatory incompetence in a male
    (D) Secondary orgasmic dysfunction in a female
    (E) Vaginismus

20. A 45-year-old woman is brought to the emergency department by ambulance after a car accident that caused injuries resulting in a significant loss of blood. The patient is conscious and informs the attending physician that her religion forbids a blood transfusion. She has an identification card in her purse that verifies her religious affiliation and her wishes not to undergo transfusion. Although the physician explains that without the transfusion she is likely to die, she still refuses the procedure. Which of the following actions should the physician take?

    (A) Declare an emergency and transfuse against the patient's wishes
    (B) Declare the patient incompetent and transfuse
    (C) Make the patient comfortable, but not transfuse
    (D) Request the hospital chaplain try to persuade the patient
    (E) Transfuse when the patient becomes comatose

21. A 34-year-old woman is brought to her family physician by her brother. He states that the patient's husband ran away with another woman the previous day. After discovering this, the patient arrived at her brother's home in a "dazed state," was unable to function appropriately the remainder of the evening, and slept fitfully all night. Early in the morning she began to talk to people who were not present, and debated whether to kill her children and herself. He denies anything like this ever happening before. Which of the following is the most likely diagnosis?

    (A) Bipolar disorder
    (B) Brief psychotic disorder
    (C) Schizoaffective disorder
    (D) Schizophrenic disorder
    (E) Schizophreniform disorder

22. A mother brings her 6-week-old infant to the pediatrician because she is concerned that her child is not babbling in response to her stimulation. Which of the following is the most likely diagnosis?

    (A) Autism
    (B) Hearing impairment
    (C) Mental retardation
    (D) Visual impairment
    (E) Within normal limits

23. A 20-year-old woman sees her baby cousin for the first time. As she attempts to play with the infant, he begins to cry incessantly. Which of the following is the most likely age of this infant?

    (A) 1-4 months
    (B) 5-8 months
    (C) 9-12 months
    (D) 13-16 months
    (E) 17-20 months

24. In a depressed patient who has threatened to commit suicide, which of the following variables is associated with a higher risk for successfully committing suicide?

    (A) Age younger than 45

    (B) Female gender

    (C) High socioeconomic status

    (D) Married

    (E) No history of major affective disorder

25. A 27-year-old swimmer who feels insecure about her athletic abilities harshly criticizes her teammates' techniques. Which of the following ego defense mechanisms is she displaying?

    (A) Displacement

    (B) Projection

    (C) Reaction formation

    (D) Repression

    (E) Sublimation

26. A 27-year-old man is brought into the emergency department by the police, who found him walking aimlessly and shouting the names of former presidents. Urine toxicology is negative, and the man appears to be oriented with respect to person, place, and time. He has had five similar admissions over the past year. Attempts to interview the patient are fruitless, as he seems easily distracted and unable to concentrate. A phone call to a friend listed in the chart provides the additional information that the man is homeless and unable to care for himself. This patient is exhibiting the signs and symptoms of

    (A) schizoaffective disorder

    (B) schizoid personality disorder

    (C) schizophrenia

    (D) schizophreniform disorder

    (E) schizotypal personality disorder

27. On the Mental Status Examination, a disruption in the sensorium section should alert the physician to explore which of the following etiologic areas?

    (A) Educational/deprivation

    (B) Familial/child-rearing

    (C) Organic/neurologic

    (D) Psychological/learned

    (E) Social/cultural

28. A couple visits their primary care physician because of sleep difficulties. The wife reports that she cannot fall asleep at night because of her obese husband's loud snoring. He complains of feeling drowsy during the day and falling asleep while driving home from work. Which of the following conditions does the husband most likely have?

    (A) Central sleep apnea

    (B) Obstructive sleep apnea

    (C) Narcolepsy

    (D) Pavor nocturnus

    (E) Somnambulism

29. An adolescent male is referred for drug abuse. He confides to the therapist that he has been taking large amounts of "reds" (secobarbital sodium) for some time and that they make him feel confident and calm. He would like to stop but says he would prefer to "do it on his own," without additional medication. The therapist should advise the patient to detoxify with medical assistance because of the danger of

    (A) insomnia

    (B) rebound anxiety

    (C) recidivism

    (D) respiratory depression

    (E) seizures

30. An urban health department reports the infant mortality rate of the city in the past year. This value corresponds to which of the following?

    (A) The number of deaths during the past year from all causes divided by the total population

    (B) The number of deaths occurring after the first 4 weeks of life and before the first birthday divided by the total number of live births

    (C) The number of deaths occurring until the first birthday divided by the total number of live births

    (D) The number of deaths occurring within the first 4 weeks of life divided by the total number of births

    (E) The number of deaths occurring within the first 4 weeks of life divided by the total number of live births

31. A 19-year-old woman, who recently moved from her family's home in another state, is hospitalized for attempting suicide by taking an overdose of antidepressant medications. On the third day of her hospital stay, she insists, under threat of a lawsuit, that her medications be stopped and that she be discharged from the hospital so she "can go home and finish the job." Her sensorium is clear. Her physician should

(A) discharge her against medical advice (AMA)

(B) honor her request and release her immediately

(C) obtain an emergency order of detention

(D) release her to go back to her parents' home

(E) sedate her

32. A female patient presents to a physician with the isolated symptom of pulling out all the hair on her head and face. She reports that there is a build up of "pressure" or tension inside her, and the hair extraction reduces the pressure/tension feeling. Which of the following is the most appropriate medication for this condition?

(A) Clozapine

(B) Diazepam

(C) Fluvoxamine

(D) Lithium

(E) Verapamil

33. A 23-year-old man arrives at the emergency department at 11:30 PM complaining of flank pain and blood in his urine. He requests Demerol to control the pain. The physician requests a urine sample, and the patient goes to the restroom, removes a pin from under his shirt collar, pricks his finger, and holds the dripping blood in the stream of urine. He returns the urine to the physician and intensifies his complaints of pain, which he now says has migrated to his ipsilateral testicle. Which of the following is the most likely diagnosis?

(A) Antisocial personality disorder

(B) Factitious disorder

(C) Malingering disorder

(D) Schizotypal personality disorder

(E) Somatization disorder

34. White coat hypertension is defined as an elevation of blood pressure resulting from the apprehension associated with visiting a physician. It is thought that the patient associates the physician's white coat with distressing experiences (e.g., being vaccinated as a child), resulting in transient hypertension. This may be viewed as a physiologic manifestation of which of the following phenomena?

(A) Classic conditioning

(B) Extinction

(C) Habit hierarchies

(D) Negative reinforcement

(E) Operant conditioning

35. Impulsive aggression has been most strongly linked to which of the following neurotransmitter systems?

(A) Dopamine

(B) Endorphin

(C) Epinephrine

(D) Gamma-amino butyric acid

(E) Serotonin

36. A young mother wishes to teach her 3-year-old son to pick up his toys when he is finished playing. A friend advises her to reward her child for completing this task. Though the approach is effective for about 1 week, the little boy returns to his previous untidy behavior. Which of the following patterns of reinforcement did she likely use?

(A) Continuous

(B) Fixed interval

(C) Fixed ratio

(D) Variable interval

(E) Variable ratio

37. A 47-year-old man is hospitalized with acute pancreatitis. His history reveals a history of episodic binge alcohol consumption. When the physician meets with the patient to discuss the condition, the patient asks: "Doctor, what caused this?" Which of the following is the most appropriate response to this question?

    (A) "I'm not sure."

    (B) "Probably a consequence of alcohol consumption."

    (C) "Probably your alcoholism."

    (D) "We need to talk about where we go from here in your long-term care."

    (E) "What do you think?"

38. An oncologist tells his patient that her laboratory results support a diagnosis of advanced malignant melanoma with multiple metastases to the liver and brain. He also advises her that the prognosis is poor. Which of the following is most likely to be the first statement that the patient will make?

    (A) "Can you keep me alive until my daughter graduates from medical school?"

    (B) "Damn you doctor, you should have caught this earlier!"

    (C) "Doctor, you must be wrong."

    (D) "I think it is time that I make a will and say goodbye to everyone."

    (E) "It's no use, I always lose and get the short end of the stick."

39. A 45-year-old woman has just given birth to her fifth child. She wishes to undergo a tubal ligation. The physician should

    (A) convince the patient to use alternative contraception until she reaches menopause

    (B) discuss the benefits and risks of the procedure with both the patient and her husband

    (C) explain to the patient that her chances of becoming pregnant are very low at her age

    (D) maintain strict confidentiality and not disclose the patient's wishes to her husband

    (E) refuse to do the procedure because of her age

40. A man brings his 45-year-old wife to the emergency department. He states she has been ill for 3 days and has had a temperature of 99.8 to 100.5 F. Today she is having difficulty staying awake, is talking to persons who are not there, and at times appears to be frightened of something. Osteopathic structural examination reveals acute somatic dysfunction at T10-L2. She is restless and somewhat combative when restrained. What is the most likely diagnosis?

    (A) Acute stress disorder

    (B) Bipolar I disorder, manic type

    (C) Brief psychotic disorder

    (D) Delirium

    (E) Dementia

41. A 40-year-old man visits a crisis counselor after a devastating explosion. Which of the following would be most likely to predispose this patient to developing emotional problems after the disaster?

    (A) Having been physically injured and trapped under rubble for 24 hours

    (B) Having lived all his life in the area where the disaster occurred

    (C) Having a previous diagnosis of post-traumatic stress disorder

    (D) Having recently been widowed

    (E) Having worked 15 miles from the site of the explosion

42. A new drug with in vitro activity against HIV is tested on a population of patients with Western-blot confirmed HIV infections. Out of the 200 individuals in the patient population, 100 individuals are chosen by lottery to receive the drug. The drug, which is tasteless, is administered in a cup of orange juice; the other patients receive pure orange juice. Neither the nurses, doctors, nor patients know which patients receive the drug. At the end of the study period, the number of CD4+ T cells is determined for all of the subjects. This is an example of a

    (A) case-control study

    (B) case report

    (C) cohort study

    (D) cross-sectional study

    (E) double-blind randomized clinical trial

43. Which of the following is the highest level of functioning that a 27-year-old person with an Intelligence Quotient (IQ) of 53 could be reasonably expected to achieve?

    (A) Live alone, work at a semi-skilled job, and maintain a totally independent lifestyle

    (B) Work in a sheltered workshop situation and maintain a totally independent lifestyle

    (C) Work in a sheltered workshop situation and be assisted during times of mild social or economic stress

    (D) Live in a controlled environment and be partially self-maintained

    (E.) Live in a nursing home environment

44. There were no new cases of Ebola virus in the United States from January 1, 1997 through January 1, 1998. Which of the following epidemiologic terms does this statement describe?

    (A) Incidence
    (B) Lifetime expectancy
    (C) Lifetime prevalence
    (D) Period prevalence
    (E) Point prevalence

45. The data presented below compare the results of a diagnostic test in the presence and absence of a disease.

	Disease present	Disease absent
Positive test	40	5
Negative test	10	95
Total	50	100

    Which of the following is the specificity of this test?

    (A) 0.05
    (B) 0.40
    (C) 0.80
    (D) 0.90
    (E) 0.95

46. A 33-year-old woman is brought into the emergency department by ambulance. She has been diagnosed as having schizophrenic disorder, disorganized type, since the age of 17. She has been on antipsychotic medications since that time, which have controlled her symptoms well. Physical examination reveals a well-nourished woman with a temperature of 103.2 F, blood pressure of 180/99/mm Hg, pulse of 97/min, and copious perspiration. She is mute, has muscular rigidity, and appears to be obtunded. Which of the following is the most likely diagnosis?

    (A) Acute dystonia
    (B) Akathisia
    (C) Neuroleptic malignant syndrome
    (D) Parkinsonism
    (E) Tardive dyskinesia

47. A 34-year-old woman complains of early morning awakenings and loss of interest in everyday activities. She is diagnosed with major depressive disorder and given fluoxetine, but does not improve. Tricyclic antidepressants and MAO inhibitors are subsequently tried without effect, and electroconvulsive therapy (ECT) is recommended. Which of the following represents the most serious side effect of ECT?

    (A) Extrapyramidal symptoms
    (B) Hearing loss
    (C) Mania
    (D) Retrograde amnesia
    (E) Rhabdomyolysis

48. A 35-year old woman lives alone. She has never been married, has a Masters of Business Administration, and has been employed as a stock broker. She was fired from her present firm because on three separate occasions over the past 2 years, without authorization from her clients, she sold all the securities in their accounts and invested the money in securities that had glossy portfolios but were worthless. On these three occasions she worked 22-24 hours per day for 10 days at a time, gorged herself on "junk food," and drank alcohol excessively. Which of the following is the most likely diagnosis?

    (A) Bipolar disorder, type I
    (B) Bipolar disorder, type II
    (C) Cyclothymic disorder
    (D) Schizophrenic disorder, paranoid type
    (E) Substance-induced delirium

49. A child who understands that the volume of a liquid poured out of a narrow glass remains the same when poured into a wider glass is at which of Piaget's stages of intellectual development?

    (A) Concrete operations
    (B) Formal operations
    (C) Preoperational
    (D) Sensorimotor
    (E) Motor sensory

50. In a restaurant, the parents of a 4-year-old child are talking with each other and not with the child. The child first says "Mommy"; when the mother does not respond, the intensity of the word "Mommy" increases. The child then begins to drop her eating utensils. When the parents still do not respond, the child knocks over her glass of milk. The parents then scold the child and busy themselves cleaning up the spilled milk and getting more for the child. This scenario is repeated 3 times before the parents angrily take the child from the restaurant. This entire scene is an example of which of the following types of learning?

    (A) Classical conditioning
    (B) Cognitive learning
    (C) Imprinting
    (D) Operant conditioning
    (E) Social learning

Behavioral Science and Biostatistics

ANSWERS AND EXPLANATIONS

1.	C		26.	C
2.	E		27.	C
3.	B		28.	B
4.	B		29.	E
5.	D		30.	C
6.	E		31.	C
7.	D		32.	C
8.	C		33.	C
9.	E		34.	A
10.	E		35.	E
11.	D		36.	A
12.	C		37.	B
13.	C		38.	C
14.	E		39.	B
15.	D		40.	D
16.	B		41.	A
17.	C		42.	E
18.	C		43.	C
19.	C		44.	A
20.	C		45.	E
21.	B		46.	C
22.	E		47.	D
23.	B		48.	A
24.	C		49.	A
25.	B		50.	D

1. **The correct answer is C.** This patient has bipolar disorder and is experiencing a manic episode. The drug of choice for this condition, lithium, can cause nephrogenic diabetes insipidus at therapeutic drug levels. Other side effects include tremor, ataxia, aphasia, and sedation.

   Agranulocytosis (**choice A**) is a side effect of clozapine, which is used for schizophrenic patients with symptoms refractory to traditional antipsychotic therapy. Unlike the standard antidopaminergics (e.g., haloperidol), clozapine rarely produces extrapyramidal side effects. Note that lithium administration causes leukocytosis, rather than leukopenia, in most cases.

   Akathisia (**choice B**), which is characterized by uncontrollable restlessness, is an extrapyramidal side effect of antidopaminergic medications used to treat schizophrenia.

   Hyperprolactinemia (**choice D**) is typically associated with antidopaminergic medications (antipsychotics), rather than with lithium.

   Urinary retention (**choice E**) is a classic anticholinergic side effect of tricyclic antidepressants.

2. **The correct answer is E.** Tardive dyskinesia is a result of long-term treatment with neuroleptic medications and is seen more frequently in older women. The condition presents with abnormal choreoathetoid movements, often involving the face and mouth in adults and the limbs in children. Once tardive dyskinesia develops, there is no known treatment to mitigate the symptoms.

   Akathisia (**choice A**), also known as restless leg syndrome, is usually well controlled by reduction of the dose of antipsychotic medication and the addition of beta-adrenergic receptor antagonists or anticholinergic drugs and benzodiazepines. It can occur early in the course of treatment.

   Anticholinergic symptoms (**choice B**), such as dry mouth, blurred vision, or constipation, usually appear early in the course of treatment, and the patient becomes tolerant to these effects.

   Dystonia of the laryngeal muscles (**choice C**) is an acute condition that is well managed with medications such as benztropine or diphenhydramine.

   Neuroleptic malignant syndrome (**choice D**) is a life-threatening condition that can occur at any point in treatment. It is characterized by muscle rigidity, hyperpyrexia, and increased blood pressure. Bromocriptine and dantrolene are used to treat this disorder.

3. **The correct answer is B.** The patient has the syndrome of inappropriate secretion of ADH (SIADH). When ADH (vasopressin) is secreted in excessive amounts, or at inappropriate times, it can cause hyponatremia as well as symptoms of nausea, vomiting, anorexia, and lethargy. Excessive release of vasopressin also results in the excretion of a concentrated urine (with a urinary osmolality usually greater than 300 mOsmol/kg) despite a subnormal plasma osmolality and serum sodium concentration. SIADH can be caused by many factors, such as ectopic ADH production and release from neoplastic tissue (small cell carcinoma of lung, pancreatic carcinoma, lymphosarcoma, Hodgkin disease, reticulum cell sarcoma, thymoma, and carcinoma of duodenum or bladder) or by drugs that release or potentiate the action of ADH, such as carbamazepine, vincristine, vinblastine, cyclophosphamide, chlorpropamide, general anesthetics, and tricyclic antidepressants.

   Baclofen (**choice A**) is a spasmolytic agent. Baclofen has not been shown to be associated with the release of ADH.

   Dantrolene (**choice C**) is a spasmolytic agent and is also used to treat malignant hyperthermia. Dantrolene has not been shown to be associated with the release of ADH.

   Phenelzine (**choice D**) and tranylcypromine (choice F) are MAO inhibitors. MAO inhibitors have not been shown to be associated with the release of ADH.

   Phenytoin (**choice E**) is an antiseizure drug and has not been shown to be associated with the release of ADH.

4. **The correct answer is B.** The model is exhibiting regression, an automatic retreat to a less mature level of behavior in times of stress (e.g., throwing temper tantrums and tattletaling).

   Reaction formation (**choice A**) involves turning a repressed impulse or unconscious wish to its opposite.

   Repression (**choice C**) occurs when conflict-provoking thoughts or feelings are hidden from the person's awareness.

   Splitting (**choice D**) refers to the unconscious inability to see an important person as having both good and bad characteristics. The characteristics are "split," such that the person is perceived as either wonderful or terrible.

   Sublimation (**choice E**) is a very mature defense mechanism that involves consciously turning socially unacceptable impulses into acceptable or more benign forms to allow their expression.

5. **The correct answer is D.** No states specifically mandate parental involvement for a minor to obtain contraception, prenatal care and delivery services, diagnosis and treatment of an STD, outpatient alcohol and/or drug treatment, or outpatient mental health services. In these situations, the physician may go ahead and treat; informing the parents is the physician's option, not a requirement.

6. **The correct answer is E.** Short-acting benzodiazepines (BZD) are the most appropriate pharmaceutical therapy for acute insomnia, including jet lag. Triazolam is the only short-acting BZD listed. It has the added benefit of not having many adverse actions (e.g., hangover effect) when taken in low doses. Higher doses, however, predispose to transient anterograde amnesia.

    Alprazolam (**choice A**) is an intermediate-acting BZD used primarily for panic attacks.

    Diazepam (**choice B**) is effective for status epilepticus and muscle spasticity. Note that lorazepam is also effective for status epilepticus.

    Flurazepam (**choice C**) is a long-acting BZD that can cause drowsiness or ataxia, rendering it a less desirable choice. It is not used as an anxiolytic, unlike many other BZDs.

    Prazepam (**choice D**) is a long-acting BZD unsuitable for the treatment of sleep disorders.

7. **The correct answer is D.** Toilet training is not possible before the age of 18 months because the long nerve fibers have not yet myelinated and sphincter control is not possible. Toilet training should be completed by 4 years of age.

8. **The correct answer is C.** Sensitivity is defined as the ability of a test to detect the presence of a disease in those who truly have the disease. It is calculated as the number of people with a disease who test positive (true positive) divided by the total number of people who have the disease (true positive + false negative). In this case, sensitivity equals the number of people with HIV antibody who test positive (100) divided by the total number of people who have HIV antibody (120). This yields 100/120 = 83% (not a very sensitive test).

    11% (**choice A**) corresponds to the prevalence of the disease in the tested population, which in this case equals the total number of people with HIV antibody (true positive + false negative = 100 + 20 = 120) divided by the total number of people tested (100 + 20 + 50 + 950 = 1120). This yields 120/1120 = 11%.

    67% (**choice B**) corresponds to the positive predictive value of the test, which equals the number of people with the disease who test positive (true positives = 100)

divided by the total number of people testing positive (all positives = 50). This yields 100/150 = 67%.

95% (**choice D**) corresponds to the specificity of the test, which equals the number of people without HIV antibody who test negative (950) divided by the total number of people without HIV antibody (1000). This yields 950/1000 = 95%.

98% (**choice E**) corresponds to the negative predictive value of the test, which equals the number of people without HIV antibody who test negative (950) divided by the total number of people testing negative (970). This yields 950/970 = 98%.

An easy way to remember these concepts is:

    Sensitivity = true positives/all diseased

    Specificity = true negatives/all normal

    PPV = true positives/all positives

    NPV = true negatives/all negatives

    Prevalence = all diseased/total population

If you prefer charts and formulas:

	(Diseased) People with HIV antibody	(Normal) People without HIV antibody
Positive test	a, true pos.	b, false pos.
Negative test	c, false neg.	d, true neg.

Sensitivity = $a/(a + c)$

Specificity = $d/(b + d)$

PPV = $a/(a + b)$

NPV = $d/(c + d)$

Prevalence = $(a + c)/(a + b + c + d)$

9. **The correct answer is E.** This is an example of social learning. That is, the father is providing the example that "big people" get their way with "little people" by using force. The son is simply modeling his father's example.

    Classical conditioning (**choice A**) is the type of associative learning in which a stimulus that did not originally elicit a given response now does. This is done by associating the stimulus with a behavior that previously did elicit the response. In this question, the child may learn to fear the principal's office because of the punitive consequences.

    Cognitive learning (**choice B**) is a type of learning that requires full attention and purposeful intent to acquire the information. This boy may learn better social interactive skills if the principal required him to write an essay on how he feels when "big people" beat up on him.

Imprinting (**choice C**) forms the basis of bonding between an infant and the mothering figure. This form of attachment is learned by association during the immediate postnatal period.

Operant conditioning (**choice D**) is learning by reinforcement of a given behavior. If the father had said to his son: "Good boy. You have to take what you want in this world," the son would be reinforced for his antisocial behavior.

10. **The correct answer is E.** This is a typical description of schizoid personality disorder. Classic clues are "night watchman" and "cold and aloof" without odd behaviors or beliefs.

Antisocial personality disorder (**choice A**) is characterized by disregard for and violation of the rights of others, deceitfulness, impulsiveness, recklessness, irresponsibility, and a lack of remorse.

People with avoidant personality disorder (**choice B**) have a fear of rejection in interpersonal relationships. They are hypersensitive and exhibit excessive concern about being completely accepted without criticism. Unlike people with schizoid personality disorders, these patients want to establish relationships with others but are terrified unless they are guaranteed acceptance.

Borderline personality disorder (**choice C**) is associated with major problems with identity (e.g., gender identity, values), anger, and impulse control. Self-destructive behavior, e.g., gambling or overspending, may be present. These patients are emotionally labile and express intense feelings inappropriately.

People with dependent personality disorder (**choice D**) allow others to assume responsibility for important areas in their lives. There is a lack of self-confidence, and the priorities of others are given the most attention.

11. **The correct answer is D.** A number of issues are involved in this situation. First, the age of majority differs from state to state. As of April 1999, only two states and the District of Columbia have laws that affirm a minor's ability to obtain an abortion on her own. Twenty-five states have laws that require consent from one or both parents. All states have an option for the minor to petition the court for permission to have the abortion. These laws obviously place pregnant minors in difficulty if the laws require consent by both parents, since one may not be available and/or their whereabouts may be unknown. Girls who live in rural areas or cannot provide their own transportation have a difficult time accessing court services. Furthermore, the court system

is usually much too complicated for the youth to manage on her own.

12. **The correct answer is C.** Proficiency bias occurs when the intervention under consideration is delivered with unusual skill (or incompetence) so that it cannot be reproduced in typical settings.

Ascertainment bias (**choice A**) occurs when patients with the suspected outcome are more extensively probed about their symptoms and histories than are patients without the suspected outcome.

Detection bias (**choice B**) occurs when more information is solicited from the treatment group than from the placebo group.

Recall bias (**choice D**) occurs in retrospective studies. Patients may not remember the severity of their symptoms or how much intervention occurred over the specified course of time.

Referral bias (**choice E**) occurs when the sample of patients used in a study is not typical of the general population. For example, if an academic medical center sees the most acutely ill patients admitted for bypass surgery, its overall bypass mortality rates will appear extraordinarily high.

13. **The correct answer is C.** Of the choices listed, only prevalence, the total number of cases of a disease in a given period of time, directly affects the positive predictive value of a test (which equals true positives/all positives).

Incidence (**choice A**) is the number of new cases of a disease given in a period of time.

The odds ratio (**choice B**), which may be calculated from case-control studies, approximates relative risk.

Relative risk (**choice D**) can reflect the incidence of a disease in a treated group divided by the incidence of a disease in a placebo group.

Duration of the disease (**choice E**) is the length of time of the disease. It affects the prevalence of the disease but not the positive predictive value.

14. **The correct answer is E.** Patients with somatization disorder have many medically unexplained symptoms in multiple body systems, causing work limitation, increased visits to the physician, needless surgery, or unnecessary medical treatments. Somatization disorder is distinguished by its ego-dystonic symptoms; that is, the patient's functioning is compromised because of the unpleasantness of symptoms. It usually begins before age 30.

Body dysmorphic disorder (**choice A**) refers to the patient who is preoccupied with the belief that some part of the body is marred in looks. It usually begins in adolescence and is equally common in males and females.

Conversion disorder (**choice B**) refers to patients with neurologic complaints that are not consistent with present-day knowledge about the nervous system (e.g., anesthesia that does not run along a nerve distribution). A classic clue to this diagnosis is that the patient reveals a relative lack of concern about the symptoms, known as "la belle indifference."

There are three types of factitious disorder (FD; **choice C**): FD with psychological symptoms, FD with medical symptoms, and chronic FD. FD with medical symptoms is different from somatization disorder. In FD, symptoms are completely fabricated, and patients often insist on hospitalization and submit to invasive procedures. They also may produce symptoms through specific acts (e.g., taking drugs). Another difference between FD and somatization disorder is that patients with FD are consciously trying to assume a sick role.

Malingering (**choice D**) refers to the situation in which a patient reports psychological or general medical symptoms to achieve some easily recognizable secondary gain. The question implied no secondary gain for the patient, therefore malingering is not the best diagnosis in this case.

15. **The correct answer is D.** Depersonalization occurs when an individual perceives that his "person" or "self" becomes detached from his body. He maintains his contact with reality and level of consciousness, as opposed to derealization (**choice E**), in which the environment seems distorted or takes on an unreal quality.

Delirium tremens (**choice A**) occurs as a withdrawal symptom in chronic alcoholics abstaining from alcohol. It is characterized by anxiety, tremor, sweating, and vivid hallucinations.

Delusions (**choice B**) are false, fixed belief systems that exist in the face of no evidence to support them and are not shared by most others.

A patient with dementia (**choice C**) has a normal level of consciousness with gradual onset of cognitive symptoms (e.g., memory disturbance) and small potential for recovery. In contrast, delirium is characterized by impaired consciousness (diminished alertness and disturbed orientation to time, place, and person), acute onset of symptoms (e.g., confusion), excessive daytime sleeping, diffuse slowing of brain waves on EEG, and full recovery in most cases.

16. **The correct answer is B.** Patients may display different expressions to different underlying emotional states based on cultural, familial, and transient circumstances. For instance, many women have been taught that they "should never be angry," so they frequently cry when they are frustrated—the natural precursor to anger.

In general, the physician should not begin by asking about specific emotional bases (**choices A, C, D, and E**). Asking the patient directly how he or she is feeling promotes patient interaction and prevents the physician from assuming a given emotion when another is present.

17. **The correct answer is C.** The rooting reflex allows puckering of the lips and sucking on objects in response to perioral stimulation. It is necessary for the child to be able to locate a nipple and ingest food. Without this reflex, the neonate cannot suckle and feed properly.

The remaining reflexes (**choices A, B, D, and E**) are crucial for later development and survival but not for immediate life.

The grasp reflex (**choice A**) is defined by when pressure is exerted on the of the neonate is stroked, it will grasp the object exerting the pressure.

The plantar reflex (**choice B**) is another name for the Babinski sign. When the lateral surface of the foot is stroked, the great toe goes up and the other toes fan.

The startle reflex (**choice D**; also called the Moro reflex) occurs when an intense sensory stimulus is received. The neonate extends and abducts the arms, then flexes and adducts them.

The tonic neck reflex (**choice E**) occurs when the head is turned; the ipsilateral leg extends and the contralateral arm and leg flex.

18. **The correct answer is C.** The reliability of a measurement refers to the ability of other researchers to reproduce the results. This can be summarized by noting that reliability = reproducibility.

The accuracy (**choice A**) of a measurement refers to the "trueness" of the measurement, i.e., how close the measured value is to the true value. It is a measure of bias. Just because another researcher could not reproduce the findings does not necessarily imply that they were inaccurate.

The power (**choice B**) of a study is best conceptualized as the probability of rejecting a null hypothesis that is in fact false. This is equal to 1 minus the probability of a type II error $(1-\beta)$, since β is the probability of failing to reject a false null hypothesis.

The sensitivity (**choice D**) of a test is a measure of its ability to detect the presence of a disease in those who truly have the disease.

The validity (**choice E**) of a measurement is an index of how well the test measures what it purports to measure. The disparate results obtained by another researcher do not necessarily mean that the results are not valid.

19. **The correct answer is C.** Primary ejaculatory incompetence means that the adult male has never developed the ability to ejaculate while engaged in sexual activity with another person. It is extremely difficult to treat.

    Dyspareunia (**choice A**) is painful intercourse and is easily treated by addressing the underlying medical causes that exist in the vast majority of cases.

    Premature ejaculation (**choice B**) is readily addressed by the "squeeze technique."

    Secondary orgasmic dysfunction (**choice D**) means there had been function but it has been lost. Any secondary sexual dysfunction is easier to treat than a primary problem.

    Vaginismus (**choice E**) is often related to fear and apprehension regarding the act of penetration and is quite easily treated by behavior modification.

20. **The correct answer is C.** The courts have repeatedly ruled that adults are free to select their religious belief system and practice the tenets of that religion. If that includes refusal of certain medical procedures, that is the individual's right to choose.

    Declaring an emergency and transfusing against the patient's wishes (**choice A**) is clearly not allowed. In fact, the physician undertaking such action is legally liable for assault and battery and is clearly open to a malpractice action.

    Declaring the patient incompetent and performing the transfusion (**choice B**) is incorrect because the ruling of incompetence must be made by the court and not the physician. Again, the physician is open to a malpractice action if such an action were taken.

    Requesting the hospital chaplain try to persuade the patient (**choice D**) is incorrect since adults in America have the right to choose their religious beliefs. Trying to dissuade them from their beliefs and impose others on them is clearly unethical.

    Performing the transfusion when the patient becomes comatose (**choice E**) clearly goes against the patient's wishes. The patient's wishes were known before she became comatose, and these wishes must be followed in delivering medical care.

21. **The correct answer is B.** Brief psychotic disorder is a thought disorder of psychotic proportion (e.g., the demonstrated auditory hallucinations). There is often a precipitating event. To make this diagnosis, the patient's symptoms must have been present for at least

1 day but not more than 1 month. This duration distinguishes brief psychotic disorder from schizophrenic and schizophreniform disorders.

Bipolar disorder (**choice A**) is defined by the presence of a manic episode (characterized by an altered, intense mood, with rapid/pressured speech and hyperactivity).

Schizoaffective disorder (**choice C**) is characterized by elements of both schizophrenia (e.g., psychotic symptoms) and mood disorders (e.g., manic or depressive symptoms).

Schizophrenic disorder (**choice D**) is a chronic recurrent thought disorder often accompanied by bizarre behaviors. It usually begins in early adulthood. To make this diagnosis, the symptoms must last 6 months or more, which distinguishes it from brief psychotic and schizophreniform disorders.

Schizophreniform disorder (**choice E**) is a thought disorder of psychotic proportion with a duration between 1 and 6 months. This duration distinguishes the condition from brief psychotic disorder and schizophrenic disorder. Often, the onset of the thought disorder is as a young adult, when the person must leave the protected environment of the home and begin to assume personal responsibility for his or her life. He or she is unable to cope with the world and his/her defenses deteriorate to the point of psychosis. Typically, patients with schizophreniform disorder were unable to maintain interpersonal relationships as adolescents.

22. **The correct choice is E.** This infant is within normal limits. Infants do not begin to vocalize in the form of babbling, particularly in response to their mother's vocalizations, until about 8 weeks of age. The mother's question and concern is probably secondary to lack of experience and a bit of insecurity about her mothering skills and aptitude.

    There is no evidence that this child is pulling away from human contact (autism, **choice A**), not responding to noises (**choice B**) or visual cues (**choice D**) in the environment, or lacking other developmental milestones (mental retardation indices in infants, **choice C**).

23. **The correct answer is B.** The baby is exhibiting stranger anxiety, which normally occurs between the ages of 5 and 9 months.

    Let's review some other social milestones that are good to be aware of during clinical work in pediatrics:

    Spontaneous smiling begins within several days after birth and disappears by 3 months. Smiling at any face occurs by 2 months, followed quickly by smiling only at familiar faces and when pleased. By 3 months, infants can imitate facial expressions. They laugh at 4 months.

Crying occurs from birth. It peaks at 6 weeks and is most frequent from 4–6 PM. Colic is defined as crying more than 3 hours a day for more than 3 days a week. It often spontaneously resolves by 4 months. Treatment includes holding, avoiding overstimulation, and antispasmodics.

Separation anxiety occurs between the ages of 10 and 18 months, when the infant is separated from the mother.

Between the ages of 2 months and 2 years, children might show preference for a comforting "transitional object" (e.g., a teddy bear), which is usually discarded by age 4, when the transition from dependence on the mother to independence is more complete.

24. **The correct answer is C.** Suicide completers tend to be male, older, and white. They typically use lethal methods (e.g., guns, jumping from high places), are recently divorced or separated, live alone, have made previous suicide attempts, have a major affective disorder (major depressive disorder or bipolar disorder), and/or are alcoholic. Patients of high socioeconomic status have a higher rate of successfully committing suicide than those of lower socioeconomic status.

25. **The correct answer is B.** Projection involves attributing one's own traits, feelings, and attitudes to someone else. This swimmer's harsh criticism of her teammates' abilities is a reflection of her personal feeling of incompetence. (Doubts about her own ability are translated into doubts about her teammates' aptitude.)

Displacement (**choice A**) involves the automatic transferring of a wish or an affect from one object to a substitute. For example, a man who is angry at his wife releases his hostility by kicking the table.

Reaction formation (**choice C**) involves turning a repressed impulse or unconscious wish to its opposite. For example, a man who is attracted to his brother's wife develops an aversion to her personality.

Repression (**choice D**) occurs when the conflicting thought or feeling is automatically hidden from the person's awareness. Forgetting an emotionally charged event is an example of repression.

Sublimation (**choice E**) is a very mature mechanism that involves consciously turning socially unacceptable impulses into acceptable or more benign forms. For example, a young college girl immerses herself in athletics rather than engage in premarital sex.

26. **The correct answer is C.** The patient has schizophrenia. The key to the diagnosis of psychosis is that there has been a marked decline in the level of functioning (i.e., the man is homeless and cannot care for himself). Although hallucinations or delusions are not mentioned

in the case history, the presence of disorganized speech and grossly disorganized behavior and the duration of symptoms (longer than 6 months) suggest a diagnosis of schizophrenia.

In schizoaffective disorder (**choice A**), alterations in mood are present during a substantial portion of the illness.

Although schizoid personality disorder (**choice B**) produces detachment from social relationships and is characterized by restriction of emotional expression, it is not accompanied by a marked decline in occupational functioning.

Schizophreniform disorder (**choice D**) is characterized by schizophrenic-like symptoms, but the duration of symptoms is, by definition, less than 6 months.

Schizotypal personality disorder (**choice E**) is characterized by eccentricities of behavior, odd beliefs or magical thinking, and difficulties with social and interpersonal relationships. Unlike schizophrenia, schizotypal personality disorder is not characterized by a formal thought disorder.

27. **The correct answer is C.** The sensorium section of the Mental Status Examination contains information on orientation, attention-concentration, memory functioning, and other related subjects. When the examining physician discovers problems in these areas, he or she should assume there is an underlying organic/neurologic process, until proven otherwise. That is, although disruptions here can result from other conditions (**choices A, B, D, and E**), the organic possibilities should always be ruled out first.

28. **The correct answer is B.** In an obese patient, loud snoring, daytime drowsiness, and falling asleep while driving are all classic clues to the diagnosis of obstructive sleep apnea. Sleep apnea is defined as the cessation of air flow for at least 10 seconds. Obstructive apnea is the most common type and is caused by muscle atonia in the oropharynx, obstruction by the tongue or tonsils, or nasal obstruction. Contributing factors include obesity, alcohol or sedative use, and hypothyroidism.

Central sleep apnea (**choice A**) occurs when the medulla does not respond to the accumulation of CO_2 in the blood. It almost always occurs in children and has been considered to be one of the causes of SIDS (sudden infant death syndrome). Typically, the child is cyanotic on awakening.

Narcolepsy (**choice C**) is a chronic disorder in which there is sudden onset of REM sleep at inopportune times. Since the patient abruptly falls asleep without warning, the condition can be dangerous. You might have considered this as part of your differential diagnosis, given the complaint of suddenly falling asleep at the wheel, but the clues provided strongly imply obstructive sleep apnea as the cause.

Pavor nocturnus (**choice D**) is the technical term for night terrors. This familial disorder often co-occurs with sleepwalking. Patients suddenly sit up in bed looking terrified. They scream, are inconsolable, cannot converse, and may run from the room. Patients generally have no recollection of the event. It is usually a childhood disorder, although it occurs in some adults.

Somnambulism (**choice E**) is the technical term for sleepwalking. This familial disorder is characterized by episodes of clumsy walking that last several minutes during sleep. The syndrome usually abates by puberty.

29. **The correct answer is E.** Secobarbital is a short-acting barbiturate with considerable dependence potential. Withdrawal from short-acting barbiturates can produce anxiety, delirium, and seizures, which may be accompanied by life-threatening cardiovascular collapse.

Insomnia (**choice A**) is a complication of barbiturate withdrawal, since barbiturates are sedative/hypnotic agents; however, this complication is not serious enough to be a contraindication to abrupt cessation of the drug.

Rebound anxiety (**choice B**) would be quite likely following abrupt cessation of the barbiturate but would not constitute a sufficient danger to the patient to preclude self-detoxification.

Recidivism (**choice C**) is quite likely in drug abusers, with or without medical intervention.

Respiratory depression (**choice D**) is common with acute administration of barbiturates but would not be expected with barbiturate abstinence.

30. **The correct answer is C.** This is one of those questions for which predicting the correct answer will facilitate your selecting the appropriate answer choice. Make sure to read each choice carefully (for example, choices D and E, though both incorrect in this case, look almost identical and could cost you points if you were not reading actively).

Choice A refers to the crude mortality rate.

Choice B refers to the postnatal mortality rate.

Choice D is an incorrect rendering of the neonatal mortality rate, since it considers the total number of births instead of the total number of live births.

Choice E refers to the neonatal mortality rate.

31. **The correct answer is C.** The physician should obtain an emergency order of detention, regardless of her threats of a lawsuit. The woman clearly still has suicidal intent, demonstrated by her expressed verbalizations, and is therefore a danger to herself.

Choices A, B, and D clearly place her in a position where she can carry out her plans to terminate her life.

Sedating her (**choice E**) is the second best choice since it will prevent her from taking her life; however, sedation does not give therapists the opportunity to address the underlying motivations for her suicidal ideation.

32. **The correct answer is C.** This woman is demonstrating the symptoms of trichotillomania, which is similar to Tourette syndrome in that the behavior of hair pulling is preceded by an impulse or pressured feeling. It is unlike obsessive compulsive disorder, which is preceded by a cognition to do something. The best medication would be fluvoxamine, a serotonin specific reuptake inhibitor.

Clozapine (**choice A**) works in the dopaminergic system and has not demonstrated potential in this disorder.

Diazepam (**choice B**) works in the GABA system and likewise has demonstrated little efficacy for trichotillomania.

Lithium (**choice D**) has demonstrated only limited success in trichotillomania.

Verapamil (**choice E**) is a calcium channel blocker that has no demonstrated efficacy in this disorder.

33. **The correct answer is C.** This man is inducing signs and reporting symptoms that are all consistent with passing a kidney stone. However, he is not seeking treatment for the condition; rather, he is requesting narcotics. This is a favorite manipulation by drug-addicted persons, particularly at a time of the evening when they cannot get to their primary care physician. By providing the information that the pain is now migrating to the testicle, the patient is increasing the pressure on the physician to provide narcotics.

Antisocial personality disorder (**choice A**) is not correct since the history provides no information about past behaviors that are against society. This man may warrant such a diagnosis if the full history is obtained and support for the diagnosis is present. His requesting narcotics suggests an addiction, and many persons with substance abuse diagnoses also have antisocial personality disorders. However, there is not enough information to warrant this diagnosis at this time.

Factitious disorder (**choice B**) is the major differential diagnosis in this man since he is actively producing symptoms to obtain something. However, in factitious disorder, the individual is seeking to enter the "sick role," that is, the person obtains primary gain. However, in the malingering person, the gain is secondary (e.g., obtaining drugs or money, hiding from the police in the hospital).

Schizotypal personality disorder (**choice D**) is incorrect because disturbed interpersonal relations are not apparent in this man's background, nor are there any other signs or symptoms of the diagnosis.

Somatization disorder (**choice E**) is incorrect since this diagnosis requires multiple symptoms in multiple systems of the body; this man is presenting with only two symptoms in one system.

34. **The correct answer is A.** Classic conditioning involves the response toward one stimulus being transferred to another stimulus. For example, a patient who fears going to the doctor experiences heightened anxiety as the physician enters the room wearing a white coat. The patient's fear then becomes associated with the white coat itself, such that future exposure to this symbol evokes similar apprehension.

Extinction (**choice B**) means that when a behavior is no longer reinforced, it will disappear.

Habit hierarchies (**choice C**) are ordered statements about the probability of occurrence of behaviors. Those behaviors that have been reinforced more strongly will be more likely to occur and will therefore be ranked higher in the response hierarchy.

Negative reinforcement (**choice D**) occurs when, in response to a behavior, an aversive condition is removed rather than a positive reward being given. For example, a teenager may finally take out the garbage to stop his mother from nagging him. This is a method involved in operant conditioning (**choice E**), which is based on the relationship between a response and the consequences (reinforcement) that follow that response.

35. **The correct answer is E.** A relationship has been found between CSF levels of 5-hydroxy indoleacetic acid (5-HIAA) and impulsive aggression. 5-HIAA is a metabolite of serotonin (5-HT). Brainstem and CSF levels of 5-HIAA are decreased in individuals exhibiting impulsive aggression. Since most neurotransmitter systems work in concert with one another, the other listed systems may have secondary roles; however, serotonin is most strongly correlated with the behavior in question.

36. **The correct answer is A.** Continuous reinforcement, which means that a person is rewarded every time he or she performs a specific behavior, is the pattern of reinforcement least resistant to extinction. This is because the person soon becomes satiated with the

reward and no longer performs the desired behavior to obtain it. On the other hand, behaviors established on the basis of partial reinforcement are most resistant to extinction. The rest of the answer choices are variants of partial reinforcement schedules.

Fixed interval (**choice B**) reinforcement means that equal amounts of time must go by before the reward can be attained (e.g., if he cleans up his toys, he'll get an ice cream cone every Sunday).

Fixed ratio (**choice C**) reinforcement means that a given number of behaviors must be done before the reward is available (e.g., he must clean up his toys at least three times before getting an ice cream cone).

Variable interval (**choice D**) means that sometimes only 1 hour must go by, sometimes 3 hours, and so forth, before the reward is available (e.g., he might receive an ice cream cone the same night he cleaned up his toys or several days later).

Variable ratio (**choice E**) means that sometimes a behavior is rewarded the first time, sometimes the third, etc. (e.g., sometimes he would get an ice cream cone after cleaning up his toys on only one occasion, sometimes after four occasions).

37. **The correct answer is B.** It is important that the patient know the association between his self-destructive behavior and the physical sequelae. However, it is also important for cooperation in long-term management to not make the patient defensive by labeling him an alcoholic (**choice C**).

Equivocating with "I'm not sure" (**choice A**) or avoiding the patient's question (**choices D and E**) does not provide a basis for cooperative and mutual trust in the doctor–patient relationship.

38. **The correct answer is C.** Kubler-Ross's Death and Dying sequence is a step-wise process with five identified stages. The order in which these stages appear is the following: 1. Denial, 2. Anger, 3. Bargaining, 4. Sadness, and 5. Acceptance. "Doctor you must be wrong" is the correct answer since it reflects the patient's inability to accept the information and indicates the denial of the first stage.

"Can you keep me alive until my daughter graduates from medical school" (**choice A**), is a statement from the 3rd, bargaining stage.

"Damn you doctor, you should have caught this earlier" (**choice B**) is a statement from the 2nd or anger phase.

"I think it is time that I make a will and say good-bye to everyone" (**choice D**) reflects the patient's acceptance of the reality and is a statement from the 5th phase (acceptance).

"It's no use, I always lose and get the short end of the stick" (**choice E**) is a statement from the 4th phase (sadness).

39. **The correct answer is B.** In most instances in which a married person seeks sterilization, the spouse's consent is also needed. Such consent is not typically extended in cases of abortion.

Convincing the patient to use alternative contraception (**choice A**) is inappropriate because it ignores the patient's will.

Explaining that the chances of becoming pregnant are very low at her age (**choice C**) is factually incorrect, especially considering that she just gave birth at age 45.

Although patient confidentiality is important, not disclosing this patient's desire for sterilization to her husband (**choice D**) violates his autonomy with regard to having children in the future. Therefore, he must be involved in the decision-making process.

Refusing to do surgery because of her age (**choice E**) would be inappropriate because she is young and healthy enough to have just given birth.

40. **The correct answer is D.** This is a psychotic level disorder (the patient is hallucinating): she has a fluctuating level of consciousness and is disoriented. Also, there is a clear history of a febrile condition that developed rather rapidly, all of which suggest delirium.

In acute stress disorder (**choice A**) a traumatic event occurs that precipitates an anxiety-type reaction, not a change in the sensorium.

In both bipolar I disorder, manic type (**choice B**) and brief psychotic disorder (**choice C**), patients may reach a level of behavioral disruption of psychotic proportion. They do not, however, demonstrate changes in level of consciousness or major disorientation.

Persons with dementia (**choice E**) demonstrate a clear sensorium with no fluctuations in the level of consciousness. Additionally, persons with dementia predominantly show symptoms of impairment of cognitive functions (e.g., memory impairment).

41. **The correct answer is A.** People who have been injured and trapped in life-threatening conditions have the highest rates of post-disaster emotional problems.

People who are new immigrants to a given area are at heightened risk (unlike **choice B**).

People with prior emotional conditions (**choice C**) also have an increased risk, as do persons who recently lost a close relative (**choice D**), but neither of these are as traumatic as being trapped and fearing for one's life.

People at a great distance from the explosion (**choice E**) are at least risk.

42. **The correct answer is E.** This is an example of a placebo-controlled, double-blind randomized clinical trial. In this type of study, subjects with a particular disorder are randomized (the lottery) to receive either the treatment in question or a placebo. The information about whether the patient receives the treatment or the placebo is not known to either the subject or the investigator (double-blind). This type of study may be used to infer causality, i.e., if the patients taking the medication have more CD4+ T cells than the other group, it is due to the drug in question.

A case-control study (**choice A**) is a retrospective study that pairs known cases of a disease with matched controls. This type of study gives information about the importance of risk factors. The lack of a prospective design makes inferences about causality difficult.

A case report (**choice B**) is a published report of a single incidence of a disease in a subject. This is usually done for rare diseases, or for rare associations of a disease with a particular risk factor.

A cohort study (**choice C**) is an observational (non-interventional) study that tracks subjects prospectively. This type of study gives a measure of incidence of a disease.

A cross-sectional study (**choice D**) samples at a selected point in time, matching individuals with the disease with controls without the disease. The lack of a prospective design makes inferences about causality difficult.

43. **The correct response is C.** An IQ of 53 places the individual in the upper level of moderate mental retardation. Such individuals would be expected to be able to work in a sheltered workshop situation and be assisted during times of mild social or economic stress. They can usually achieve self-maintenance in unskilled or semiskilled work under sheltered conditions. However, they do need supervision and guidance when under mild social or economic stress. As a consequence, they may do better living in a group home where there are "house-parents" on whom they can depend.

Choices A and B reflect expectations that are too high for a person of this IQ. However, persons with mild mental retardation can function at these levels.

Choices D and E are the highest expectations for severe and profound mental retardation, respectively.

44. **The correct answer is A.** Incidence is the number of new cases of a disease in a given period of time.

Lifetime expectancy (**choice B**) is the total probability of a person having a particular condition in his or her lifetime.

Lifetime prevalence (**choice C**) is the number of people who state that they have had a particular condition in their lifetime (e.g., 10% of adults state they have been alcoholic at some time in their life).

Period prevalence (**choice D**) is the number of people who have a disorder during a specified time period (longer than a calendar day or point in time).

Point prevalence (**choice E**) is the total number of cases of a condition at a given point in time.

45. **The correct answer is E.** Specificity is the proportion of persons who do not have the disease and are correctly identified by the test as being disease-free. It is given by TN/(FP + TN), where TN stands for true negatives (people who do not have the disease and test negative) and FP stands for false positives (people who do not have the disease but test positive). In this case, 95/(5 + 95) = 95/100 = 0.95.

46. **The correct answer is C.** Neuroleptic malignant syndrome (NMS) is a potentially fatal condition that can occur at any time during the course of treatment with neuroleptics. The exact etiology is unknown. Excessive muscle contraction produces muscular rigidity and is also responsible for the high temperature. The obtunded mental state and mutism are characteristic. Muscle relaxants, such as dantrolene, and dopamine agonists, such as bromocriptine, are used in the treatment of NMS.

Acute dystonia (**choice A**; prolonged contractions of muscle groups), akathisia (**choice B**; "restless legs"), and parkinsonism (**choice D**; pill-rolling tremor and rigidity) are all extrapyramidal side effects that occur early during neuroleptic treatment.

Tardive dyskinesia (**choice E**) is a late-appearing complication of neuroleptic therapy characterized by perioral and athetoid movements.

47. **The correct answer is D.** Although electroconvulsive therapy (ECT) is highly efficacious in treating major depressions that are refractory to tricyclic antidepressants and selective serotonin reuptake inhibitors, it produces retrograde amnesia as its major side effect.

Extrapyramidal symptoms (**choice A**) are commonly produced by acute administration of antipsychotic drugs, such as phenothiazines or butyrophenones, not ECT.

Hearing loss (**choice B**) is not a common side effect of ECT.

Mania (**choice C**) is not a recognized side effect of ECT.

Rhabdomyolysis (**choice E**) does not generally occur with ECT when it is performed correctly, with the administration of skeletal muscle relaxants.

48. **The correct answer is A.** Bipolar disorder, type I, is the appropriate diagnosis because she has had repeated manic episodes. The inappropriate grandiose activity with her clients' accounts (without the benefit of consultation), decreased need for sleep, and involvement in potentially self-destructive behavior (e.g., excessive alcohol consumption) support this diagnosis.

There is no history of depressive episodes, which is mandatory for the diagnosis of bipolar disorder, type II (**choice B**).

Since her behavior is of psychotic proportion, and there is no history of depressive episodes, cyclothymic disorder (**choice C**) is incorrect.

Persons with schizophrenic disorder, paranoid type (**choice D**), have a major thought and affect disorder, and characteristically hallucinate. During an episode, they are unable to function in reality, e.g., selling and buying securities on the stock market. She demonstrates no such behavior.

The hallmark of delirium (**choice E**) is a fluctuating level of consciousness. There are no indications in the history that she is manifesting this symptom.

49. **The correct answer is A.** The concrete operational period (ages 7-11 years) is defined by the child's awareness of the conservation of volume, which demonstrates that the child is able to reason in a logical way in terms of the physical world. Note that the child does not develop understanding of abstract concepts until he or she has reached the formal operational stage (**choice B**), at age 11 to adulthood.

The preoperational stage (**choice C**), ages 2 to 7 years, is associated with significant language development. However, the child has not yet developed the ability to take the perspective of others; thus, the child's thinking tends to remain egocentric.

The sensorimotor stage (**choice D**) corresponds to ages 0 to 2 years and is characterized by the infant developing increasingly sophisticated sensorimotor skills and behavior patterns.

Piaget's theory of the development of cognition does not include motorsensory (**choice E**), which is a "look-alike" distractor.

50. **The correct answer is D.** This is a case of operant conditioning, or learning by reinforcement. In this example, the child's behavior is the operant, which is being reinforced by the parents. That is, the child wants parental attention and is rewarded by the parents only when her disruptive behavior escalates to the point at

which the parents must pay attention. The parents are using a "fixed-ratio" of reinforcement, since every time the child gets to the truly disruptive point, they reinforce the behavior.

Classical conditioning (**choice A**) is the type of associative learning in which a stimulus that did not originally elicit a given response now does. This occurs secondary to association of the stimulus with a behavior that previously did elicit the response. For example, a cat does not normally come to its owner if the owner rings a bell. However, if the bell is rung while the cat is eating, the cat associates the bell with food and learns to come to the owner when the bell is rung.

Cognitive learning (**choice B**) requires full attention and purposeful intent to acquire the information.

Imprinting (**choice C**) forms the basis of bonding between an infant and the mothering figure. This form of attachment is learned by association during the immediate postnatal period.

Social learning (**choice E**) involves modeling or imitation. For instance, a child learns familial values by modeling the parental example.

1. A 50-year-old woman presents with back pain. On examination of her lumbar spine, T1-T4 all have posterior right transverse processes. When testing side-bending you also notice that the left shoulder depresses more easily as compared with the right. The most likely diagnosis is

   (A) type I somatic dysfunction; T1-T4 rotated right, sidebent left

   (B) type I somatic dysfunction; T1-T4 rotated right, sidebent right

   (C) type II somatic dysfunction; T1-T4 rotated right, sidebent right

   (D) type II somatic dysfunction; T1-T4 rotated right, sidebent left

   (E) type I somatic dysfunction; T1-T4 rotated left, sidebent left

2. A 63-year-old woman with COPD will have chronically tender hypomobile and fibrotic paraspinal musculature at which of the following segments?

   (A) C3-C5

   (B) T2-T4

   (C) T9-T12

   (D) L1-L2

   (E) L3-L5

3. A 56-year-old man with ulcerative colitis has ropy and fibrotic paraspinal musculature on the left at T12-L2 spinal segments. These tissue texture changes represent

   (A) somatic dysfunction resulting from visceral symptoms by way of parasympathetic autonomic fibers

   (B) somatic dysfunction resulting from abnormal stimuli from the lateral corticospinal tract (fix 120)

   (C) somatic dysfunction resulting from visceral dysfunction by way of visceral afferent fibers

   (D) visceral dysfunction resulting from abnormal stimuli from the ventral corticospinal tract (fix 121)

   (E) visceral dysfunction resulting from visceral symptoms by way of parasympathetic autonomic fibers

4. A 33-year-old patient with a history of acute right-sided low back pain presents to your office. He states the back pain worsens when he stands erect. The pain lessens with flexion of the lumbar spine. Pain is localized to the low back and does not radiate. Structural examination reveals a tender point medial to the right ASIS, L1 flexed, rotated, and sidebent to the right. Leg lengths are equal. ASISs and PSISs appear equal. The sacrum is symmetrical and springs freely. Neurologic evaluation is normal. X-rays demonstrate an increased lumbo-sacral (Ferguson's) angle, but there is no evidence of degenerative joint disease. Given the patient's symptoms, which of the following is most likely to be true?

   (A) This patient will have a positive seated flexion test.

   (B) This patient will have a positive Thomas test.

   (C) This patient is most likely to have a herniated lumbar disc.

   (D) This patient has a bilateral sacral extension and therefore will have a false-negative seated flexion test.

   (E) This patient is likely to have a somatic dysfunction in the right lower extremity.

5. The above patient (in Question 4) will most likely benefit from which of the following treatments?

   (A) Muscle energy to the sacrum

   (B) Therapeutic stretching to the hip extensors

   (C) Muscle energy to the pelvis

   (D) Counterstrain to the iliopsoas

   (E) OMT is contraindicated due to the likelihood of a herniated disc

6. Examination of a 40-year-old woman reveals tender points over the right articular pillar of the third cervical segment. Using the principles of strain/counterstrain, which of the following positions is most likely to decrease the pain?

   (A) Extension, left sidebending, and left rotation

   (B) Extension, right sidebending, and right rotation

   (C) Flexion, left sidebending, and left rotation

   (D) Flexion and right sidebending

   (E) Flexion only

Questions 7-9

CASE A

A 71-year-old man comes to the emergency department complaining of abdominal pain and a temperature of 39.0 C (102.2 F). On examination he has left lower quadrant tenderness with some guarding and rebound tenderness. He states that recently he has been constipated, but denies any rectal bleeding.

7. At which of the following locations would you expect to find a Chapman point?

   (A) Anterior left thigh in the rectus femoris muscle

   (B) Tip of the left twelfth rib

   (C) Left ischial tuberosity

   (D) Lateral left thigh in the iliotibial band

   (E) Left of the spinous process of T12

8. The pain generated from this patient's condition is caused by nociceptive afferents by way of which nerve?

   (A) Greater splanchnic nerve

   (B) Lesser splanchnic nerve

   (C) Least splanchnic nerve

   (D) Vagus nerve

   (E) Phrenic nerve

9. A 56-year-old woman presents to your office with right-sided neck and shoulder pain. Occasionally, the pain radiates to her elbow and hand. The pain started last week after she finished painting her guest bedroom ceiling. She states that the pain is now associated with any movement of her right arm over her head. Pain is relieved with rest and Tylenol. On examination she has a tender point at the insertion of the anterior scalene on the right. C3 is flexed and rotated right, rib 1 is elevated on the right, and T1 is extended and sidebent left. She has full active range of motion in her shoulder without any signs of impingement. Abduction and extension of the shoulder with external rotation of the arm produces radiation of the pain down the shoulder and hand. The patient's right arm is then abducted with palpation of the radial pulse. She then is instructed to turn her head to the right side; there is an absent radial pulse. X-rays of the cervical spine show mild degenerative joint disease. Given all of this information, which of the following statements is most accurate?

   (A) C3 should be placed in extension, right rotation, and left sidebending, to correct the dysfunction using rotatory HVLA thrust

   (B) This patient most likely has supraspinatus tendonitis

   (C) Under the principles of postisometric relaxation muscle energy, the right anterior scalene can be used to correct the dysfunction at rib 1

   (D) This patient has compression of the neurovascular bundle as it exits the thoracic outlet

   (E) This patient most likely has C6 radiculopathy from cervical stenosis

Questions 10 and 11

<u>CASE B</u>

A 23-year-old male was working on his car when suddenly he burnt his hand, causing him to extend his lumbosacral spine suddenly. He immediately felt back pain. He presented to your office the following day hyperextended and laterally flexed to the left. There is an increased lumbar lordosis. He is comfortable lying supine, but the pain significantly worsens when seated or with forward flexion. There is a positive hip drop test.

10. Spasm of what muscle most likely caused this somatic dysfunction?

   (A) Lumbar paraspinals
   (B) Piriformis
   (C) Iliopsoas
   (D) Gluteus medius
   (E) Quadratus lumborum

11. Articular mobility of the muscle spasm (in the previous question) is most likely to cause somatic dysfunction of what structure?

   (A) 12th rib
   (B) Lumbar
   (C) Sacrum
   (D) Leg
   (E) Innominate

12. A 49-year-old female has the "worst headache of her life." It started suddenly without a history of trauma. She has a left facial droop, and she has developed weakness and parasthesias in her left arm. Which of the following osteopathic treatments is indicated initially to improve the patient's symptoms?

   (A) Occipital condylar decompression to improve the patient's headache
   (B) Cervical fascial release
   (C) Thoracic inlet release to promote lymphatic drainage from the head and neck
   (D) Sympathetic chain ganglion inhibition to normalize sympathetics to the face and upper extremity
   (E) All osteopathic treatment is contraindicated in this patient due to the acute nature of this illness.

Questions 13-15

<u>CASE C</u>

13. A 14-year-old male presents with nausea, vomiting, and abdominal pain for 48 hours. His temperature is 101 C. The pain originally started in the midepigastric area, but now the pain is localized to the right lower quadrant. There is rebound tenderness and guarding. The WBC count is 18,000 with a left shift. Flat and upright of the abdomen is negative. This patient is most likely to have somatic dysfunction in which of the following muscles?

   (A) Piriformis
   (B) Iliopsoas
   (C) Paraspinals
   (D) Gluteus maximus
   (E) Rectus abdominus

14. Where would you expect to find small facial or "ganglioform" contractions?

   (A) The tip of the 12th rib
   (B) Umbilicus
   (C) One cm lateral to the L1 spinous process
   (D) One cm superior to the umbilicus
   (E) Rib angle of Ribs 10-12

15. At which structure would you most likely find a somatic dysfunction?

   (A) C5
   (B) T1
   (C) T5
   (D) T12
   (E) L5

16. An 11-year-old presents to your office for a routine sports physical and scoliosis screen. Neurologic examination is normal. On musculoskeletal examination, there is no evidence of joint instability. The most cost-effective way to screen for scoliosis is:

    (A) Ask the patient to stand while you examine for lateral spinal curves.

    (B) Ask the patient to stand, then bend over to touch his toes while you look for a paraspinal hump.

    (C) Order standing postural X-rays to evaluate for sacral base unleveling.

    (D) Order lumbar spine views (anterior-posterior and lateral views).

    (E) Perform a standing flexion test to evaluate sacral base unleveling.

17. A 3-year-old male with a persistent fever, stridor, severe sore throat, and cough for two days presents to the emergency room. The mother states that the child refuses to take any solids or liquids. She also states that he has this "barking" type of cough. Physical examination demonstrates a well developed male in no respiratory distress; however, lung auscultation reveals bilateral rhonchi. Osteopathic manipulation to which of the following structures will most likely influence parasympathetic tone in the lungs?

    (A) AA

    (B) T1

    (C) T5

    (D) L2

    (E) S3

18. A 27-year-old female is post-op Day 2 from a cesarean section. She is reluctant to get out of bed secondary to pain. She has not had a bowel movement since surgery. Which osteopathic technique is most likely to relieve her constipation?

    (A) Thoracic rib raising and paraspinal inhibition

    (B) Myofascial release to the thoracolumbar fascia

    (C) Muscle energy and HVLA to her thoracic and lumbar somatic dysfunctions

    (D) Thoracoabdominal diaphragm release to improve abdominal lymph return

    (E) Liver and spleen lymphatic pump

19. A 24-year-old nonsmoking male presents to your office with fever, congestion, sore throat, and rhinorrhea for 24 hours. On examination, his throat is slightly erythem-atous with tonsil enlargement and exudates. His lungs are clear, and there is no evidence of ego-phony. Monospot (test for mononucleosis) is negative. After appropriate treatment with antibiotics, which osteopathic treatment would you perform initially to improve lymphatic drainage from the head and neck?

    (A) Lymphatic pump techniques

    (B) Thoracic inlet fascia release

    (C) Release of the pelvic diaphragm

    (D) Counterstrain to the cervical tenderpoints

    (E) Decrease lateral curvature of the spine

20. A patient presents to your office with a "stitch in her right side." She states that it occurred yesterday while she was gardening. The pain worsens with deep inspiration, and there is a tender point at the inferior border of the 12th rib. On examination, you notice Rib 12 has limited motion in inhalation. You decide to treat the patient with osteopathic manipulation. In addition to treating the thoracolumbar junction, you wish to perform counterstrain on the tender point. Which muscle would your treatment be directed toward?

    (A) Psoas major

    (B) Serratus anterior

    (C) Quadratus lumborum

    (D) Levator costarum

    (E) Transversus abdominis

21. A patient presents to your office with low back pain. While lying prone, the lumbar spine appears to have a lateral convexity to the left, and all appear to have transverse processes posterior on the left. What would your diagnosis be?

    (A) Type II mechanics with the lumbar spine sidebent left, rotated left

    (B) Type II mechanics with the lumbar spine sidebent right, rotated right

    (C) Type I mechanics with the lumbar spine sidebent right, rotated left

    (D) Type I mechanics with the lumbar spine sidebent left, rotated right

    (E) There is not enough information given to make a correct diagnosis.

22. A 27-year-old female presents to your office with gluteal pain. The pain started immediately after picking up her five-year-old son. The pain is sharp and is localized to the sacroiliac area. On examination, you find a positive seated flexion test on the right, her left ILA is posterior compared to her right, and her superior sulcus is deeper on the right than the left. The lumbosacral spring test is negative. And you notice her lumbar curve is convex to the right. Assuming the patient has a sacral torsion, what would be the somatic dysfunction at L5?

    (A) L5 NS_LR_R

    (B) L5 FR_LS_L

    (C) L5 ER_RS_R

    (D) L5 NS_RR_L

    (E) L5 FR_RS_R

23. A 25-year-old female is complaining of gluteal pain. She states that the pain started after biking several miles. She appears mildly obese and is not physically active. On examination, you notice that the sacral sulci are equal in depth, but there is no springing at the sacral base. The seated and standing flexion tests are both negative. Based on the information given, what is the most likely diagnosis?

    (A) Unilateral extended sacrum on the right

    (B) Anterior sacral base

    (C) Unilateral extended sacrum on the left

    (D) Posterior sacral base

    (E) Forward sacral torsion on a left oblique axis

24. A patient has a posterior transverse process on the right when he bends backwards. Flexion yields no asymmetry. Which of the following is the correct treatment position for a direct technique?

    (A) Flexed, rotated left, sidebent left

    (B) Flexed, rotated right, sidebent right

    (C) Extended, rotated right, sidebent right

    (D) Extended, rotated left, sidebent left

    (E) Neutral, rotated right, sidebent left

25. A 25-year-old medical student is complaining of right-sided low back/sacroiliac pain. The pain started one week ago while studying for board exams. On examination, you notice tenderness over the right SI joint, a positive seated flexion test on the left, the sacral sulcus on the left is anterior, whereas the right ILA is posterior. Based on the information given, what is the most likely diagnosis?

    (A) Left sacral rotation on a left oblique axis (L on L)

    (B) Left sacral rotation on a right oblique axis (L on R)

    (C) Right sacral torsion on a left oblique axis (R on L)

    (D) Right sacral torsion on a right oblique axis (R on R)

    (E) Unilateral sacral flexion on the right (USF_R)

26. A 30-year-old male runner presents with left-sided low back pain and left hip pain. The pain started yesterday after a five-mile run. It is sharp but does not radiate into the lower extremities. On examination, you notice he has a positive standing flexion test on the left, his left ASIS is inferior, the left PSIS is superior, sacral sulci appear symmetrical, and it is freely mobile. Based on the information given, what is the most likely diagnosis?

    (A) Left superior innominate shear

    (B) Left anterior innominate

    (C) Left posterior innominate

    (D) Unilateral sacral flexion on the left (USF_L)

    (E) Left sacral rotation on a right oblique axis (L on R)

27. A patient recently fell forward on an outstretched arm. Unfortunately, he hyperextended his wrist during the fall. Now he is experiencing wrist pain. The wrist is warm, slightly edematous, and there is significantly decreased range of motion of the wrist and forearm. There is pain to palpation on the volar aspect of the wrist. Pulses are normal and sensation is intact to the wrist and hand. X-rays of the wrist are negative. Which of the following statements is true regarding this patient's injury?

    (A) Despite the negative X-rays, this patient most likely has a fracture of the scaphoid bone.

    (B) Due to the decreased range of motion and edema, this patient has a somatic dysfunction of the wrist.

    (C) Due to the severely decreased range of motion, this patient has a complete ligament tear.

    (D) The extent of his injuries is limited only to his wrist.

    (E) Due to the likelihood of a nondisplaced fracture of the scaphoid, this patient should be empirically treated with closed reduction and external fixation with percutaneous pinning.

28. A 65-year-old male with a 10-year history of osteoarthritis presents to your office for a routine physical. He states that his arthritis mostly affects his right knee. Overall, he states that he is currently in good health, but his right knee is still causing him some pain, especially in the morning when he notices that it is very stiff. He denies any recent trauma to the knee, and asks you if you could examine it. What are some findings you would expect to see when examining his knee?

    (A) Edematous, boggy tissue with palpation; full range of motion of the knee with some crepitus

    (B) Erythema of local tissues; significant effusion; decreased range of motion of the knee with some crepitus

    (C) Severe, sharp pain with palpation; hypertonic muscles; decreased range of motion of the knee with no crepitus

    (D) Little to no edema or erythema; cool, dry skin to palpation; ropy and fibrotic muscles; decreased range of motion of the knee with some crepitus

    (E) Severe sharp pain with palpation; anterior laxity; significant effusion; and a positive bounce home test

29. A patient has a posterior transverse process on the right at the second thoracic segment; symmetry is restored when the segment is flexed. When treating with muscle energy, which of the following is the best statement?

    (A) Treatment is directed at the apex of the group dysfunction.

    (B) T2 would have to be laterally flexed to the left and rotated to the right to correctly reverse all three planes of motion.

    (C) T2 would have to be placed in a neutral position, rotated, and sidebent to the left.

    (D) With the patient's right arm behind his head and his left arm holding his right elbow the practitioner can manipulate his torso so that extension, rotation, and sidebending is isolated at T2.

    (E) T2 should be extended, rotated, and sidebent toward the restrictive barrier.

30. When examining a patient you notice thoracic segments T3-T5 are rotated right. Which of the following is the best statement regarding this somatic dysfunction?

    (A) T3 is rotated right, sidebent right.

    (B) Ribs 3-5 are limited in inhalation on the right.

    (C) T4's right transverse process is more caudad.

    (D) T5 is limited in right sidebending compared with T6.

    (E) T4's right transverse process is more anterior.

31. When evaluating range of motion of a patient's neck, you ask the patient to rotate his head to the right and then to the left as far as he can. He demonstrates that he is unable to fully rotate his head to the right without causing pain, but he is able to rotate his head 90° to the left without pain. You assess his range of motion to be approximately 45° to the right and 90° to the left. Which of the following statements is true regarding this patient's range of motion?

    (A) This patient demonstrated that he has limited passive range of motion with right rotation.

    (B) The patient demonstrated full left rotation to his physiologic barrier.

    (C) The patient has limited passive range of motion with right rotation, but he may have full active range of motion with right rotation.

    (D) Since the patient has limited right rotation, he must have limited left sidebending.

    (E) Since the patient has limited right rotation, he must have limited right sidebending.

32. While evaluating a patient's neck pain, you notice that when the head is in the forward flexed position to 45°, you can only turn his head approximately 75° to the left, whereas you can turn his head 90° to the right. Given this information, what else would you expect to find on this patient?

    (A) His occiput would resist left translation.

    (B) Using the index and middle fingers in the suboccipital triangle, the occiput will resist anterior glide on the right.

    (C) Segments C2-C4 will resist right sidebending.

    (D) The lower cervical segments will be rotated to the right to compensate for the somatic dysfunction of the upper segments.

    (E) The atlas will resist left rotation.

33. While evaluating a patient's upper back pain, you notice that T3's transverse process is posterior on the right. Flexing T3 worsens the asymmetry, while extension returns T3 to the neutral plane. What can be said regarding the somatic dysfunction of T3?

(A) Somatic dysfunction at T3 is consistent with that of type II mechanics where rotation and sidebending are in opposite directions.

(B) Due to the biomechanics of the thoracic spine, flexion of the patient's head will cause relative extension of T2 on T3.

(C) T3 will resist left rotation in the extended position.

(D) Extension of the spine will allow T3 to return to type I mechanics where sidebending and rotation are to opposite sides.

(E) Flexing T3 will limit its rotation to the left.

34. In a patient with low back pain, L3 seems to have a dysfunction that moved in a sagittal plane and around a vertical axis. Which of the following dysfunctions best describes the position of L3?

(A) L3 is neutral, sidebent right, rotated left.

(B) L3 is extended, rotated right, sidebent right.

(C) L3 is rotated right.

(D) L3 is sidebent left.

(E) L3 is extended.

35. A patient with knee pain presents to your office. In addition to medication and osteopathic treatment, you decide to facilitate the patient's recovery with exercises that would strengthen the knee. You instruct the patient to lie supine with the knees extended. You tell the patient that while in this position, tighten the quadriceps with the knee in full extension; hold for five seconds and relax. Which one of the following statements correctly describes this type of exercise?

(A) Isotonic contraction, in which there is an increase in quadriceps tension

(B) Eccentric contraction, in which there is no increase in quadriceps tension

(C) Isometric contraction, in which there is an increase in quadriceps tension

(D) Concentric contraction, in which there is no increase in quadriceps tension

(E) Isometric contraction, in which there is no increase in quadriceps tension

36. A patient complaining of back pain is found to have midthoracic paraspinal tender points, as well as a somatic dysfunction of T4. Further examination of T4 reveals restriction in extension and right rotation. You decide to use a direct, active technique. Which of the following best describes the treatment position for this patient?

(A) Extend, rotate, and sidebend T4 to the right until there is tension. Then ask the patient to rotate to the left for 3-5 seconds. Repeat this 3-5 times.

(B) Extend, rotate, and sidebend T4 to the left until there is an ease of motion. Then ask the patient to breathe deeply and relax. Wait approximately 90 seconds, then return the patient to the neutral position.

(C) Extend, rotate, and sidebend T4 to the right until there is tension. Then wait for a release in muscular tension and slowly return to the neutral position.

(D) With the patient supine and arms crossed, place your thenar eminence under the posterior transverse process and flex the patient's until tension is built up at T4. Have the patient take a deep breath in and exhale. At end exhalation direct an HVLA thrust downward (toward the table).

(E) Locate a tender point within the paraspinals. Extend, rotate, and sidebend the patient so that there is relief of tenderness. Wait approximately 90 seconds. Then slowly return the patient to the neutral position.

37. An 86-year-old female with coronary artery disease, congestive heart failure, diabetes mellitus, COPD, and hypertension is recovering from a bilateral pneumonia. She was intubated for two weeks in the intensive care unit. After a long hospitalization, she was transferred to a skilled nursing facility. Since her infection she has been bedridden. She now complains of back pain. Understanding her fragile state, you decide to ease her back pain with osteopathic manipulation. Which one of the following treatment protocols is best suited for this patient?

    (A) Myofascial release to the thoraco-lumbar junction, followed by gentle high-velocity low-amplitude treatment

    (B) Indirect treatments to the lumbar fascia, followed by direct gentle articulatory techniques

    (C) Rib raising to help with respiration, followed by muscle energy to the pelvis and lumbar somatic dysfunctions

    (D) Myofascial release of the sacrum, followed by isotonic exercises to strengthen the lumbar spine

    (E) Low-velocity moderate-amplitude techniques, followed by gentle isometric exercises to strengthen the lumbar spine

38. A 26-year-old female was in a motor vehicle accident 24 hours ago. She was a restrained driver, but now she is complaining of neck pain. She states that she has severe sharp pain on the right side of the neck, and it does not radiate. She does not have any numbness or tingling in her extremities. Spurling's maneuver is negative. Neurologic exam, including muscle strength testing, is normal. She has limited range of motion with right rotation of the neck and paraspinal tenderness. Tissues are edematous, erythematous, boggy with increased moisture, and muscles are hypertonic. X-rays show a straightening of the cervical lordosis but no fracture. Given the above information, what osteopathic treatment is most appropriate for this patient?

    (A) Muscle energy to the cervical spine to increase her range of motion

    (B) Thoracic inlet release

    (C) Counterstrain to cervical tender points

    (D) High-velocity low-amplitude techniques to her cervical spine

    (E) Direct myofascial release to her cervical spine

39. A 76-year-old male with a history of coronary artery disease, diabetes, and prostate cancer is complaining of back pain. He noticed that the back pain started about two months ago. The pain developed gradually and has persisted, despite over-the-counter ibuprofen and heating pads. On examination, he has mild paraspinal tenderness; the tissue is ropy and fibrotic. The thoraco-lumbar vertebrae appear to be rotated right and side-bent left. He has tight hamstrings on the left, as well as a left on left sacral torsion. In addition to ordering laboratory work and lumbar spine X-rays, you decide to do osteopathic manipulation. Which treatment protocol is best suited for this patient?

    (A) Myofascial release to the sacrum, followed by HVLA to the thoracolumbar junction

    (B) Myofascial release to the thoracolumbar fascia, followed by a pelvic diaphragm release

    (C) Counterstrain on the lumbar paraspinals with the lumbar spine in hyperextension, followed by gentle indirect myofascial release to the pelvis

    (D) Pelvic diaphragm release, followed by HVLA to the thoracolumbar junction

    (E) Indirect myofascial treatment to the thoracolumbar vertebrae and sacrum, followed by gentle stretching of the tight hamstrings

40. A 28-year-old male is in the intensive care unit after a motorcycle accident. He has an unstable pelvic fracture, for which he had surgery 24 hours ago. He has been extubated and despite severe pain, he offers no complaints. Which one of the following is the best statement regarding osteopathic treatment for this patient?

    (A) This patient should receive osteopathic manipulation daily until he is transferred out of the unit.

    (B) This patient should receive direct active forms of treatment such as muscle energy.

    (C) This patient can be treated more frequently as compared with a person twice his age with similar circumstances.

    (D) Pedal pump would be of no use in this patient.

    (E) Osteopathic treatment is contraindicated in this patient due to the acute nature of the illness.

41. A patient presents with chronic neck pain. Osteopathic evaluation of the neck uses the articular pillars as palpatory landmarks for diagnosis. Which one of the following statements regarding the articular pillars of the cervical spine is true?

    (A) They are located anterior to the transverse processes.

    (B) They are located between the vertebral body and the cervical lamina.

    (C) They are the portion of bone located immediately posterior to the facet joints.

    (D) They are located between the cervical lamina and the spinous processes.

    (E) The vertebral artery courses through the articular pillars.

42. A 29-year-old female is complaining of left-sided chest pain associated with deep inspiration. On structural examination, you notice limited inhalation of Ribs 2-5 on the left and upper thoracic paraspinal tenderness. After ruling out emergent causes of chest pain, you decide that this pain is due to a musculoskeletal abnormality. Which of the following muscles or muscle groups would be most useful in correcting this somatic dysfunction using a direct method?

    (A) Serratus anterior

    (B) Anterior scalene

    (C) Posterior scalene

    (D) Pectoralis minor

    (E) Lattissimus dorsi

43. A 64-year-old male comes to your office complaining of headaches. The headaches are associated with neck pain and stiffness. They are exacerbated at times of stress and are relieved with the use of NSAIDS. He is coming to your office for osteopathic manipulation. On examination, you notice right-sided fullness in the suboccipital triangle, and the occiput resists anterior motion at this region. The lower cervical spine has a lateral convexity to the right, and it resists translation to the left. Given the above information, which of the following structural abnormalities is true?

    (A) The occiput is flexed.

    (B) The occiput is rotated right.

    (C) The atlanto-axial joint is sidebent right.

    (D) C2 is rotated left.

    (E) The lower cervical spine is rotated to the right.

44. In a patient with neck pain, the second cervical segment is found to resist translation to the left with the head in the flexed position. There is ease of translation to the left in the extended position. Given this information, what is the diagnosis of this somatic dysfunction?

    (A) C2 is flexed, sidebent right, rotated right.

    (B) C2 is flexed, sidebent left, rotated left.

    (C) C2 is extended, sidebent right, rotated right.

    (D) C2 is extended, sidebent left, rotated left.

    (E) There is insufficient information to make a diagnosis.

45. An MRI on a patient experiencing neck pain with numbness and tingling in his upper extremity shows a disc herniation that is extending through the C7/T1 intervertebral foramen on the left. It appears to be compressing the nerve that runs through this foramen but does not seem to be interfering with any other neural structure. Which of the following symptoms do you expect this patient to have?

    (A) Numbness of the lateral aspect of the forearm

    (B) Weakness with the intrinsic muscles of the hand

    (C) Weakness with arm abduction

    (D) Weakness with elbow flexion

    (E) Winging of the scapula

46. A patient with limited rotation of the neck is most likely to have a dysfunction at which structure?

    (A) The occiput

    (B) The sphenoid

    (C) The axis

    (D) The atlas

    (E) The fifth cervical segment

47. A patient presents with thoracic back pain. An osteopathic structural examination of the thoracics is performed. Which of the following is true regarding the anatomy and physiology of the thoracic region?

    (A) When a patient is standing with his arms at has side, the inferior angle of the scapula is immediately lateral to the spinous process of T10.

    (B) The spinous processes of the thoracic region point increasingly downward, such that T12's spinous process is approximately at the level of the body of L1.

    (C) Inhalation causes a pressure gradient within the thoracic cavity that promotes venous and lymph return.

    (D) The ribs limit lateral flexion of the spine; therefore, thoracic vertebrae move most easily about a transverse axis.

    (E) The third rib is immediately lateral to the Angle of Louis.

48. A 7-year-old child presents with shortness of breath and wheezing to the ER. His mother states that the symptoms started two hours ago. He has been hospitalized for asthma once in the past when he was four years old. His asthma is usually controlled with an albuterol inhaler; however, this time it did not help. On examination, he is in mild respiratory distress. There is bilateral rhonchi on auscultation with an increase in expiratory phase and evidence of accessory muscle use. Which of the following is true concerning accessory (secondary) muscles of respiration?

    (A) The pectoralis minor facilitates bucket-handle motion of ribs.

    (B) The middle scalene is responsible for elevating Rib 2 during inspiration.

    (C) Accessory muscles are responsible for more than 60% of respiration with normal breathing.

    (D) Injury to the long thoracic nerve will limit pump-handle and bucket-handle motion of the ribs.

    (E) Diaphragmatic fatigue will inevitably result in respiratory failure.

49. A patient has a somatic dysfunction of Rib 1. The patient has pain with inhalation. On examination, the rib seems to lag in inhalation and move easily into exhalation. Which of the following is true concerning Rib 1?

    (A) Clavicle influence on Rib 1 is limiting motion of Rib 1.

    (B) Rib 1 has bucket-handle motion.

    (C) Rib 1 lacks a tubercle and is therefore considered an atypical rib.

    (D) Hypertonicity of the anterior scalene is most likely limiting motion of Rib 1.

    (E) Rib 1 does not directly attach to the sternum.

50. A 24-year-old female is complaining of chest pain. The pain started after working in her garden yesterday. The pain is right-sided, it does not radiate, and she denies any shortness of breath or chest pressure. She denies any syncope or dizziness. Further questioning reveals no cardiac risk factors. EKG is normal. On examination, you notice an exhalation dysfunction of Ribs 2-6 on the right. Which of the following statements is true regarding treatment of this somatic dysfunction?

    (A) Using muscle energy, treatment would be directed at Rib 6.

    (B) Using muscle energy, the pectoralis minor would be contracted to help Rib 6 move into inhalation.

    (C) Using muscle energy, the posterior scalene should be contracted to influence Rib 2 cephalad.

    (D) An indirect treatment would be directed at Rib 6.

    (E) An indirect treatment would try to influence the cervico-thoracic fascia caudad.

OMM

ANSWERS AND EXPLANATIONS

1.	A	26.	B
2.	B	27.	B
3.	C	28.	D
4.	B	29.	E
5.	D	30.	D
6.	C	31.	B
7.	D	32.	E
8.	C	33.	E
9.	D	34.	B
10.	A	35.	C
11.	B	36.	A
12.	E	37.	B
13.	B	38.	C
14.	A	39.	E
15.	D	40.	C
16.	B	41.	B
17.	A	42.	C
18.	A	43.	B
19.	B	44.	D
20.	C	45.	B
21.	C	46.	D
22.	A	47.	C
23.	D	48.	D
24.	D	49.	B
25.	D	50.	C

1. **The correct answer is A.** This patient with back pain has a somatic dysfunction of her thoracic spine. Because the transverse processes of the thoracic vertebrae are posterior on the right side, they must be rotated to the right. Left shoulder depression will induce left sidebending. Therefore, these segments must be sidebent left. If a group of segments are rotated and sidebent to opposite sides, they are said to follow type I mechanics.

   Right rotation and right sidebending is an example of type II mechanics (**choice B**). This typically occurs with single vertebral somatic dysfunction. In addition, T1-T4 in this question are sidebent left.

   Right rotation and right sidebending is an example of type II mechanics (**choice C**). This typically occurs with single vertebral somatic dysfunction. Because the left shoulder depresses more easily than the right, these segments must be sidebent left.

   T1-T4 rotated right, sidebent left would be an example of type I mechanics (not type II) (**choice D**).

   Left rotation and left sidebending would be an example of type II mechanics (**choice E**). This typically occurs with single vertebral somatic dysfunction. The transverse processes of the thoracic vertebrae, however, are posterior on the right side; they must be rotated to the right, not the left.

2. **The correct answer is B.** Chronic tender hypomobile fibrotic paraspinal musculature results from chronic abnormal visceral stimuli from autonomic afferents. The respiratory system receives sympathetic innervation from segments T2-T7. Therefore, this patient is most likely to have chronically tender hypomobile and fibrotic paraspinal musculature at these segments.

   C3-C5 (**choice A**) has no influence on autonomic tone in the lungs. It is of note that the occiput, atlas, and axis influence the lungs by way of the vagus nerve.

   Chronic respiratory dysfunction does not result in paraspinal muscle changes at T9-T12 (**choice C**) or at L1-L2 (**choice D**). These segments receive autonomic innervation from viscera below the diaphragm.

   No autonomic influences stem from L3-L5 (**choice E**).

3. **The correct answer is C.** The patient in this question has a somatic dysfunction resulting from a visceral dysfunction (a viscerosomatic reflex). Nociceptive input from visceral afferent fibers enters the dorsal horn of the spinal cord and facilitates these segments. This initiates vasomotor changes and alters the output to somatic musculature.

   This patient has somatic dysfunction resulting from visceral symptoms by way of sympathetic, not parasympathetic (**choice A**), autonomic fibers.

The lateral corticospinal tract (**choice B**) originates in the cerebral cortex, traverses through the spinal cord, and terminates by way of interneurons on the dorsal horn. Its function is volitional skilled motor activity.

The ventral corticospinal tract (**choice D**) is similar to the lateral corticospinal tract in origin and termination; however, it is concerned with control of axial muscles.

Ropy and fibrotic paraspinal musculature on the left at T12-L2 represents somatic dysfunction, not visceral dysfunction (**choice E**).

4. **The correct answer is B.** The above patient has a flexion contracture of the iliopsoas. Signs and symptoms of iliopsoas syndrome include increased pain with standing or walking, a positive Thomas test, a tender point medial to the ASIS, and a non-neutral dysfunction of L1 or L2.

   A positive seated flexion test (**choice A**) is positive in sacral somatic dysfunction. The above patient had a symmetrical sacrum that springs freely, and a sacral somatic dysfunction is not possible.

   A bilateral sacral extension (**choice D**) will result in a falsely negative seated flexion test, but the sacrum will not spring freely (a positive lumbosacral spring test).

   A lumbar herniated disk (**choice C**) is often associated with radiation of the pain, and the pain often gets worse with flexion of the lumbar spine.

   Although this patient *may* have a somatic dysfunction in the right leg (**choice E**), leg lengths are equal, and the pelvis appears equal. Therefore, this is not the statement that is most likely to be true.

5. **The correct answer is D.** Counterstrain to the iliopsoas is often very effective when treating a flexion contracture of the iliopsoas.

   The sacrum in the above patient is symmetrical and springs freely and has no somatic dysfunction. Therefore, **choice A** would not be correct.

   Therapeutic stretching (**choice B**) to the hip extensors will be of no benefit to a flexion contracture to the iliopsoas. However, therapeutic stretching of the hip flexors would be of benefit. The above patient does not have a herniated disc for reasons stated in the previous explanation. Most cases of herniated discs can be treated conservatively with bed rest initially, then OMT will help decrease and improve the structure-function relationship of the lumbosacral spine.

6. **The correct answer is C.** Cervical tender points that are located on the articular pillars are considered anterior tender points. Anterior tender points are best treated in flexion. According to the principles of strain/counter-

strain, cervical tender points typically are treated with the head sidebent and rotated away from the tender point. Therefore, the head should be placed in flexion, left sidebending, and left rotation.

If this patient had a posterior tender point on the third cervical segment on the right (i.e., at the spinous process on the right), then the head would be placed in extension, left sidebending, and left rotation (**choice A**).

If this patient had a posterior tender point on the third cervical segment on the left (i.e., at the spinous process on the left), then the head would be placed in extension, right sidebending, and right rotation (**choice B**).

Typical treatment positions for the cervical spine include all three planes of motion, not just flexion and sidebending (**choices D and E**).

7. **The correct answer is D.** This patient has diverticulitis. Ninety-four percent of diverticula disease in elderly patients occurs in the sigmoid colon. The Chapman point for the sigmoid colon is on the left femur; in particular, it is on the lateral femur within the iliotibial band.

There are no reported Chapman points in the rectus femoris muscle (**choice A**).

There is no Chapman point at the tip of the left twelfth rib (**choice B**).

The left ischial tuberosity is the Chapman point for the hemorrhoidal plexus (**choice C**).

The posterior Chapman point for the kidney is located just left of the spinous process of T12 (**choice E**).

8. **The correct answer is C.** This patient has diverticulitis. Ninety-four percent of diverticula disease in elderly patients occurs in the sigmoid colon. The visceral afferent travels along the least splanchnic nerve into T12-L2 segments of the spinal cord and could facilitate these segments.

The greater splanchnic nerve (**choice A**) enters the spinal cord at T5-T9; these segments are responsible for autonomic innervation to the upper gastrointestinal tract.

The lesser splanchnic nerve (**choice B**) enters T9-T12; these segments are responsible for autonomic innervation to the middle gastrointestinal tract.

The vagus nerve (**choice D**) is responsible for autonomic (parasympathetic) innervation for the entire gastrointestinal tract, except for the descending sigmoid colon and the rectum.

The phrenic nerve (**choice E**) innervates skeletal muscle and does not have visceral afferent fibers.

9. **The correct answer is D.** This patient has thoracic outlet syndrome (TOS). TOS can result in neck and shoulder pain and often can radiate pain into the upper extremity. The patient has a positive Adson test, which is a screening maneuver for TOS.

C3 should be placed in extension, *left* rotation, and *right* sidebending to correct the dysfunction using rotatory HVLA thrust. Therefore, **choice A** is incorrect.

This patient is unlikely to have supraspinatus tendonitis (**choice B**). Although the patient has some pain with overhead activity, she does not have any pain with impingement of the greater tuberosity of the humerus against the acromion (signs of impingement), which would be positive in supraspinatus tendonitis.

Direct muscle energy (postisometric relaxation) with the anterior scalene could be used to correct an exhalation dysfunction of Rib 1 (**choice C**). This patient has an inhalation dysfunction of Rib 1. Before treating any rib dysfunction, however, you must address any thoracic dysfunctions first.

This patient is not likely to have a radiculopathy at C6 (**choice E**) for several reasons. First, a cervical radiculopathy caused by spinal stenosis is often associated with moderate or severe degenerative changes seen on x-ray. In addition, the patient is likely to have more frequent, if not continuous, pain or numbness radiating into her elbow or hand.

10. **The correct answer is A.** The above patient has a spasm of the lumbar paraspinals. Lumbar paraspinals are responsible for extending and sidebending (laterally flexing) the spine. Often the patient will complain of pain that increases with forward flexion.

The piriformis (**choice B**) may cause gluteal pain and is responsible for externally rotating the leg.

The iliopsoas (**choice C**) is the primary flexor of the hip and is often associated with back pain, but usually the patient will complain of pain while standing erect. Further, the pain will usually subside in the seated position.

The gluteus medius (**choice D**) may refer pain to the low back; however, due to the origin (ilium) and insertion (greater trochanter), spasm of this muscle will not directly cause lumbar extension and lateral flexion.

Spasm of the quadratus lumborum (**choice E**) can cause low back pain, but a pure quadratus lumborum spasm is not as common as a lumbar paravertebral spasm. Therefore, this is not the most likely answer.

11. **The correct answer is B.** Although the lumbar paravertebrals attach to the ribs and the sacrum, they exhibit the greatest influence on the lumbar segments.

Spasm of the quadratus lumborum may cause 12th rib dysfunction (**choice A**).

The psoas may cause innominate dysfunction (**choice E**).

The piriformis may cause sacral and leg somatic dysfunction (**choices C** and **D**, respectively).

And the gluteus medius may cause innominate (**choice E**) and leg dysfunction.

12. **The correct answer is E.** The above patient has an acute subarachnoid bleed. Osteopathic treatment is absolutely contraindicated for any acute intracranial bleed or any condition where there is increased intracranial pressure.

Occipital condylar decompression (**choice A**) and cervical fascial release (**choice B**) may improve a patient's headache, especially if it is a tension headache.

A thoracic inlet release (**choice C**) can promote lymphatic drainage, but it has no role in an acute bleed.

The neurologic deficit the patient is experiencing is due to blood crossing the blood-brain barrier; it is not due to an autonomic dysfunction.

13. **The correct answer is B.** The above patient has an acute appendicitis. Iliopsoas dysfunction is the most common musculoskeletal condition associated with appendicitis. This is probably because of the close proximity of the iliopsoas to the appendix.

The piriformis (**choice A**) and gluteus maximus (**choice D**) are pelvic muscles and are not irritated in appendicitis. The rectus abdominus (**choice E**), although a muscle in the abdomen, because of its position in relation to the appendix is an unlikely candidate to be irritated in appendicitis.

The paraspinals (**choice C**) are too superficial to be irritated in appendicitis.

14. **The correct answer is A.** Small fascial contractions (i.e., Chapman's reflexes) represent viscero-somatic reflexes. The Chapman's point for acute appendicitis is located at the tip of the 12th rib. This is probably the most tested Chapman's reflex on the COMLEX boards. Other Chapman's points are as follows:

   Bladder: umbilicus (**choice B**)

   One cm lateral to the L1 spinous process (**choice C**): kidneys

   One cm superior to the umbilicus (**choice D**): kidneys or bladder

15. **The correct answer is D: T12.** Appendicitis is most likely to cause a somatic dysfunction in the lower thoracic area. This is due to the fact that T9-T12 receive input from and supply visceral efferents to the lower GI tract (including the appendix). T5-T9 (**choice C**) supply the upper GI tract (stomach through the pancreas). T12-L2 supply the distal 1/3 of transverse colon to rectum.

16. **The correct answer is B.** The best way to screen for scoliosis is to ask the patient to bend forward while you look for a paraspinal hump.

Scoliosis may be evident while looking for lateral curves of the spine while the patient is standing (**choice A**); however, subtle scoliosis will be missed this way.

Standing postural X-rays to evaluate for sacral base unleveling (**choice C**) are part of the workup of scoliosis; however, X-rays are costly and are not used for screening. Therefore, **choice D** is also unnecessary.

A standing flexion test (**choice E**) will not detect scoliosis and will not detect sacral base unleveling.

17. **The correct answer is A:** AA. The patient described in the question above is most likely to have croup. Croup is an infection that affects the respiratory system. The vagus nerve is the parasympathetic innervation to the lungs; therefore, any segment that affects the vagus nerve may influence the lungs.

Parasympathetic innervation stems from the cranial nerves 3, 7, 9, and 10 and from S2-S4 (**choice E**).

The vagus nerve exits the cranium and is influenced by three vertebral segments (OA, AA, and C2).

Sympathetic innervation stems from the thoracolumbar column. The sympathetic innervation to the respiratory system stems from T2-T7. Because the question asks for parasympathetic influence (not sympathetic), any segment in the thoracolumbar area must be wrong.

18. **The correct answer is A.** The patient in the above question is suffering from a paralytic ileus from her surgery. An ileus is a common complication following surgery and it is seen in a hypersympathetic state. In order to restore normal function to her sympathetics, rib raising would be the best technique. Rib raising helps "normalize" sympathetics.

Although both myofascial release (**choice B**) and a thoracoabdominal diaphragm release (**choice D**) can be used in this patient, it will not directly affect her constipation.

Muscle energy (**choice C**) is contraindicated in post-surgical cases.

And a liver and spleen pump (**choice E**) should not be used on a patient with recent abdominal surgery.

19. **The correct answer is B.** Treatment of the thoracic inlet fascia should be done initially to help drain the head and neck structures.

Lymphatic pump techniques (**choice A**) will improve lymphatic return; however, the lymphatic pumps can be used more effectively once the thoracic diaphragm is released.

The patient has cervical tenderness; however, this may be due to cervical adenopathy. Therefore, counterstrain (**choice D**) may not help this patient.

Releasing the pelvic diaphragm (**choice C**) will facilitate drainage of lymph from the pelvic structures, not the head and neck.

Decreasing lateral spinal curves (**choice E**) may benefit the patient symptomatically, but it will not greatly influence lymph return. Therefore, it is not the best answer.

20. **The correct answer is C:** quadratus lumborum. The quadratus lumborum originates from the medial half of the inferior border of the 12th rib and tips of the lumbar transverse processes and aids in deep inspiration. A tender point for quadratus lumborum can be found throughout the belly of the muscle from the origin to insertion.

   The psoas major (**choice A**) attaches to the transverse processes of T12-L4 (and sometimes L5), and the serratus anterior (**choice B**) attaches to Ribs 1-8. Neither attaches to Rib 12 and could not limit its range of motion or cause a tender point to exist there.

   The transverse abdominis (**choice E**) does attach to Rib 12, but it is not involved with respiration and therefore would not limit its range of motion.

   Levator costarum (**choice D**) are small muscles that elevate the ribs during inspiration; however, they attach to the superior border of the ribs and therefore will not cause a tender point on the inferior border.

21. **The correct answer is C**. The patient has a lateral convexity to the left (i.e., the lumbar spine is sidebent to the right). He is also noted to have his transverse processes to the left (i.e., the lumbar spine is rotated to the left).

   When the spine sidebends and rotates in opposite directions, we call this type I mechanics. Type I mechanics occur when the spine is in the neutral position (no flexion or extension). Type II mechanics occur when the spine is either flexed or extended. In this case, sidebending and rotation are in the same direction.

22. **The correct answer is A: $L5\ NS_LR_R$.** The above patient has a left sacral rotation on a left oblique axis (L on L). A positive seated flexion test indicates that the oblique axis would be on the left. A shallow (posterior) ILA on the left and a deep sulcus on the right indicate left rotation. The lumbosacral spring test will be negative with a forward torsion. Stating that the lumbar curve is convex to the right is a clue that the lumbar spine is sidebent

to the left (so this could help you eliminate a couple of your answers). Following the rules of L5 on the sacrum will help us narrow down the answer. Rule #1: When L5 is sidebent, a sacral oblique axis is engaged on the same side as the sidebending. Working backwards: if we have a *left* oblique sacral axis, then we must have L5 sidebent *left*. Rule #2: When L5 is rotated, the sacrum rotates in the opposite direction. Again working backwards: if we have left rotation of the sacrum, then L5 must be rotated right. Now using Fryette's law: if L5 is sidebent left and rotated right (i.e., opposite directions), then it must be in the neutral plane (i.e., $L5\ NS_LR_R$).

23. **The correct answer is D.** The above patient has a posterior sacral base (i.e, sacral base posterior or a bilateral sacral extension). This type of dysfunction can occur after any activity that applies anterior pressure at the sacral apex or posterior pressure at the sacral base (e.g., childbirth). The examiner will notice that the sacral sulci are equal in depth, and there is no springing at the sacral base (i.e., the lumbosacral spring test is negative). The seated flexion test will be *falsely* negative. Why? Both SI joints are restricted, and asymmetry will not be appreciated.

   In a unilateral extended sacrum on the right (**choice A**), the sulci on the right will appear more posterior than those on the left, and the seated flexion test will be positive on the right.

   In a unilateral extended sacrum on the left (**choice C**), the sulci on the left will appear more posterior than those on the right, and the seated flexion test will be positive on the left.

   In an anterior sacral base (**choice B**), the findings will be the same as above, except that the sacral base would spring.

   A forward sacral torsion (**choice E**) (left on left or right on right), the seated flexion test would be positive, the sulci would appear asymmetric, and the lumbosacral spring test would be negative.

24. **The correct answer is D.** When the patient bends backward, the segment rotates to the right. When the patient flexes, the segment returns to the neutral position; therefore, the segment must be rotated right sidebent right, and because it gets better with flexion (you name it for the way it wants to go), it must be flexed. A direct treatment entails positioning the segment so that it approximates its restrictive barrier (i.e., reversing all planes of motion). An indirect treatment entails positioning the segment away from its restrictive barrier (i.e., taking the segment where it wants to go). So if the segment is flexed rotated right and sidebent right, the correct treatment position for a direct technique is extended, rotated left, and sidebent left.

25. **The correct answer is D:** right sacral rotation on a right oblique axis. In a sacral torsion, the seated flexion test (the test that checks for sacral dysfunction) is positive on the opposite side of the axis. A left anterior sulcus with a posterior ILA indicates right rotation.

    In an L on L (**choice A**), R on L (**choice C**), and a unilateral sacral flexion on the right (**choice E**), the seated flexion test would be positive on the right. Therefore, it is easy to immediately eliminate those answers.

    Left sacral rotation on a right oblique axis (**choice B**) would present with different palpitory findings. The sacral sulcus would be posterior (or shallow) on the left and the ILA would be anterior.

26. **The correct answer is B.** A positive standing flexion test indicates that the patient has a somatic dysfunction of the pelvis. Therefore, we can immediately eliminate any sacral dysfunctions (**choices D and E**).

    With a posterior innominate (**choice C**), the left ASIS would be superior, and the left PSIS would be inferior.

    With a superior innominate shear (upslip innominate) (**choice A**), both the left ASIS and the PSIS would be superior. Therefore, this is not the correct answer.

27. **The correct answer is B.** A somatic dysfunction is defined as an impairment or altered function of related components of the somatic (body framework) system: skeletal, arthroidial, and myofascial structures and related vascular, lymphatic, and neural elements. The patient in the above question has a restricted range of motion (altered function) and has edema (impairment of myofascial structures).

    All of the other statements are not necessarily true regarding this injury. Yes, a patient can have a fracture of the scaphoid with negative X-rays (**choice A**); however, only 10 to 20% of patients will have an occult fracture, and usually pain will be present in the anatomic snuff box (not the volar aspect).

    Severely decreased range of motion will occur with several injuries to the wrist, not just a complete ligament tear (**choice C**).

    When a patient falls on an outstretched arm, he is likely to affect his radial head at the elbow. This is further eluded to by stating that he has decreased range of motion at his forearm (pronation and supination). A nondisplaced fracture of the scaphoid can usually be treated with a spica thumb splint, not surgery.

28. **The correct answer is D.** The above patient has an impairment (i.e., somatic dysfunction) in his right knee in the form of osteoarthritis. Osteoarthritis can present itself in many ways, but the key to the above question is to understand that the condition has been present for ten years, and there is no recent history of trauma. Therefore, when you examine his knee you would expect to find chronic changes. There are some key phrases used to describe chronic somatic dysfunctions: cool, dry skin, decreased or no edema or erythema, flaccid, ropy and fibrotic tissues, little to no pain that may be burning, achy, or dull on nature.

    Acute somatic dysfunctions usually present with severe or sharp pain, hypertonic muscles, boggy edematous tissues with increased moisture. **Choice A** is wrong because edematous and boggy tissues are associated with acute somatic dysfucntions. Also, osteoarthritis usually has decreased range of motion with crepitus, but in some mild cases a patient may have near full or full range of motion with little or no crepitus.

    Choice B is wrong because there is erythema with significant effusion—again, signs of acute changes.

    Choice C is wrong because severe, sharp pain with hypertonic muscles is associated with acute changes.

    Choice E is wrong because anterior laxity (positive anterior drawer or Lachman's test) with an effusion and a positive bounce home test (confirming that there is an effusion present) are all findings that describe an acute ACL tear.

29. **The correct answer is E.** The patient in the above question has a somatic dysfunction at T2. The segment is flexed rotated right and sidebent right. When using muscle energy as a treatment, you should reverse all planes of motion, and in doing so, you move the segment in the direction of the restrictive barrier.

    Choice A is wrong because the patient does not have a group dysfunction (it is a single segmental dysfunction).

    Choice B is wrong because laterally flexing (sidebending) to the left and rotating to the right would not correctly reverse the planes of motion—not to mention it doesn't say anything about extending the segment.

    Choice C is wrong because T2 would have to be placed in an extended position, rotated left, and sidebent left to reverse all planes of motion.

    Choice D is wrong because the head should be used as a lever to induce motion at T1-T4. The practitioner uses the torso to manipulate T5-L5 into the correct position.

30. **The correct answer is D.** If T3-T5 are rotated right, then according to Fryette's laws, they should be in the neutral plane and sidebent left (T3-T5 NS_LR_R). Remember, group dysfunctions are typically in the neutral plane, and in that case, they sidebend and rotate

to opposite sides. Also remember that when describing a somatic dysfunction, we describe motion of the superior segment in relation to the inferior one (in this case T5 on T6).

Choice A is wrong because it is describing a non-neutral dysfunction rotated right, sidebent right.

Choice B is wrong because a thoracic dysfunction does not always preclude a rib dysfunction.

Choice C is wrong because if T4 is sidebent to the left, then its right transverse process would be more cephalad.

Choice E is wrong because if T4 is rotated to the right, then its right transverse process would be more posterior.

31. **The correct answer is B.** When you ask a patient to actively move a joint to its end points, you are asking the patient to demonstrate active range of motion. Passive range of motion is when a physician (or any other person for that matter) moves a joint. Any person can actively move a joint to its physiologic barrier (if there is no somatic dysfunction present). Any other person can move someone else's joint to its anatomic barrier (if there is no somatic dysfunction present). When there is somatic dysfunction present, that person or physician can only go to the restrictive barrier. So the above patient has a restrictive barrier at 45° at right rotation, and a physiologic barrier to the left at 90°.

Choice A is wrong because the patient is demonstrating active range of motion.

Choice C is wrong because he has limited active range of motion (and given the somatic dysfunction, he'll have limited passive range of motion also).

Choices D and E are both wrong for many reasons:

You cannot comment on vertebral somatic dysfunction without actually palpating a dysfunction.

A strained muscle in the neck may cause somatic dysfunction, but what muscle? And how does it act upon the cervical spine?

You don't know whether or not the somatic dysfunction is neutral or non-neutral.

32. **The correct answer is E.** Flexing the patient's head will lock out rotation of C2-C7 and will almost completely limit rotation to the AA. It is apparent that the AA (or the atlas on the axis) is rotated to the right and limited to the left. If the atlas is rotated right, it will resist left rotation.

Choices A and B are wrong because the AA will not necessarily effect the occiput (OA). It is of note that pushing anterior on the right at the OA will cause left rotation of the occiput (again, another way to evaluate motion at the OA).

Choices C and D are wrong because motion at the AA will not necessarily cause compensation or somatic dysfunction of the lower cervical units.

33. **The correct answer is E.** The patient in the above question has T3 extended, rotated right, and sidebent right. Due to the biomechanics of the thoracic and lumbar spine, rotation and sidebending are toward the same sides when the spine is in the non-neutral position. Conversely, rotation and sidebending are toward opposite sides when the spine is in the neutral position. If the spine is flexed, a restrictive barrier is introduced; this restrictive barrier includes rotation and sidebending to the left. Therefore, flexing T3 will limit its rotation to the left.

Choice A is wrong because type II mechanics occur when sidebending and rotation are to the same sides.

Choice B is wrong because flexion of T3 on T4 will cause relative extension of T4 on T3. Flexion of the patient's head will cause T2 to be flexed on T3.

Choice C is wrong because if T3 is extended, symmetry is restored and rotation is no longer apparent. Therefore, dynamic testing of T3 will demonstrate T3 with no restriction while in the extended position (think of translating the cervical spine in the neutral, flexed, and extended positions to find out where the asymmetry lies).

Choice D is wrong because even though you are eliminating the asymmetry in the extended position, as soon as you extend the thoracic spine, you induce type II mechanics.

34. **The correct answer is B.** Vertebral motion in a sagittal plane is flexion or extension. So L3 must be either flexed or extended. Vertebral motion about a vertical axis is rotation. Therefore, L3 must also be rotated understanding Fryette's principles; one must conclude that if a vertebra is flexed or extended and rotated it must be sidebent toward the same side. The only answer above in which L3 is non-neutral, rotated, and sidebent toward the same side is choice B.

Choice A describes a neutral dysfunction that is rotated and sidebent toward opposite sides.

Choice C states nothing about flexion or extension (i.e., motion in a sagittal plane).

Choice D states nothing about motion of either a sagittal plane or vertical axis.

Choice E states nothing about motion around a vertical axis.

35. **The correct answer is C.** The patient in the above question is doing a type of isometric contraction. The definition of an isometric contraction is a contrac-

tion that results in the increase in tension without an approximation of muscle origin and insertion.

An isotonic contraction (**choice A**) is one in which there is an approximation of muscle origin and insertion without an increase in muscle tension.

Concentric (**choice D**) and eccentric (**choice B**) contractions are contractions in which there is an approximation (concentric) or lengthening (eccentric) of muscular origin and insertion. Tension is not related to this type of contraction.

36. **The correct answer is A.** The treatment calls for a direct active technique. The only type of treatment that falls into this category is muscle energy and myofascial release. Therefore, we should look for answers that describe these techniques, then figure out the correct position. First, let's eliminate the techniques that are not muscle energy or myofascial release.

    Choice D describes an HVLA (direct and passive) technique, and **choice E** describes a counterstrain (indirect and passive) technique, so these two choices can be eliminated. A direct technique is a type of treatment in which the segment or tissue is moved toward the restrictive barrier. An active treatment is a technique in which the patient participates in the treatment.

    Choice B is describing a type of myofascial release; however, since you are moving away from the restriction, this is an indirect form of treatment. Therefore, this choice is wrong.

    Choice C is describing another type of myofascial release. You are moving the body toward the restriction (a direct treatment); however, you are waiting for a release of muscle tension, a passive technique.

37. **The correct answer is B.** The elderly patient in the above question is recovering from a severe disease. She has been bedridden (i.e., she has osteoporosis) and has coronary disease. As noted in the *Foundations of Osteopathic Medicine,* elderly patients and hospitalized patients typically respond better with indirect techniques or gentle direct techniques such as articulatory techniques. Therefore, **choice B** is the correct answer.

    Since this patient has osteoporosis, high-velocity low-amplitude techniques are contraindicated; therefore, **choice A** is wrong.

    Choice C is wrong because this patient will not be able to tolerate muscle energy because of her low vitality, and rib raising, although it will help the patient's respiratory status, is not the best choice for reducing low back pain.

    Choice D is wrong because the patient will not be able to tolerate isotonic exercises, even though myofascial release of the sacrum would help this patient.

Choice E is wrong because this patient could not tolerate isometric exercise because of her low vitality.

38. **The correct answer is C.** The above patient has an acute cervical sprain. The patient has no evidence of neurologic impingement. According to the *Foundations of Osteopathic Medicine* (p. 486), acute neck strains/sprains are often better treated with indirect techniques to prevent further strain. Therefore, C is the correct answer. Counterstrain is an indirect, passive treatment that will allow the patient and musculature to relax, thus decreasing her pain.

    Muscle energy (**choice A**) is a direct and active form of treatment. This type of treatment may actually worsen the patient's pain and probably should not be used within 48 hours of injury.

    Thoracic inlet release (**choice B**) is a gentle technique, but its primary purpose is to increase lymphatic flow.

    HVLA (**choice D**) is contraindicated in acute cervical sprains and should not be used because it may worsen the patient's symptoms.

    Direct myofascial release (**choice E**) is not the best choice because ideally an indirect form should be used.

39. **The correct answer is E.** Because this patient is elderly with several comorbidities, the only suitable treatment protocol is gentle direct or indirect methods. **Choice E** is the best answer because indirect myofascial release will correct the dysfunctions at the thoracolumbar junction and sacrum without causing the patient discomfort. And gentle stretching of the hamstrings may help prevent pelvic dysfunction and improve flexibility.

    The patient in the above question has a history of prostate cancer and we are unaware of the extent of his cancer. The cancer could have metathesized to the vertebral column and caused his back pain (especially since the pain did not improve with NSAIDS or heating pads). HVLA could cause a pathologic fracture.

    Also, patients with advanced stages of cancer should not be treated with lymphatic techniques, such as a pelvic diaphragm release (**choice B**) due to an increased risk of lymphogenous spread. Given this information, we can eliminate **choices A, B,** and **D.**

    Because this patient is elderly, the patient may not be able to tolerate lumbar hyperextension (**choice C**). The patient must remain comfortable during the treatment in order for it to be effective. Also, since we haven't ruled out bone metatheses, hyperextension may cause a pathologic fracture (although chances are slim, the consequences are severe).

40. **The correct answer is C.** As a general rule, younger patients can be treated more frequently; their bodies tend to heal quicker. An older person will not heal as quick and often needs more time to respond to the osteopathic manipulation. Therefore, **choice C** is correct.

This patient may develop postoperative complications and may not be able to tolerate osteopathic manipulation daily, so therefore **choice A** is not the best answer.

Muscle energy (**choice B**) is relatively contraindicated in postsurgical patients and patients in the intensive care unit; therefore, this is not the best answer.

Pedal pump (**choice D**) would certainly help this patient prevent DVTs, and it will also help promote lymph flow since this patient suffered a pelvic fracture and will have limited motion in his lower extremities.

Osteopathic treatment (**choice E**) is not contraindicated in acute illnesses. Typically, once the patient has been stabilized and there is no life-threatening issue, osteopathic treatment can be used to promote healing.

41. **The correct answer is B.** Understanding the location of the articular pillars is important because osteopathic physicians use them to induce cervical motion to check for somatic dysfunctions.

The articular pillars (or lateral masses) are a portion of bone that lies between the superior and inferior facets (therefore, **choice C** is wrong).

They are located posterior to the transverse processes (therefore, **choice A** is wrong) and connect the vertebral body to the cervical lamina (thus, **choice B** is the right answer and **choice D** is wrong). The vertebral artery courses through the foramen tranversarium located in the transverse processes.

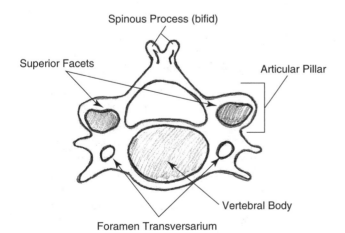

A typical cervical vertebrae

42. **The correct answer is C.** The patient in the above question has a group exhalation dysfunction of Ribs 2-5. As you inhale, the ribcage moves. Ribs 1-5 generally move in a pump-handle manner, whereas Ribs 6-10 move in a bucket-handle fashion. And Ribs 11 and 12 move in a caliper motion. As you inhale, Ribs 1-5 elevate anteriorly (pump-handle motion). If a person is found to have limited inhalation of Ribs 2-5, these ribs are thought to be "stuck" down. Ribs that are "stuck" down are said to have an exhalation dysfunction (the older terminology is "inhalation restriction"). In order to treat a rib dysfunction, it is imperative to understand which rib is the "key" rib. The "key" rib is the rib that treatment is directed toward. When an exhalation dysfunction is present, the "key" rib is the highest rib in the dysfunction. When an inhalation dysfunction is present, the "key" rib is the lowest rib in the dysfunction. In the above question the "key" rib is Rib 2. When treating ribs using a direct treatment, such as muscle energy, you would move the rib into its restrictive barrier (in this case, into inhalation). You would use a muscle that attaches to the "key" rib. Therefore, the muscle that attaches to the key rib (Rib 2) is the posterior scalene. The following chart shows what muscles should be used when treating exhalation dysfunctions utilizing the muscle energy technique.

Ribs	Muscles
Rib 1	Anterior and middle scalenes
Rib 2	Posterior scalene
Ribs 3-5	Pectoralis minor
Ribs 6-9	Serratus anterior
Ribs 10-12	Latissimus dorsi

43. **The correct answer is B.** A common way to test for rotation in the cervical spine is to push anteriorly on the lateral mass of the cervical spine at each segment. If there is resistance on one side compared with the other, then the segment is rotated toward that side. To test rotation at the OA (occipito-atlantal joint), the practitioner would push anterior at the level of the suboccipital area. The above patient has suboccipital fullness on the right, and the occiput resists anterior motion—this indicates that the occiput on the atlas is rotated to the right. Therefore, **choice B** is the right answer.

Since the OA is rotated right, it must be sidebent left (the OA follows type I mechanics); however, because we did not test the OA in flexion and extension, we do not know whether the OA is flexed, extended, or neutral. Therefore, **choice A** is wrong.

The above question makes no mention about the direction of the atlanto-axial joint (C1 on C2) or C2; therefore, **choices C** and **D** are wrong.

The lower cervical spine in the patient described above has a lateral convexity to the right, and it resists translation to the left. This indicates that this area of the spine is sidebent left and must be rotated left (since this section of the spine follows type II mechanics). Therefore, **choice E** is wrong.

44. **The correct answer is D.** As a general rule in osteopathic medicine, one names the somatic dysfunction in the direction of ease (in this case, name the dysfunction for the way the segment wants to go). In the above question, the patient's cervical spine resists translation to the left. Left translation induces right sidebending. Therefore, the cervical spine resists right sidebending. If it resists right sidebending, then it must be sidebent left. Due to facet orientation, the second cervical segment always sidebends and rotates to the same side. Therefore, if it is sidebent left, it must be rotated left. This resistance is worse when the head is in the flexed position and eases with the head in the extended position. Since you name the dysfunction for where the segment wants to go, C2 must be extended, sidebent left, and rotated left.

45. **The correct answer is B.** The nerve that exits the C7/T1 intervertebral foramen is C8. In the cervical spine the nerve root exits above its corresponding vertebra. Although there is some overlap between the nerve roots, the C8 nerve root supplies sensation to the little finger and medial forearm. It also supplies motor innervation to the wrist flexors and interossi (another name for interossi are the intrinsic muscles of the hand).

Numbness to the lateral aspect of the forearm (**choice A**) will be due to impingement of the C5 nerve root.

Weakness with arm abduction (**choice C**) and elbow flexion (**choice D**) will be due to impingement of the C5 or C6 nerve root.

Winging of the scapula (**choice E**) is classically seen with injury to the long thoracic nerve, which innervates the serratus anterior. The C5, C6, and C7 nerve roots make up the long thoracic nerve.

46. **The correct answer is D.** As a general rule, when referring to segmental motion or restriction, it is traditional to refer to motion (or restriction) of the segment above in a functional vertebral unit (two vertebrae). For example, when describing the motion (or restriction) of C1, it is the motion of C1 on top of C2. As the neck rotates, most of the rotation comes from the atlas rotating around the dens of the axis, thus the atlanto-axial

(C1-C2) joint is responsible for most of the rotation of the neck. Therefore, restriction with neck rotation will most likely stem from the atlas. Facet orientation determines vertebral motion.

Due to the orientation of the occipital condyles on the atlas, this joint (**choice A**) (the occiputo-atlantal joint) typically prefers flexion and extension.

The sphenoid bone (**choice B**) is not directly related to rotation restriction of the neck.

The axis (**choice C**) (C2) prefers rotation; however, most of the rotation of the neck comes from the atlas.

The fifth cervical segment (**choice E**) (again, due to facet orientation) prefers sidebending.

47. **The correct answer is C.** The fibers in the diaphragm are arranged such that when it contracts in inspiration, the vena caval opening dilates, permitting more venous blood to pass from the abdomen to the thorax. Also, the negative pressure created by inspiration promotes lymph and venous return back to the heart. This is further evidenced by the splitting of the second heart sound during inspiration. The splitting of the second heart sound occurs when there is more inflow into the right ventricle, causing delayed closure of the pulmonic valve.

When a patient is standing with his/her arms at his/her side (**choice A**), the inferior angle of the scapula is immediately lateral to the spinous process of T7, not T10.

Although the spinous processes point increasingly downward (**choice B**), they only do so from T1-T9. From T10-T12, the spinous processes quickly revert so that the spinous process of T12 is located at the body of T12.

The ribs limit lateral flexion (sidebending) (**choice D**); however, the thoracic vertebrae move most easily in rotation (a transverse plane), not in flexion and extension (a transverse axis).

The second rib (not the third [**choice E**]) is immediately lateral to the Angle of Louis. This is important because this is often used as a landmark for counting ribs.

48. **The correct answer is D.** Secondary muscles of respiration are as follows: scalenes, pectoralis minor, serratus anterior and posterior, quadratus lumborum, and latissimus dorsi. The long thoracic nerve innervates the serratus anterior. Serratus anterior originates at the medial border of the scapula and attaches to Ribs 2-9, and it aids in respiration of these ribs. As a person inhales, the person's ribcage elevates. Ribs 1-5 primarily move in a pump-handle fashion, and Ribs 6-10 primarily move in a bucket-handle fashion. Since the serratus anterior attaches to Ribs 2-9, it will affect these ribs and limit motion of these ribs.

The pectoralis minor (**choice A**) attaches to Ribs 3-5 and therefore will facilitate pump-handle motion, not bucket-handle motion.

The middle scalene (**choice B**) attaches to Rib 1, and therefore is responsible for elevating Rib 1 during inspiration.

When the body is breathing normally, the diaphragm (not accessory muscles [**choice C**]) bears most to all of the work. Accessory muscles are only used when a person is in acute distress or breathes deeply.

Diaphragmatic fatigue (**choice E**) can result in respiratory failure; however, the diaphragm is not an accessory muscle of respiration (it is a primary muscle of respiration).

49. **The correct answer is B**. Although Rib 1 primarily moves in a pump-handle fashion, it does have some bucket-handle motion. All ribs have varying proportions of pump-handle, bucket-handle, and caliper motion. However, Ribs 1-5 primarily move in a pump-handle fashion, Ribs 6-10 primarily move in a bucket-handle fashion, and Ribs 11-12 primarily move in a caliper motion.

The clavicle typically does not limit motion of Rib 1 (**choice A**), and therefore, it typically will not cause an exhalation dysfunction. However, if the clavicle does have a somatic dysfunction, this statement is possible. However, the above patient does not have a clavicle dysfunction; therefore, one cannot assume that its influence is causing the exhalation dysfunction of Rib 1.

Rib 1 is considered an atypical rib (**choice C**), but it is because it has no angle (it does have a tubercle that attaches to T1). The above patient has an exhalation dysfunction because he has limited motion of Rib 1 in inhalation, and the rib eases into exhalation (you name the dysfunction in the direction of ease).

The anterior scalene does attach to Rib 1 (**choice D**); however, hypertonicity of this muscle will cause an inhalation dysfunction because the anterior scalene will pull the anterior portion of Rib 1 cephalad (into inhalation).

Rib 1 (**choice E**) does directly attach to the sternum.

50. **The correct answer is C**. A group exhalation dysfunction of Ribs 2-6 indicates that these ribs moved caudad. To correct this dysfunction, treatment would have to be directed at the "key" rib: this rib is the uppermost rib in an exhalation dysfunction (in this case Rib 2). A direct technique, such as muscle energy, would utilize the posterior scalene to pull Rib 2 cephalad.

Choice A is wrong because Rib 6 is not the "key" rib; therefore, directing a muscle energy treatment toward this rib will not correct this dysfunction.

Choice B is wrong for two reasons: first, as already explained, treating Rib 6 with muscle energy is futile; and second, the pectoralis minor is used to treat exhalation dysfunction of Ribs 3, 4, or 5. In this exhalation dysfunction, Ribs 2-6 have moved caudad.

Regardless of the treatment type (direct or indirect), treatment should always be directed at the key rib; in this case, Rib 2.

Manipulation of the cervico-thoracic fascia (**choice E**) will not directly influence an exhalation dysfunction of Ribs 2-6.

1. A 23-year-old female comes to your office complaining of right-sided thoracic pain. The pain started after a fall approximately one week ago. The severity of the pain has decreased throughout the week; however, it is still present, especially at maximum inhalation. Naproxen sodium two times daily seems to decrease the pain. The patient has no cardiac risk factors. X-rays in your office reveal no fracture. EKG reveals normal sinus rhythm with no evidence of an abnormality. On examination, you notice that Ribs 6-9 on the right are restricted in inhalation. The thoracic vertebrae, T5-T9, have a lateral convexity to the left, and the transverse processes of these vertebrae are posterior on the left. The seventh cervical vertebrae is sidebent left when in the neutral and flexed position, but this asymmetry seems to resolve in the extended position. Which of the following statements is true?

    (A) The above patient has an inhalation dysfunction, T5-T9 is neutral, sidebent right, rotated left.

    (B) The patient would be asked to rotate her torso to the right when correcting T5-T9 using muscle energy.

    (C) Muscle energy treatment of the rib dysfunction should be directed at Rib 9.

    (D) With the head flexed, sidebent left, and rotated right, a high-velocity low-amplitude rotational thrust would be directed at C7 to correct this dysfunction.

    (E) The pectoralis minor could be used to correct the rib dysfunction.

2. A patient has an exhalation dysfunction of Rib 6 on the right. Which of the following is the best statement concerning this somatic dysfunction?

    (A) This patient will have limited cephalad motion of Rib 6 at the midaxillary line.

    (B) This patient will have a tender point in the pectoralis muscle.

    (C) This patient will display a winging of his scapula.

    (D) The six thoracic vertebrae are non-neutral, sidebent right, and rotated right.

    (E) The six thoracic vertebrae are non-neutral, sidebent left, and rotated left.

3. A patient is noted to have a somatic dysfunction of T2-T6 that is neutral, sidebent right, and rotated left. Also, this patient demonstrates an inhalation dysfunction of Ribs 2-6. Which of the following is the best statement regarding treatment of these somatic dysfunctions?

    (A) Muscle energy treatment should be directed toward Rib 6, using the serratus anterior.

    (B) Muscle energy treatment should be directed toward Rib 2, using the posterior scalene.

    (C) A high-velocity low-amplitude thrust should be directed at the angle of Rib 4.

    (D) A high-velocity low-amplitude thrust should be directed at the right transverse process of T4.

    (E) Muscle energy treatment should be directed at the thoracic spine with the head sidebent left and rotated right.

4. A patient complains of low back pain. Evaluation shows dysfunction in the lumbar region. Which of the following is the best statement regarding the anatomy and biomechanics of the lumbar spine?

(A) Weakness in the lateral portions of the posterior longitudinal ligament makes high-lumbar disc herniations more common than low-lumbar herniations.

(B) A straightening of the lumbar lordosis will always result in a decrease in the lumbosacral angle.

(C) The L5 nerve root typically exits superior to the intervertebral disc of the L5 and S1 vertebrae.

(D) The lumbar spine moves easiest about a sagittal axis.

(E) Sacralization of the lumbar spine reinforces the lumbosacral unit, decreasing the likelihood of degenerative joint disease.

5. A patient complains of pain in the lower extremities. After an osteopathic structural examination, the patient is diagnosed with claudication. Which of the following is commonly seen in neurogenic claudication caused by spinal stenosis but is not typically seen in peripheral vascular disease with vascular claudication?

(A) Increased lower extremity pain with walking

(B) Pain relief with sitting

(C) Posterior calf pain

(D) Relief of pain by using a shopping cart

(E) Absence of parasthesias

6. A 24-year-old male presents to your office complaining of low back and gluteal pain. The pain is localized to the back and is dull and achy. Structural examination reveals L1 and L5 FS_RR_R. Two tender points are noted: one approximately one centimeter lateral to the pubic symphysis on the right side of the superior ramus and the other approximately one inch medial to the ASIS on the right. The lumbosacral junction springs freely. He has a positive standing flexion test on the right. His left PSIS is more inferior, and his left ASIS is more superior when compared with the right. Which of the following statements holds true?

(A) This patient has a right sacral torsion on a left oblique axis.

(B) This patient is likely to have a positive Thomas test.

(C) The tender point near the pubic symphysis identifies a somatic dysfunction at L1.

(D) The correct position to correct L5 with a direct technique is sidebent right, rotated right.

(E) This patient has a posteriorly rotated innominate on the right.

7. A 39-year-old male presents to your office with severe low back pain radiating to his lower extremities. The pain started yesterday while he was working on his car. The pain came suddenly: It was first localized to the low back, then progressed to sharp burning pain down both legs; worse on the right than the left. Now both of his legs feel numb and weak. He also states that he had difficulty holding his urine this morning. He denies dysuria or hematuria but does have a history of renal stones. Neurologic examination of his lower extremities reveals absent Achilles reflex bilaterally and diminished knee jerk reflex bilaterally. Muscle strength is approximately 3/5 throughout his lower extremities. Which one of the following statements describes the correct course of treatment?

(A) Immediate transportation by EMS to the hospital for neurosurgic evaluation

(B) Indirect OMT techniques to decrease restrictions, along with prescriptions for muscle relaxants and narcotic analgesics to be used as needed

(C) Physical modalities, such as ultrasound and electrical stimulation, to the low back

(D) NSAIDS and referral to MRI clinic if pain not improved in one week

(E) Comprehensive osteopathic manipulation starting with gentle indirect techniques, then direct techniques one week later after muscle spasm has subsided

8. A 72-year-old male presents with chronic back pain that has been worsening over the past several months. He describes a dull ache in his low back with pain radiating down the back of his legs. Aggravating factors include standing or walking, especially when walking downstairs. Alleviating factors include sitting and NSAIDS as needed. On examination, pulses are strong in the lower extremities, and capillary refill is adequate. He has a decreased lumbar lordosis and severely limited range of motion of the lumbar spine. There is a decreased sensation in the posterior aspect of his thighs—otherwise, neurologic examination is normal. Considering this patient's symptoms, what is the most likely finding this patient will have on radiologic studies?

(A) A herniated nucleus propulsis impinging the caudal sac on magnetic resonance imaging

(B) A fracture of the pars interarticularis of a lumbar vertebra

(C) An anterior displacement of L5 on S1, resulting in entrapment of the cauda equina

(D) Degenerative changes within the intervertebral disc and narrowing of the intervertebral foramina

(E) Compression fracture of the lumbar vertebrae

9. A 20-year-old man complains of acute lower back pain. He has a sacral dysfunction. Which of the following is the best answer regarding sacral biomechanics?

(A) As a person inhales, the lumbosacral angle increases.

(B) The primary respiratory mechanism (PRM) influences sacral motion about an inferior sacral axis.

(C) The sacrum nutates with craniosacral flexion.

(D) During ambulation, weight-bearing on the left leg will cause a left oblique axis to be engaged.

(E) A positive seated flexion test on the right will indicate sacral dysfunction on a left oblique axis.

10. A 40-year-old female presents to your office with severe low back pain of acute onset. The pain started soon after lifting a 17-lb turkey out of the oven. She is unable to stand up straight, sit, or laterally flex to the right without severe pain radiating down the back of her right leg. On physical examination, there is no neurologic deficit. Structural examination reveals a positive seated flexion test on the right. The left inferior lateral angle of the sacrum is anterior when compared with the right There is limited springing at the lumbosacral junction. Given the above information, what is the sacral diagnosis?

(A) Left sacral rotation on a right oblique axis

(B) Right sacral rotation on a right oblique axis

(C) Right sacral rotation on a left oblique axis

(D) Right unilateral sacral flexion

(E) Flexed sacral base

11. A 34-year-old male truck driver presents to you with a chief complaint of moderate to severe low back pain. He gives a history of falling off a loading dock three days prior. Examination of the patient in the prone position reveals a deep sacral sulcus on the left, a posterior inferior lateral angle (ILA) on the right when compared with the opposite side, and lumbosacral junction that springs freely upon compression. What is the most likely diagnosis?

(A) A forward sacral torsion on a right oblique axis

(B) A forward sacral torsion on a left oblique axis

(C) A backward sacral torsion on a left oblique axis

(D) A left unilateral sacral flexion

(E) Bilateral sacral extension

12. A 20-year-male presents with low back pain after falling onto a concrete floor when he slipped on a puddle of oil. The patient gives a history of episodic aching of the lumbar region prior to the fall. With the patient standing, there is noticeable absence of the lumbar lordosis. With the patient prone, the ILAs are equal in depth. Motion testing reveals no motion at the lumbosacral junction. What is the most likely diagnosis?

(A) Bilaterally flexed sacrum

(B) Sacral base extension

(C) A forward sacral torsion on a left oblique axis

(D) A backward sacral torsion on a left oblique axis

(E) Right unilateral sacral flexion

Questions 13-14

<u>CASE A</u>

Evaluation of a patient with hip and groin pain reveals a positive standing and seated flexion test on the left. The right ASIS appears more caudad on the right, and the right PSIS is more cephalad when compared with the left. The lumbosacral junction springs freely. The left sacral sulcus is more anterior when compared with the right.

13. Which of the following is the best answer?

   (A) This patient will have an apparent short leg on the right.

   (B) This patient has a posterior rotated innominate on the left.

   (C) AP compression of the pelvis on the left will demonstrate adequate resiliency.

   (D) This patient will have a positive Thomas test.

   (E) The above patient is likely to have tight quadriceps.

14. If a sacral torsion is present in the above question, what would be the diagnosis at the fifth lumbar vertebrae?

   (A) L5 NS_LR_R

   (B) L5 NS_RR_L

   (C) L5 ER_RS_L

   (D) L5 FR_LS_L

   (E) L5 FR_RS_L

15. A 45-year-old male presents to your office with intermittent right shoulder and arm pain and numbness. He states that the symptoms occur primarily when his arm is raised above his head. This started about one month ago and has gotten progressively worse. He does not recall any precipitating factors or recent trauma. He has no past medical history and has no cardiac risk factors. On examination, the patient has tender points at the anterior scalene and trapezius on the right. There is some restriction to left rotation of the lower cervical spine, and Rib 1 on the right has limited exhalation motion. There is full active range of motion of the glenohumeral joint with no pain elicited. Adson's test is positive. Capillary refill is normal in the right upper extremity. X-rays of the cervical spine show mild degenerative joint disease. Given the above information, which of the following statements is most accurate?

   (A) This patient will have a positive Allen's test.

   (B) This patient's condition is most likely due to a partial tear of the supraspinatus tendon.

   (C) Using muscle energy, the anterior scalene should be contracted to influence motion at Rib 1.

   (D) This patient will have an absent or diminished brachioradialis reflex on the right.

   (E) This patient's condition is most likely due to a slight compression of the subclavian artery and brachial plexus.

16. A 79-year-old female presents to your office with complaints of shoulder pain with arm movement. The patient's left arm is in a sling. Two months prior, she fell in her home and hit her shoulder on the coffee table. She went to the emergency room where X-rays were negative for a fracture or dislocation. She states that the pain from the initial injury has resolved but her shoulder now hurts with movement of the upper extremity. She was instructed by the ER physician to use the sling for the initial injury; however, because she is having pain with arm movement, she thought it would be best to continue the use of the sling. On examination, there appears to be atrophy of the supraspinatus and deltoid muscles on the left. There is some tenderness at the tip of the acromion. There is also a positive drop arm test. Abduction of the left shoulder demonstrates limited left glenohumeral motion. Internal and external rotation of the upper extremity is severely diminished. Given the above information, which of the following statements is most accurate?

(A) This patient will benefit from continued use of the shoulder sling and weekly osteopathic treatment to improve shoulder range of motion.

(B) The patient's condition is due to chronic impingement of the supraspinatus tendon.

(C) This patient is likely to have a positive Adson's test.

(D) Early mobilization following the injury with osteopathic treatment directed at freeing up restrictions of the glenohumeral area would have prevented complications of the initial injury.

(E) This patient needs immediate referral to an orthopedic surgeon for evaluation of a complete rotator cuff tear.

17. A 23-year-old male is complaining of wrist and elbow pain. Physical examination reveals limited supination of the affected forearm, and the radial head resists anterior glide. X-rays are negative for fracture. Which of the following statements is most accurate?

(A) This condition is associated with an increased carrying angle.

(B) The ulna will resist medial glide.

(C) This type of dysfunction can be caused by falling on an outstretched pronated arm.

(D) The patient's hand will appear more abducted on the affected side.

(E) The affected wrist will have limited flexion.

Questions 18-19

CASE B

A patient complains of neck and shoulder pain after a motor vehicle accident in which she was wearing a seatbelt.

18. Injury to the posterior cord of the brachial plexus will have the greatest effect on which movement?

(A) Wrist flexion
(B) Abduction of the fingers
(C) Elbow flexion
(D) Shoulder extension
(E) Thumb abduction

19. Injury to the upper portion of the brachial plexus will have the least effect on which of the following?

(A) Sensation to the middle finger
(B) Sensation to the lateral portion of the forearm
(C) Brachioradialis reflex
(D) Arm abduction
(E) Movement of the intrinsic muscles of the hand

20. A 25-year-old marathon runner presents to your office with ankle and knee pain. He states that the pain started several months ago and has gotten progressively worse. A thorough history and physical examination indicates that the patient has a posterior proximal fibular head dysfunction and a tender point at the posterior aspect of the proximal fibular head. Which of the following statements is true?

(A) The ankle will resist inversion.
(B) The ankle will move freely into supination.
(C) The proximal fibular head will resist posterior glide.
(D) The distal fibular head will move posterior with supination of the ankle.
(E) The tender point is best treated with the knee extended, foot inverted, and the tibia internally rotated.

21. A 25-year-old male is complaining of severe low back pain radiating into the foot. The pain started immediately after lifting a heavy object. He describes a lightening type of pain shooting into his left foot. He denies any bowel or bladder problems. There is a positive straight-leg raising test. A cursory osteopathic structural examination of this patient demonstrates bilateral paraspinal hypertonicity. The lumbar spine moves freely into right sidebending and left rotation at segments L2-L5. The sacrum has forward rotation along a right oblique axis. Which of the following statements is the best answer?

    (A) HVLA should be directed at the lumbar spine with L2-L5 rotated right and sidebent left.
    (B) This patient will have a positive lumbosacral spring test.
    (C) This patient is likely to have a positive hip drop test.
    (D) This patient will most likely need surgery to remove the herniated disk.
    (E) This patient's injury would have been prevented with weekly osteopathic treatment.

22. After two weeks of conservative management, the patient in the above question comes to your office still having significant pain. An MRI shows a posterio-lateral disc herniation at the L4/L5 disc space that appears to impinge the thecal sac. Which of the following findings is this patient most likely to have on examination?

    (A) Weak hip flexors
    (B) Weak quadriceps
    (C) Babinski's reflex
    (D) Decreased sensation to the dorsum of the foot
    (E) Decreased sensation at the ishial tuberosity

23. During a cranial sacral treatment, internal rotation of the temporal bones is diagnosed. Internal rotation of the temporal bones is associated with which of the following?

    (A) Caudad motion of the dura
    (B) TMJ dysfunction
    (C) External rotation of the occiput
    (D) Tender points in the temporalis muscle
    (E) Nausea

24. A football player complains of foot pain when he runs. Which of the following statements is true regarding the biomechanics of the foot?

    (A) Posterior glide of the talus provides talocrural (tibiotalar) stability.
    (B) Tenderness on the plantar surface of the foot at the lateral portion of the transverse arch may indicate somatic dysfunction of the navicular bone.
    (C) Resistance of ankle plantarflexion is likely to indicate a somatic dysfunction of the talocalcaneal joint.
    (D) Excessive pronation of the ankle will most likely result in a strain of the anterior talofibular ligament.
    (E) Somatic dysfunctions of the ankle most commonly occur when the foot is dorsiflexed.

25. A patient complains of constant ringing in her ears. Tinnitus may result from a dysfunction of which of the following bones?

    (A) Frontal
    (B) Maxillae
    (C) Zygoma
    (D) Temporal
    (E) Parietal

26. While performing cranial sacral treatment, a restriction is noted at the occipito-temporal suture. Tension along the occipito-temporal suture is most likely to result in which of the following?

    (A) Dysphagia
    (B) Diplopia
    (C) Tender point in the sternocleidomastoid at the attachment of the clavicle
    (D) Decreased venous drainage of the cranium
    (E) Bell's palsy

27. Palpation of the cranial vault on a patient with cephalgia demonstrates a left sidebending/rotation sphenobasilar strain pattern and a five-cycle per minute cranial rhythmic impulse (CRI) with decreased amplitude and vitality. Which of the following is the most effective technique to normalize the CRI on this patient?

    (A) Frontal lift
    (B) Temporal rocking
    (C) CV4 decompression
    (D) Vault hold
    (E) V-spread

CASE C

A 66-year-old diabetic male came to the ER via EMS with chest tightness. He states the pain started half an hour ago, and it was not relieved with nitroglycerine sublingually times three. The pain radiates to his left shoulder, and he states this is a similar type of pain he had when he experienced his last myocardial infarction. He is currently diphoretic and has dyspnea. His vitals are stable. On examination, he appears in mild distress, and there is a grade 2 systolic ejection murmur on auscultation. The abdomen is soft and nontender. There is no clubbing cyanosis or edema on extremities, but there is tenderness in the left deltoid.

28. Which of the following structures will have the least effect on this patient's cardiac function?

   (A) The occiput
   (B) The second cervical vertebrae
   (C) The fifth cervical vertebrae
   (D) The second thoracic vertebrae
   (E) The fourth thoracic vertebrae

29. Tenderness in the left deltoid is most likely to represent:

   (A) Chapman's point
   (B) A somatic-visceral reflex
   (C) A viscero-somatic reflex
   (D) Travell's trigger point
   (E) Jones counterstrain point

CASE D

You are asked to evaluate a 24-year-old female for a severe unrelenting headache. She was admitted to ICU through the ER three days ago for an acute GI bleed. She states the pain has been present for three days and describes the pain as a steady, dull (occasionally sharp) pain, located at the base of the head and radiating to the right eye. It occasionally extends across the forehead. She denies having pain from bright lights and she does not have nausea, vomiting, or sinus congestion. She reports having had similar symptoms in the past, particularly at the end of a "stressful day." Osteopathic structural examination demonstrates tenderness, muscular tension, and fullness in the suboccipital region (R > L). Deep palpation at the right occipito-atlantal (OA) joint radiates pain to the area of the right temporalis region.

30. Which of the following statements best explains the tenderness at the OA junction?

   (A) The dysfunction is due to a vasodilitation of the cranial blood supply.
   (B) It is likely the result of hypertonicity of the temporalis muscle.
   (C) Treatment may consist of myofascial release or spray and stretch using vapocoolant spray.
   (D) Treatment may consist of counterstrain to the temporalis muscle.
   (E) Treatment should initially begin with muscle energy directed at the OA to decrease muscle tension in the suboccipital region.

31. What is the rationale for using rib raising on this patient?

   (A) It will improve VQ function.
   (B) It will reduce cardiac output.
   (C) It will reduce sympathetic hypertonicity.
   (D) It will stimulate the diaphragm and improve lymphatic flow.
   (E) It should not be done because it is contraindicated in a person with an acute GI bleed.

32. Current treatment for headache often indicates use of anti-inflammatory medication. Most medication from this class would be absolutely contraindicated in this case because there is a risk of what?

    (A) Tinnitus

    (B) Gastric bleeding

    (C) Nausea and vomiting

    (D) Tenderness and fullness in the subxiphoid space

    (E) Tissue texture changes in the midthoracic paraspinal region

33. The following morning you recheck this patient. She reports that her headache has resolved and she was able to get some rest after your OMT treatment yesterday. Which of the following best indicates follow-up care?

    (A) Since symptoms have resolved, no follow-up is necessary.

    (B) Re-evaluate your patient today and determine if further intervention is necessary.

    (C) Re-evaluate the patient in one week.

    (D) Repeat the same OMT treatment two more times to insure adequate resolution of somatic dysfunction.

    (E) Refer to physical therapy for initiating ultrasound therapy to the suboccipital area.

Questions 34-37

CASE E

A 62-year-old man was admitted to the hospital with a diagnosis of congestive heart failure. He appears slightly anxious. History reveals that he is noncompliant with his medications. He admits to a 20-lb weight gain, has developed swelling of the legs, and has nocturia. This progressed to dyspnea on exertion and then to severe orthopnea. He had emergent medical care upon admission to the hospital, which included diuresis. On examination, he is 5'11 and weighs 270 lbs. BP 140/70, HR 105, RR 22 and shallow, temp. 98.6. There is an S3 gallop rhythm, rales in the lungs, soft and enlarged liver, and grade 2 pretibial edema.

34. In this patient, treatment of which area would be most likely to decrease excessive sympathetic tone to the heart?

    (A) O-A

    (B) C3-C5

    (C) T2-T4

    (D) T10-T12

    (E) L3-L5

35. In this patient, treatment of which area would have the greatest effect on renal function?

    (A) O-A

    (B) T2-T4

    (C) T10-T12

    (D) L4-L5

    (E) The sacrum

36. In this patient, what should you do prior to instituting lymphatic pump treatments?

    (A) CV4 technique

    (B) Treat thoracic inlet

    (C) Liver pump

    (D) Kirksville Krunch to the midthoracic spine

    (E) Cervical HVLA

37. Which lymphatic technique would be the most effective for this severely debilitated patient?

    (A) Liver pump

    (B) Pectoral traction

    (C) Classic thoracic pump

    (D) Ischial rectal fossa technique

    (E) Effleurage of the legs

Questions 38-40

CASE F

A 54-year-old secretary, with a history of type 2 diabetes complains of pain and paresthesia in her right thumb, index, and middle fingers for one month. She describes the pain as an ache that is intermittent and worse at night. Shaking or rubbing the hands seems to help. The symptoms are reproduced while driving her car and typing. She also describes some weakness in opening jars of food. Osteopathic structural examination reveals a tender point in the right anterior scalene. There is an inhalation dysfunction of the right first rib. There is myofascial tenderness and trigger points in the forearm flexors. There is loss of sensation of the thumb, index, and middle fingers of the right hand. Right thumb abduction was weak without any muscle atrophy.

38. In this patient, treatment of which area would most likely decrease excessive sympathetic tone to the upper extremity?

    (A) O-A
    (B) C2-C3
    (C) C5-T1
    (D) T2-T7
    (E) T10-L2

39. In this patient, treatment of which area would have the greatest effect on lymphatic drainage from the upper extremity?

    (A) Rib raising to Ribs 4-7
    (B) Myofascial release to the cervico-thoracic junction
    (C) Condylar decompression
    (D) Effleurage to the upper extremity
    (E) Superior cervical ganglion inhibition

40. A patient complains of wrist pain. Structural examination shows a wrist flexion dysfunction. The forearm flexors have their origin from which anatomic structure?

    (A) Medial epicondyle
    (B) Radial head
    (C) Olecranon process
    (D) Humeral condyle
    (E) Phalanges

41. A 24-year-old male presents with hand numbness. The symptoms started one week ago and has gotten progressively worse. Examination reveals decreased sensation over the fourth and fifth digits. Sensation to the first three digits and medial portion of the forearm is normal. Biceps, triceps, and brachioradialis reflexes are 2/4 and symmetric. Manual muscle testing reveals weakness with wrist adduction, as well as weakness with the hypothenar muscles. At what location would Tinel's test most likely be positive in the above patient?

    (A) Between the flexor digitorum profundus and flexor digitorum superfiscialis
    (B) Distal to the flexor retinaculum
    (C) Over the transverse carpal ligament
    (D) At the cubital tunnel
    (E) One centimeter proximal to the tunnel of Guyon

42. A 55-year-old male presents to your office with frequent-burning epigastric pain associated with nausea. The pain has been present for several months but has gotten worse over the past several weeks. He gives a history of gastric reflux. He states that the pain appears midmorning; it is relieved by food, but the symptoms return two to three hours after a meal. A palpatory structural examination of this patient may reveal somatic dysfunction of which of the following areas?

    (A) T1-T4
    (B) T5-T9
    (C) T10-T12
    (D) T11-L1
    (E) L2-L3

43. A patient is seeking nonpharmacologic treatment for asthma. You recommend osteopathic manipulative treatment intended to normalize autonomic stimulation to the lungs. Which of the following areas would you direct your treatment?

    (A) Suboccipital area

    (B) C3-C5

    (C) Thoracic inlet

    (D) T8-T12

    (E) Ribs 8-12

44. A 64-year-old smoker with chronic bronchitis has a productive cough with thick green mucus. What is the goal behind OMT treatment directed at the autonomic nervous system?

    (A) It will stimulate the vagus nerve and cause bronchodilation.

    (B) It will inhibit the cough reflex, providing symptom relief.

    (C) It will thin the mucus by decreasing sympathetic tone.

    (D) It will mechanically cause a flattening of the diaphragm, which increases negative intrathoracic pressure.

    (E) It will directly stimulate the phrenic nerve and cause better diaphragm motion.

45. When examining a patient with COPD, you note an increased AP diameter of his chest. Which of the following is the best reason for a COPD patient to have an increased AP diameter of his/her chest?

    (A) The destruction of elastic fibers and chronic air trapping results in permanent inhaled rib positions.

    (B) Chronic increased sympathetic tone causes a bronchoalveolar expansion and results in an increase in total lung capacity.

    (C) Poor oxygenation to the diaphragm causes fibrosis and muscle shortening, resulting in a flattened diaphragm and an increased AP diameter.

    (D) The chronic overuse of scalenes and intercostal muscles pulls the ribs superiorly, resulting in an expanded thoracic cage.

    (E) Chronic viscerosomatic input to the pleura causes fibrosis and expansion of the thoracic cage.

Questions 46-48

<u>CASE G</u>

A 52-year-old male is in the cardiovascular ICU after undergoing a triple coronary artery bypass graft using mammary artery and saphenous vein autografts. Postoperative course was uneventful, other than persistent chest pain.

<u>Pertinent physical findings on the second postoperative day:</u>

- Patient appears to be in moderate distress.

- Vital signs: BP 140/90, HR 62, RR 22 and shallow, temperature 98.

- Heart: regular rate and rhythm at 62. No rubs, clicks, or murmurs.

- Lungs: decreased respiratory effort and excursion throughout the lung fields; few scattered bibasilar crackles.

- Chest: midline sternal dressing and sutured sternotomy incision is present; there is no apparent drainage and the wound has a mild erythema.

- Extremities: strong peripheral pulses. Dressing and surgical wound on left medial lower limb; no evidence of infection. There is no edema.

- Musculoskeletal examination: T1-T4 left-sided tissue texture changes. Ribs exhibit decreased excursion, numbers 3-5 left exhalation dysfunction is present (inhalation restriction). Diaphragm excursion is decreased and thoracoabdominal fascias prefer right rotation and right sidebending. Shoulders are drawn up toward ears. Scalene muscles are tight bilaterally and firm to touch. Thoracic inlet rotation to the right. OA is flexed, sidebent left, and rotated right.

46. Which of the following manipulative techniques would be most harmful to this patient?

    (A) Indirect myofascial release of cervicothoracic junction
    (B) Costochondral approach for diaphragm release
    (C) Rib raising
    (D) CV4 bulb decompression
    (E) Occipito-atlantal suboccipital release

47. What is the most likely etiology of the bibasilar crackles in this patient?

    (A) Pneumothorax
    (B) Postoperative pneumonia
    (C) Pulmonary embolism
    (D) Postoperative atelectasis
    (E) Congestive heart failure

48. Which of the following manipulative techniques is the most appropriate technique for treating the cause of the bibasilar crackles?

    (A) Rib raising
    (B) Occipito-atlantal suboccipital release
    (C) Thoracic lymphatic pump
    (D) Muscle energy to Ribs 3-5
    (E) Paraspinal inhibitory soft tissue technique

49. A 52-year-old male presents to your office with erectile dysfunction. He states that he has trouble maintaining his erection during intercourse. He denies any dysuria, hematuria, or difficulty voiding. Physical examination reveals a normal prostate, and his PSA level is 0.4. Which of the following osteopathic treatments will most likely improve this patient's symptoms via an alteration of the autonomic nervous system?

    (A) Treatment of T11-L2 vertebral segments
    (B) Paraspinal inhibition of the thoraco-lumbar fascia
    (C) Rib raising to Ribs 11 and 12
    (D) Occipito-atlantal release
    (E) Balancing the sacrum

50. A 77-year-old female with known colon cancer at the cecum undergoes a hemicolectomy with end-to-end anastomosis. Histologic diagnosis is consistent with adenocarcinoma Duke's B classification. Given the above information, at what location is this patient likely to have tissue texture abnormalities?

    (A) T1-T3
    (B) T5-T9
    (C) T10-T12
    (D) L1-L3
    (E) Sacrum

ANSWERS AND EXPLANATIONS

1.	D		26.	D
2.	A		27.	C
3.	E		28.	C
4.	C		29.	C
5.	D		30.	C
6.	B		31.	C
7.	A		32.	B
8.	D		33.	B
9.	D		34.	C
10.	C		35.	C
11.	A		36.	B
12.	B		37.	B
13.	B		38.	D
14.	B		39.	B
15.	E		40.	A
16.	D		41.	D
17.	C		42.	B
18.	D		43.	A
19.	E		44.	C
20.	B		45.	A
21.	C		46.	B
22.	D		47.	D
23.	A		48.	A
24.	A		49.	E
25.	D		50.	C

1. **The correct answer is D.** The patient in the above question has the following dysfunctions: *1)* an exhalation dysfunction of Ribs 6-9, *2)* T5-T9 neutral, sidebent right, and rotated left, and *3)* C7 extended, rotated left, and sidebent left. Since Ribs 6-9 have limited inhalation motion, then they must ease into exhalation. Since you name the dysfunction in the direction of ease, it must be an exhalation dysfunction. Thoracic convexity to the left implies that T5-T9 are sidebent right. Since the transverse processes are posterior on the left, this implies that these vertebrae are rotated left. According to the laws of Fryette, if a vertebra is sidebent and rotated in opposite directions, it must be in the neutral position. The question also states that C7 is extended and sidebent left. Due to facet orientation, C7 always rotates and sidebends in the same direction; therefore, C7 must be rotated right.

    Choice A is wrong because, as stated above, there is an exhalation dysfunction of Ribs 6-9. When using muscle energy, the thoracic vertebrae will be rotated and sidebent toward the restrictive barrier, and the patient is asked to move in the opposite direction.

    In this case, the thoracic vertebrae should be sidebent left and rotated right, and the patient would then be asked to rotate to the left (not the right [**choice B**]).

    Muscle energy treatment of the ribs (**choice C**) should be directed toward the "key" rib. In exhalation dysfunctions, the uppermost rib is the "key" rib (i.e., Rib 6). When using an HVLA rotational thrust to correct the dysfunction, the cervical spine would be in the flexed position, rotated toward the restrictive barrier, and sidebent away (to lock out the facets above C7). A rotational thrust toward the restrictive barrier (to the right) will correct this dysfunction.

    The pectoralis minor (**choice E**) is used to correct an exhalation dysfunction of Ribs 3, 4, and 5. The serratus anterior is used for Ribs 6-9.

2. **The correct answer is A.** Rib 6 moves primarily in a bucket-handle fashion (the lateral aspect of Rib 6 moves cephalad with inhalation and caudad with exhalation). Since Rib 6 has an exhalation dysfunction, it will have limited inhalation motion (you name the dysfunction in the direction it wants to go). This means that Rib 6 will have limited cephalad motion at the midaxillary line.

    The pectoralis muscle originates at the coracoid process and inserts onto Ribs 3-5. A tender point in this muscle (**choice B**) would be due to a somatic dysfunction of Ribs 3-5, not Rib 6.

    Winging of the scapula (**choice C**) will cause weakness in the serratus anterior, and it is a result of injury to the long thoracic nerve. It is not related to a somatic dysfunction of Rib 6.

    Although a rib dysfunction and thoracic dysfunction can easily be seen together, these dysfunctions are not always associated with one another. Therefore, **choices D and E** are not necessarily true and thus not the best answers.

3. **The correct answer is E.** The patient has both a rib dysfunction and a thoracic dysfunction. It is customary to treat the thoracic spine before treating rib dysfunctions because often a rib dysfunction can be due to a thoracic dysfunction.

    Choices A, B, and **C** are all wrong because these treatments are directed at the rib dysfunction.

    In order to correct the thoracic dysfunction with HVLA, the thrust should be directed at the *left* transverse process of T4 (**choice D**).

    When treating with muscle energy, the restrictive barrier should be engaged. Since the vertebrae are rotated left and sidebent right, the correct treatment position is neutral, sidebent left, rotated right (**choice E**).

4. **The correct answer is C.** In the thoracic and lumbar regions, the nerve root will exit the intervertebral foramina below its corresponding segment. For example, the L5 nerve root will exit between L5 and S1. Since the spinal cord ends at L1 and L2, the remaining nerve roots become longer as they approach the lower segments. This causes the lumbar nerves to exit the superior aspect of their intervertebral foramina, just above the intervertebral disc.

    The posterior longitudinal ligament narrows as it approaches the sacrum. This results in a posterio-lateral weakness making disc herniations more common in the lower lumbar region (**choice A**).

    The lumbosacral angle is formed by the intersection of a horizontal line and the line of inclination of the sacrum. If straightening of the lumbar lordosis results in a sacrum that is more vertical, it will decrease the lumbosacral angle and **choice B** would be true. However, slight spinal flexion can straighten the lumbar lordosis and not affect the line of inclination of the sacrum, thus not affecting the lumbosacral angle.

    The lumbar spine moves easiest through flexion and extension. This is motion about a transverse axis and in a sagittal plane (**choice D**).

    Sacralization may alter the structure-function relationship of the lumbosacral junction, leading to early disc degeneration (**choice E**).

5. **The correct answer is D.**

   Calf pain that worsens with walking (**choice A**) and is relieved with sitting (**choice B**) occurs with both neurogenic claudication and vascular claudication.

   The absence of parasthesias (**choice E**) is more typical with vascular claudication. The symptoms of lumbar stenosis with neurogenic claudication can be relieved by flexion of the spine, such as pushing a shopping cart while walking. This is not seen with vascular claudication.

6. **The correct answer is B.** The above patient has several dysfunctions; let's start by eliminating some of the answers. A right sacral torsion on a left oblique axis (i.e., a backward sacral torsion): A backward sacral torsion will result in a positive lumbosacral spring test (i.e., the lumbosacral junction will not spring freely). Also, if a sacral torsion is present, it would follow the "rules of L5 on the sacrum."

   According to these rules, L5 rotates in the opposite direction of the sacrum, and sidebending of L5 is in the same direction as the oblique axis of the sacrum. Therefore, a right sacral torsion (rotated right) on a left oblique axis would coincide with L5, which is rotated left and sidebent left. L5 in the above question is FS_RR_R. Thus, **choice A** is the wrong answer.

   A tender point approximately 1 cm lateral to the pubic symphysis on the superior ramus will coincide with an L5 dysfunction; therefore, **choice C** is wrong. An L1 anterior tender point is located approximately 1 cm medial to the ASIS. A tender point approximately one inch medial to the ASIS on the right indicates probable tension in the right iliopsoas and can clue you in about a flexion contracture of this muscle.

   In order to treat L5 with a direct technique, one must move the vertebrae toward the restrictive barrier. Since L5 is flexed, rotated right, and sidebent right, one must extend, rotate left, and sidebend left to engage the restrictive barrier. Therefore, **choice D** is wrong.

   The patient's left PSIS is more inferior, and his left ASIS is more superior when compared with the right, so the left innominate appears to be rotated posterior in relation to the right (**choice E**). However, since the above patient has a positive standing flexion test on the right, the pelvic dysfunction is present on the right. This must mean that he has a right innominate rotated anteriorly.

   This leaves our final answer, **choice B.** How can we confirm this answer? A positive Thomas test is associated with a flexion contracture of the iliopsoas. This dysfunction is consistent with some of the findings this patient has. First of all, as mentioned above, a tender point one inch medial to the ASIS indicates an iliopsoas

   contracture. And a flexion contracture of the iliopsoas is associated with a high lumbar dysfunction, flexed, rotated toward, and sidebent toward the ipsilateral side.

7. **The correct answer is A.** The patient in the above question has a suspected cauda equina syndrome (CES). CES is usually the result of a large central disc herniation compressing the roots of the cauda equina. Symptoms include low back pain with weakness and numbness in the lower extremities; particularly, the patient will have "saddle anesthesia," which is numbness along the "saddle" area (the sacral) dermatomes. The hallmark of CES is bladder and bowel incontinence or dysfunction with neurologic deficits. This patient gives no indication to have bladder dysfunction (a history of kidney stones is not sufficient reason to have bladder dysfunction in the face of a new neurologic deficit). Because this patient indicates difficulty holding his urine, CES must be ruled out. If CES is present, neurologic decompression must be done within 48 hours or irreversible neurologic damage may occur.

   The remaining answers would be indicated if the patient initially presented with low back pain, but due to the acute nature of possible CES, an immediate neurosurgic evaluation must be done first to rule out CES.

8. **The correct answer is D.** The patient's aggravating factors (standing and walking, especially when walking downstairs) and alleviating factors (sitting and NSAIDS as needed), along with the physical findings should indicate to the test taker that this patient is most likely to have lumbar spinal stenosis. Lumbar stenosis is narrowing of the spinal canal and/or entrapment of the nerves as they exit the intervertebral foramina because of the narrowing of these foramina. Radiographically, degenerative changes are present with narrowing of the intervertebral foramina. As the patient extends his lumbar spine (by standing or walking, especially downstairs), the intervertebral foramen physiologically become more narrowed. If a patient has narrowing of this area already (i.e., lumbar spinal stenosis), neural impingement can occur. The patient's symptoms will usually improve with flexion of the lumbar spine (sitting).

   It is very unlikely for a 72-year-old male to have a disc herniation (**choice A**). As people age, their nucleus propulsis dries up, losing its gel-like properties. Because it dries up, there is nothing to herniate.

   A fracture in the pars interarticularis without anterior slippage is called spondylolysis (**choice B**). If anterior slippage is present, this is referred to as spondylolisthesis (**choice C**). Both of these choices occur much less frequently; therefore, these answers are incorrect.

A 72-year-old male may get a compression fracture of the lumbar (**choice E**), but this also is not common. Also, a lumbar compression fracture is less likely to result in a neurologic deficit, and the pain would not be alleviated with sitting, but rather by lying supine.

9. **The correct answer is D.** Postural motion, craniosacral motion, respiration, ambulation, and L5 motion all influence sacral motion. When a person is ambulating, the innominates rotate about a transverse axis, while the sacrum rotates about two oblique axes. Weight bearing on the left leg will cause a left oblique axis to be engaged, and the opposite is true for the right leg. This explains why **choice D** is the correct answer.

As a person inhales, the diaphragm pushes downward, decreasing the lumbar lordosis, causing the sacral base to move posterior. This motion will decrease the lumbosacral angle; therefore, **choice A** is the wrong answer.

The PRM influences sacral motion about a superior sacral axis.

Nutation and counternutation are terms used for motion at the sacral base associated with craniosacral motion. Flexion of the cranial bones will cause the sacral base to extend (move posterior). This is called counternutation. Extension of the cranial bones will cause the sacral base to flex (move anterior). This is called nutation. Therefore, **choice C** is wrong.

A positive seated flexion test on the right will indicate sacral dysfunction on a left oblique axis, if and only if a sacral torsion is present. Other sacral dysfunctions (sacral shears, bilateral sacral flexions, extension, etc.) do not move about an oblique axis. Therefore, **choice E** is not the best answer.

10. **The correct answer is C.** The above question gives two facts about sacral dysfunction: *1)* The left inferior lateral angle of the sacrum is anterior when compared with the right, and *2)* there is limited springing at the lumbosacral junction. The first fact indicates that either the left ILA has moved anterior or the right ILA has moved posterior. The possibilities include a right sacral rotation on a left oblique axis, a right unilateral sacral flexion, or a right margin posterior. The second fact indicates that part of the sacral base has moved posterior (a positive lumbosacral spring test). The only dysfunction of the three possibilities in which the sacrum moves posterior is a right sacral rotation on a left oblique axis. Therefore, **choice C** is the only possible answer.

A left sacral rotation on a right oblique axis (**choice A**) would cause a left ILA to be posterior compared with the right.

A right sacral rotation on a right oblique axis (**choice B**), a right unilateral sacral flexion (**choice D**), and a flexed sacral base (**choice E**) will all result in a sacral base that springs freely (i.e., a negative lumbosacral spring test).

11. **The correct answer is A.** The above question gives three findings about sacral dysfunction: *1)* a deep sacral sulcus on the left, *2)* a posterior inferior lateral angle (ILA) on the right when compared with the opposite side, and *3)* a lumbosacral junction that springs freely.

The first fact indicates that the sacral base on the left has moved anterior (it does not say "when compared with the right," so you can't be sure about anything at the right sacral sulcus). The third fact does give you some idea about the right sulcus. Since the lumbosacral junction can spring, the right sulcus could not have moved posterior. Thus, either both sulci moved anterior or just the left moved anterior.

Given this information, the possible diagnoses could be a forward sacral torsion, a unilateral sacral flexion, and a bilateral sacral flexion. We can eliminate **choices C and E** because both of these answers will result in a sacrum that does not spring freely at the lumbosacral junction (a positive lumbosacral spring test).

The last fact indicates that the right ILA has moved posterior. The only possibility (given the choices) is a forward sacral torsion on a right oblique axis (**choice A**). A forward sacral torsion on a left oblique axis (**choice B**) and a left unilateral sacral flexion (**choice D**) both will result in a left ILA that is posterior.

12. **The correct answer is B.** The above question gives two facts about sacral dysfunction: *1)* the ILAs are equal in depth, and *2)* there is no motion at the lumbosacral junction.

The second fact indicates that there is a positive lumbosacral spring test (i.e., the sacral base has moved posterior). Given this fact alone we can eliminate **choices A, C**, and **E**. All of these dysfunctions will result in a sacral base that springs freely.

Let's take a look at the last fact: the ILAs are equal in depth. A sacral torsion will result in ILAs that are not equal in depth. A backward sacral torsion on a left oblique axis (i.e., a right sacral rotation on a left oblique axis) (**choice D**) will result in a left ILA that is anterior when compared with the right. Thus, the only possible correct answer is a sacral base extension; this can also be called a bilateral sacral extension.

13. **The correct answer is B.** The patient in the above question has a positive standing flexion test (SFT) on the left (i.e., the patient has a pelvic somatic dysfunction on the left). Since the right ASIS is more caudad and the right

PSIS is more cephalad, the right innominate has rotated anterior when compared with the right.

However, since the SFT indicates a somatic dysfunction on the left, the left innominate must have rotated posteriorly. This typically results in a shorter leg ipsilaterally (on the left). Therefore, **choice A** is incorrect.

Since the somatic dysfunction is on the left, the pelvis will resist AP compression and will not demonstrate adequate resiliency (**choice C**).

A flexion contracture of the iliopsoas will result in a positive Thomas test (**choice D**).

Tight quadriceps are associated with an anteriorly rotated innominate (**choice E**). Tight hamstrings are associated with a posteriorly rotated innominate.

14. **The correct answer is B.** If a sacral torsion is present in the above question, the diagnosis would be right sacral rotation on a right oblique axis. Using the rules of L5 on the sacrum and Fryette's principles, one can deduce the dysfunction of L5.

Rule of L5

- When L5 is rotated, the sacrum rotates in the opposite direction. Sacrum rotated right, L5 must be rotated left.
- When L5 is sidebent, a sacral oblique axis is engaged on the same side as the sidebending. Sacrum has a right oblique axis, L5 must be sidebent right.

Fryette's Principle I

If L5 is rotated right and sidebent left, L5 must be in the neutral plane (L5 NS_RR_L).

15. **The correct answer is E.** The patient in the above question has thoracic outlet syndrome (TOS). TOS is due to a compression of the neurovascular bundle as it enters the upper extremity. Symptoms include neck ache and parasthesias radiating into the upper extremity. On examination, the patient will have a positive Adson's test and possibly myofascial tenderness at the cervicothoracic junction (in this case, the anterior scalene). The anterior scalene is in close proximity to the subclavian artery, vein, and brachial plexus, and hypertonicity of this muscle can result in TOS. Allen's test is positive if there is claudication of the radial or ulna arteries.

Capillary refill would be prolonged (**choice A**).

A partial tear in the supraspinatus tendon is essentially a rotator cuff tear. This is usually the result of trauma (**choice B**).

This patient has an inhalation dysfunction of Rib 1. Using muscle energy to contract the anterior scalene could be used to treat an exhalation dysfunction of Rib 1 (**choice C**).

And although TOS will result in compression of the neurovascular bundle, it typically does not alter the reflexes; therefore, **choice D** is not the most accurate answer.

16. **The correct answer is D.** The patient in the above question injured her supraspinatus tendon, resulting in a tear of the rotator cuff. Clues here would be the atrophy of the supraspinatus and deltoid, along with tenderness at the tip of the acromium and a positive drop arm test. Her arm has been immobile for two months. A complication of shoulder immobility is frozen shoulder syndrome (adhesive capsulitis). Symptoms include severely limited glenohumeral motion with end-range pain. Osteopathic treatment should be directed at freeing up restrictions at the glenohumeral area. Prevention of this is early mobilization.

Continued use of a sling will result in worsening of the frozen shoulder (**choice A**).

This patient's condition was due to trauma; chronic impingement may lead to supraspinatus tendonitis, not necessarily a tear (**choice B**).

Adson's test will be positive in thoracic outlet syndrome (**choice C**).

It is unlikely that the patient suffered a complete rotator cuff tear; however, even if she did, the injury is two months old. There is no need for immediate referral (**choice E**).

17. **The correct answer is C.** As a person supinates his forearm, the radial head will glide anterior. Conversely, pronation will cause the radial head to glide posterior. Because the patient has limited supination and the radial head resists anterior glide, the patient had a posterior radial head dysfunction. Symptoms include wrist and elbow pain, and it is often caused by a fall on an outstretched pronated arm.

Another common somatic dysfunction of the upper extremity includes an abducted or adducted ulna. An increased carrying angle (**choice A**) and resistance to medial glide of the ulna (**choice B**) are associated with an abducted ulna. A hand that appears more abducted is associated with an adducted ulna (**choice D**).

Motion of the ulna, carrying angle, position of the hand, and wrist flexion (**choice E**) are not directly related to a radial head dysfunction.

18. **The correct answer is D.**

The median nerve is primarily responsible for wrist flexion and thumb abduction; it stems from the medial and lateral cords (**choices A and E**).

The ulnar nerve is responsible for abduction of the fingers; it stems from the medial cord (**choice B**).

The musculocutaneous nerve is primarily responsible for elbow flexion; it stems from the lateral cord (**choice C**).

The brachioradialis also flexes the elbow, but to a lesser degree it is innervated by the radial nerve. The latissimus dorsi is the primary shoulder extender. The triceps also helps with shoulder extension. The latissimus dorsi is innervated by the thoracodorsal nerve, and the triceps is innervated by the radial nerve—both of which stem from the posterior cord (**choice D**).

19. **The correct answer is E.** The brachial plexus is composed of nerve roots C5-C8 and T1. Injury to the upper portion will usually affect C5, C6, and sometimes the C7 nerve roots. The hand has 18 intrinsic muscles (7 interossi, 4 lumbricles, 3 hypothenar, and 4 thenar muscles), thirteen of which are innervated by the ulnar nerve (C8 and T1 nerve roots). The rest are innervated by the C8 portion of the median nerve.

Sensation to the middle finger is supplied by the C7 nerve root (**choice A**).

Sensation to the lateral portion of the forearm is supplied by the musculocutaneous nerve (C5 and C6) (**choice B**).

The brachioradialis is innervated by the radial nerve (C5, C6, and C7) (**choice C**).

The deltoid is primarily responsible for arm abduction (axillary nerve: C5, C6). The supraspinatus also helps with arm abduction (suprascapular nerve: C5, C6) (**choice D**).

20. **The correct answer is B.** Under normal physiologic conditions, the fibular head moves anterior with pronation of the ankle and posterior with supination of the ankle. If the fibular head gets stuck posteriorly, the ankle will move freely into supination (plantar flexion and inversion and internal rotation) (**choice B**) and will resist pronation (dorsiflexion, eversion, and external rotation).

Because the fibular head is stuck in the posterior position, it will resist anterior glide (**choice C**).

The movement of the distal fibular head is almost reciprocal to that of the proximal fibular head (with the exception of some minor movements). If the proximal fibular head moves posterior with supination, the distal fibular head will move anterior (**choice D**).

The counterstrain position for a tender point at the posterior proximal fibular head is knee flexed, foot inverted, and tibia externally rotated. Thus, **choice E** is not correct.

21. **The correct answer is C.** The above patient is likely to have an acute herniated disc. However, most herniated discs do not require surgery (approximately 95% can be treated conservatively). Therefore, **choice D** is not the most suitable answer.

HVLA (**choice A**) should not be used in this case because the symptoms indicate a possible herniated disc. HVLA is relatively contraindicated in acute herniated discs.

The purpose of the hip drop test is to evaluate side-bending of the lumbar spine. If the lumbar spine is sidebent right, the hip drop test is likely to be positive (**choice C**). The sacrum has forward rotation on a right oblique axis (i.e., the sacrum is rotated right on a right oblique axis).

The lumbosacral test will be positive in all dysfunctions in which the sacral base has moved posterior. In a right rotation on a right oblique axis the sacral base has moved anterior, not posterior (**choice B**).

Currently there is no literature stating that weekly osteopathic manipulation prevents a herniated disc (**choice E**).

22. **The correct answer is D.** A herniated disc at the level of the L4 and L5 interspace is most likely to interfere with the L5 nerve root; nevertheless, depending on the exact location and the size of the herniation, the L4 and S1 nerve roots may be affected. Since the patient denies any bowel or bladder dysfunction, it is unlikely that the disc herniation affected S2-S4 nerve roots. Cutaneous distribution of the L5 nerve root involves the dorsum of the foot; therefore, the patient will have greatest neurologic deficit in this area.

The hip flexors include the iliacus and psoas. These muscles are innervated by the L1 and L2 nerve roots (**choice A**). The quadriceps are innervated by L2 to L4 nerve roots; because this muscle is innervated by several nerve roots, injury to the L5 (and maybe L4) will not have a profound effect on the quadriceps (**choice B**).

Babinski's reflex is an indication of an upper motor neuron injury. A disc herniation at L4/L5 is below the cord and will not result in a Babinski's reflex (**choice C**).

Sensation to the ishial tuberosity is supplied by the S3 nerve root (**choice E**).

23. **The correct answer is A.** The inherent motility of the brain and spinal cord is responsible for cranial bone motion. The cranial bones move about the sphenobasilar synchondrosis (SBS). The SBS is moved through a biphasic cycle (flexion and extension). During flexion, the midline bones (sphenoid, occiput, ethmoid, and vomer) move through a flexion phase, while the paired bones (temporal, parietal, frontal, etc.) move through

an external rotation phase. The converse is true for extension of the midline bones (internal rotation of the paired bones). Since the dura mater is the inelastic membrane that attaches firmly to the cranial bones and the sacrum, motion of the cranial bones will cause motion at the sacrum. Extension of the cranium is associated with flexion of the sacrum. During extension of the cranial bones, the dura moves caudad to allow for sacral flexion.

TMJ dysfunction may be related to a dysfunction of the temporal bone, not physiologic motion of this bone (**choice B**).

Internal rotation of the temporal bone is related to flexion of the occiput (the occiput is a midline bone and only flexes or extends). Therefore, **choice C** is incorrect.

As the temporal bone internally rotates (several times a minute), the temporalis muscle does not develop tender points (**choice D**).

Nausea (**choice E**) is associated with occiput, C1, or C2 dysfunction, not temporal internal rotation.

24. **The correct answer is A.** The talocrural joint (or tibiotalar joint) is the articulation of the tibia and fibula on the talus (the ankle mortise). The main motion of this joint is plantar and dorsiflexion. With plantarflexion, the talus glides anteriorly. With dorsiflexion, the talus glides posteriorly, and the ankle becomes more stable.

The cuboid composes the lateral portion of the transverse arch. Therefore, tenderness on the plantar surface of the foot at the lateral portion of the transverse arch may indicate somatic dysfunction of the *cuboid* bone (**choice B**).

Resistance to ankle plantarflexion is likely to indicate a somatic dysfunction of the talocrural or tibiotalar joint. The talocalcaneal joint (subtalar joint) is the main shock absorber of the foot and allows internal and external rotation of the leg while the foot is fixed (**choice C**).

Excessive supination of the ankle is likely to result in a strain of the anterior talofibular ligament (**choice D**).

Somatic dysfunctions of the ankle occur most commonly when the foot is plantarflexed (**choice E**).

25. **The correct answer is D.** The balance of the temporal bone plays a key role in the function of cranial nerve 8. If the temporal bone is significantly restricted (i.e., if there is a somatic dysfunction of the temporal bone), then the function of the vestibulocochlear nerve will be affected. Symptoms of CN VIII dysfunction include tinnitus, vertigo, and hearing loss. Please note that the balance of the sphenoid and occiput can also alter the effect on CN VIII (however, most authors believe it is to a much lesser effect).

Somatic dysfunction of the frontal bone may alter the effect of CN I only (**choice A**).

Somatic dysfunction of the maxillae may alter the effect of the second division of CN V (**choice B**).

Somatic dysfunction of the zygoma or the parietal may result in facial pain or cephalgia, but they do not have a key role in cranial nerve well-being (**choices C and E**, respectively).

26. **The correct answer is D.** Tension along the occipito-temporal suture can cause many symptoms due to proximity of many vital nerves, arteries, and veins. However, the jugular foramen lies right along the suture, so tension of this suture line may alter the function of the jugular foramen. What exits (or enters) the jugular foramen? CN's IX, X, XI, the inferior petrosal sinus, the sigmoid sinus, and the posterior meningeal artery. The two sinuses drain most of the blood from the cranium, so altered function of the jugular foramen will result in decreased venous drainage from the cranium.

Dysphagia may be due to an alteration in the function of CN XII; it exits the hypoglossal canal located in the occiput (**choice A**).

Diplopia may be due to an alteration in the function of CN's III, IV, and VI. They exit the superior orbital fissure (**choice B**).

Tension along the occipito-temporal suture certainly can result in tender points of the neck musculature; however, most of the tender points would be located within the posterior occipital muscles and the SCM at the attachment of the mastoid process (**choice C**).

Tension along the occipito-temporal suture will not result in Bell's palsy. Bell's palsy is due to a compression of the facial nerve (CN VII) as it exits the stylomastoid foramen located in the temporal bone (**choice E**).

27. **The correct answer is C.** The CV4 decompression technique can be used to increase the amplitude of the CRI, first by resisting the flexion and extension of the occiput until a "still point" is reached, then allowing restoration of normal flexion and extension.

A lift technique is often used to balance ligamentous tension. This is typically performed on the frontal or parietal bones (**choice A**).

Temporal rocking can help eliminate restrictions in the temporal bone or nearby areas. It does not have a significant effect on the amplitude of the CRI (**choice B**).

The vault hold is typically used to diagnose dysfunctions at the sphenobasilar symphysis. However, it can be used to balance membranous tension (**choice D**).

The V-spread is used to free restrictions of impacted sutures (**choice E**). It can be applied to any suture in the cranium, but it does not have a significant role in increasing the amplitude or vitality of the CRI.

28. **The correct answer is C.** The fifth cervical vertebra has the least impact on cardiac function.

    Why? Let's look at the other answers first. The occiput, the first cervical vertebra, and the second cervical vertebra have a direct effect on vagus nerve function. Since the vagus nerve supplies parasympathetic fibers to the heart, somatic dysfunction of any of these structures can have an impact on cardiac function (**choices A and B**).

    Sympathetic fibers from T1 to T5 innervate the heart. Therefore, somatic dysfunction of any of these structures can have an impact on cardiac function (**choices D and E**).

    The fifth cervical vertebra has no direct autonomic or structural link to the heart.

29. **The correct answer is C.** A viscero-somatic reflex occurs when localized visceral stimuli produce patterns of reflex response, in segmentally related somatic structures. In other words, abnormal visceral stimuli from the heart enter the spinal cord. Then, through a process called facilitation, interneurons get "sensitized" and produce an exaggerated motor response, causing increased muscular tension. In this patient, abnormal visceral stimuli from the myocardium sensitize interneurons, and this results in deltoid pain.

    A somato-visceral reflex occurs when abnormal somatic stimuli (from something that irritates the somatic structure) enter the spinal cord and result in altered function of the visceral structure (**choice B**).

    A Chapman reflex point (**choice A**) is a smooth, firm, discretely palpable nodule approximately 2-3 mm in diameter and is located within the deep fascia or on the periostium of the bone. Chapman's points are manifestations of viscero-somatic reflexes; however, the specific Chapman's points for the heart are at the spinous process of T3 and the intercostal space of Ribs 2 and 3 at the sternum.

    A Jones tender point (**choice E**) is a small, tense area usually in the belly of a muscle that is used to diagnose and treat somatic dysfunctions. The above patient has some deltoid tenderness, the question does not describe a specific point; therefore, it cannot be assumed that this patient has a Jones tender point.

    A trigger point (**choice D**) is "a hypersensitive focus, usually within a taut band of skeletal muscle or in the muscle fascia." A trigger point classically refers pain when it is compressed. The above question makes no mention of

focal tenderness in the deltoid, and it makes no mention of a referral to pain when the tenderness in the deltoid is compressed. Therefore, one cannot conclude that the tenderness in the deltoid is a trigger point.

30. **The correct answer is C.** The patient in the above question has a tension headache. She has suboccipital tension, as well as a trigger point at the OA joint. (It is a trigger point because pain radiates to the temporalis region with deep palpation.) Trigger points can be treated with spray and stretch technique and myofascial release. Other treatments include injection with local anesthetic, dry needling muscle energy techniques, ultrasound, high voltage galvanic stimulation, reciprocal inhibition, and ischemic compression.

    Yes, muscle energy can be used; however, in this patient, initial treatment should be directed at the cervical and thoracic spine to help decrease suboccipital tension followed by indirect treatments to the suboccipital region (**choice E**).

    Trigger points give rise to a characteristic referral pattern. Posterior cervical and suboccipital trigger points often refer pain to the temporal region or the orbit. The problem lies within the posterior cervical and suboccipital musculature, not within the referral area (**choice B**).

    Likewise, counterstrain to the temporalis muscle will help eliminate tenderness within the temporalis. It will not eliminate pain from the referral area (**choice D**).

    The pain from a migraine is from cerebral vasodilation. In migraine patients, local vasodilation of cerebral vessels seems to be produced when platelets line up in a portion of a cerebral artery and release humoral vasodilating substances. The vasodilatation is not autonomic—it is humoral. Migranes may be associated with nausea and vomiting, as well as photophobia. Migranes are not typically associated with cervical tension; therefore, this patient likely has a tension headache (**choice A**).

31. **The correct answer is C.** Anxiety and physical or emotional stress increases sympathetic tone and can result in increased muscle tension. Rib raising will normalize sympathetic tone and will result in decreased muscle tension.

    Rib raising will improve VQ function, reduce cardiac output, and stimulate the diaphragm; however, these techniques will not resolve this patient's headache (**choices A, B, and D**).

    Rib raising is not contraindicated in an acute GI bleed. It is contraindicated in poststernotomy patients and those patients with fractured ribs (**choice E**).

32. **The correct answer is B.** The most common serious side effect of anti-inflammatory medication (NSAIDS) is an acute GI bleed. Because this patient is in the ICU because of an acute GI bleed, the use of NSAIDS for this patient would be absolutely contraindicated.

Tinnitus (**choice A**) is a side effect of aspirin use, but it would not be contraindicated in this patient because its effects are benign and reversible when the medication is stopped.

Nausea and vomiting (**choice C**), as well as tenderness (**choice D**), in the subxiphoid space (epigastric space) are side effects of NSIADS; however, both are not life-threatening and neither would warrant an absolute contraindication for this patient.

Tissue texture changes in the midthoracic and paraspinal region (**choice E**) may indicate visceral somatic dysfunction. However, this also is not life-threatening and would not warrant an absolute contraindication for this patient.

33. **The correct answer is B.** Although the patient's symptoms have resolved, the patient still may have some suboccipital tenderness and some somatic dysfunction. If somatic dysfunction is found, treatment may prevent further headaches. Therefore, it is best to evaluate this patient again.

As mentioned in the question, this patient suffers from chronic headaches from "stress." Chronic problems need chronic treatment, making follow-up necessary (**choice A**).

If you wait one week to evaluate the patient, the tension headache may return; thus, this is not the best answer (**choice C**).

Blindly treating the patient with the same OMT treatment is not benefiting the patient because you cannot assume the same dysfunctions are present (especially since the symptoms have resolved) (**choice D**).

Ultrasound was not used initially; therefore, you do not know if the patient will benefit from it (**choice E**).

34. **The correct answer is C.** The sympathetic innervation stems from the thoracic and lumbar region. The cardiovascular system receives sympathetic innervation from segments T1-T5. Therefore, treatment of T2-T4 would be most likely to decrease excessive sympathetic tone to the heart.

The OA (atlanto-occipital) joint has a direct influence on the function of the vagus nerve (parasympathetic innervation to the heart). Therefore, treatment of the OA joint may alter parasympathetic tone to the heart (**choice A**).

The phrenic nerve innervates the diaphragm and it arises from the C3-C5 nerve roots. The phrenic nerve is not responsible for sympathetic innervation to the heart (**choice B**).

The kidneys receive sympathetic innervation from T10-T12 (nothing above the diaphragm is sympathetically innervated from below T8) (**choice D**).

Because the spinal cord ends at about L2, nothing can possibly receive sympathetic innervation from L3-L5 (**choice E**).

35. **The correct answer is C.** The sympathetic innervation stems from the thoraco-lumbar region. The kidneys receive sympthetic innervation from segments T10-L1. Therefore, treatment of these segments would be most likely to decrease excessive sympathetic tone to the kidneys.

The OA (atlanto-occipital) joint has a direct influence on the function of the vagus nerve (parasympathetic innervation to the kidneys). Therefore, treatment of the OA joint may alter parasympathetic tone to the kidneys (**choice A**).

The heart, lungs, head and neck structures, and the esophagus receive sympathetic innervation from segments T2-T4 (**choice B**).

Because the spinal cord ends at about L2, nothing can possibly receive sympathetic innervation from L3-L5 (**choice D**).

The pelvic splanchnic (S2-S4) nerve is responsible for parasympathic innervation to some pelvic structures (within the GI system, the pelvic splanchnic innervates the lower ureter and bladder, not the kidney). Manipulation of the sacrum could alter the function of the pelvic splanchnic (**choice E**).

36. **The correct answer is B.** Before initiating lymphatic pump techniques, it is imperative that restrictions are removed from all pertinent diaphragms. Lymphatic pumps are intended to improve lymphatic return to the heart, and in this patient, it is to decrease the patient's peripheral edema. Lymphatic pump techniques will not be as effective if there are diaphragmatic restrictions. There are four diaphragms in the body:

1) The tentorium cerebelli

2) The thoracic inlet

3) The thoraco-abdominal diaphragm

4) The pelvic diaphragm

Removing restriction within the thoracic inlet will improve lymphatic treatment response.

The CV4 technique may stimulate respiratory centers—respiratory centers are located at the base of the fourth ventricle—but stimulation of the thoraco-abdominal diaphragm will not remove its restrictions (**choice A**).

The liver pump is a lymphatic technique that will enhance lymph return, but again, restrictions must be removed first before starting lymphatic pumps (**choice C**).

The Kirksville Krunch to the thoracic region is relatively contraindicated (**choice D**) because it will increase intra-abdominal pressure.

Cervical HVLA (to the OA, C1, and C2 joints only) will alter vagal tone to the viscera but it will not affect restrictions in the diaphragm (**choice E**).

37. **The correct answer is B.** Pectoral traction should be used in this patient because it is gentle and will not result in sudden changes in abdominal pressure. Also, the most appropriate lymphatic technique would most influence lympathic return to the heart. Lymphatic techniques that concentrate their effects directly on the thoraco-abdominal areas would work best.

The liver pump and classic thoracic pumps are all too vigorous in this patient because the liver may be friable in this type of patient. Thus, any increase in intra-abdominal pressure should be avoided in this patient (**choices A and C**).

An ischial rectal fossa release will decrease restrictions within the pelvic diaphragm but it will not directly affect lymphatic return to the heart without a thoraco-abdominal diaphragm release (**choice D**).

Effleurage of the legs will decrease edema of the lower extremities; however, because of the distance from the heart, a release of proximal diaphragms are more appropriate (**choice E**).

38. **The correct answer is D.** The above patient has carpal tunnel syndrome (CTS). This condition is a result of compression of the median nerve, usually at the flexor retinaculum; however, cervical or rib dysfunction, as well as anterior scalene hypertonicity, may further complicate CTS. Ipsilateral upper thoracic and rib dysfunctions will result in increased upper extremity sympathetic tone and produce arm and hand symptoms. Decreasing sympathetic tone is an intergral part of OMT treatment for CTS.

The upper thoracic segments supply sympathetics to the upper extremity. Kuchera reports T2-T8, whereas other texts (*Foundation of Osteopathic Medicine*) report T5-T7 (**choice D**).

Sympathetic innervation arises from the thoracic and lumbar regions. There are no sympathetics arising from the cranium or the cervical regions; thus OA and C2-C3 are wrong (**choices A and B**).

C5-T1 make up the brachial plexus; however, sympathetics originate from the upper thoracic region. Thus, treatment of these areas will most likely decrease sympathetic tone to the arm (**choice C**).

T10 to L2 supply sympathetics to the lower extremity (**choice E**).

39. **The correct answer is B.** This is the best answer for two reasons: *1*) Decreasing restrictions within the thoracic inlet (cervico-thoracic junction) will enhance lymphatic drainage, and *2*) because upper thoracic and rib dysfunction will result in increased upper extremity sympathetic tone, myofascial release may improve the rib dysfunction, thus decreasing sympathetic tone in the upper extremity.

Increased sympathetic influences to the lymphatics cause a reduction in the size of lymphatic channels, producing tissue congestion. Therefore, rib raising will enhance lymphatic drainage but it is only addressing sympathetic tone, whereas myofascial release will affect sympathetic tone and muscular tension at the cervico-thoracic junction (**choice A**).

Condylar decompression may decrease tension in the upper cervical musculature. However, it will not have a great effect on the cervico-thoracic junction (**choice C**).

Effleurage of the upper extremity will mechanically decrease upper extremity edema; regardless, edema is likely to return because the thoracic inlet and sympathetic tone would not be addressed (**choice D**).

The superior cervical ganglion supplies sympathetics to the head. Inhibition will not alter the sympathetics of the upper extremity (**choice E**).

40. **The correct answer is A.** The forearm flexors are innervated mostly by the median nerve (hence trigger points within these muscles with median nerve compression). They originate from the medial epicondyle and insert into the carpal bones and the phalanges.

The radial head is located on the lateral aspect of the forearm, near the extensor muscles of the forearm (**choice B**).

The olecranon process is the posterior portion of the ulna that articulates with the humerus. The triceps insert onto this structure (**choice C**).

The humeral condyle articulates between the olecranon process and the coranoid process of the ulna (**choice D**).

The forearm flexors insert onto (not originate from) the phalanges (**choice E**).

41. **The correct answer is D.** The patient in the above question is likely to have an ulnar nerve entrapment at the elbow. This is also called cubital tunnel syndrome.

Entrapment occurs at the elbow, and the patient will complain of numbness of the medial part of the palm and the fourth and fifth digits. Distal to the cubital tunnel, the ulnar nerve innervates the flexor carpi ulnaris (adduction of the wrist) and the hypothenar muscles; therefore, entrapment at the cubital tunnel will cause weakness in these muscles. Sensation to the forearm is preserved because it is innervated by the medial antibrachial nerve. The biceps, triceps, and brachioradialis reflex will all be normal in peripheral ulnar nerve neuropathy. Tinel's test is performed by tapping over the nerve at a location where the nerve is near the skin. It is positive if symptoms are exacerbated with tapping over the nerve.

Typically, in the upper extremity, Tinel's test is done over the carpel tunnel (flexor retinaculum and transverse carpal ligament) for peripheral median nerve neuropathy (**choices B** and **C**) and the cubital tunnel for peripheral ulnar neuropathy (**choice D**).

The ulnar nerve does pass between the two flexor digitorum muscles; however, tapping over the belly of muscles is not a Tinel's test—not to mention it would not reproduce symptoms (**choice A**).

The tunnel of Guyon is a structure at the wrist, which the ulnar nerve and artery pass through. This can be a site for ulnar nerve compression. Nonetheless, the above patient has weakness of the flexor carpi ulnaris; therefore, entrapment must be proximal to the wrist (**choice E**).

42. **The correct answer is B.** The patient in the above question likely has a duodenal ulcer. Typically, a duodenal ulcer improves with eating and worsens two to three hours postprandial, unlike a gastric ulcer that often worsens with eating. Chronic abnormal stimuli from the duodenal bulb will enter the spinal cord in the midthoracic level (T5-T9) and facilitate these segments. This may result in abnormal efferents to somatic structures. This will result in a viscero-somatic reflex and palpatory findings at these levels (T5-T9). T5-T9 innervate the following structures: stomach, liver, gallbladder, spleen, and portions of the duodenum and pancreas.

T1-T4 innervate structures above the diaphragm (**choice A**).

T10-T12 innervate the jejunum, ileum, and proximal 2/3 of the transverse colon (**choice C**).

T11-L1 and L2-L3 innervate portions of the colon and pelvic structures (**choices D** and **E**).

43. **The correct answer is A.** The lungs receive autonomic innervation from the vagus nerve (parasympathetic) and T2-T7 paraspinal sympathetic ganglia. Therefore,

osteopathic treatment directed at either of these structures would alter autonomic tone. Vagus nerve function is altered by the temporal bone, the occipital bone, the atlas (C1), and the axis (C2). The occiput, C1, and C2 are located in the suboccipital area; therefore, manipulation of this area will alter the vagus nerve and affect autonomic tone in the lungs.

C3-C5 manipulation may alter the diaphragm but it will not alter the autonomic tone in the lungs (**choice B**).

Manipulation of the thoracic inlet may improve lymphatic return and may improve myofascial restrictions at the cervico-thoracic junction. However, this will not directly affect autonomics (**choice C**).

Manipulation of T8-T12 and rib raising to Ribs 8-12 will alter the sympathetic nervous system below the diaphragm (**choices D** and **E**).

44. **The correct answer is C.** Increased sympathetic tone results in hypertrophy of the mucosa with an increase in the number of its goblet cells. This results in increased secretion of mucus. Sustained sympathetic tone results in the production of a sticky, thick mucus, which is difficult to clear. Decreasing sympathetic tone will result in production of a thinner mucus from the respiratory epithelium.

Stimulation of the vagus nerve will result in bronchoconstriction not bronchodilatation (**choice A**).

Inhibiting the cough reflex would worsen the patient's condition. It will result in decreased excretion of mucus and may promote mucus plugging and air trapping (**choice B**).

Flattening the diaphragm will also be detrimental to this patient. A COPD patient already has an increased total lung capacity and a flattened diaphragm. Further flattening will result in decreased diaphragmatic excursion, increased work by accessory muscles, and poor lymphatic return (**choice D**).

Manipulation directed at the autonomic nervous system will not directly stimulate the phrenic nerve; however, treatment of C3-C5 will directly affect the phrenic nerve and result in improved diaphragmatic excursion (**choice E**).

45. **The correct answer is A.** Years of cigarette smoking results in a destruction of elastic fibers of the lung (an emphysema type of COPD). Irritation of the lung parenchyma may result in an overproduction of mucus, causing obstruction and air trapping (chronic bronchitis and asthma type of COPD). These two factors expand the chest cavity and can result in an increased lung capacity, thus permanently positioning the ribs in inhalation.

Increased sympathetic tone will cause bronchodilation and will result in bronchoalveolar expansion; however, this is not the primary reason why there is an increased AP diameter of a person with COPD (**choice B**).

Patients with COPD will have impaired oxygenation; nonetheless, it will not result in a fibrosis of the diaphragm. If this were true, all skeletal muscles in the body would be fibrosed (**choice C**).

Both the scalenes and intercostals will help elevate the ribs into inhalation, yet these muscles are not strong enough to overcome the natural recoil of the lungs (**choice D**).

The lung send visceral affect stimuli to T2-T7 segments, which may become facilitated and affect the pleura. However, this will not result in fibrosis or expansion of the lungs (**choice E**).

46. **The correct answer is B**. The above patient is critically ill. OMT should be used sparingly. And only gentle techniques should be used. Be careful not to overtreat these types of patients. They can handle only very little OMT. There are several costochondral approachs for diaphragm release, most of which entails the practitioner to apply a significant amount of pressure on the thoracic cage. This type of treatment in a patient that just underwent a sternotomy may cause more harm, and so it is relatively contraindicated.

An indirect thoracic inlet release will promote lymphatic drainage and is gentle enough for this patient (**choice A**).

Rib raising, although a direct technique, is a gentle, low velocity, moderate (to low) amplitude treatment that will not disrupt the sternal incision (**choice C**).

The CV4 technique will enhance the amplitude of the CRI. Like all cranio-sacral treatment, it is a gentle technique and can be used in a postsurgical patient (**choice D**).

An occipito-atlantal suboccipital release is a gentle direct technique that will help normalize parasympathetic function (prevent bradyarrthmias) and it is not contraindicated in this patient (**choice E**).

47. **The correct answer is D.** In a patient who just underwent major surgery, including a sternotomy, it is very common to have limited chest-wall motion. Limited chest-wall motion will lead to atelectasis. Atelectasis is the most common etiology of bibasilar crackles in any postsurgical patient. Bibasilar crackles are a sign of alveolar collapse or pleural effusion. Pnuemothorax, pneumonia, pulmonary embolus, and congestive heart failure are all possible in this patient, but all of these diagnoses are less common in the post-op patient, especially given the history and physical findings.

A pneumothorax would result in an absent breath sound in a section of the lung fields (**choice A**).

Pulmonary emboli are more common approximately four days after surgery and usually present with sinus tachycardia (**choice C**).

Pneumonia would be more likely if this patient had a fever (**choice B**).

The above patient does not have an S3 gallop or peripheral edema; this makes congestive heart failure a less likely possibility (**choice E**).

48. **The correct answer is A.** The bibasilar crackles are due to limited chest-wall motion. This patient has recently undergone a sternotomy. Deep breathing is likely to cause chest pain. Pain medication may limit respiratory effort. Therefore, any manipulative treatment that will enhance respiration will be beneficial to this patient. Rib raising is an excellent technique to help increase chest-wall motion. This will have many beneficial effects. It will directly increase chest-wall motion, and increasing chest-wall motion will enhance diaphragmatic excursion. Increasing diaphragmatic excursion will enhance lymphatic return. Also, rib raising will help normalize sympathetic influence on the viscera (**choice A**).

An occipito-atlantal release will not directly increase chest-wall motion (**choice B**).

A thoracic lymphatic pump entails the practitioner to rapidly push and release the thoracic cage, causing pressure gradients within the thoracic cavity. This motion is contraindicated in a poststernotomy patient (**choice C**).

Muscle energy will eliminate the left exhalation dysfunction and thus will increase motion of these ribs. However, muscle energy is a direct active technique. This type of treatment is too aggressive in a critically ill patient and therefore is not the best treatment approach (**choice D**).

Paraspinal inhibitory techniques will normalize sympathetics to the viscera (which would be beneficial) but they will not increase chest-wall motion (**choice E**).

49. **The correct answer is E.** The patient in the above question has difficulty maintaining an erection. The parasympathetic nervous system is responsible for maintaining erection. Therefore, osteopathic treatment should be geared at influencing or normalizing the parasympathetic nerves that supply the erectile tissue of the penis. The pelvic splanchnic nerve (S2-S4) supplies parasympathetic fibers to the genitalia. Treatment, therefore, should be directed at the sacrum.

Treatment of T11-L2 vertebral segments, rib raising to Ribs 11 and 12, and paraspinal inhibition of the thoracolumbar fascia will alter the sympathetic- influence on the genitals; in this case, ejaculation (**choices A, B, and C**).

An occipito-atlantal release will alter parasympathetics via the vagus nerve; however, the vagus nerve does not innervate the erectile tissue of the penis (**choice D**).

50. **The correct answer is C.** Abnormal and continuous stimuli from the right side of the colon will enter the spinal cord at the T10-T12 level. This will result in segmental facilitation (i.e., sensitized interneurons) at these segments. Normal sensory input from general afferents at T10-T12 will become amplified at the sensitized interneurons, resulting in an exaggerated motor response. This will cause an increase in tension of the paraspinal musculature and tissue texture abnormalities at T10-T12.

Visceral receptors in the head and neck, the heart, and the lungs send stimuli to T1-T3 (**choice A**).

Visceral receptors in the upper GI tract (stomach, liver, gallbladder, spleen, and portions of the duodenum and pancreas) send stimuli to T5-T9 (**choice B**).

Visceral receptors in the lower GI tract (transverse colon to rectum) send stimuli to L1-L3 (**choice D**).

The sacrum receives visceral stimuli from the lower GI tract (transverse colon to rectum) via the pelvic splanchnic nerve (S2-S4) (**choice E**).

STANDARD REFERENCE LABORATORY VALUES

	REFERENCE RANGE	SI REFERENCE INTERVALS
BLOOD, PLASMA, SERUM		
* Alanine aminotransferase (ALT, GPT at 30°C)	8-20 U/L	8-20 U/L
Amylase, serum	25-125 U/L	25-125 U/L
* Aspartate aminotransferase (AST, GOT at 30°C)	8-20 U/L	8-20 U/L
Bilirubin, serum (adult) Total // Direct	0.1-1.0 mg/dL // 0.0-0.3 mg/dL	2-17 μmol/L // 0-5 μmol/L
* Calcium, serum (Total)	8.4-10.2 mg/dL	2.1-2.8 mmol/L
* Cholesterol, serum	140-250 mg/dL	3.6-6.5 mmol/L
Cortisol, serum	0800 h: 5-23 μg/dL // 1600 h: 3-15 μg/dL	138-635 nmol/L // 82-413 nmol/L
	2000 h: 50% of 0800 h	Fraction of 0800 h: ≤ 0.50
Creatine kinase, serum (at 30°C) ambulatory	Male: 25-90 U/L	25-90 U/L
	Female: 10-70 U/L	10-70 U/L
* Creatinine, serum	0.6-1.2 mg/dL	53-106 μmol/L
Electrolytes, serum		
Sodium	135-147 mEq/L	135-147 mmol/L
Chloride	95-105 mEq/L	95-105 mmol/L
* Potassium	3.5-5.0 mEq/L	3.5-5.0 mmol/L
Bicarbonate	22-28 mEq/L	22-28 mmol/L
Estriol (E_3) total, serum (in pregnancy)		
24-28 weeks // 32-36 weeks	30-170 ng/mL // 60-280 ng/mL	104-590 // 208-970 nmol/L
28-32 weeks // 36-40 weeks	40-220 ng/mL // 80-350 ng/mL	140-760 // 280-1210 nmol/L
Ferritin, serum	Male: 15-200 ng/mL	15-200 μg/L
	Female: 12-150 ng/mL	12-150 μg/L
Follicle-stimulating hormone, serum/plasma	Male: 4-25 mIU/mL	4-25 U/L
	Female: premenopause 4-30 mIU/mL	4-30 U/L
	midcycle peak 10-90 mIU/mL	10-90 U/L
	ostmenopause 40-250 mIU/mL	40-250 U/L
Gases, arterial blood (room air)		
pO_2	75-105 mm Hg	10.0-14.0 kPa
pCO_2	33-44 mm Hg	4.4-5.9 kPa
pH	7.35-7.45	[H^+] 36-44 nmol/L
Glucose, serum	Fasting: 70-110 mg/dL	3.8-6.1 mmol/L
	2-h postprandial: < 120 mg/dL	< 6.6 mmol/L
Growth hormone – arginine stimulation	Fasting: < 5 ng/mL	< 5 μg/L
	provocative stimuli: > 7 ng/mL	> 7 μg/L
Immunoglobulins, serum		
IgA	76-390 mg/dL	0.76-3.90 g/L
IgE	0-380 IU/mL	0-380 kIU/mL
IgG	650-1500 mg/dL	6.5-15 g/L
IgM	40-345 mg/dL	0.4-3.45 g/L
Iron	50-170 μg/dL	9-30 μmol/L
Lactate dehydrogenase (L → P, 30°C)	45-90 U/L	45-90 U/L
Luteinizing hormone, serum/plasma	Male: 6-23 mIU/mL	6-23 U/L
	Female: follicular phase 5-30 mIU/mL	5-30 U/L
	midcycle 75-150 mIU/mL	75-150 U/L
	postmenopause 30-200 mIU/mL	30-200 U/L
Osmolality, serum	275-295 mOsmol/kg	275-295 mOsmol/kg
Parathyroid hormone, serum, N-terminal	230-630 pg/mL	230-630 ng/L
* Phosphatase (alkaline), serum (p-NPP at 30°C)	20-70 U/L	20-70 U/L
* Phosphorus (inorganic), serum	3.0-4.5 mg/dL	1.0-1.5 mmol/L
Prolactin, serum (hPRL)	< 20 ng/mL	< 20 μg/L
* Proteins, serum		
Total (recumbent)	6.0-7.8 g/dL	60-78 g/L
Albumin	3.5-5.5 g/dL	35-55 g/L
Globulins	2.3-3.5 g/dL	23-35 g/L
Thyroid-stimulating hormone, serum or plasma	0.5-5.0 μU/mL	0.5-5.0 mU/L
Thyroidal iodine (^{123}I) uptake	8-30% of administered dose/24 h	0.08-0.30/24 h
Thyroxine (T_4), serum	5-12 μg/dL	64-155 nmol/L
Triglycerides, serum	35-160 mg/dL	0.4-1.81 mmol/L
Triiodothyronine (T_3), serum (RIA)	115-190 ng/dL	1.8-2.9 nmol/L
Triiodothyronine (T_3), resin uptake	25-35%	0.25-0.35
* Urea nitrogen, serum (BUN)	7-18 mg/dL	1.2-3.0 mmol urea/L
* Uric acid, serum	3.0-8.2 mg/dL	0.18-0.48 mmol/L

(*) Included in the Biochemical Profile (SMA-12)

	REFERENCE RANGE	SI REFERENCE INTERVALS

CEREBROSPINAL FLUID

	REFERENCE RANGE	SI REFERENCE INTERVALS
Cell count	0-5 cells/mm^3	0-5 x 10^6/L
Chloride	118-132 mmol/L	118-132 mmol/L
Gamma globulin	3-12% total proteins	0.03-0.12
Glucose	40-70 mg/dL	2.2-3.9 mmol/L
Pressure	70-180 mm H$_2$O	70-180 mm H$_2$O
Proteins, total	< 40 mg/dL	< 0.40 g/L

HEMATOLOGIC

	REFERENCE RANGE	SI REFERENCE INTERVALS
Bleeding time (template)	2-7 minutes	2-7 minutes
Erythrocyte count	Male: 4.3-5.9 million/mm^3	4.3-5.9 x 10^{12}/L
	Female: 3.5-5.5 million/mm^3	3.5-5.5 x 10^{12}/L
Hematocrit	Male: 41-53%	0.41-0.53
	Female: 36-46%	0.36-0.46
Hemoglobin, blood	Male: 13.5-17.5 g/dL	2.09-2.71 mmol/L
	Female: 12.0-16.0 g/dL	1.86-2.48 mmol/L
Hemoglobin, plasma	1-4 mg/dL	0.16-0.62 µmol/L
Leukocyte count and differential		
Leukocyte count	4500-11,000/mm^3	4.5-11.0 x 10^9/L
Segmented neutrophils	54-62%	0.54-0.62
Band forms	3-5%	0.03-0.05
Eosinophils	1-3%	0.01-0.03
Basophils	0-0.75%	0-0.0075
Lymphocytes	25-33%	0.25-0.33
Monocytes	3-7%	0.03-0.07
Mean corpuscular hemoglobin	25.4-34.6 pg/cell	0.39-0.54 fmol/cell
Mean corpuscular hemoglobin concentration	31-36% Hb/cell	4.81-5.58 mmol Hb/L
Mean corpuscular volume	80-100 µm^3	80-100 fl
Partial thromboplastin time (nonactivated)	60-85 seconds	60-85 seconds
Platelet count	150,000-400,000/mm^3	150-400 x 10^9/L
Prothrombin time	11-15 seconds	11-15 seconds
Reticulocyte count	0.5-1.5% of red cells	0.005-0.015
Sedimentation rate, erythrocyte (Westergren)	Male: 0-15 mm/h	0-15 mm/h
	Female: 0-20 mm/h	0-20 mm/h
Thrombin time	< 2 seconds deviation from control	< 2 seconds deviation from control
Volume		
Plasma	Male: 25-43 mL/kg	0.025-0.043 L/kg
	Female: 28-45 mL/kg	0.028-0.045 L/kg
Red cell	Male: 20-36 mL/kg	0.020-0.036 L/kg
	Female: 19-31 mL/kg	0.019-0.031 L/kg

SWEAT

	REFERENCE RANGE	SI REFERENCE INTERVALS
Chloride	0-35 mmol/L	0-35 mmol/L

URINE

	REFERENCE RANGE	SI REFERENCE INTERVALS
Calcium	100-300 mg/24 h	2.5-7.5 mmol/24 h
Chloride	Varies with intake	Varies with intake
Creatinine clearance	Male: 97-137 mL/min	
	Female: 88-128 mL/min	
Estriol, total (in pregnancy)		
30 weeks	6-18 mg/24 h	21-62 µmol/24 h
35 weeks	9-28 mg/24 h	31-97 µmol/24 h
40 weeks	13-42 mg/24 h	45-146 µmol/24 h
17-Hydroxycorticosteroids	Male: 3.0-10.0 mg/24 h	8.2-27.6 µmol/24 h
	Female: 2.0-8.0 mg/24 h	5.5-22.0 µmol/24 h
17-Ketosteroids, total	Male: 8-20 mg/24 h	28-70 µmol/24 h
	Female: 6-15 mg/24 h	21-52 µmol/24 h
Osmolality	50-1400 mOsmol/kg	
Oxalate	8-40 µg/mL	90-445 µmol/L
Potassium	Varies with diet	Varies with diet
Proteins, total	< 150 mg/24 h	< 0.15 g/24 h
Sodium	Varies with diet	Varies with diet
Uric acid	Varies with diet	Varies with diet